Flaps and Grafts in Dermatologic Surgery

Flaps and Grafts in Dermatologic Surgery

SECOND EDITION

Thomas E. Rohrer, MD
SkinCare Physicians
Chestnut Hill, Massachusetts
Clinical Associate Professor
Dermatology
Brown University Alpert School of Medicine
Providence, Rhode Island

Jonathan L. Cook, MD
Professor of Dermatology
Assistant Professor of Surgery
Duke University Medical Center
Durham, North Carolina

Andrew J. Kaufman, MD, FACP
The Center for Dermatology Care
Thousand Oaks, California
Clinical Associate Professor of Dermatology
Keck School of Medicine at USC
Los Angeles, California

ELSEVIER

ELSEVIER

1600 John F. Kennedy Blvd.
Ste 1800
Philadelphia, PA 19103-2899

FLAPS AND GRAFTS IN DERMATOLOGIC SURGERY, SECOND EDITION   ISBN: 978-0-323-47662-1

Copyright © 2018 by Elsevier, Inc. All rights reserved.

No part of this publication may be reproduced or transmitted in any form or by any means, electronic or mechanical, including photocopying, recording, or any information storage and retrieval system, without permission in writing from the publisher. Details on how to seek permission, further information about the Publisher's permissions policies and our arrangements with organizations such as the Copyright Clearance Center and the Copyright Licensing Agency, can be found at our website: www.elsevier.com/permissions.

This book and the individual contributions contained in it are protected under copyright by the Publisher (other than as may be noted herein).

Notices

Knowledge and best practice in this field are constantly changing. As new research and experience broaden our understanding, changes in research methods, professional practices, or medical treatment may become necessary.

Practitioners and researchers must always rely on their own experience and knowledge in evaluating and using any information, methods, compounds, or experiments described herein. In using such information or methods they should be mindful of their own safety and the safety of others, including parties for whom they have a professional responsibility.

With respect to any drug or pharmaceutical products identified, readers are advised to check the most current information provided (i) on procedures featured or (ii) by the manufacturer of each product to be administered, to verify the recommended dose or formula, the method and duration of administration, and contraindications. It is the responsibility of practitioners, relying on their own experience and knowledge of their patients, to make diagnoses, to determine dosages and the best treatment for each individual patient, and to take all appropriate safety precautions.

To the fullest extent of the law, neither the Publisher nor the authors, contributors, or editors, assume any liability for any injury and/or damage to persons or property as a matter of products liability, negligence or otherwise, or from any use or operation of any methods, products, instructions, or ideas contained in the material herein.

Previous edition copyrighted 2007.

Library of Congress Cataloging-in-Publication Data

Names: Rohrer, Thomas E., editor. | Cook, Jonathan L., editor. | Kaufman, Andrew J., editor.
Title: Flaps and grafts in dermatologic surgery / [edited by] Thomas E. Rohrer, Jonathan L. Cook, Andrew J. Kaufman.
Description: Second edition. | Philadelphia, PA: Elsevier, [2018] | Includes bibliographical references and index.
Identifiers: LCCN 2017034158 | ISBN 9780323476621 (hardcover : alk. paper)
Subjects: | MESH: Dermatologic Surgical Procedures–methods | Surgical Flaps | Skin Transplantation | Reconstructive Surgical Procedures
Classification: LCC RD121 | NLM WR 670 | DDC 617.4/770592–dc23
LC record available at https://lccn.loc.gov/2017034158

Senior Content Strategist: Charlotta Kryhl
Content Development Specialist: Lisa M. Barnes
Publishing Services Manager: Catherine Jackson
Senior Project Manager: Daniel Fitzgerald
Designer: Brian Salisbury

Printed in China.

Last digit is the print number: 9 8 7 6 5 4 3 2 1

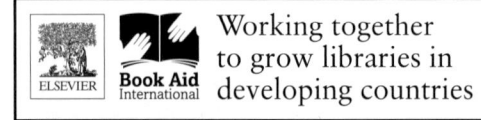

Contents

1. **Anatomy,** 1
   STUART J. SALASCHE and STEPHEN H. MANDY

2. **Basic Principles in Flap Reconstruction,** 16
   ASHLEY WYSONG and SHAUNA HIGGINS

3. **Second Intention Healing and Primary Closure,** 34
   MICHAEL COSULICH, JEREMY ETZKORN, THUZAR MYO SHIN, and CHRISTOPHER J. MILLER

4. **Advancement Flaps,** 50
   CHRISTIE R. TRAVELUTE and ROBERTA SENGELMANN

5. **Rotation Flaps,** 71
   GLENN D. GOLDMAN

6. **V-Y Flaps and Island Flaps,** 82
   JOEL COOK

7. **Transposition Flaps,** 99
   ASHISH C. BHATIA, JOE OVERMAN, and THOMAS E. ROHRER

8. **Staged Interpolation Flaps,** 116
   TRI H. NGUYEN and JANET LI

9. **Skin Grafts,** 132
   GERARDO MARRAZZO and JOHN ALBERTINI

10. **Scalp Reconstruction,** 145
    JUSTIN J. LEITENBERGER and KEN K. LEE

11. **Forehead and Temple Repair,** 155
    MARY L. STEVENSON and JOHN A. CARUCCI

12. **Periocular Reconstruction,** 165
    ANDREA WILLEY

13. **Cheek Reconstruction,** 183
    RICHARD G. BENNETT

14. **Ear Reconstruction,** 210
    HAYES B. GLADSTONE and GREG S. MORGANROTH

15. **Nasal Reconstruction,** 223
    JONATHAN L. COOK

16. **Perioral Reconstruction,** 258
    JOSEPH F. SOBANKO

17. **Neck Reconstruction,** 289
    ANNA BAR and SPRING GOLDEN

18. **Surgical Complications and Revision of Scars,** 300
    CHERYL JANENE GUSTAFSON and C. WILLIAM HANKE

Index, 311

Video Contents

All reconstructive techniques were performed by Tri H. Nguyen, MD.

Production and postproduction for all of the videos were performed by Michael R. Migden, MD.

3 *Second Intention Healing and Primary Closure*

Video 3.1	Geometric Broken Line Closure - Design and Execution
Video 3.2	Z-Plasty - Design and Execution
Video 3.3	M-Plasty

4 *Advancement Flaps*

Video 4.1	Advancement Burow Advancement Introduction
Video 4.2	Advancement Burow Advancement 2 Flap Creation
Video 4.3	Advancement Burow Advancement 3 Flap Closure
Video 4.4	Advancement Burow Advancement 4 Final

5 *Rotation Flaps*

Video 5.1	Rotation Cervical Facial 1 Introduction
Video 5.2	Rotation Cervical Facial 2 Introduction
Video 5.3	Rotation Cervical Facial 3 Flap Closure
Video 5.4	Rotation Cervical Facial 4 Final
Video 5.5	Rotation Dorsal Nasal 1 Introduction
Video 5.6	Rotation Dorsal Nasal 2 Flap Creation
Video 5.7	Rotation Dorsal Nasal 3 Flap Closure
Video 5.8	Rotation Dorsal Nasal 4 Final

6 *V-Y Flaps and Island Flaps*

Video 6.1	Island Pedicle IPF Classic 1 Introduction
Video 6.2	Island Pedicle IPF Classic 2 Flap Creation
Video 6.3	Island Pedicle IPF Classic 3 Flap Closure
Video 6.4	Island Pedicle IPF Classic 4 Final
Video 6.5	Island Pedicle IPF Transposed 1 Introduction
Video 6.6	Island Pedicle IPF Transposed 2 Flap Creation
Video 6.7	Island Pedicle IPF Transposed 3 Flap Closure
Video 6.8	Island Pedicle IPF Transposed 4 Final

7 *Transposition Flaps*

Video 7.1	Transposition Bilobed 1 Introduction
Video 7.2	Transposition Bilobed 2 Flap Creation
Video 7.3	Transposition Bilobed 2 Flap Closure
Video 7.4	Transposition Bilobed 3 Flap Closure
Video 7.5	Transposition Bilobed 4 Final
Video 7.6	Transposition Melolabial 1 Introduction
Video 7.7	Transposition Melolabial 2 Flap Creation
Video 7.8	Transposition Melolabial 3 Flap Closure
Video 7.9	Transposition Melolabial 4 Final
Video 7.10	Transposition Rhombic W-Z Plasty 1 Introduction
Video 7.11	Transposition Rhombic W-Z Plasty 2 Flap Creation
Video 7.12	Transposition Rhombic W-Z Plasty 3 Flap Closure
Video 7.13	Transposition Rhombic W-Z Plasty 4 Final

8 *Staged Interpolation Flaps*

Video 8.1	Paramedian Forehead Flap - Design and Execution
Video 8.2	Paramedian Forehead Flap - Thinning of Flap, Closure of Secondary Defect, and Securing Flap to Surgical Defect
Video 8.3	Cheek-to-Nose Interpolation Flap - Design of Flap
Video 8.4	Cheek-to-Nose Interpolation Flap - Harvesting of Cartilage Graft and Design and Creation of Flap
Video 8.5	Cheek-to-Nose Interpolation Flap - Closure of Secondary Defect and Securing Flap in Surgical Defect
Video 8.6	Cheek-to-Nose Interpolation Flap - Immediately Postrepair
Video 8.7	Cheek-to-Nose Interpolation Flap - Division and Inset of Pedicle
Video 8.8	Lip Switch Flap - Design of Flap (1)
Video 8.9	Lip Switch Flap - Creation of Flap (2)
Video 8.10	Lip Switch Flap - Closure of the Secondary Defect and Completion of Flap (3)
Video 8.11	Lip Switch Flap - Immediate Postrepair (4)
Video 8.12	Lip Switch Flap - Correction at Half-Way Point (5)
Video 8.13	Lip Switch Flap - Division and Inset of Pedicle (6)
Video 8.14	Lip Switch Flap - Healed View (7)

9 *Skin Grafts*

Video 9.1	Burow Graft on Nasal Supratip - Healed View (3)
Video 9.2	Full-Thickness Skin Graft - Evaluation and Introduction (Nasal Ala Recipient) (1)
Video 9.3	Full-Thickness Skin Graft - Harvesting and Preparing Graft for Nasal Ala (2)

Video 9.4	Full-Thickness Skin Graft - Suturing Inc. Tacking Sutures - Nasal Ala (3)	Video 16.4	Lip Wedge 4 Final
Video 9.5	Bolster Dressing for Skin Graft - Nasal Ala (4)	Video 16.5	Lip Advancement 1 Introduction
		Video 16.6	Lip Advancement 2a Crescentic Advancement Crescent
Video 9.6	Burow Full-Thickness Skin Graft Nasal Supratip - Introduction (1)	Video 16.7	Lip Advancement 2b Crescentic Advancement Crescent
Video 9.7	Burow Graft - Nasal Supratip - Execution (2)	Video 16.8	Lip Advancement 3a Crescentic Advancement Mucosal FL

16 Perioral Reconstruction

Video 16.1	Lip Wedge 1 Introduction	Video 16.9	Lip Advancement 3b Crescentic Advancement Mucosal FL
Video 16.2	Lip Wedge 2 Creation	Video 16.10	Lip Advancement 4 Final
Video 16.3	Lip Wedge 3 Complex Closure		

Contributors

John Albertini, MD
Private Practice
The Skin Surgery Center
Clinical Associate Professor (Volunteer)
Department of Plastic and Reconstructive Surgery
Wake Forest Baptist Health
Winston Salem, North Carolina

Anna Bar, MD
Assistant Professor
Department of Dermatology
Oregon Health and Science University
Portland, Oregon

Richard G. Bennett, MD
Clinical Professor of Dermatology
Keck School of Medicine
University of Southern California
Clinical Professor of Medicine (Dermatology)
David Geffen School of Medicine
University of California, Los Angeles
Los Angeles, California

Ashish C. Bhatia, MD
DuPage Medical Group
Naperville, Illinois

John A. Carucci, MD, PhD
Professor of Dermatology
Chief
Mohs Micrographic and Dermatologic Surgery
Program Director
Micrographic Surgery and Dermatologic Oncology Fellowship
The Ronald O. Perelman Department of Dermatology
New York University Langone Medical Center
New York, New York

Joel Cook, MD
Professor of Dermatology and Dermatologic Surgery
Professor of Otolaryngology
Medical University of South Carolina
Charleston, South Carolina

Jonathan L. Cook, MD
Professor of Dermatology
Assistant Professor of Surgery
Duke University Medical Center
Durham, North Carolina

Michael Cosulich, MD
Chief Resident
Department of Dermatology
University of Mississippi Medical Center
Jackson, Mississippi

Jeremy Etzkorn, MD
Assistant Professor
Department of Dermatology
Hospital of the University of Pennsylvania
Philadelphia, Pennsylvania

Hayes B. Gladstone, MD
President
Gladstone Clinic
San Ramon, California

Spring Golden, MD
Golden Dermatology
Honolulu, Hawaii

Glenn D. Goldman, MD
Professor and Chief of Dermatology
University of Vermont College of Medicine
Burlington, Vermont

Cheryl Janene Gustafson, MD
Dermatologist
Laser and Skin Surgery Center of Indiana
Carmel, Indiana

C. William Hanke, MD, MPH, FACP
Dermatologist
Laser and Skin Surgery Center of Indiana
Carmel, Indiana

Shauna Higgins, MD
Skin Cancer Research Fellow
Department of Dermatology
University of Southern California
Los Angeles, California

Ken K. Lee, MD, PC
Portland Dermatology Clinic, LLP
Portland, Oregon

Justin J. Leitenberger, MD
Assistant Professor
Department of Dermatology
Oregon Health & Science University
Portland, Oregon

Janet Li, MD
University of Texas Department of Dermatology
Houston, Texas

Stephen H. Mandy, MD
Volunteer Professor
Dermatology and Cutaneous Surgery
Miller School of Medicine University of Miami
South Beach Dermatology
Miami, Florida

Gerardo Marrazzo, MD
Private Practice
The Skin Surgery Center
Hickory, North Carolina

Christopher J. Miller, MD
Director of Dermatologic Surgery
Assistant Professor
Department of Dermatology
Hospital of the University of Pennsylvania
Philadelphia, Pennsylvania

Greg S. Morganroth, MD
CEO
California Skin Institute
Mountain View, California

Tri H. Nguyen, MD
Texas Surgical Dermatology PA
Spring, Texas

Joe Overman, MD
Resident
Dermatology
Boston Medical Center
Boston, Massachusetts

Thomas E. Rohrer, MD
SkinCare Physicians
Chestnut Hill, Massachusetts
Clinical Associate Professor
Dermatology
Brown University Alpert School of Medicine
Providence, Rhode Island

Stuart J. Salasche, MD
Private Practice
Tucson, Arizona

Roberta Sengelmann, MD
Skin Cancer (Mohs) & Cosmetic
Dermatology/Surgery
Santa Barbara, California

Thuzar Myo Shin, MD, PhD
Assistant Professor
Department of Dermatology
Hospital of the University of Pennsylvania
Philadelphia, Pennsylvania

Joseph F. Sobanko, MD
Assistant Professor of Dermatology and Director of
    Dermatologic Surgery Education
Department of Dermatology
University of Pennsylvania
Philadelphia, Pennsylvania

Mary L. Stevenson, MD
Assistant Professor
Stewart J. Rahr Young Investigator
Mohs Micrographic Surgery and Dermatologic Surgery
The Ronald O. Perelman Department of Dermatology
NYU Langone Medical Center
New York, New York

Christie R. Travelute, MD
Professor
Department of Dermatology
Penn State Milton S. Hershey Medical Center
Hershey, Pennsylvania

Andrea Willey, MD
Surgical & Aesthetic Dermatology
Mohs & Reconstructive Surgery
Sacramento, California

Ashley Wysong, MD, MS
Assistant Professor and Director of Mohs and
    Dermatologic Surgery
Department of Dermatology
University of Southern California
Los Angeles, California

Foreword

"If it ain't broke...don't fix it."
Bert Lance (Jimmy Carter Administration)

I am both humbled and honored to have been asked to write the foreword to the second edition of *Flaps and Grafts in Dermatologic Surgery*. The initial volume has been a valued "go-to" resource for reconstructive surgeons and has fostered the education and skill set of specialists in dermatology, plastic surgery, facial plastic surgery, and oculo-plastic surgery. The obvious "elephant in the room" question arises—why a new edition? The answer is simply growth and expansion of material and evolution of thought. The knowledge base of cutaneous reconstructive surgery is far from static. The progress and change since the initial edition is exponential. The second edition builds on the classic teaching foundation of the first, both expanding on immutable principles where appropriate and introducing new approaches and concepts developed since the initial publication.

The format of the initial edition has been maintained. Introductory chapters review concepts in anatomy and basic principles in tissue movement. The chapter detailing primary closure has been enhanced with coverage of the appropriate and valued use of second intent healing. Subsequent chapters introduce and expand upon the design and mechanics of the various flap and graft variations, followed by discussion of the application of reconstructive options to relevant anatomic sites.

As in the prior edition, this book does not fit in the mold of a "dry" textbook presentation. The contributors discuss their topics in a very personal way, as if directly addressing a colleague, detailing pearls and caveats, and relating the wealth of information through experience that has accumulated throughout their careers. In this way, the second edition introduces modifications and changes that parallel the growth of the specialty. Former authors bring the reader up to date with their current reconstructive philosophy while contributors new to the book allow some very different perspectives to be introduced. As in the prior edition, the text is enhanced by high-quality expertly narrated videos that detail many of the described reconstructive techniques.

The pioneering physicians who first coined the phrase "dermatologic surgery" would find the current specialty almost unrecognizable and would be in awe of the talent and skill of the educators and clinicians who have led this field to its present state of advancement. The contributors to this book are clearly individuals who are not content with the status quo and who realize that even things that are not "broken" can be reexamined, improved, modified, and enhanced. It is with great enthusiasm that I welcome this current edition and look forward to many future editions to come.

Leonard M. Dzubow, MD
Media, Pennsylvania

Preface

This latest edition of our textbook presents an in-depth regional approach to facial reconstruction with an emphasis on surgical anatomy. The best way to learn dermatologic surgery is to observe it. Accordingly, this new text contains a multitude of detailed figures and an accompanying Expert Consult website with very high-definition video demonstrations of the flaps and grafts described within the text. Presenting written explanations, line drawings, preoperative, intraoperative, and postoperative photographs, figure animations, and video presentations give the reader an opportunity to learn elegant surgical repairs from many different perspectives.

We, the editors of this text, have spent our careers teaching dermatologic surgery to residents, fellows, and colleagues. This is reflected in the thorough step-wise nature of this latest textbook. The opening chapter gives the reader an in-depth and practical presentation of the surgical anatomy of the face. Important structures and landmarks are clearly described, delineated, and exposed. How the facial anatomy changes with age and why this is important in aesthetic procedures are also discussed in this chapter to give the dermatologic surgeon even greater perspective.

The next set of chapters in the text concentrate on the principles and biomechanics of flap design and give elegant examples of how these are used in practice. Dr. Dzubow's important text, *Facial Flaps: Biomechanics and Regional Application*, was one of the first comprehensive looks at the intricacies of tissue movement in facial reconstruction, and his text has long been a cornerstone of our teaching materials. By incorporating sophisticated explanations of the nature of tissue movement into this current text, these contemporary authors have reviewed the general principles of aesthetic surgical closures and the specific biomechanics of tissue advancement, rotation, transposition, and interpolation in a detailed, orderly manner. Illustrations and video presentations are used to guide the reader through a wide variety of flaps and grafts used for facial reconstruction.

The following chapters present a regional approach to the repair of facial wounds. This text is designed to give the dermatologic surgeon insight into the multiple surgical options available for the reconstruction of variously sized facial defects. Seeing and reading about the different options for the repair of a wide variety of surgical wounds help the physician learn how thoughtful surgical planning and meticulous operative technique contribute to aesthetically pleasing and functional results. Because considerable emphasis is placed on understanding the thought process behind the selection and execution of reconstructive procedures, the surgeon's ability to adapt and modify repair options to even challenging surgical wounds will be greatly enhanced.

The straightforward principles outlined in this textbook govern modern dermatologic surgery. The techniques of dermatologic surgery have advanced far beyond a simple "fill the hole" mentality. The goals of any reconstructive surgical procedure should be to maintain function, to restore appearance, and to protect the health of the patient. The psychologic ramifications of facial surgery can have a profound impact on patients' quality of life, and virtually all patients, regardless of age, have some underlying concerns about how they will appear after undergoing facial surgery. Obtaining consistently aesthetic results in reconstructive surgery following skin cancer removal is a goal that can only be achieved with a firm understanding of the surgical principles espoused in this text. Successful reconstructive surgery is as much an art form as it is a science or technique. While general surgical principles must be rigorously followed, design creativity and operative flexibility are often the differences between good and great surgeons. It is our sincere hope that this text, created from the generous contributions of some of the leaders in our field, helps all dermatologic surgeons become great by improving the care of their patients.

Thomas E. Rohrer, MD
Jonathan L. Cook, MD
Andrew J. Kaufman, MD, FACP

*To my wonderful children, Harrison, Sam, and Emma,
who give me a continual influx of energy
and enthusiasm for life.
To my wife, Margot, for her love, friendship,
and daily inspiration.
And to my mentors, Len Dzubow, Don Grande, Barbara
Gilchrest, William J. O'Malley, and my parents, Bob and
Marilyn Rohrer.*
—Thomas E. Rohrer

*To my patients, whose continued belief in the value of
trust in the doctor-patient relationship has brought me
immeasurable happiness and satisfaction.*
—Jonathan L. Cook

*To my parents for their love and guidance. To my
brother, Bobby, a true warrior and friend, and my other
brother, Michael, for his support and friendship.
To Barbara, Kelly, and the girls, and to my wife, Jayme,
and children, Madeline and Ethan, for their patience,
love, and inspiration.*
—Andrew J. Kaufman

1 Anatomy

STUART J. SALASCHE, MD, and STEPHEN H. MANDY, MD

Introduction

A working knowledge of anatomy is essential to perform any of the myriad of procedures in dermatologic surgery. Most surgical skills, even the basic ones, such as scar orientation and level of undermining, are predicated on a basic command of anatomy. More complicated tasks, such as nerve block anesthesia, designing tissue flaps and grafts for advanced repair of surgical defects, and the placement of botulinum toxin and fillers, require an even more intimate understanding. Without an in-depth working understanding of the pertinent anatomy, there is a real potential for the surgeon to cause damage by cutting into a vital structure or to be so insecure as to not progress in one's acquisition of sophisticated surgical skills.

Surface Landmarks and Surface Anatomy

Being a keen observer of the surface anatomy of the face enables the surgeon to assess the patient for the vagaries of aging, to identify the reservoirs of redundant skin available for repairs, and to identify optimal placement of scars. It also allows the surgeon to project and visualize the course or location of the deeper vital structures onto the surface.

MASSETER MUSCLE AND MIDPUPILLARY LINE

The masseter muscle is a good starting point. It is the large muscle of mastication that occupies the lateral portion of the cheek below the zygomatic arch (Fig. 1.1). The parotid gland rests on this muscle. At its anterior border on a line drawn from the tragus to the middle of the upper cutaneous lip, the parotid duct can be identified as it dips inward, piercing the buccinator muscle to open into the mouth at the level of the second upper molar. Also, at the jaw line, just at the anterior border of the lower masseter muscle, the facial artery and vein enter onto the face. Pulsation of the artery is often possible at this location. The superficial temporalis artery pulse can be felt just anterior to the ear at its superior attachment. Just beyond this, it splits into superior and parietal branches.

The midpupillary line is identified with the patient sitting up and gazing straight ahead. Three important openings in the skull can be located. The superior orbital foramen is located at the superior orbital rim, often palpable as a notch along the rim. Through it exits the important supraorbital neurovascular complex. Similarly, the infraorbital foramen, about 1 cm below the inferior orbital rim, contains the infraorbital neurovascular artery, vein, and sensory nerve. Finally, the mental foramen, located in the alveolar bone of the mandible in the midpupillary line and just below the canine tooth, contains the mental artery, vein, and nerve. All three foramena may be somewhat medial to the midpupillary line. The exact location of all three of these orifices is important when performing respective nerve blocks of the sensory nerves exiting them.

RELAXED SKIN TENSION LINES

The lines and wrinkles that develop with age and sun exposure become an easily recognizable road map of the face. These wrinkles and creases, first noted as hyperanimation smile lines or frown (scowl) lines, may become permanently etched as elastic tissue degenerates and becomes ineffective in resisting the pull of the underlying muscles of facial expression. These are referred to as the relaxed skin tension lines (RSTLs; Fig. 1.2) and run perpendicular to the exertion of the mimetic muscles below. These lines are often the best choice for the placement of elective scar lines on the face. When they are readily apparent, no problem is posed in designing scar orientation. In younger people, having them animate by grimacing, wrinkling the forehead, smiling, or puckering will usually expose the RSTLs sufficiently to make the correct choice. Similarly, pinching the skin from various directions will also reveal the flow of the RSTLs. Scars not oriented within or parallel to the RSTLs are generally more noticeable, as they do not go with "flow" of the region. This is especially apparent when the patient is smiling or going through some other active form of dynamic emotional expression.

COSMETIC UNITS AND JUNCTION LINES

One of the major conceptual advances over the past decade or so in reconstructive and aesthetic surgery is the refinement and widespread acceptance of the junction lines and cosmetic (aesthetic) units of the face (Fig. 1.3). Cosmetic unit junction lines are the lines on the face at the borders of the cosmetic units. They include the well-defined melolabial fold that separates the cheek from the lip, the mentallabial crease that divides the chin from the cutaneous lower lip, the hairline, and the jaw line. More subtle junction lines separate the cheek from the nose (nasofacial) and lower eyelid from the cheek. The nose has several subunits defined by the alar groove, the dorsal crests, and the nasofacial line. Collectively these are the outlines that caricaturists use along with exaggerated features (broad forehead, wide-set eyes, protruding nose) to rapidly define an individual's countenance and personality. They are also the best location for camouflaging scars. Since lines and shadows are

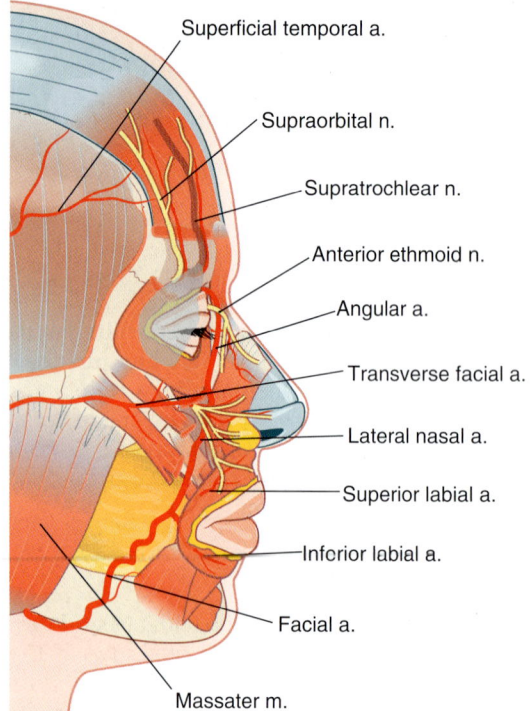

Fig. 1.1 Regional anatomy based on masseter muscle and arterial system of the face.

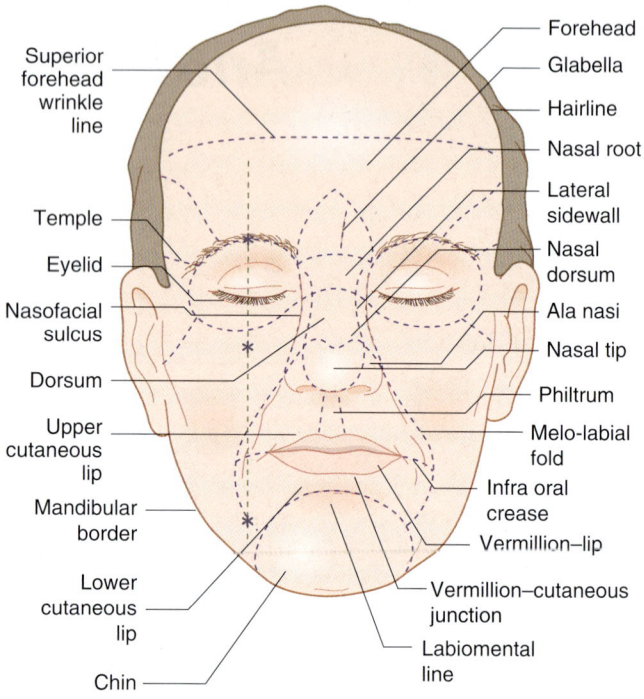

Fig. 1.3 Cosmetic units and junction lines.

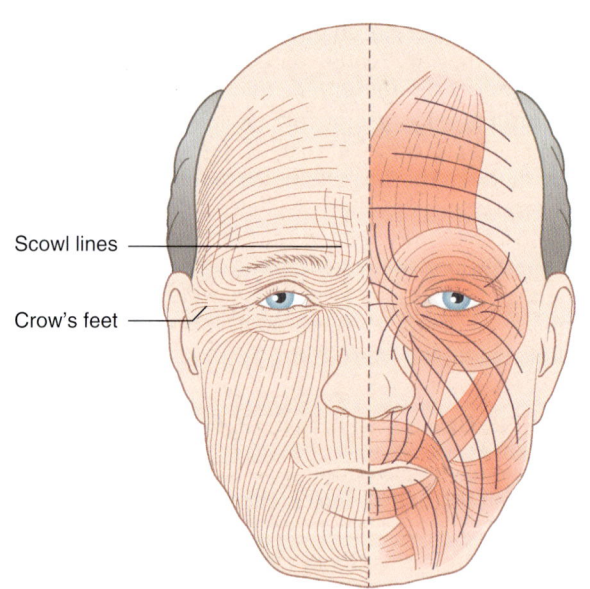

Fig. 1.2 Relaxed tension lines of the face.

anticipated in these areas, scars tend to visually disappear when placed within them. Conversely, scars crossing junction lines stand out as noticeable.

Cosmetic units are the areas cordoned off by the junction lines. They share common characteristics of skin color and texture, pore size, elasticity, thickness, presence or absence of hair, and shading. The cheek, temple, chin, and eyelids are their own well-defined units, whereas the nose, cheek, and ear are subdivided into smaller units. The nose in particular has been defined to include the root, dorsum, lateral side walls, paired alae nasi, soft triangles, columella, and tip.

Several useful principles of closure have been derived from the conceptualization scheme noted previously. These include:

- Scars should be oriented within junction lines or within or parallel to the RSTLs.
- Closures should be confined to a single cosmetic unit when possible.
- When closure is not possible within a single cosmetic unit, skin should be recruited from adjacent units and scar lines oriented so they lie within the intervening junction lines and within or parallel to the RSTLs.
- When a defect involves several cosmetic units, consider repairing each unit individually.
- When most of a cosmetic unit or subunit is missing, consider sacrificing the remaining portion and replace the entire unit.[1]

FREE MARGINS: CONCEPT OF TENSION VECTOR OF CLOSURE

Another important concept when performing facial surgery is that of the free margins—the eyebrows, eyelids, lips, and nostril rims. These structures are extremely important, as they offer little resistance to the forces of wound closure and can be easily distorted by excess tension. This can occur from the immediate direct exertion of tension by a side-to-side closure or the delayed application of tension as a second intention healing wound or split-thickness graft site contracts. The resulting asymmetries can be both cosmetically unsettling and functionally disabling. Ectropion of the lower lid can lead to permanent visual problems, while eclabion and lack of a proper oral seal can cause problems with phonation, eating, and drinking, in addition to being aesthetically unpleasing.

Tension vectors of closure can be favorably manipulated by one of several techniques:

- *Offset bias suturing:* Each suture is skewed a bit from its anticipated placement 90 degrees to the long axis. The cumulative effect is to favorably alter the tension vector the requisite number of degrees to avoid pulling the free margin in question out of position.
- *Flaps:* Tissue rearrangement is designed so the tension vector is favorably disposed and avoids pulling on free margins.
- *Suspension or anchoring suture:* Instead of directing buried suture toward the free margin, a suture is placed from the undersurface of the closure down to and anchored to the underlying periosteum or perichondrium of the area. All tension is then directed downward toward these strong, unyielding structures, and away from the eyelid or eyebrow at risk of being distorted.
- *Full-thickness skin graft:* Placement of a full-thickness graft prevents wound contraction and the development of a tension vector of closure in any direction.

Concavities and Convexities: Implications for Second Intention Healing

The face is not a flat structure. Rather, it is composed of undulating well-defined elevations and depressions that need to be taken into consideration when planning closures. Scar lines that traverse from convexity to concavity may contract in an unbecoming manner and may require preplanning with an S-plasty configuration for appropriate closure. However, the major effect of whether an area is flat, concave, or convex determines how well defects resolve when allowed to heal by second intention. Although the size and depth of the defect have some impact on the final healing, defects on concave surfaces such as the temple, the medial canthus, and the alar groove do well, whereas defects on convex surfaces such as the malar eminence, the tip of the nose, and the chin generally heal poorly with webbed or elevated scars. Defects on flat surfaces, such as the forehead or cheek, typically respond somewhere in between.

The Aging Face

With time, predictable wrinkles and sagging take place. This is compounded by changes related to overexposure to ultraviolet radiation in sunlight. Up until 30 years of age, people do not have wrinkles at rest (Glogau I). The RSTLs first appear as hyperanimation lines perpendicular to the pull of the underlying muscles of facial expression (Glogau II). Crow's feet lines and small crinkles under the eyes when smiling are often the first to become noticeable. With time, the elastic tissue and collagen fascicles that traverse the

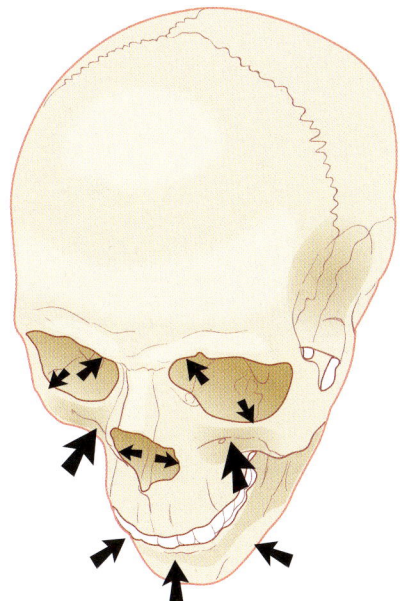

Fig. 1.4 Facial skeletal resorption with arrow size indicating degree.

subcutaneous fat compartment and bind the muscles of facial expression to undersurface of the dermis degenerate and the RSTLs become permanently etched on the face (Glogau III). If the patient has significant photo-damage with deposition of solar elastosis within the papillary dermis, the lines become even more prominent, usually with a pronounced roadmap of lines all over the face (Glogau IV).

Aging has a profound effect upon the facial skeleton, the greatest on the bones of dental origin, the maxilla and mandible. These recede in their anterior projection and height beginning at a relatively early age. Regression of the orbital rim creates inferolateral and superomedial enlargement of the orbit causing loss of support for the periorbital soft tissues (Fig. 1.4). Enlargement of the piriform aperture deepens the nasolabial groove, and these changes, previously attributed to gravity, create laxity of restraining fascial tissues and a generalized sagging of the skin that manifests as brow ptosis, dermatochalasis of the upper eyelids, hollowing under the eyes, vertical lines in the preauricular area, deepened melo-labial folds, rhytids of the perioral area, and pronounced jowls. These areas of redundant and excess, along with the temple and the glabella, constitute the reservoirs of skin available for recruitment for tissue rearrangements.

Generalized lipodystrophy of subcutaneous fat and specific resorption of the facial fat compartments and particularly the buccal fat pad (Figs. 1.5 and 1.6) leads to a volume depletion of the face, resulting in a sunken appearance of the cheeks and a hollowing of the temples.[4] What used to be thought of as a simple act of gravity creating a sagging face is now known to be a much more complicated interaction of fat atrophy, bone resorption, dynamic musculature, and changes in collagen and elastin.

Damage also results in splotchy hyperpigmentation and hypopigmentation; vascular changes in the form of telangiectasia of the cheeks and poikiloderma of the neck and

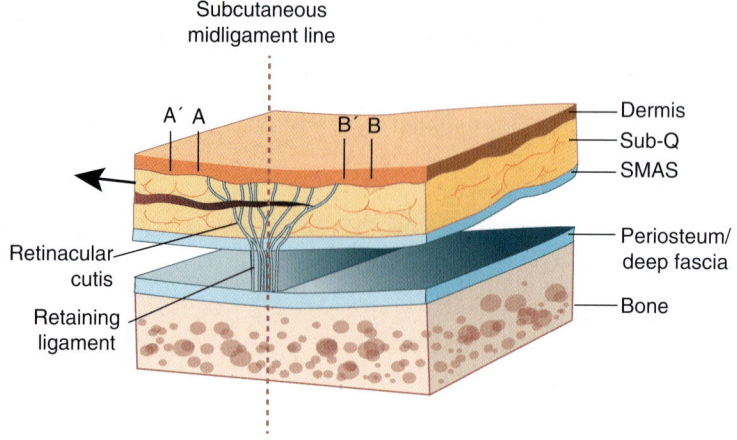

Fig. 1.5 *SMAS*, Superficial musculoaponeurotic system.

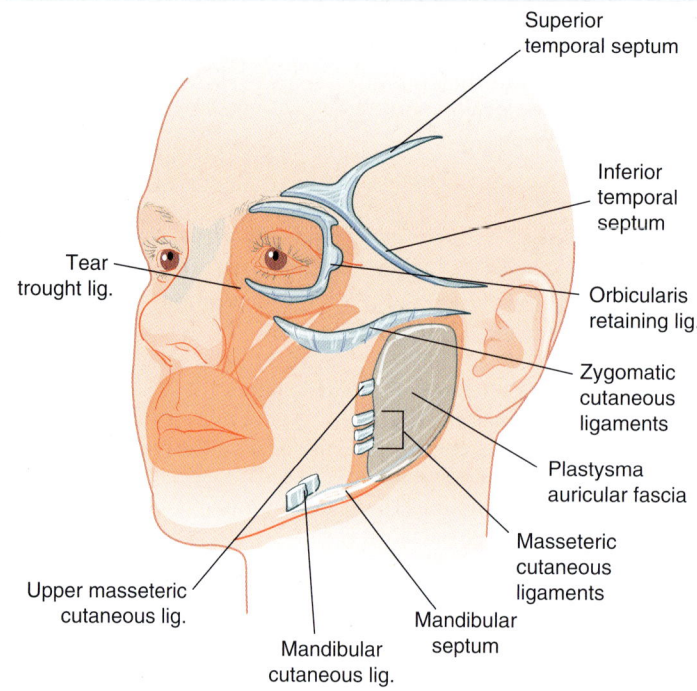

Fig. 1.6 Retaining ligament.

rims of the ears; and the signature damage of ultraviolet radiation, the deposition of solar elastotic material in the papillary dermis, giving the skin a yellowish, thickened, and leathery appearance.

An accurate assessment of the aging face is important not only in correctly judging where there is available skin for recruitment in tumor defect repair but also for determining which cosmetic procedure is most applicable for any particular patient. An upper lid blepharoplasty may only compound severe brow ptosis if that condition is not also addressed. Similarly, it is important to recognize if a resurfacing (ablative laser, chemical peel, etc.), revolumizing (fillers), or tissue tightening procedure (radiofrequency, ultrasounds, etc.) would offer a particular patient the greatest benefit.

The Musculoaponeurotic System

INTRODUCTION

Humans communicate by use of the muscles of facial expression (the mimetic muscles). By use of this silent mode of interacting, human discourse is enriched by nuance and subtlety. Shades of annoyance, reverie, indifference, skepticism, sarcasm, and so on are molded onto the spoken word.

Muscles of facial expression are unique in that they are the only muscles to insert into the skin. They do so via fibrous septae that connect the superior portion of the muscle to the undersurface of the dermis and are part of the branching network of fibers known as the retinacular cutis. This is part of a larger complex system of fibrous septa

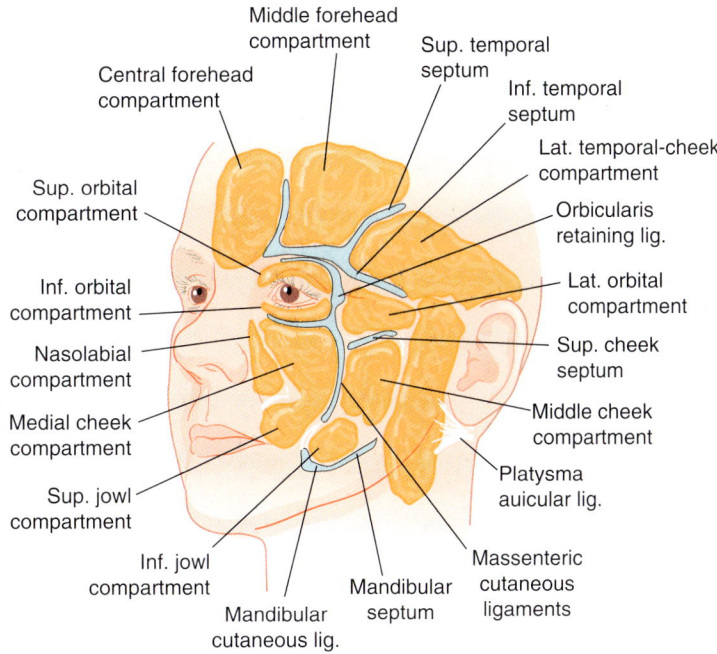

Fig. 1.7 Retaining ligaments and fat compartments of the face.

in the subcutaneous layer of the face that connect to the retaining ligaments and contribute to the septa that create the fat compartments of the face. They also insert or interdigitate with the other mimetic muscles. So while the frontalis muscle wrinkles the forehead and raises the eyebrow, it helps open the eye widely by partially inserting into the upper fibers of the orbicularis oculi muscle (Fig. 1.7).

Innervation of the muscles is exclusively by branches of the facial or cranial nerve VII. This occurs at the lateral undersurface of the muscle. The muscles are most effective and concentrated in the midplane of the face and exert their major effect around the two major orifices of the face—the eyes and the mouth.

The aponeurotic component is made up of retaining ligaments that are strong and deep fibrous attachments that originate from the periosteum or deep fascia and travel perpendicularly through the facial layers to insert in the dermis (Figs. 1.8 and 1.9). These ligaments act as anchor points, retaining and stabilizing the skin and superficial fascia (superficial musculoaponeurotic system [SMAS]) to the underlying deep fascia and skeleton. They tend to be more laterally displaced on the face in the SMAS of the cheek and the superficial temporalis fascia of the temple, which has a superior temporal septum and an inferior temporal septum. The orbicular retaining ligament surrounds the orbit connecting medially to the tear trough ligament (Fig. 1.10). The other major components of the aponeurotic system are the zygomatic cutaneous, masseteric, and mandibular ligaments, and the galea aponeurotica is spread over the expanse of the skull, connecting the anteriorly displaced frontalis muscle with the occipitalis muscle of the neck.[3] These ligaments and fascial components restrict cutaneous mobility and may be necessary to surgically disrupt in order to mobilize tissue for closures. It is also important to recognize that these retaining ligaments often share intimate relationships with branches of the facial nerve, so knowledge of their anatomic relationship is essential to avoid nerve damage during dissection.

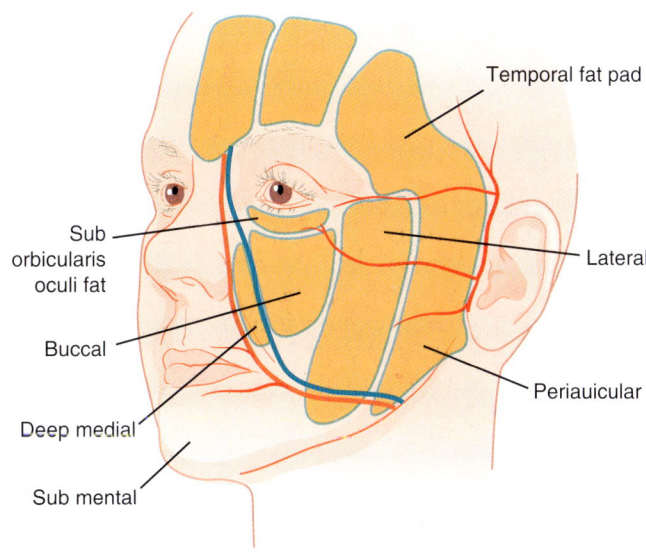

Fig. 1.8 Fat compartments.

MUSCLES ACTING AROUND THE EYELIDS

The frontalis muscle is the primary muscle of the forehead, and its main function is to wrinkle the skin of the forehead and elevate the eyebrow. Accordingly, it has been called the "surprise" muscle. Through its interdigitations with the upper fibers of the orbicularis oculi muscle, it also assists in opening the eye widely. Injury to the temporalis muscle results in flattening the skin of the forehead, brow ptosis,

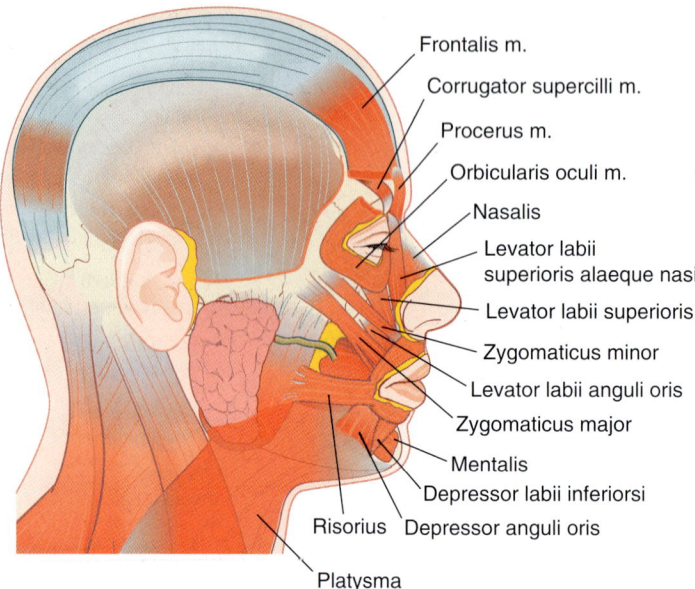

Fig. 1.9 Muscles of facial expression.

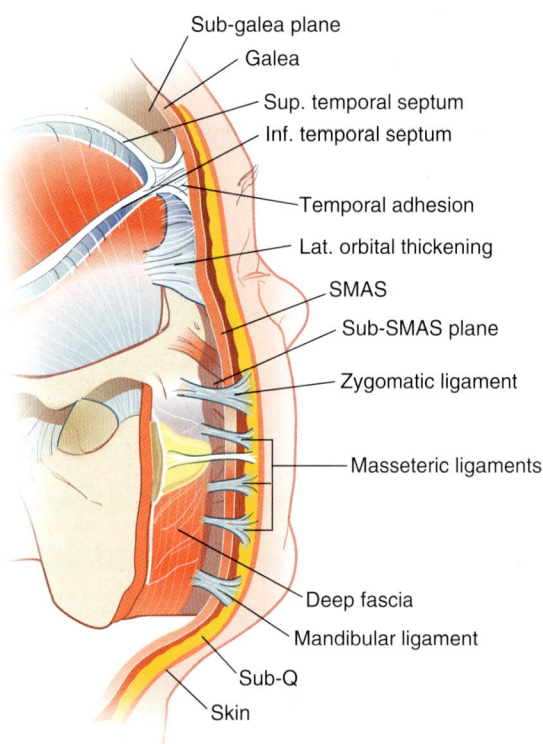

Fig. 1.10 Sagittal section of the retaining ligaments. *SMAS,* Superficial musculoaponeurotic system.[3]

and the larger transverse head that runs laterally to insert widely into the skin of the eyebrow. It functions mainly to pull the eyebrow medially and slightly downward, and creates the vertical scowl lines of the glabella. Recently the depressor supercilii has been described. It arises just above and deep to the corrugator supercilii and extends vertically superior to also attach into the skin of the medial eyebrow. It appears that there are three muscles that act in concert to depress the medial eyebrow: the most deeply placed depressor supercilii, the middle oblique head of the corrugator supercilii, and the vertically oriented fibers of the medial/superior orbicularis oculi muscle.

The key to the orbital region is the large, sphincter-like circumferential orbicularis oculi muscle. It has both outer orbital and inner palpebral portions. The orbital portion originates broadly from the superior and inferior bony orbital rims and inserts into the medial and lateral canthal tendons, as well as the superficial temporalis fascia. It also interdigitates with fibers from the frontalis, corrugator supercilii, and procerus muscles. The orbital division is under voluntary control and acts to close the eye tightly and depress the eyebrow. Unilateral contraction results in a wink. The palpebral portion over the orbital septum and tarsal plate acts to gently close the eye (voluntary) or blink (involuntary). The muscle is innervated by fibers of the temporal and zygomatic branches of the facial nerve.

MUSCLES ACTING AROUND THE NOSE

The nose is relatively devoid of musculature when compared with the eyes and lips. The muscles consist mainly of the procerus muscle that extends down from the frontalis vertically onto the upper nose across the root and into the aponeurosis of the nasalis muscle on the nasal dorsum. Contraction, usually in concert with the adjacent lip elevators, "scrunches" up and shortens the nose and causes the transverse RSTLs across the root. The levator labii superioris alaeque nasi arises from the maxilla under the medial orbicularis oculi and descends vertically to the mid-upper

and accentuation of the effects of dermatochalasis and upper visual field gaze.

The corrugator supercilii muscle has come under intense interest with widespread popularity of botulinum toxin injections. The muscle originates from the frontal bone of the medial orbit in line with and just above the medial canthal tendon insertion. It has two slips—the oblique head that runs a short distance superiorly to insert into the skin of the medial eyebrow and helps depress the medial brow, lip, but also sends slips to the lateral ala nasi. In concert with alar fibers of the nasalis muscle, it aids in dilating the nostril with each inspiration. The broad thin nasalis muscle is the intrinsic nasal muscle with alar fibers just discussed, transverse fibers over the dorsum that just tense the skin over the dorsum, and the depressor septi portion that pulls down the septum and aids in deep inspiration.

MUSCLES ACTING AROUND THE MOUTH

As noted earlier, the mouth is the most expressive part of the face. This is due to the myriad number of muscles that not only insert into the overlying skin but also insert and exert motion from every possible direction into the sphincter-like orbicularis oris muscle. Further modulation of fine muscular movement is aided by a structure called the modiolus (hub, Latin), from which the orbicularis originates. Lying about 1 cm lateral to the oral commissure, it is a muscular platform-like confluence of several of the muscles inserting into the orbicularis and acting on the corner of the mouth, including the zygomaticus major, levator anguli oris, risorius, depressor anguli oris, buccinator, and platysma muscles. Actions are amplified or muted by fine-tuning of the synergistic and antagonistic muscles. The action of the orbicularis muscle itself is to draw the lips together and to pucker the lips.

There are four lip elevators. From most medial to lateral, they include the levator labii superioris alaeque nasi, levator labii superioris, zygomaticus major, and zygomaticus minor. They are all important in smiling, sneering, and snarling movements. The upper lip and corner of the mouth are retracted and elevated by the risorius and levator anguli oris muscles. The buccinator muscle, beloved by trumpet players, plays an important role in chewing by keeping food tucked inward between the teeth.

The muscles working on the lower lip include the mentalis muscle, which wrinkles the skin of the chin and also helps pouch out and protrude the lower lip (sniveling); the depressor anguli oris, which retracts and depresses the corner of the mouth; and the depressor labii inferioris muscle, which, as the name implies, depresses the lower lip. The depressor anguli oris can be injected with botulinum toxin to improve the down turning of the corner of the mouth that occurs with age. The latter two are important (along with the upper lip elevators and angle retractors) in attaining the wide, happy, toothy grin associated with laughing. The marginal mandibular nerve innervates all three muscles. Finally, the platysma muscle, innervated by the cervical nerve, stretches broadly from the chest upward across the expanse of the neck over the jaw line to blend with the angle of the mouth depressors. Despite being thin in some people, it helps cover and protect the marginal mandibular nerve at the anterior border of the masseter muscle at the jaw line.

Motor Nerves

INTRODUCTION

There are two kinds of muscles of the face: the muscles of facial expression and the skeletal muscles of mastication (pterygoid, masseter, and temporal muscles). The former are innervated entirely by the facial (VIIth cranial) nerve, whereas the latter are supplied by motor fibers of the trigeminal (Vth cranial) nerve. The facial nerve has the greatest clinical relevance to dermatologic surgeons and will be the topic of this section.

FACIAL NERVE (CRANIAL NERVE VII)

The facial nerve is a complex structure with an anatomy that varies from patient to patient. The possibility of injuring or severing one of the branches of this nerve is of paramount importance in every procedure performed on the face, whether extirpating a tumor, repairing the defect after removing the tumor, or performing cosmetic "lifting" procedures. The consequences of such a dire event can be cosmetically and functionally devastating for the patient and a source of medical–legal concern for the surgeon. It is important to know the projected pathway and expected depth within the skin of all the motor nerves within the surgical field, so one can not only attempt to avoid them, but also include during the informed consent process a discussion of the potential consequences of injuring them.

After leaving the interior skull at the stylomastoid foramen, the facial nerve classically divides into two major trunks within the substance of the parotid gland, the superior temporofacial and the inferior cervicofacial, which in turn divide into the five major branches: the temporal, zygomatic, buccal, marginal mandibular, and cervical branches (Fig. 1.11). In reality, the temporal and marginal mandibular branches are single terminal rami in about 85% of the population; the other branches cross-arborize and have multiple rami, making the muscles by these latter nerves less prone to permanent paresis. Obviously the former are at greater risk for lasting damage if severed or injured during surgery.

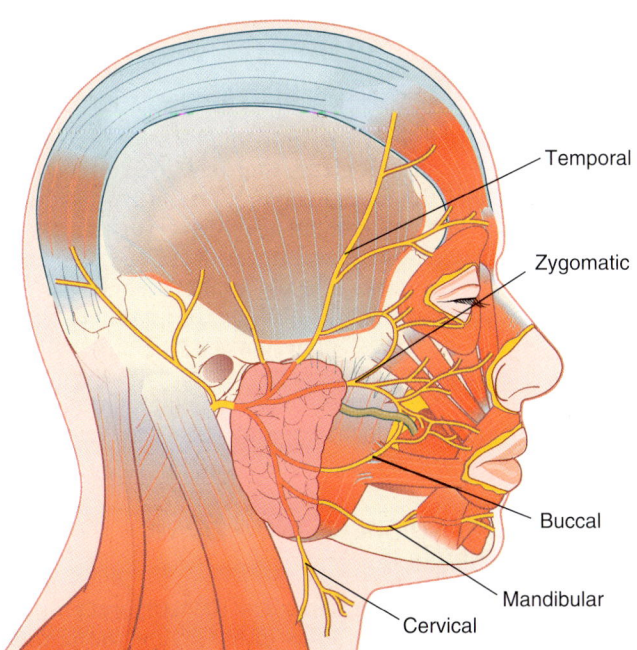

Fig. 1.11 Facial nerve.

TEMPORAL NERVE

The temporal nerve can be roughly projected onto the skin from a line connecting a point 0.5 cm below the tragus of the ear to a point 2 cm above the lateral eyebrow, where it innervates the frontalis muscle. Some fibers go to the upper orbicularis muscle. Like the other branches, it is protected in its initial course by the parotid gland through which it runs. It is most vulnerable at the zygomatic arch and the temple, where it resides deep in superficial temporal fascia below the inferior temporal septum (see Fig. 1.5). Remember that the neurovascular bundle containing the sensory auriculotemporal nerve and superficial temporalis artery and vein are more superficial in the lower subcutaneous fat above the superficial temporal fascia. The temporal nerve is most vulnerable during extirpative surgery involving invasive or recurrent skin tumors that frequently occur in this area. Imprecise undermining in the wrong plane may also damage the nerve. It is prudent to recognize that motor nerves, as myelinated nerves, are also subject to the effects of local anesthesia, and repeat injections, as may occur in Mohs micrographic surgery, can cause deep, long-lasting nerve blocks. This can cause the unwary surgeon and the patient needless concern for the 10 or more hours it takes nerve function to return. In general, if the surgery has exposed a fascial plane that moves easily in a side-to-side manner to the probing (gloved) finger, the superficial temporal fascia and the temporal nerve are probably intact. If the tissue is an immovable, tightly bound-down glistening membrane, the temporal fascia over the temporal muscle of mastication has been reached, and the nerve has a much higher probability of having been severed.

Damage to the temporal nerve results in paresis of the frontalis, with an ipsilateral inability to wrinkle the forehead, raise the eyebrow, and open the eye widely. The asymmetry is discomforting, and functional upper visual field problems may ensue if the resulting brow ptosis is compounded by significant dermatochalasis of the upper lid skin.

ZYGOMATIC AND BUCCAL NERVES

The zygomatic nerve divides into many arborizing rami after leaving the parotid gland, and has interconnections with branches of the buccal nerve. It primarily innervates the orbicularis oculi muscle but also the corrugator supercilii and procerus muscles and upper fibers of the levator labii superioris complex. The zygomatic branches travel deep to the zygomatic ligaments along the zygomatic arch. The buccal nerve shares connections with the zygomatic nerve, but primarily innervates the levator labii superioris, levator labii superioris alaeque nasi, buccinator, zygomaticus major and minor, levator anguli oris, and orbicularis oris muscles.

MARGINAL MANDIBULAR AND CERVICAL NERVES

The marginal mandibular nerve, like the temporal branch, is most often a solitary ramus after leaving the parotid gland. It innervates the lip depressors, the risorius muscle, and the mentalis muscles. It is particularly prone to injury because it is relatively superficial and covered by only a variable platysma muscle at the jaw line at the anterior border of the masseter muscle. It may be at, above, or below the jaw line between its exit from the parotid and the anterior border of the masseter muscle. Skin cancers as well as deep acne scars occur frequently in these locations, making surgery dangerous for the unwary. The marginal mandibular nerve is just posterior to the mandibular ligament and about 10 mm anterior to the anterior margin of the masseter muscle. Injury to the nerve results in an inability to retract or depress the corner of the mouth when smiling. The unopposed pull from the unaffected side causes the damaged-side lower lip to flatten and rotate inward upon smiling (see Fig. 1.11).

The cervical branch innervates the platysma muscle and is rarely a clinical consideration.

Sensory Nerves of the Head and Neck

The major sensory nerves of the head and neck run independently of the motor nerves. In general, they course as part of neurovascular bundles consisting of the nerve, an artery, and a vein. Compared with the motor nerves, they are more superficial and hence more prone to surgical injury and/or involvement with invasive skin cancers. Invasive skin cancers can envelop the nerve or travel along it beyond the main tumor mass by perineural invasion. This sometimes results in paresthesia and dysesthesia, but more importantly in larger subclinical extensions, larger defects, and a higher incidence of recurrences and metastases. On the other hand, injury to a sensory nerve is not as serious as cutting a motor nerve. Damage is usually not permanent, and there is often a full reversal of anesthesia or dysesthesia with time. The latter is dependent upon the distance regeneration has to occur from the sensory ganglion to point of injury. Sensory nerves generally regrow but very slowly. Patients must realize that it may take up to a year for sensation to return, and in some cases regrowth is not complete. The major nerves of the face are the trigeminal (Vth cranial) nerve and the neck branches of the cervical plexus (C2, C3).

With a good grasp of the anatomy of the sensory nerves, one can perform specific nerve blocks (mental, infraorbital, supratrochlear, and supraorbital) or regional blocks, which use combinations of nerve blocks to anesthetize whole areas for surgical procedures, such as on the nose, ear, and forehead/scalp. Unfortunately, much of the cheek is innervated by small terminal branches and requires local anesthesia, often with multiple injection sites.

TRIGEMINAL NERVE (CRANIAL NERVE V)

As the nerve of the embryonic first branchial arch, the trigeminal nerve supplies motor fibers to the muscles of mastication, secretory fibers to the lacrimal, parotid, and mucosal glands, and sensory innervation to the face and anterior scalp. It has three main sensory branches originating from the middle cranial fossa-situated trigeminal or gasserian ganglion, which divide the face and scalp both horizontally and vertically (Fig. 1.12). These nerve

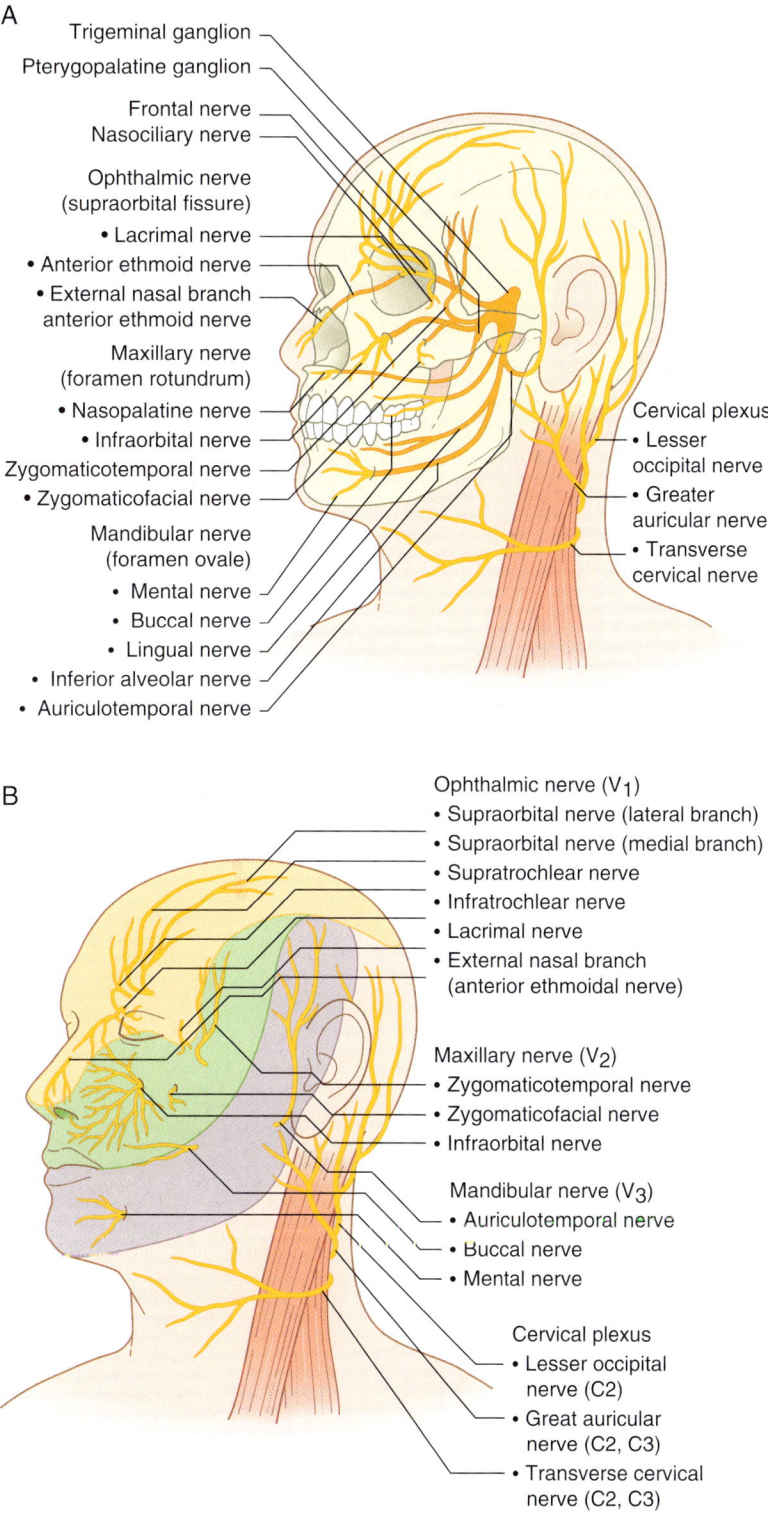

Fig. 1.12 Sensory nerves. (A) Deep. (B) Cutaneous.

divisions have been classically designated as the ophthalmic (V1), maxillary (V2), and mandibular (V3) nerves.

Ophthalmic Nerve (V1)

The ophthalmic nerve (V1) exits the skull at the supraorbital fissure. It has three main branches: the nasociliary, the frontal, and the lacrimal nerves. The nasociliary further divides into the infratrochlear nerve to the medial canthus and the root of the nose, and the external nasal branch of the anterior ethmoidal nerve. The latter reaches the surface of the nose between the nasal bones and the upper lateral cartilage to supply the dorsum, tip, and columella of the nose. Blisters of herpes zoster in its distribution require ophthalmic examination, as the cornea is supplied by a common nerve origin. The frontal nerve divides into the supratrochlear nerve, which reaches the surface via the supratrochlear notch in the supraorbital rim about 1 cm lateral to midline to supply the medial upper eyelid and forehead/scalp and the supraorbital nerve, which surfaces at the supraorbital foramen about 2.5 cm from midline in the midpupillary line to supply the upper eyelid and the forehead/scalp. Finally, the lacrimal nerve supplies the lateral upper eyelid.

Maxillary Nerve (V2)

The maxillary nerve (V2) emerges from the foramen rotundum and also divides into three main branches. The largest, the infraorbital nerve, exits the infraorbital foramen 0.5 to 1 cm below the infraorbital rim in the midpupillary line to innervate the upper lip, medial cheek, lateral nose, and lower eyelid. The smaller zygomaticofacial supplies the malar eminence, and zygomaticotemporal innervates the temple region.

Mandibular Nerve (V3)

The mandibular nerve (V3) is the largest of the three trigeminal divisions and the only one to carry motor fibers to the muscles of mastication. Like the others, it has three main branches: the auriculotemporal, buccal, and mental nerves. The auriculotemporal runs deeply beneath the mandible and reaches the cutaneous surface superior to the parotid gland in company with the superficial temporal artery and vein to supply the lateral ear, temple, and parietal/temporal scalp. The buccal nerve divides into many branches in the region of the buccinator muscle before reaching and supplying the medial cheek. It is not available for nerve block. The mental nerve exits the mental foramen of the alveolar bone in the midpupillary line, along with the mental artery and vein to supply the chin and lower lip.

The infraorbital and mental nerves are prime candidates for nerve block anesthesia. These two nerves, along with the infratrochlear, supratrochlear, and supraorbital, can be blocked in various combinations for regional blocks of the nose and forehead/scalp.

Vascular System

The incredibly rich blood supply to the face is responsible for the wide array of surgical procedures that can be carried out there. The vascular system to the face is unique in being supplied by two separate artery complexes, the external and the internal carotid systems (see Fig. 1.5). These systems have rich anastomoses, and there is also an extremely rich cross-anastomosis involving paired bilateral arteries such as the superior labial arteries and the supratrochlear arteries. Furthermore, unlike the blood supply on the trunk and extremities, where perfusion of the surface is via vertically oriented perforating vessels from the underlying skeletal muscles, the final perfusion of the skin of the face is through the horizontally displaced subdermal plexus that lies high in the subcutaneous fat just under the reticular dermis. This allows for wide undermining of side-to-side closures and the seemingly endless number of random flaps (no named artery in pedicle) that have been designed to repair defects of the face. Proper design of axial pattern flaps (ones that depend on a named artery), such as the paramedian forehead flap, is dependent on knowledge of the location of the major vessels of the face—in this case, the supratrochlear artery.

EXTERNAL CAROTID SYSTEM

The external carotid system is the main blood supply to the lower face, temple, and posterior scalp.

The main branch of the external carotid artery to the central face, the facial artery, enters onto the face after exiting the submandibular gland at the anterior border of the masseter muscle at the jaw line (see Fig. 1.1). It runs obliquely superior within the substance of the lip depressor muscle complex toward the commissure of the lip. Within the substance of the orbicularis oris muscle, it first gives off the inferior labial artery that runs medially through the lower lip to meet its pair from the other side. Next, at the level of the upper lip, the similarly disposed superior labial artery is given off and runs transversely through the upper lip to meet its contralateral partner.

After giving off the superior labial artery, the facial artery becomes known as the angular artery as it makes its way up toward the alar base and consequently upward alongside the nose to anastomose with the dorsal nasal artery, a branch of the ophthalmic artery of the internal carotid system. This anastomotic complex at the medial canthal level is an important vascular pedicle for the dorsal nasal or Rieger flap. Recent anatomic studies revealed that the angular artery has four variations that occur with nearly equal frequency. The illustration (Fig. 1.13) depicts the variations.[2] The complex anastomotic vascular arrangement in

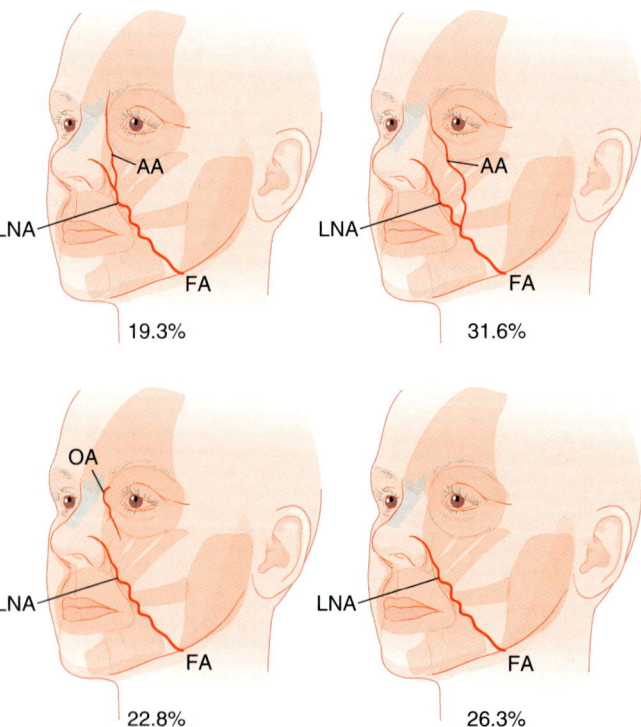

Fig. 1.13 Variations of the angular artery. *AA*, Angular artery; *FA*, facial artery; *LNA*, lateral nasal artery.

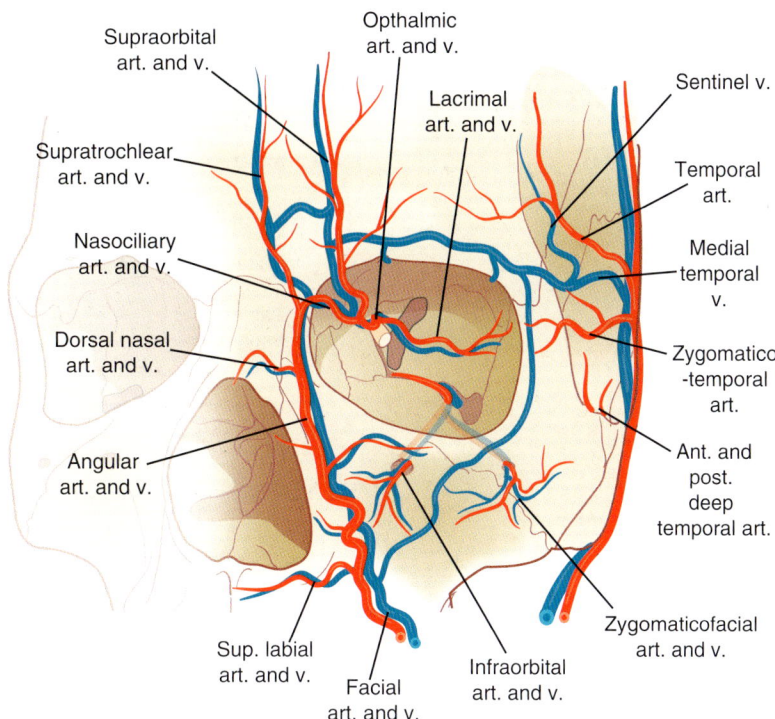

Fig. 1.14 Periocular vascular anatomy. (Carruthers JD, Fagien S, Rohrich RJ, Weinkle S, Carruthers A. Blindness caused by cosmetic filler injection: a review of cause and therapy. *Plastic and Reconst Surg*. 2014;134:1197–1201.)

the periocular area is cause for concern, as many arteries connect directly or indirectly to the retinal and internal carotid arteries and have resulted in blindness and strokes when injected with particulate material such as intradermal fillers (Fig. 1.14).[5]

Other main branches off the external carotid include the occipital artery that courses posteriorly and superiorly in company with the sensory occipital nerve between the trapezius and sternocleidomastoid muscles, to run just above the occipital muscle to supply the posterior scalp. The postauricular artery arches around the styloid process to a groove between the mastoid process and the external ear to supply the posterior ear and portions of the adjacent scalp above and behind the ear.

After giving off the facial and occipital arteries, the external carotid artery divides into its two terminal branches, the superficial temporal artery and the internal maxillary artery. The latter branch is primary internal to the mouth and nose, but after several divisions does supply terminal vessels that exit the infraorbital and mental foramen as same-named arteries, along with their respective veins and sensory nerves. They provide important anastomoses with the facial artery.

The more important division to dermatologic surgeons is the superficial temporal artery. This runs superiorly in front of the ear within the substance of the parotid gland, along with the same-named vein and the auriculotemporal nerve, a sensory branch of the mandibular nerve of the trigeminal (Vth cranial) nerve. As the neurovascular bundle exits the superior pole of the parotid gland, the artery is palpable at the level of the superior attachment of the ear. At this point, it splits into anterior and parietal branches to supply the temple/lateral forehead and parietal scalp, respectively.

INTERNAL CAROTID SYSTEM

The main volume of blood from the internal carotid system is dedicated to supplying the brain. A portion is allotted to the face, predominantly to the ophthalmic artery whose terminal branches exit the skull as the supraorbital and supratrochlear arteries, as part of the same-named neurovascular bundles (see Fig. 1.14). They exit their respective foramen and pierce the overlying frontalis muscle to run superiorly. At this point, they are displaced deep in the subcutaneous fat above the frontalis fascia and subsequently over the galea aponeurotica as they course superiorly over the scalp. They supply the forehead and anterior scalp (see Fig. 1.14). As noted earlier, the supratrochlear artery is recruited for the classic and extremely useful axial midline and paramedian forehead flap. Both arteries partake in the rich anastomotic network over the scalp by connecting with branches of the superficial temporalis and occipital arteries. This network is so powerful that traumatic scalping can be repaired by vascular reconnection of even one of these major vessels that supply the scalp.

The other major branch off the ophthalmic artery is the dorsal nasal branch (in some studies noted as the infratrochlear artery) at the medial canthus. It runs inferiorly along the side of the nose in the medial canthal region to supply the bridge of the nose and to connect with the angular artery of the external carotid system.

It is interesting that above the zygomatic arch, the neurovascular bundles containing the major arteries and veins all course in the deep subcutaneous plane above the fascia or muscles of facial expression. Conversely, below the arch, the vessels are usually within the substance of the mimetic muscles and do not course in the company of the major

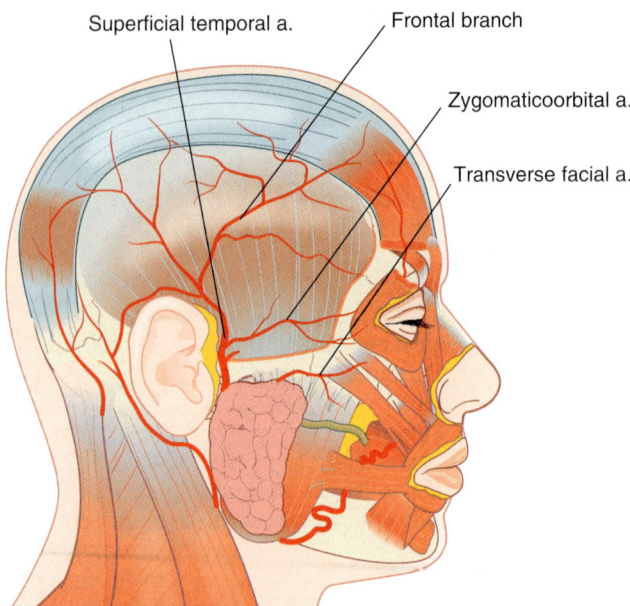

Fig. 1.15 Venous system of the face and corresponding arteries.

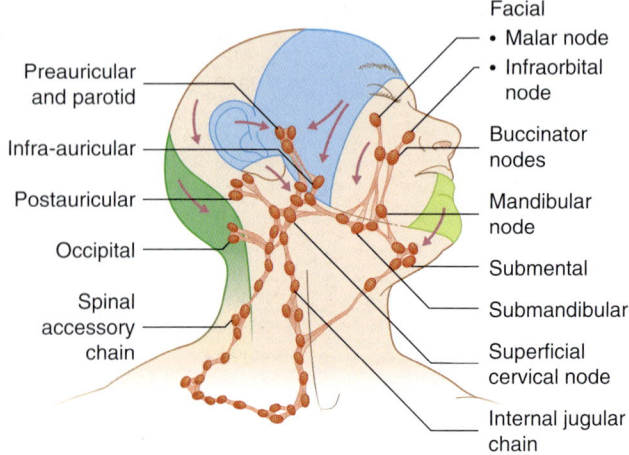

Fig. 1.16 Lymphatic drainage.

sensory nerves. Knowledge of the route and depth of the vessels will aid in preserving them during a procedure in the region. On the other hand, when they have to be cut, as in a lip wedge excision, knowing that the labial artery is located in the very posterior portion of the distal orbicularis oris allows the surgeon to locate and clamp it off immediately before it retracts into the substance of the muscle.

VENOUS SYSTEM

The vascular drainage of the face, for the most part, parallels the arterial supply. Generally, the veins have a straighter, less tortuous path than their counterpart arteries (Fig. 1.15).

LYMPHATIC SYSTEM

The advent and widespread use of lymphoscintigraphy have at once confirmed and expanded much of what we know about the lymphatics of the head. The system is certainly much more variable than once believed. The impetus for this interest is that melanoma, squamous cell carcinoma, and Merkel cell carcinoma all tend to metastasize first to primary echelon nodes, and a complete examination for these tumors includes evaluation of the draining lymph nodes either by manual palpation or by histopathologic evaluation, following sentinel lymph node biopsy.

Some generalities apply to the lymphatic system of the head and neck. First, the central face and scalp are usually devoid of lymph nodes, except for a few inconsistent, ectopic nodes found above the mimetic muscles in the subcutaneous fat. Generally they are encountered by accident during surgery or found in the pathology specimen. Next, afferent drainage is organized in flow patterns that proceed in a superior to inferior, diagonal direction toward the collecting, primary echelon nodes in the upper neck region. These include the submental, submandibular, jugulodigastric, and occipital lymph nodes (Fig. 1.16). Drainage from these superficial nodes then proceeds to the deeper cervical systems in the neck (the spinal accessory, internal jugular, and transverse cervical lymph node basins).

The real wild cards in the system are the lymph nodes within the substance of the parotid gland. These nodes are difficult to assess clinically, and even lymphoscintigraphy may prove troublesome due to the proximity of the parotid gland. They drain a wide area, including portions of the anterior scalp, forehead, lateral eyelids, cheeks, nose, and upper lip. Subsequent drainage is to the deeper neck node basins.

Special Structures: Lip, Nose, Eyelids, and Ear

LIP

The lips are the guardians of the oral seal that is required for phonation and mastication. On a social level, the marvelously expressive lips convey our nonverbal communication. As such, they are at once the least complicated and the most mobile of the special structures of the face. The two are related; by not having a constricting solid structure such as the bony/cartilaginous frame of the nose or the form-shaping tarsal plate of the eyelid, the lips are quite flexible, stretchable, and elastic. Having only a very thin subcutaneous fat layer in the cutaneous portion also facilitates this ability.

Internally, the lips consist solely of the orbicularis oris muscle and the myriad muscular insertions attached to it. They are covered on the outside by skin, on the inside by a wet mucosa, and at the vermilion by a dry modified mucosa (Fig. 1.17). The submucosa contains many salivary glands on the oral portion.

The lips may be divided into vermillion and cutaneous cosmetic units. The cutaneous upper lip is the most complicated section, having a small triangular portion that extends superior and lateral to the alar base and a central subunit, the philtrum. Two convex philtral crests (columns, ridges) define the midline concave philtral bowl. The lower portion of the latter is the beautiful downward-curving Cupid's

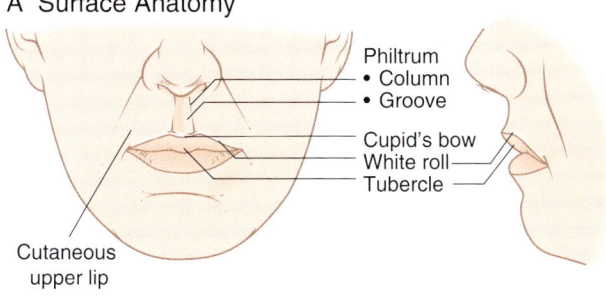

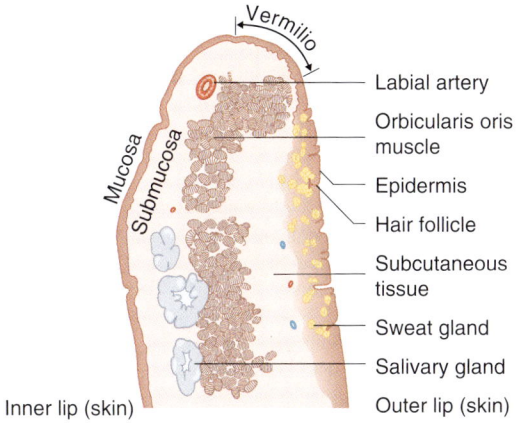

Fig. 1.17 Structures of the lip and cross section.

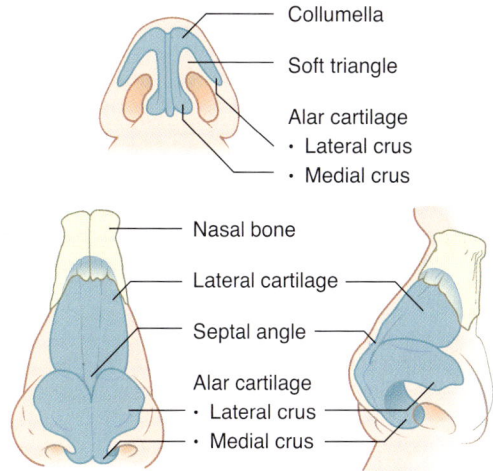

Fig. 1.18 Structures of the nose.

bow. The philtrum is a reservoir of extra skin and interdigitating orbicularis muscle that allows for the dramatic stretching and vertical shortening of the upper lip when smiling or opening the mouth wide. In many people, the sharp cutaneous/vermilion junction line has a superimposed white roll. This 1- to 2-mm, glabrous strip of skin is due to an anterior bulging of the orbicularis oris muscle. It can be quite prominent, especially in younger patients, and is an important consideration in placing transverse scar lines.

NOSE

The nose is an extremely complex, aesthetically and functionally important midline structure that is all too often the site of invasive skin cancers. It is supported by a bony/cartilaginous infrastructure that features the inflexible paired nasal bones superiorly and the highly mobile paired upper lateral/alar cartilage complex inferiorly (Fig. 1.18). Conversely, the skin over the rigid bony upper portion is highly movable (zone 1), while the skin over the mobile cartilage portion is thick, sebaceous, and bound down (zone 2).

On the surface the nose can be broken down into several cosmetic subunits. These include the root of the nose that extends from medial canthus to medial canthus. The skin lines in this concave unit run transversely across it. Obliteration of the concave nature of this area during repairs causes the profile to be dramatically altered and the nose to appear very large on the frontal view. The paired lateral sidewalls separate the nose from the cheek and are in turn separated from each other by the midline dorsum of the nose unit. The heart-shaped convex tip of the nose is the most prominent feature of the nose and is bounded by the paired alae nasi. The columella is the midline structure below the tip separating the nostril apertures and culminating in the upper philtrum of the lip. The RSTLs of the upper nose run obliquely out from the medial canthus down the dorsum and lateral sidewall. They end part-way down, as there are no skin lines on the lower nose. As noted earlier, they run transversely across the root.

The lower nose is supported by the paired, upper lateral cartilages, which act as extensions of paired nasal bones. The paired, lower lateral, or alar cartilages begin as medial crura that form the columella. As they swing back and curve, they form an arch that is the tip of the nose. As the lateral crura diverge obliquely upward and laterally away from the midline vertical nasal septum cartilage, they support the ala nasi. It is important to recognize that the ala nasi are composed of fibro-fatty muscular tissue and are devoid of cartilage. Their ability to flare (and not collapse) with each inspiration is due to the involuntary contraction of the levator labii superioris alaeque nasi and nasalis muscles. If these latter muscles have been removed during tumor extirpation, then a cartilage strut must be included in the surgical repair or the nostril will collapse during inspiration.

The upper portion of the nose is innervated by the infratrochlear (V1) of the trigeminal, whereas the anterior branch of the external ethmoid nerve (also V1) supplies the tip. The lateral portions of the nose are innervated by the infraorbital nerve (V2).

EYELIDS

The eyelid is perhaps the most complicated structure on the face and of extreme functional importance. Successful repair of the unique structures that compose the eyelids are contingent on thorough knowledge of the anatomy, as it is so closely related to function. The eyelids guard the globe and orbit and are structured on the orbicularis oculi muscle, whose orbital and palpebral components have been discussed earlier in this chapter. As noted, the orbicularis is

1 • Anatomy

A Cross Sectional Anatomy

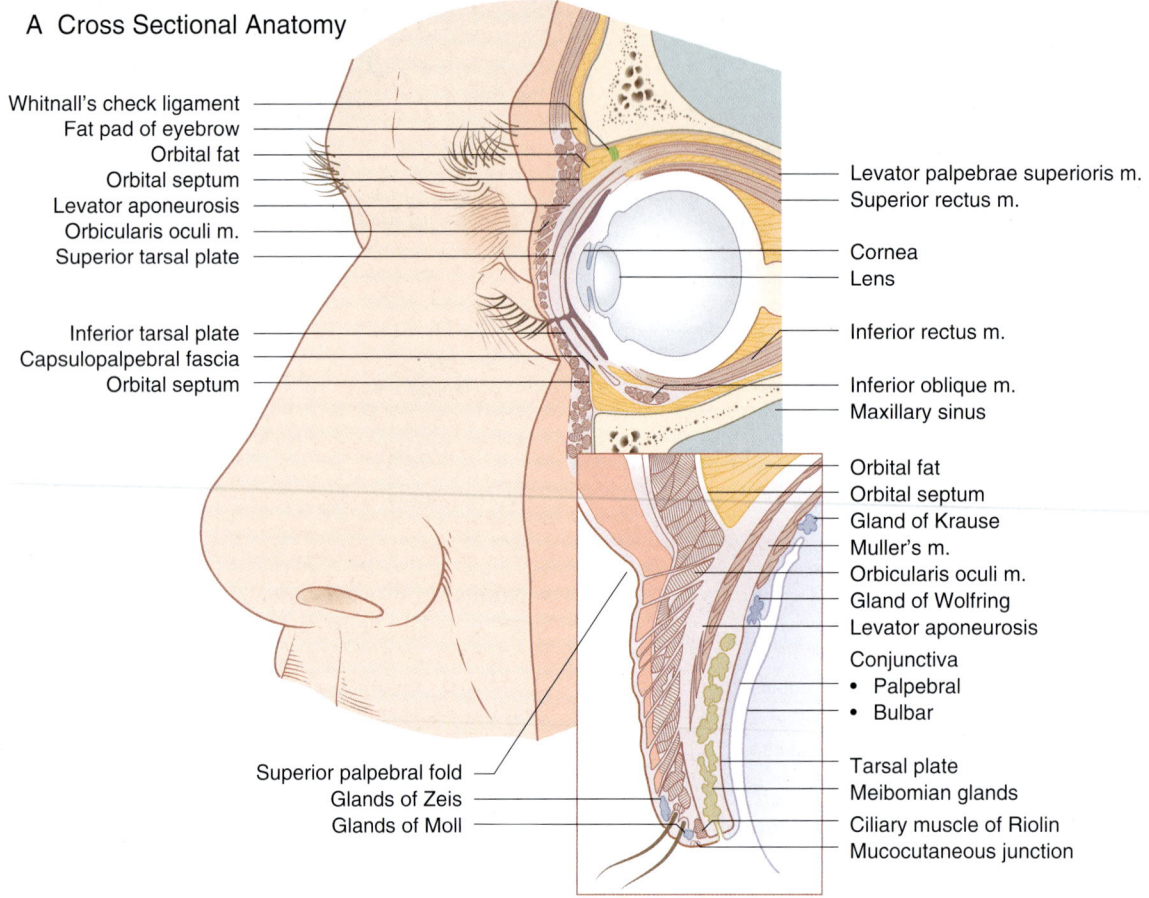

B Surface Landmarks

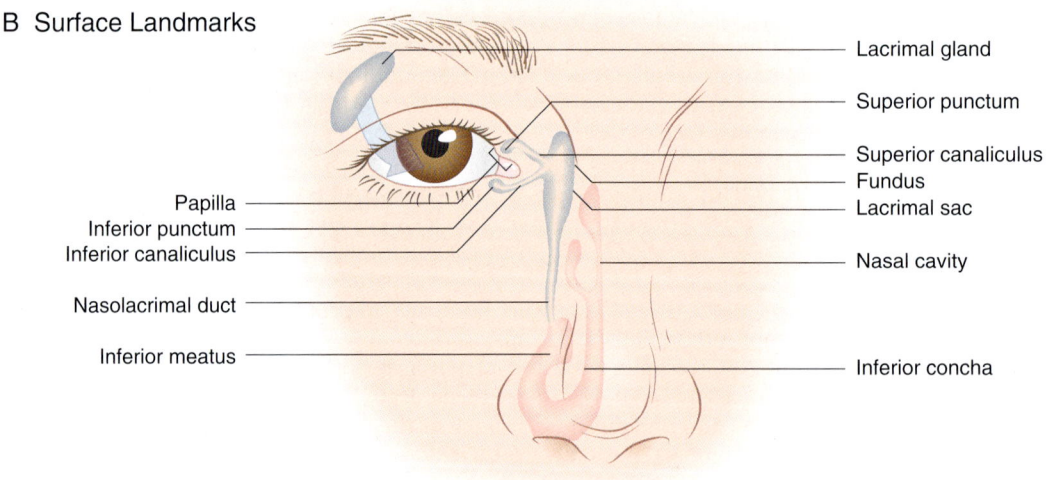

Fig. 1.19 Structures of the eye and lachrimal apparatus.

responsible for closing the lid. The levator palpebrae superioris muscle and aponeurosis is responsible for opening the eye (Fig. 1.19). It is innervated by the oculomotor or third cranial nerve. It arises from the superior orbit and divides into two components: Muller's muscle, which attaches into the superior margin of the tarsal plate under sympathetic nerve control, and the levator aponeurosis, which fuses with the orbital septum to form the superior palpebral fold about 10 mm above the lid margin and then continues downward to attach to the anterior surface of the tarsal plate. It also sends fibers through the pretarsal orbicularis to insert into the lid skin. This is why the skin in the pretarsal area is bound down, whereas it is loose and eventually redundant in the preseptal area above the superior palpebral fold. The space between the orbital septum and the levator aponeurosis contains the orbital fat pads. The skin of the eyelids is the thinnest and most elastic in the body. It contains little subcutaneous fat.

The posterior portion of the eyelid closest to the globe contains the tarsal plate that consists of dense fibrous tissue. This gives form to the lids and also contains the sebaceous Meibomian glands. The conjunctiva covers the posterior eyelids as well as the globe. Hair follicles of the eyelashes (cilia), with both sebaceous glands (Zeis) and sweat glands (Moll) exit onto the lid margin below the muscular layer, while the Meibomian glands exit onto the lid closer to the conjunctival surface.

The lacrimal system is important to eye homeostasis (see Fig. 1.19). The lacrimal gland is situated in the postseptal space lateral to the fat pads. The lacrimal collecting system consists of the upper and lower lacrimal puncta at the medial eyelid margins, which open into the lacrimal canaliculi at the medial margin of the tarsi. The upper and lower canaliculi converge under the medial canthal tendon as the common canaliculus, to run horizontally into the nasolacrimal duct on the side of the nose opposite the medial canthus, and drains as the nasolacrimal canal into the nose beneath the inferior turbinate.

EAR

The ear appendage is essentially skin stretched over a rather intricately molded cartilage infrastructure. It is important to the dermatologic surgical, as it has a high risk for both basal cell (BCC) and squamous cell carcinomas (SCC). Invasive SCC tumors of the helical rim tend to reach the larger lymphatic and venular vessels of perichondrium at a shallower depth than elsewhere on the body, making metastases from this area a real threat.

The outer rim of the ear is the convex helix that extends upward from the lobule to curve around, and ending as the crus of the helix that divides the concha bowl into the upper cymba and the lower cavum (Fig. 1.20). Opposite the cavum and guarding the external auditory meatus is the small protuberance, the tragus. Also superior to the lobule is the convex antihelix. This structure parallels the helix in its vertical dimension and is separated from it by the depression between them, the scapha. The antihelix splits at its superior end into two crura to form a central concavity, the triangular fossa. Only the lobule is not supported by cartilage.

The sensory innervation of the ear is complicated. The anterior surface closest to the cheek as well as the anterior-

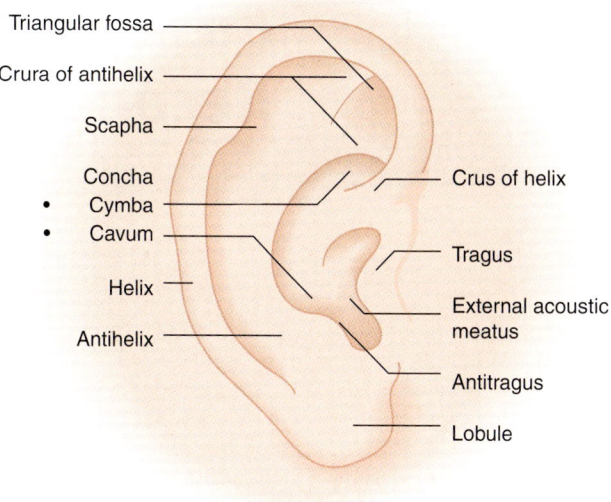

Fig. 1.20 The ear.

superior portion of the external auditory canal is supplied by branches of the auriculotemporal branch of the mandibular division (V3) of the trigeminal nerve. The lower posterior surface, as well as the lower anterior helical portion, is innervated by the great auricular nerve (C2, C3), while the upper posterior portion and the upper vertical portion of the anterior helical area are supplied by the lesser occipital nerve (C2, C3). Variable contributions of the cranial nerves IX and X supply the remaining portions of the external auditory canal. Understanding this innervation pattern is required for regional nerve block of the ear.

References

1. Salasche SJ. Anatomy. In: Rohrer TE, Cook JL, Nguyen TH, et al, eds. *Flaps and Grafts in Dermatologic Surgery*. Philadelphia: Elsevier; 2007: 1-14.
2. Kim Y, Choi D, Gil Y-C, Hu KS, Tansatit T, Kim HJ. The anatomic origin and course of the angular artery regarding its clinical implications. *Dermatol Surg*. 2014;40(10):1070-1076.
3. Alghoul M, Codner M. Retaining ligaments of the face: review of anatomy and clinical implications. *Aesthet Surg J*. 2013;33(6):769-782.
4. Rohrich RJ, Pessa JE. The fat compartments of the face: anatomy and clinical implications for cosmetic surgery. *Plast Reconstr Surg*. 2007; 119(7):2219-2227.
5. Carruthers JD, Fagien S, Rohrich RJ, Weinkle S, Carruthers A. Blindness caused by cosmetic filler injection: a review of cause and therapy. *Plast Reconstr Surg*. 2014;134(6):1197-1201.

2 Basic Principles in Flap Reconstruction

ASHLEY WYSONG, MD, MS, and SHAUNA HIGGINS, MD

The reconstruction of wounds has long been a challenge to surgeons. Whereas some wounds may be left to heal by second intention or closed in a simple side-to-side linear fashion, others require more complex movement of local or distant tissue to restore functional and anatomic relationships, and to optimize the cosmetic outcome.

Surgeons have used skin flaps to repair wound defects for centuries. The term "flap" was derived from the Dutch word "flappe" during the 16th century. "Flappe" referred to something that was fastened by one side and hung broad and loose. As early as 700 BCE, the Sushruta Samhita first documented a technique of reconstructing a large nasal tip defect with a cheek flap.[1] Since that time, surgeons' knowledge of biology, anatomy, and physiology has greatly increased. This understanding allows us to significantly decrease the likelihood of surgical complications such as hemorrhage, hematoma, infection, and flap failure. This chapter addresses some basic principles of flap reconstruction including flap design, construction, classification, and practical tips.

Basic Terminology

A **skin flap** is a construct typically consisting of skin and subcutaneous tissue with a partially intact vascular supply that is transferred or repositioned from an adjacent or more distant donor site to a recipient site. The recipient site is called the **primary defect** and, in dermatologic surgery, is usually the wound resulting from the removal of a cutaneous tumor (Fig. 2.1). The **secondary defect** is defined as the wound that is created by cutting, lifting, or sliding the flap to fill the primary defect (see Fig. 2.1). The **base** of the flap is the area that remains attached to the skin adjacent to the defect. It is this base, also known as the pedicle of the flap, that contains the vascular supply necessary for initial flap survival. The tip of the flap is the portion of the flap furthest from the flap's base.

Flaps Defined by Blood Supply

There are many classification schemata for reconstructive flaps. One common method of defining flaps is to determine the flap's perfusion sources. Flaps may be categorized based on vascular supply as musculocutaneous, fasciocutaneous, axial, or random. A musculocutaneous flap includes muscle tissue in the base of the flap, whereas a fasciocutaneous flap includes only the fascial covering of the muscle in the pedicle. An example of a musculocutaneous flap used in dermatologic surgery is the Keystone flap, which relies on musculocutaneous and fasciocutaneous vascular perforators taken together with venous and neural connections within the flap's base, which may increase the perfusion, and thus the reliability, of any flap.

The most common flaps used in dermatologic surgery, composed of primarily of subcutaneous tissue and skin (and sometimes superficial muscular fascia), are axial and random perfusion flaps. Axial flaps (also called arterial flaps) have a relatively large-diameter, named artery present within the pedicle of the flap, which directly provides nutrients to the full extent of the flap. This named artery typically lies in the subcutaneous layer superficial to the muscle fascia. On the face, the most commonly used axial flap is the paramedian forehead flap, which depends on the supratrochlear artery (and occasionally branches of the supraorbital artery) for survival. A random flap, the most commonly used flap design in reconstructive dermatologic surgery, depends on the small, unnamed perfusion plexus of highly anastomotic vessels in the dermis to provide nutrients to the flap. Because the arterial input of random pattern flaps is much less predictable, attention to proper flap design and delicate surgical technique is required to ensure surgical success.

Blood flow is the most crucial factor for flap viability. Vascular perfusion pressure is a description of the force of blood flow through a vessel. Perfusion pressure and blood flow in the body's vessels are analogous to water flowing from a faucet through a garden hose. The greatest pressure and highest flow will be at the faucet head. As water travels farther away from the faucet, its pressure and flow decrease in strength. To maintain sufficient flow to the distal tip of the hose, the perfusion pressure within the hose must exceed the resistance of the hose. Similarly, in the human body, the perfusion pressure of any vessel that supplies blood and nutrients to the skin must exceed the capillary resistance in order to maintain vessel patency and preserve continued blood flow. A critical pressure is required to maintain patency of capillaries. Below this certain pressure, the capillaries will close, and insufficient blood will be supplied to the distal portions of the flap. The greater the distance from the feeding artery or arteriole, the lower the perfusion pressure will be (Fig. 2.2). Thus beyond a certain distance, the flap tip will no longer receive blood nutrients, and it will thus necrose.[2,3]

An understanding of perfusion pressures has dictated that flaps be designed with appropriate flap length to pedicle width ratio. Until 1970, it was widely believed that the viable length of a flap was directly proportional to the width of the base. Surgeons believed that in order to double the

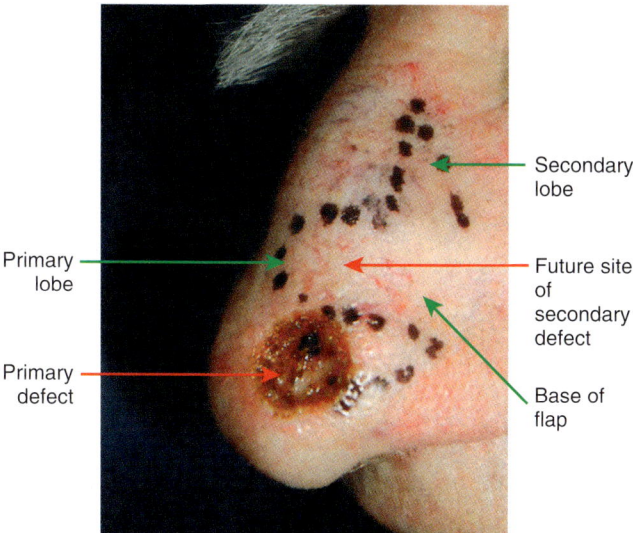

Fig. 2.1 The wound resulting from the extirpation of the tumor is the primary defect. The secondary defect is defined as the wound created by cutting, lifting, and sliding the flap to fill the primary defect. Here, the secondary defect will be filled by the second lobe of the flap. The base of the flap is that area that remains attached to the contiguous skin adjacent to the defect.

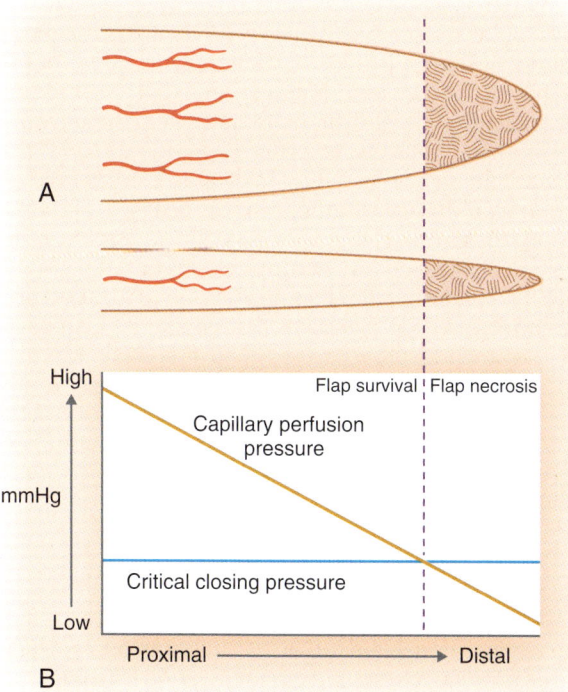

Fig. 2.2 Flap perfusion pressures necessary for flap survival. The graph shows how perfusion pressure decreases the greater the distance that the blood must flow from the feeding artery or arteriole. (A and B) Show that despite greater recruitment of random arterioles, there is a point where perfusion pressure is less than the capillary resistance. At this point of no flow, the flap will necrose.

length of the flap, one would simply need to double the width of the flap base, thereby including a sufficient number of vessels in the pedicle to sustain the flap tip. Many felt that there was no ultimate limit to flap length. In 1970 Milton disputed this conventional hypothesis by publishing his research on axial flaps in the pig model. He discovered that "flaps made under the same conditions of blood supply survive to the same length regardless of width."[8] Daniel and Williams confirmed Milton's research on axial flaps and further studied survival of random pattern flaps. Although they concluded that "an increase in width did not result in an increased length of survival,"[4] their data showed a trend toward wider pedicles allowing greater flap length survival. Studies by Stell in a pig model and confirmed when extrapolated to humans suggested that viable flap length was not directly proportional to pedicle width, and that beyond a certain pedicle width, greater recruitment of random vessels cannot support the flap tip (see Fig. 2.2).[3] Clinical experience with random flap survival has echoed this survival trend.

Overall, perfusion pressure limits the ultimate length of both axial and random flaps. The greater the perfusion pressure in the flap's pedicle, the longer the flap can be without undergoing necrosis. Moreover, the greater the perfusion pressure at the flap's base, the more narrow the pedicle may be. Arteries always have greater perfusion pressures than distal arterioles and capillaries. Accordingly, the longest viable flaps with the narrowest bases (largest length-to-base ratios) are arterial flaps. Therefore a paramedian forehead flap that uses the supratrochlear artery may be at least four times as long as the flap's pedicle width (at least a 4:1 ratio; Fig. 2.3). Musculocutaneous flaps have the next greatest blood supply in the pedicle, followed by fasciocutaneous and random flaps in descending order.

The commonly used random pattern flaps are largely supported by the redundant subdermal vascular plexus in the skin. Fig. 2.4 highlights the innate vasculature of the skin, upon which flap survival depends. The deeper, muscular-based arteries supply the subdermal plexus, which subsequently perfuses the intradermal plexus. The intradermal vasculature alone is usually unable to support tissue viability, due to low perfusion pressures and blood flow within these distal capillaries.[2,6,7] However, the subdermal plexus, found in the mid to superficial subcutaneous fat, contains both arterioles and capillaries with sufficient perfusion pressure to sustain tissue viability following flap movement. This anatomy is critical to understand when undermining (dissecting under the flap and its surrounding area to allow tissue movement) a cutaneous flap. If undermining is performed superficial to the subdermal plexus (i.e., within the dermis), the flap has a significantly increased chance of undergoing tissue ischemia.

The perfusion pressures of random cutaneous flaps vary with the flaps' locations on the body.[3,4,6,8–13] As soon as a random pattern flap is incised and raised, there is a significant decrease in the perfusion pressure to the distal, disrupted skin.[14,15] Fortunately at normal skin temperature, the amount of blood flowing through the facial skin is 10 times greater than that needed to supply the skin's basic metabolic needs.[16–19] Other areas of the body are not as well supplied with this redundancy of blood supply. A general rule is that the more distant the surgical flap is located from

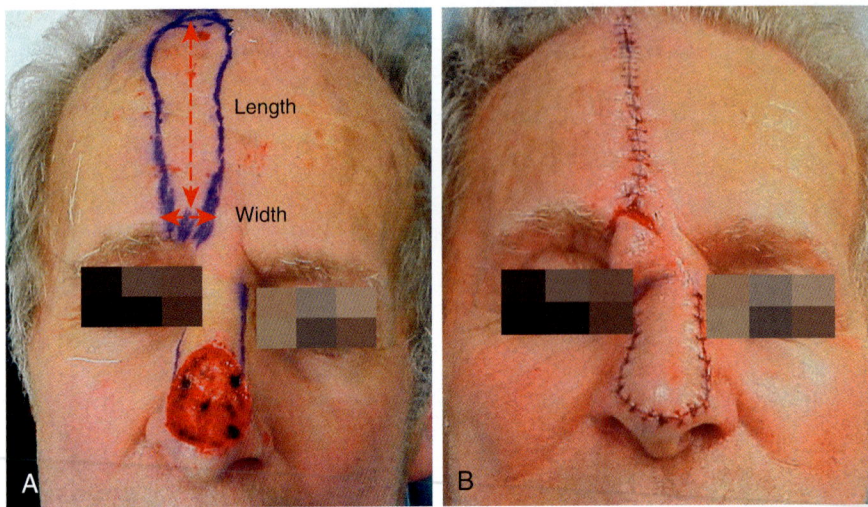

Fig. 2.3 Measuring the flap length to width. By including a large bore artery (the supratrochlear artery) in the flap pedicle, the ratio may be at least as great as 4:1 as shown in the preoperative photo (A) and after suturing (B).

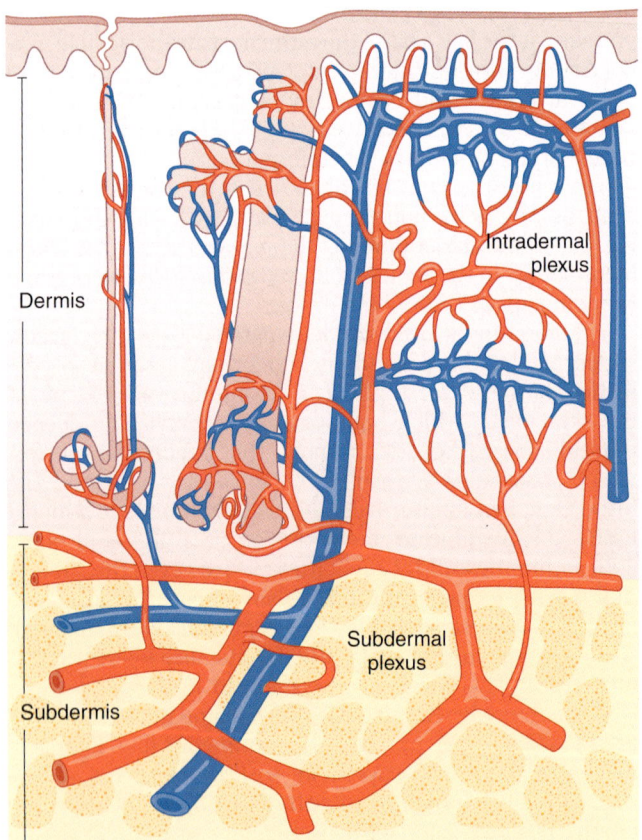

Fig. 2.4 The support of commonly used random pattern flaps by the redundant subdermal vascular plexus in the skin. The deeper, muscular-based axial arteries (not shown) supply the subdermal plexus, which subsequently perfuses the intradermal plexus. The intradermal vasculature alone is usually unable to support tissue viability because of low perfusion pressures and blood flow within these distal capillaries. The subdermal plexus, found in the mid- to superficial subcutaneous fat, contains both arterioles and capillaries with sufficient perfusion pressure to sustain tissue viability following flap movement. Therefore undermining of a random pattern flap must occur below the subdermal plexus.

the heart, the less the perfusion pressure will be. Hence a flap on the leg should be designed with a smaller flap length-to-pedicle width ratio when compared with a flap on the face.

As previously discussed, there is a point at which no matter how many extra vessels are recruited at the base, the distal perfusion pressure will be less than the critical closing pressure of the arterioles and capillaries (see Fig. 2.2).[3,6,8,15,20] When the perfusion pressure is less than this intravascular resistance, the flap receives diminished nutrients and necrosis can ensue. Generally, random cutaneous flaps of the face with a maximum length-to-base ratio of 3:1 survive.[21–23] On the trunk and legs, the maximum length-to-base ratio is considered to be 2:1.[12,21,22,24,25] An axial flap on the face may have a 4:1 or greater ratio depending on the arterial supply of the pedicle.[21,26] Remember that these ratios are only guidelines. Patient-related factors must be taken into account when contemplating the feasibility and design of a flap. In addition to location of the body, local perfusion pressures can be altered by a variety of factors such as tobacco use, history of radiation to the area, medical comorbidities (i.e., atherosclerosis, high or low blood pressure, arrhythmias), and use of vasoconstrictors. In addition, flap design must take into account variations in skin laxity based on location, age, and comorbid conditions.

Flap Physiology

Flap survival is dependent on various factors, including blood flow, angiogenesis and vascularization, edema, wound closure tension, postoperative complications such as hematoma/seromas, and infection. Prior to the first incision, the flap skin is fully vascularized and viable using the definition of normal skin. Once the flap is raised, it is immediately ischemic, since the normal vessels supplying that skin are cut and the flap now depends on decreased circulation from the collateral vessels. A flap is always initially viable, since the skin can survive up to 12 to 13 hours of avascularity at 37°F.[27–29] An ischemic flap can survive even longer, since the blood flow needed to sustain skin is only 2 to 8 cc per 100 g per minute, and normal flow to the skin is 10 times greater than this minimum.[16,27] Thus Meyers[27] was correct when he commented that a fresh flap is always ischemic but viable.

Once incised and relocated, the flap receives its nutrients from both the cutaneous pedicle and the base of the primary defect. Sufficient blood flow through the base of the flap is essential in the initial 24 to 48 hours after the initial flap creation. In both axial and random flaps, blood flow immediately drops as the flap is elevated. For axial flaps, microvascular flow actually increases to a level greater than the preoperative state within 5 hours.[15,30] Flow in random pattern flaps, however, starts to improve differentially for up to 4 weeks. Marks used the rat model to show that flow improved on a gradient; flow increased within 14–16 hours to the skin closest to the pedicle, within 24–48 hours to the skin 1 cm distal to the pedicle, and within 96 hours 3 cm distal to the pedicle.[15] All sites recovered approximately 30% of their blood flow per day, with the proximal most portion recovering full blood flow by the end of 7 days and the most distal tip by the end of 14 days. Until 14 days, recovery of blood flow occurred on a gradient that depended on the distance of the skin from the base of the flap. Microvascular flow grew to higher than preoperative levels from 14 to 21 days, and then gradually returned to baseline during the fourth week. The opening of collateral vessels appears to allow this sequential recovery of blood flow. However, there appears to be a limit on how fast these collaterals can open.[15]

This time-dependent opening of collateral vessels may be partially explained by arteriovenous (AV) shunts. These shunts control blood supply to the capillary network that supplies the flap. There are pre-AV shunt sphincters under the control of the sympathetic nervous system. When the flap is incised and undermined, local sympathetic nerve fibers are disrupted and release catecholamines. As a result, there is local vasoconstriction for up to 48 hours, by which time the nerve's supply of norepinephrine is exhausted.[27,31] Once sympathetic tone is relaxed, the blood flow to the capillary collaterals is increased to help supply the flap with nutrients.[14] However, this effective sympathectomy cannot fully explain why random flaps have a graded flow recovery. Upon incision, the entire flap should have equal catecholamine release and subsequent equal flow recovery.[32] Other humoral factors such as prostaglandin release may come into play.[33]

Local tissue conditions resulting from surgical trauma also decrease flap perfusion and subsequent survival. Following any local injury, the inflammatory cascade releases the powerful vasoconstrictor thromboxane A2.[34,35] In addition, free radicals are released, causing direct injury to the flap.[36,37] Finally, the edema inevitably associated with surgical trauma causes further capillary vessel resistance by increasing manual compression on the skin's smaller caliber perfusion sources.[38] In addition, fluid collection under the flap in the form of a postoperative hematoma or seroma can further decrease blood flow. All of these negative factors decrease perfusion to the flap and can threaten flap survival.

Conversely, the flap may also benefit from surgical trauma. Relative local hypoxemia and increased levels of metabolic by-products induce opening of precapillary sphincters, thereby promoting increased local blood flow.[27,31,39] Moreover, adhesion molecules, such as E-selectin, are activated following exposure to released coagulation cascade molecules such as endotoxin, interleukin-1, and tumor necrosis factor alpha.[40] These adhesion molecules recruit molecules including neutrophils to the flap to clear debris and anabolic waste products. Finally, ischemic tissue attracts endothelial progenitor cells, which allow for the ingrowth of new vascular channels to supply the flap.[41] Flap survival is dependent on the balance of all these factors, ultimately influencing pedicle blood flow.

The nascent flap not only receives nutrients from the pedicle, but it also gains nutrition from the base of the primary defect through angiogenesis, revascularization, and neovascularization.[41–44] Within the first two days of flap placement, a fibrin layer develops below the flap and provides a suitable environment for angiogenesis.[36] Endothelial cells and macrophages release angiogenic cell factors important in neovascularization, the local growth of new blood vessels into the surgically manipulated skin.[41,44–46] Neovascularization is seen as early as 3 days in the rat model,[47] and at 4 days in rabbit[48] and pig[42] models. In staged, pedicled flaps in humans, revascularization adequate for division of the flap pedicle has been demonstrated by the seventh postoperative day.[42,49,50] This new vascular growth works in conjunction with the preexisting collateral vessels to nourish the flap.

Tissue edema, wound closure tension, and infection also negatively affect flap blood supply and survival. Although none of these factors can solely lead to necrosis of a well-vascularized flap, each can contribute to further ischemia in a marginally perfused flap. Postoperative tissue edema places external force on small capillaries,[38] resulting in increased capillary resistance. Thus there must be greater perfusion pressure at the pedicle to counter this resistance and ensure flap tip survival. Recent studies in the rat model revealed that significant postoperative edema will not solely cause flap necrosis.[51] However, it can be an additive factor, along with high wound closure tensions and/or infection.

Closing wounds under large amounts of tension can place undue vascular stress on the wound edges and tip of the flap. It is typically recommended that one undermine 2 to 4 cm,[52] or 50% to 100% of the defect width,[53] beyond the wound edge to decrease wound tension. Undermining beyond this distance may be detrimental, since there may be unnecessary vascular compromise, more bleeding, and greater dead space, all of which can lead to surgical complications. High closure tension leads to dehiscence and wound edge necrosis, but it does not usually lead to entire flap necrosis.[54–56] Wound infection can cause partial or complete flap necrosis. With local infection, there is release of toxic free radicals and greater tissue edema.[57] Infection can also lead to vessel thrombosis.[58] In addition to local tissue destruction and vascular compromise, collagen production and deposition are hindered.[59] Therefore flap adhesion to the wound bed and overall tensile strength are affected. Overall, there are many factors involved in the initial period of wound healing that are critical to the flap's survival. Predictably acceptable flap results depend on proper flap design, gentle operative technique, and the avoidance of surgical complications.

Flap Biomechanics

In addition to understanding the skin's vascular supply and physiology, the surgeon must also appreciate the unique biomechanical properties of the skin if flap surgery is to be successful. All materials have characteristic biomechanical properties: stress, strain, creep, and stress relaxation. In regard to skin, stress is the force applied per cross-sectional area, and strain is the change in length divided by the original length of the given tissue, to which a given force is applied. The stress–strain relationship of skin shows that skin, unlike some other materials, is not truly elastic (Fig. 2.5). As a small amount of stress (or tension) is placed on the skin, there is a corresponding change in the skin's length (strain). At a certain point on the stress–strain curve (see zone III in Fig. 2.5), even a large amount of applied force will not result in further incremental skin stretch.[26] This nonelastic property of skin is mainly due to its structural constituents—collagen and elastin. In relaxed skin, collagen is randomly oriented, and elastin is loosely wrapped around and attached to multiple points on the collagen bundles.[60–64] When a small amount of force is initially applied to skin, the elastin network is first deformed[63,65] and the skin is easily lengthened (see zone I in Fig. 2.5). With sun exposure and intrinsic aging, there is a progressive decrease in the functional elastic fiber network.[65] As a result, the stress–strain curve is shifted to the right so that when applied to aged or sun-damaged skin, less applied force results in greater lengthening. As continued force is applied, the collagen fibers begin to reorient parallel to the direction of the force (rapid transition of the curve; see zone II in Fig. 2.5).[64] At the point where the elastin and collagen fibers are maximally stretched, even a large amount of force will only minimally stretch the skin (see zone III in Fig. 2.5).

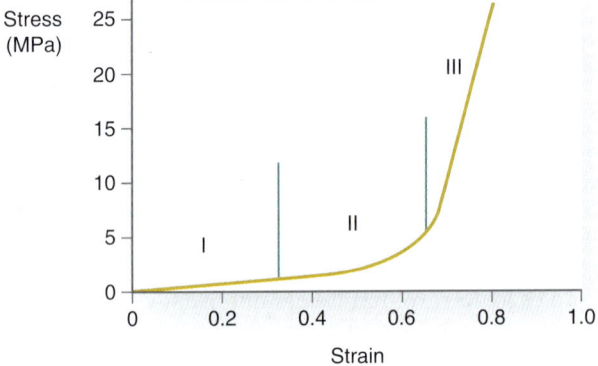

Fig. 2.5 Stress–strain curve demonstrating the nonlinear properties of skin when stretched (vertical axis). When a small amount of force is initially applied to skin, the elastin network is first deformed and the skin is easily lengthened (horizontal axis; zone I). As progressive continued force is applied, the collagen fibers begin to reorient parallel to the direction of the force (zone II). At the point where the elastin and collagen fibers are maximally stretched, even a large amount of force will only minimally stretch the skin (zone III). With sun exposure and intrinsic aging, the stress–strain curve is shifted to the right.

Thus the skin is not truly elastic at all levels of applied tension.

Creep refers to the increase in strain seen when skin is under constant stress. When the skin is held at sufficient tension, elastic fibers fragment and collagen fibers will align parallel to the applied force. As a result of this reorganization of the elastic and collagen fiber networks, interstitial fluid will be displaced and can be seen with the naked eye.[66] Creep typically begins to occur within several minutes of constant force application. While skin demonstrates elastic properties with low loads, skin exhibits "stress relaxation" and creep when larger forces are applied for longer periods of time. Stress relaxation occurs when skin is held under constant tension. In this case the amount of force (stress) required to maintain this tension decreases with time. The skin's relaxation under stress is closely related to its ability to increase in length when placed under a constant stress (the creep phenomenon). In the case of a cutaneous flap, if held steadily at high tension for 5 to 10 minutes, the skin will lengthen and relax. Surgeons with an understanding of this property may use an intraoperative pulley stitch to take advantage of this mechanical property. As a result of intraoperative creep, a smaller flap can be used to fill a larger defect, but the potential reliance upon secondary motion around the surgical defect must be recognized. When skin is held at a constant tension for several days, stress relaxation occurs. There is a decrease in stress due to an increase in skin cellularity and the permanent stretching of skin components.[64] In clinical practice, serial excision and tissue expansion use the principles of creep and stress relaxation. When a large lesion is partially excised and reconstructed under tension, the skin relaxes and lengthens, allowing further staged excisions.

Understanding the stress–strain curve is essential for optimal wound closure. When reviewing reconstructive options, it is important to avoid any excessive stress on the defect edges that would force the involved skin into the third part of the stress–strain curve; this involves minimizing tension on the wound closure. Unfavorably high wound closure tensions limit recruitment of skin laxity and can be detrimental to wound healing. Specifically, high tension may lead to wound edge necrosis, wound dehiscence, and cosmetically unacceptable scars (i.e., widened, atrophic, or hypertrophic scars). Wound edge tension may be minimized by appropriate undermining; however, care must be taken to understand and minimize the underlying mechanism of stress or restriction. For example, a galeotomy may be used to release galeal fascial restraint and allow for additional movement of the skin and subcutaneous tissue on the scalp; careful dissection of the skin from the underlying orbicularis muscle in the periocular area creates movement of the skin to allow for tension redistribution away from the free margin; and separating the vertical connections within the subcutaneous tissue of the cheek from the underlying superficial muscular aponeurotic system (SMAS) drastically reduces tension on closures and allows for substantial movement of tissue for closure of large cheek defects.

In addition to understanding the role of tension reduction on wound closure, it is important to identify situations where tension redistribution is required. Specifically, when side-to-side linear closure is not possible due to excessive tension or stress on the primary closure, or when linear wound closure abuts a free margin or crosses a cosmetic subunit boundary, the vector of tension may need to be redistributed in the form of a rotation or transposition flaps, discussed later. Overall, by taking advantage of the above-mentioned mechanical properties of skin and designing appropriate flaps, the surgeon takes tension off the wound edges, and returns the skin to the first or second zone of the stress–strain curve.[64] Understanding these principles, as well as mastering techniques for tension reduction and redistribution, allows the closure of skin flaps under low or moderate tension. As a result, wound edges can survive, and a good cosmetic result can be obtained.

Flaps Defined by Movement

In addition to classifying flaps by their vascularity, flaps are often also categorized by their primary movement directions. The three basic flap movements are advancement, rotation, and transposition. With advancement flaps, the major motion of the flap is largely along a single linear direction toward the primary defect (Fig. 2.6). Rotation flaps are those flaps that are rotated in an arc or curvilinear fashion along a pivot point to fill the adjacent primary defect without crossing any intervening skin (Fig. 2.7). A transposition flap is incised and lifted over intact skin and then placed into the wound (Fig. 2.8). A distinct type of transposition flap is called the interpolation flap. An interpolation flap is a flap, potentially with a predictable, axial vascular supply, that involves two steps or stages. The first stage of the flap is transposing the tissue into the wound with the pedicle overlying the intervening skin. The second stage is separating the flap from its origin and therefore dividing its pedicle.

In addition to classifying flaps by their unidirectional motion, some authors, noting the inherent limitations of such schemata, categorize flaps as sliding or lifting flaps.[67,68] Sliding flaps include advancement and rotation flaps, where tissue is pushed into the primary defect. A lifting flap is the typical transposition or interpolation flap, in which tissue must be lifted over normal skin to fill the wound. These more general classifications recognize that very few flaps move tissue along a single, predictable path. For example, most rotation flaps also incorporate a significant degree of tissue advancement, and vice versa.

As alluded to previously, when discussing the motion of these flaps, the surgeon must understand the tension vector created by the flap's closure. This vector depends on the primary and secondary motion of the flap. The primary motion of the flap is the tension placed on the flap tissue as it is moved to fill the wound (primary defect) (Fig. 2.9). The secondary motion, created by the movement of the flap into the defect, is the force placed on the tissue surrounding the primary defect (see Fig. 2.9). The combined force created by the primary and secondary motions causes a new tension vector that must be anticipated by the surgeon when deciding which flap can best be used for repair. This final tension vector varies, depending on the flap chosen, and may be appreciated when placing the key stitch. The key stitch is the stitch placed to initially move the flap and accurately place it into the primary defect.[69] If not properly planned, the flap's final tension vector may cause undesirable pulling on free margins such as the eyelid, alar rim, and mouth.

ADVANCEMENT FLAP

The advancement flap has long been used in facial reconstruction. Its first description has been attributed to Celsus

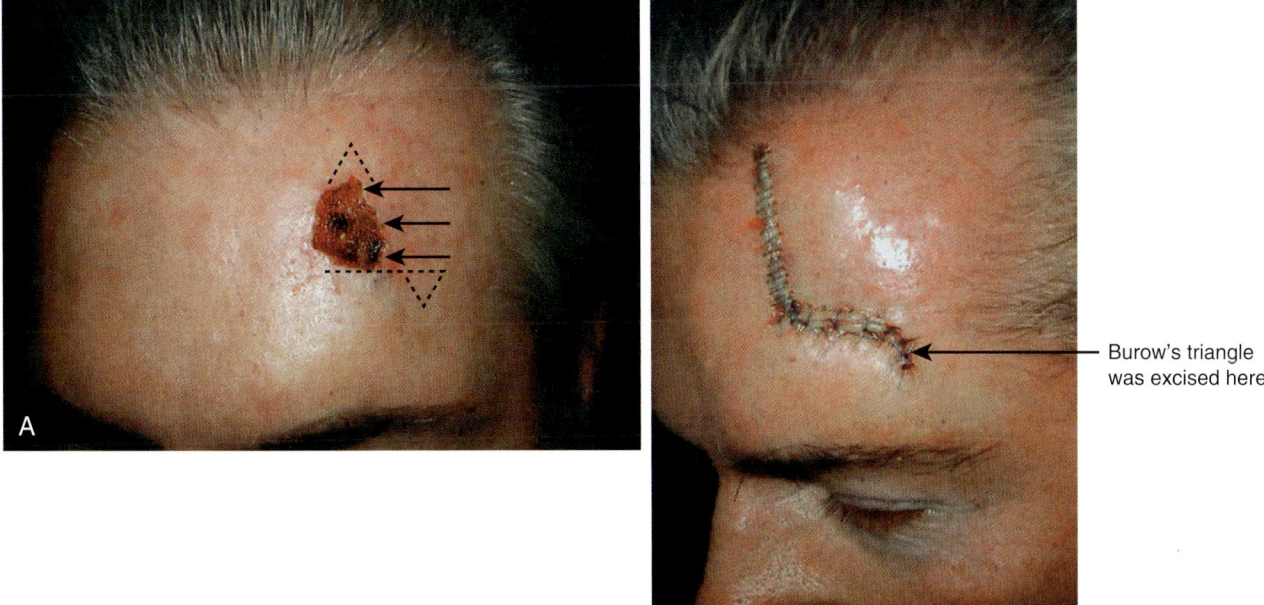

Fig. 2.6 The lateral forehead skin laxity was used in this unilateral advancement flap. (A) The arrows indicate the direction of the flap movement. (B) The arrow indicates where the Burow's triangle was removed.

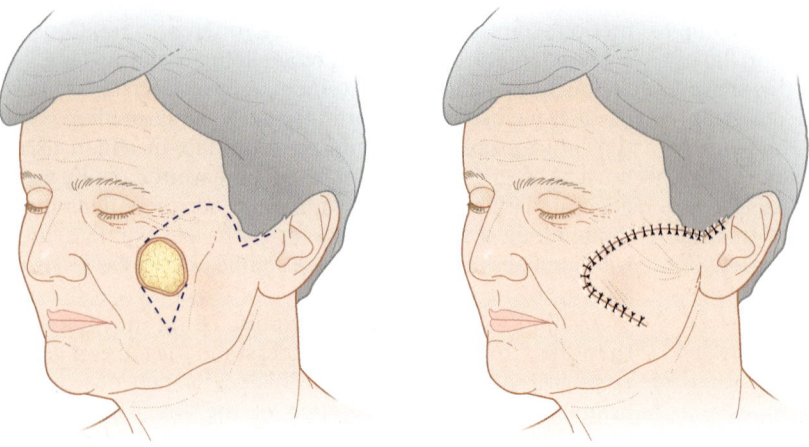

Fig. 2.7 This lateral cheek rotation flap illustrates how the flap is rotated in an arc along a pivot point to fill the adjacent primary defect without crossing any other intervening skin.

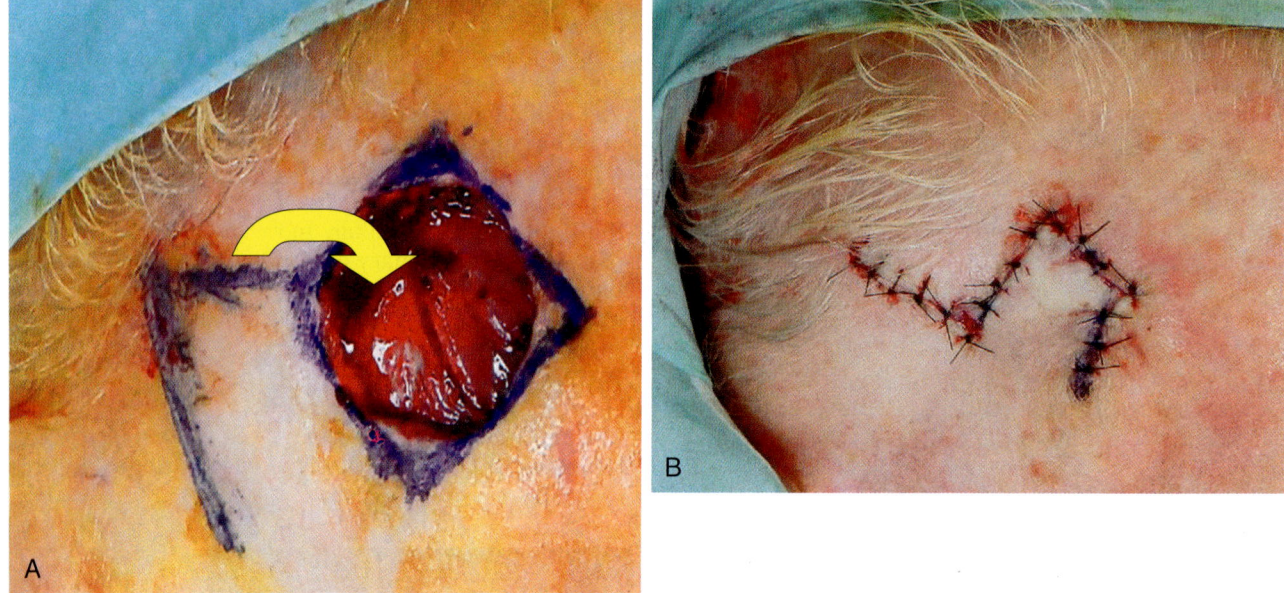

Fig. 2.8 A rhombic transposition flap. The flap must be transposed over intact skin to be placed into the defect. The flap must be transposed over intact skin (A) to be placed into the defect (B).

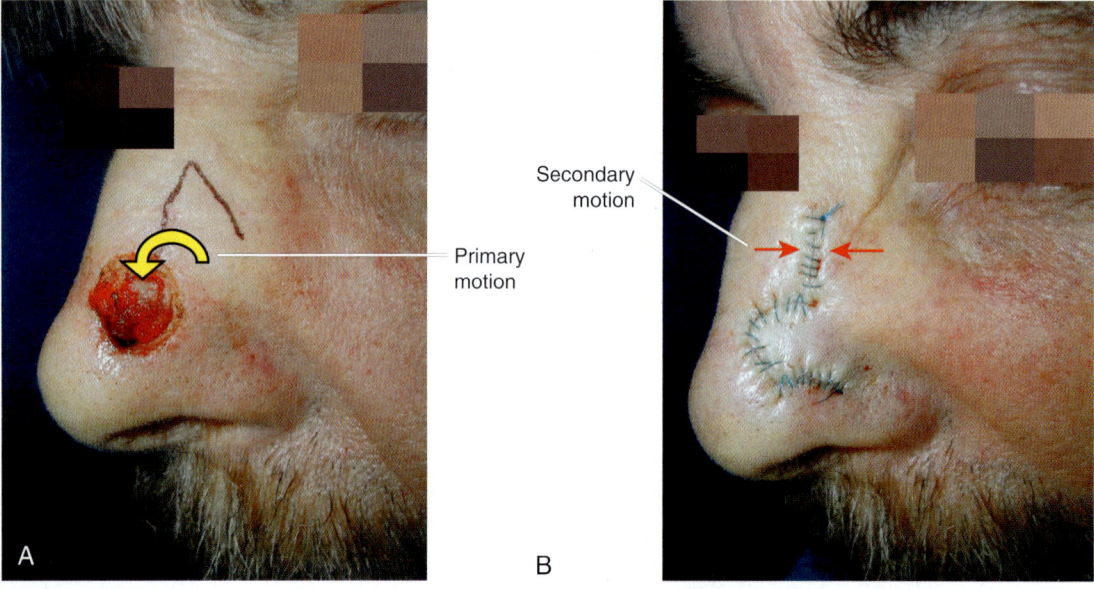

Fig. 2.9 (A) The primary motion of the flap *(yellow arrow)*. (B) As a result of this motion, tension will be redistributed and the secondary motion tension can be seen on the lateral nasal bridge *(red arrows)*.

of ancient Rome, who used the flap for the reconstruction of the cheek and ears.[70,71] In the 1800s, French surgeons advocated the use of "lambeau par glissement" (sliding flaps) for facial reconstruction.[72] In 1885 Burow modified and further described the advantages of this flap in reconstruction.[73]

The unilateral, bilateral, and V to Y advancement flaps are the most commonly used advancement flaps in dermatologic surgery. The primary and secondary motions, and thus the resulting tension vectors of these flaps, are usually in a simple linear line along the direction of the flap movement (see Fig. 2.6).[73] The key stitch typically brings the leading edge of the flap to the opposite wound edge to close the primary defect. As the tissue is advanced and sutured into place, a standing cone (or cones) develop(s). These standing cone deformities, or dog ears, are caused by the pouching of excess, compressed skin near the flap's base when tissue is advanced under tension.[74]

The standing cone may be corrected by either extending the incision line to remove the excess tissue or using an M-plasty (Fig. 2.10A).[75,76] By truncating one end of the closure, the M-plasty flap has the advantage of providing a shorter final wound length. If the wound cannot be extended due to a free margin or approaching cosmetic subunit boundary, tissue protrusions can be anticipated. As the length of the flap base is longer than the edge of the flap itself, uneven lengths of tissue requiring approximation are created (see Fig. 2.10B). The inequality of tissue lengths can be accounted for by removing a triangle of skin, called a Burow's triangle,[77] from anywhere along the skin surrounding the flap (see Figs. 2.6 and 2.10B). In addition, the unequal lengths can be accounted for by removing a curvilinear segment of skin from the limb of the flap itself, thereby lengthening the overall arm of the flap to equal that of the flap base and redistributing the redundant tissue along the length of the incision (see Fig. 2.10C). This is particularly useful on the upper cutaneous lip and eyebrow areas.

When using bilateral advancement flaps to correct a circular defect, the repair may be described as an A-to-T (T-plasty) or an O-to-H flap (H-plasty). These unilateral and bilateral advancement flaps are most commonly used in repairs on the forehead, scalp, and eyelids. The V-to-Y advancement flap[78] uses a subcutaneous pedicle that perfuses a triangular flap that advances along a single direction (see Fig. 2.10D). All borders of the flap are incised to the subcutaneous fat, and the resulting island of tissue, now liberated from lateral dermal attachments, is advanced to fill the defect. The pedicle is underneath rather than at the edge of the flap and may include muscle.[79–81] Various modifications,[82,83] such as parallel release incisions of the pedicle base, allow significant advancement of the flap with predictable flap survival.[84] Because the flap's muscular-containing, thick pedicle ensures liberal blood flow, this flap is the most likely of all flaps to survive in patients with tobacco use, which can result in decreased perfusion. The flap can be used anywhere on the face, but the authors find this flap to be particularly useful for repairs of the upper cutaneous lip, the alar–cheek sulcus, and the lateral eyebrow, with alopecic defects to help restore medial hair-bearing areas. Of note, the V-to-Y advancement flap was previously synonymous with the "island pedicle flap"; however, this terminology now refers exclusively to flaps in which a portion of the donor tissue is deepithelialized and tunneled or passed beneath the skin to a distant recipient site. It is important to differentiate the island pedicle flap from a V-to-Y advancement flap for both clinical documentation and coding purposes.

ROTATION FLAPS

In 1842 Pancoast described using rotation flaps to close facial wounds.[85] Like most random pattern flaps, rotation flaps recruit tissue adjacent to the primary defect. An arc or semicircle flap is incised and pivoted into the wound (Fig. 2.11). Thus the primary motion is rotation. Similar to advancement flaps, the secondary motion of the flap causes a standing cone deformity at the base of the flap. This Burow's triangle may be excised from anywhere along the arc of the flap from the nonpedicle side (see Fig. 2.11A). Another similarity between rotation and advancement flaps is the placement of the key stitch. This first stitch closes the primary defect.

The surgeon must pay particular attention to the size of the designed rotation flap. Because it is rotated along an arc, the functional flap length is shorter than the actual length of the flap's incision (see Fig. 2.11B). Hence the planned length must be longer than the diameter of the wound.[86] Dzubow recommends that the planned height of the flap be greater than the height of the defect to account for this functional loss of length.[87] One advantage of the rotation flap is that its base is typically broad, and therefore the flap's length-to-width ratio may be as long as 6:1.[88] This makes the flap particularly useful when closing inelastic areas such as the scalp.

To increase the movement of the rotation flap, a back-cut or Z-plasty may be employed. A back-cut is when an incision is placed into the pedicle of the flap to allow greater forward movement (see Fig. 2.11C). Although the back-cut can increase flap mobility, this maneuver cuts into the flap's base, thereby increasing the risk of tip ischemia. In areas with excellent vascularity, such as the gabella, the back-cut is often incorporated into the rotation flap's design. Another technique used to increase flap movement and reduce the primary tension vector is the use of a Z-plasty at the tail of the rotation flap (see Fig. 2.11D).

Rotation flaps are most often used for repairs of the scalp, forehead, cheek, and nose. The Rieger flap,[89] or dorsal nasal rotation flap, uses a back-cut in its design to allow closure of small- to medium-sized defects of the distal third of the nose. In 1985 Marchac and Toth modified the flap design by defining an axial pedicle for the flap based on the angular artery.[90] This modification allows a greater flap length-to-pedicle base ratio because of a reliable blood supply. Multiple rotation flaps may be used to repair large defects on the chin, forehead, and nasal tip. When two mirror-image rotation flaps are designed to repair the defect, the closure is called an O-to-Z repair. There are a few specialized forms of bilateral rotation flaps that have also been reported: the Peng flap for the nose and the bilateral vermillion flap on the lip.[91,92] When three or more rotation flaps are used, it is often referred to as a pinwheel flap.

TRANSPOSITION FLAPS

Transposition flaps were documented in the pre–Common Era. In about 2000 BC, Indians committing adultery were

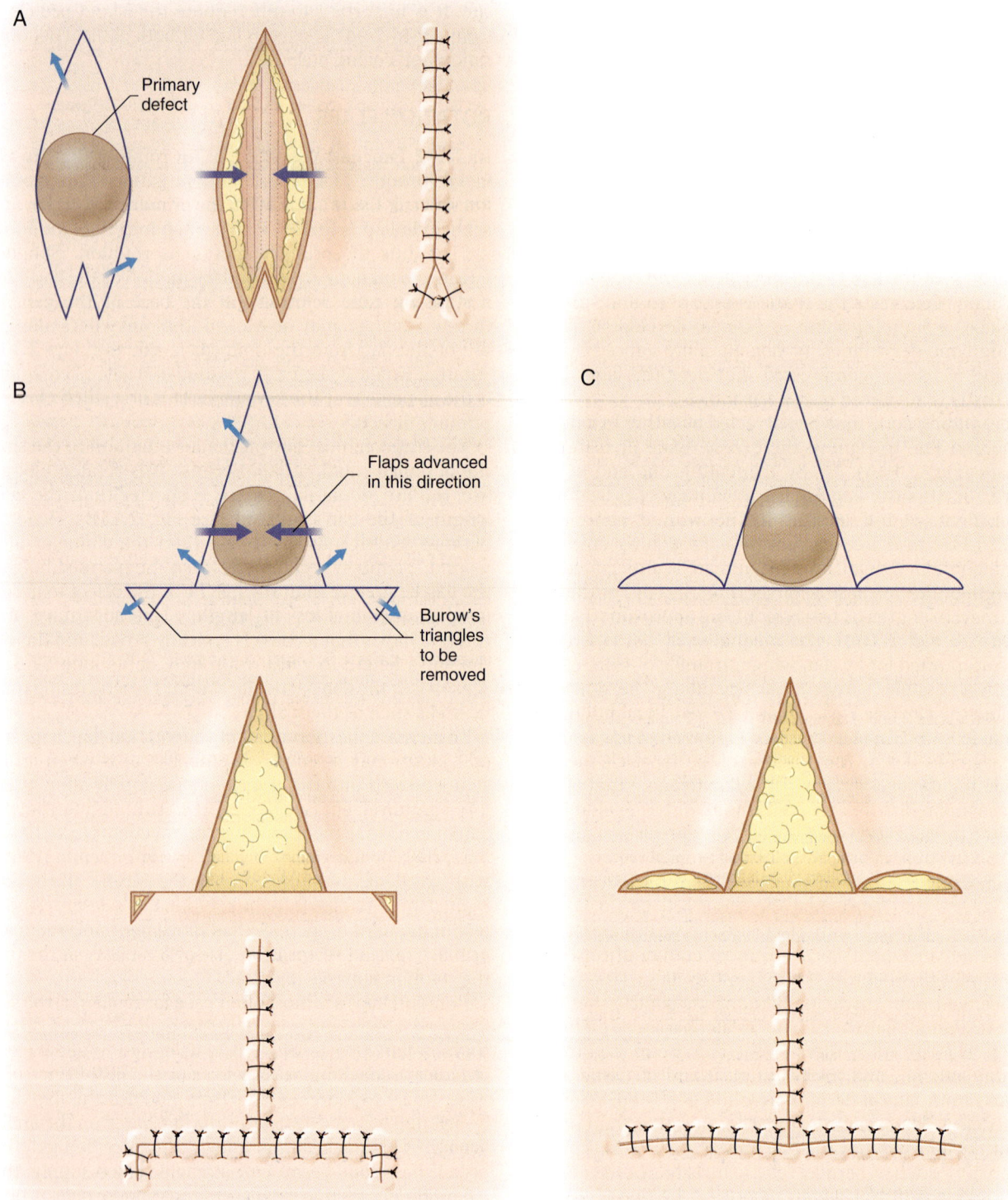

Fig. 2.10 (A) The M-plasty, a variant of a linear closure, is depicted at the inferior wound margin. This technique is useful in shortening overall wound length and can be particularly useful when attempting not to cross facial subunit boundaries. (B) Here, an A-to-T repair (bilateral advancement flap) is used to correct the circular defect. The thick arrows indicate the direction of advancement. The smaller arrows indicate the tissue that must be removed to avoid standing cone deformities. (C) On certain anatomic locations where it would be disadvantageous to take inferior Burow triangles into other cosmetic subunits, such as on the upper cutaneous lip or on the forehead along the eyebrow, a crescentic dog ear can be taken to form the flap tissue itself, which serves to elongate the flap length, avoiding standing cones.

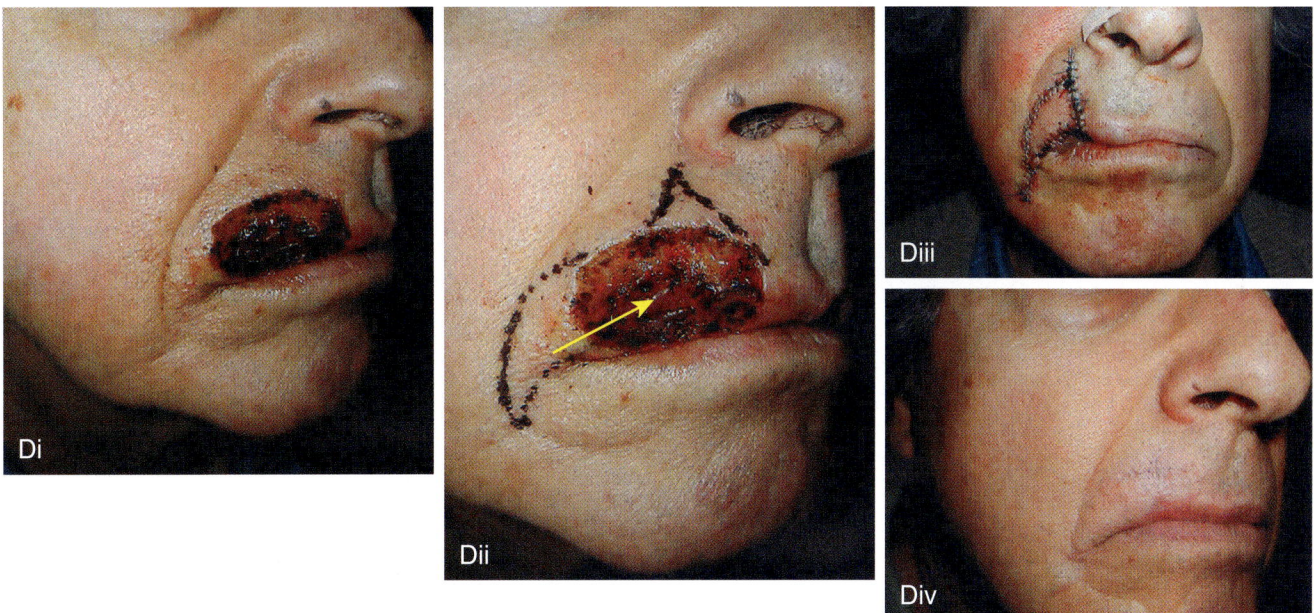

Fig. 2.10, cont'd An island pedicle flap is used (D) to correct this defect (Di) following removal of an infiltrative basal cell carcinoma. All borders of the flap are incised to the subcutaneous flap and the resulting island of tissue is advanced (Dii, Diii) to fill the defect. Panel Div shows the result at 3 months.

punished by nasal tip amputation. Although reconstructive procedures may have occurred even at that time, the Indian text Sushruta Samhita of the 8th century BC is credited with first describing nasal reconstruction using a cheek transposition flap.[1] By approximately 1000 AD, the "Indian flap," a forehead flap used to cover nasal defects, was introduced. By the 15th century, this surgical technique found its way to Europe, and the flap's use continues today.[93]

Many transposition flaps use both advancement and rotation as a component of their tissue motion. As it is raised and pivoted into the wound, the transposition flap is also advanced to close the primary defect. These flaps, like some pure rotation flaps, borrow tissue that might lie at a considerable distance from the primary defect. In addition, there is a three-dimensional lifting of the flap over intervening, intact skin as the flap is placed into the wound, rather than the two-dimensional pushing of the rotation or advancement flap tissue into the adjacent wound. Finally, the transposition flap's axis of tension is linear rather than the curvilinear axis seen in rotation flaps.

Understanding this tension vector is essential to proper transposition flap design. The secondary motion of the flap is a direct consequence of the tension that occurs with closure of the secondary defect. This vector can be visualized by placing a key suture to close the flap's donor defect. With the key stitch in place, the flap is effectively pushed into the primary wound. Incorrect planning of the transposition flap can adversely affect free margins of the face, as the wound closure tensions required to repair the flap's donor site can result in significant anatomic distortion if the flap's donor site is not carefully selected.

Dermatologic surgeons most commonly use the rhombic, bilobed, and melolabial transposition flaps. The rhomboid, or Limberg,[94] flap uses the geometry of two equilateral triangles placed base to base to form the shape of an equilateral parallelogram (rhombus; Fig. 2.12A). The typically circular primary defect can be modified to resemble a rhombus where all sides are equal in length, two interior angles are 60°, and two interior angles are 120°. The first flap incision is designed along the short diagonal and will equal the length of each side of the rhombus. As Fig. 2.12A depicts, the angle of the flap incision will equal 60°, and four different rhombic flaps can be potentially created. A variation of the traditional Limberg flap is the Dufourmentel[95] rhomboid flap, which uses a 60° interior flap angle (see Fig. 2.12B) and the Webster flap, which uses a 30° interior flap angle (see Fig. 2.12C). This smaller angle at the flap's apex can minimize the possibility of a distracting tissue bulge near the peak of the flap's donor site. The rhombic flap is extremely versatile and can be used anywhere on the face, provided that the secondary motion at the flap's donor site is carefully considered.

Another variant of the transposition flap is the bilobed flap, a useful flap that allows tissue mobilization in areas where closure of the secondary defect is difficult. Esser first described this flap in 1918 for nasal tip reconstruction in three case reports (Fig. 2.13A).[96] In the bilobed design, there are actually two flaps that share a common pedicle. The primary flap is designed to close the primary defect, and the second flap fills the secondary defect (see Fig. 2.13B). Because the secondary lobe's donor site is typically located in an area of relative skin excess, this tertiary defect can be closed in a simple side-to-side manner. Although the design nuances of the bilobed flap can be initially confusing, the movement of the flap can be accurately predicted if the basic principles of transposition flaps are well understood.

A third commonly used transposition flap in dermatologic surgery is the melolabial transposition (one-staged) flap. With this type of flap, the base may be located on the inferior or superior[97] cheek, depending on the coverage needed (Fig. 2.14A and B). The base contains a highly

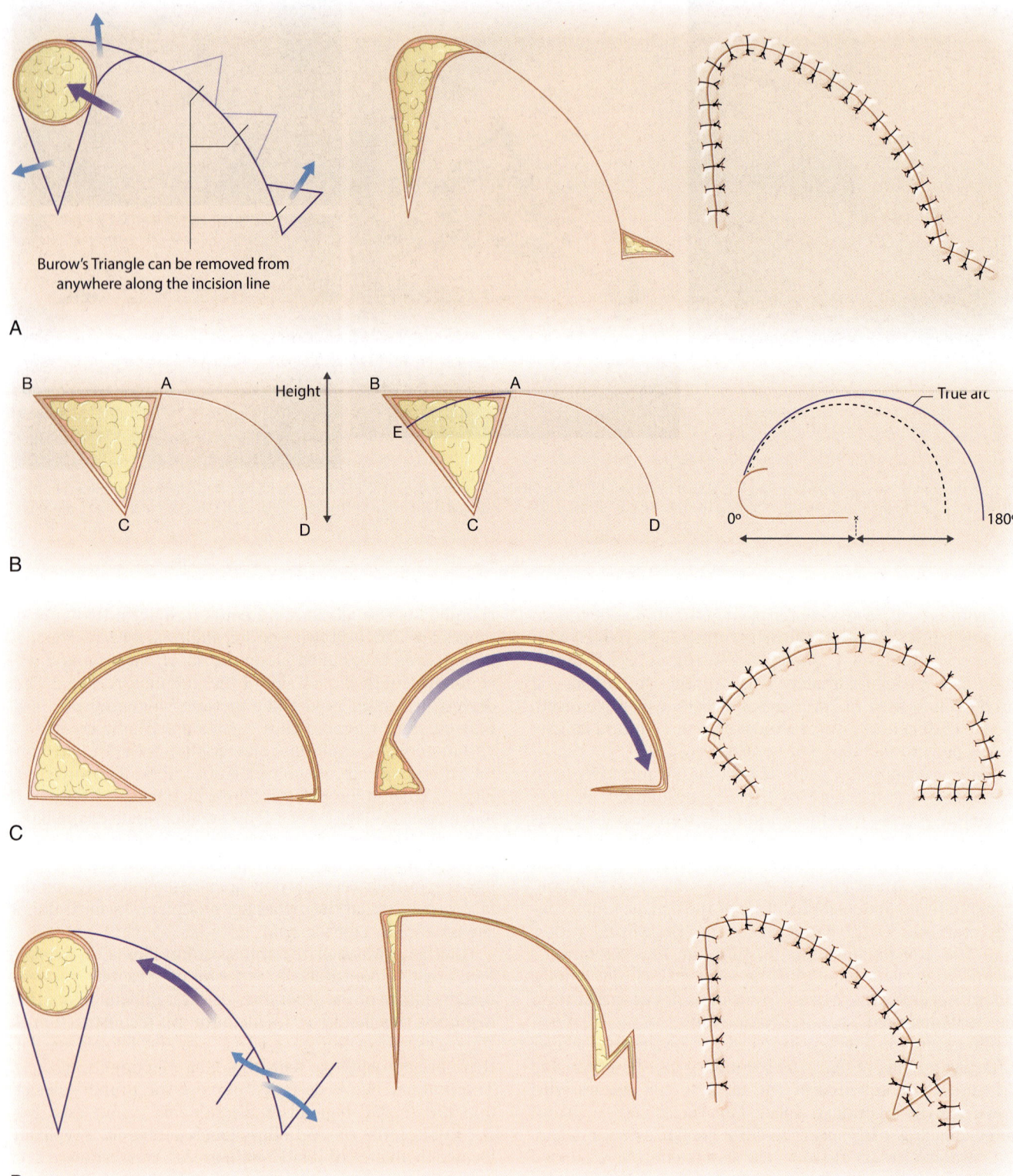

Fig. 2.11 Rotation flaps. (A) Rotation flaps use tissue adjacent to the primary defect. The semicircular flap is incised and pivoted along one axis into the wound. The Burow's triangle may be excised from anywhere along the tissue arc of the flap to prevent a standing cone deformity and allow easier flap movement into the defect. (B) When the rotation flap AD is rotated along its pivot point C, it will only reach point E and fill the triangle ACE without tension. The effective length of any flap is shortened when rotating on a fixed point (seen on right). To compensate for this functional length loss, Dzubow recommends that the planned height actually be greater than the defect height.[86] (C) To increase the forward rotation of the flap, a back-cut may be employed. Although there is improved movement, there is increased risk of distal flap ischemia, since the back-cut decreases the size of the vascular pedicle. (D) A Z-plasty can also be employed to lengthen the flap and extend its reach.

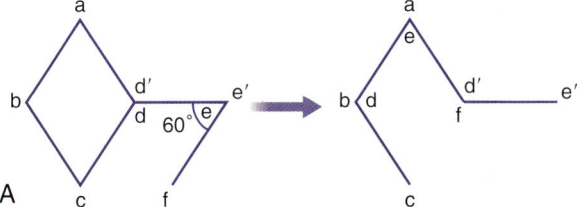

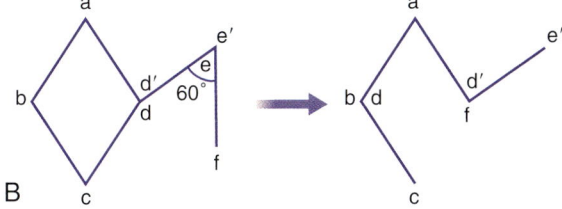

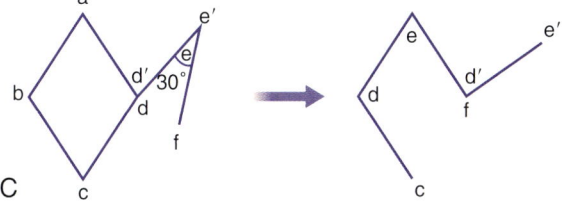

Fig. 2.12 Rhomboid transposition flaps. (A) The classic Limberg flap is shown. The circular primary defect can be modified to resemble a rhomboid where all sides are equal in length, and two interior angles are 60 degrees, and the other two interior angles are 120 degrees. The first flap incision is designed along the short diagonal and will equal the length of each side of the rhomboid rhombus. Four rhomboid flaps can potentially be designed by extending from any of the corners of the rhomboid. The Dufourmental flap (B) is more versatile than the Limberg and can be easier to close as there is less normal tissue over which to transpose (d′). The Webster modification (C) uses a 30-degree interior flap angle instead of Limberg's traditional 60-degree interior angle to minimize the standing cone deformity usually located at the peak of the flaps donor site. It is also helpful to use when there is less tissue laxity at the donor site. It depends on some secondary movement from the edges of the defect in order to close the flap under minimal tension. The Webster also may combine an M-plasty at the defect base to minimize a standing cone at the turning point of the flap.

vascular array of perforating vessels derived from the angular artery. As a result of this excellent perfusion, the melolabial flap may be designed significantly longer than the typically acceptable 3:1 length-to-base ratio and still survive. The secondary defect at the flap's donor site is easily closed due to the laxity of medial cheek tissue.

INTERPOLATION FLAPS

The interpolation flap is often considered a variant of the transposition flap involving multiple surgical stages. The first stage of the flap is transposing the donor tissue over normal tissue into the wound with a resulting temporary pedicle overlying the intervening skin. The second stage is separating the flap from its origin, dividing its pedicle, and insetting the flap into the recipient site. The flap division is traditionally performed at 3 weeks; however, division may be performed earlier or later depending on patient-specific factors. Commonly used interpolation flaps in dermatologic surgery are the melolabial interpolation flap (two-staged; see Fig. 2.14C–E) and the paramedian forehead flap (see Fig. 2.3).

Practical Points

The surgeon must always consider the following four options for repairing a wound: second intention healing, primary linear closures, skin grafts, and skin flaps. With each alternative, functional and cosmetic outcomes must be realistically anticipated. For example, if a lower eyelid defect is allowed to granulate or is closed horizontally, the unacceptable wound closure tensions horizontally oriented and parallel to the free margin can place the patient at risk for an ectropion and subsequent corneal irritation. A full-thickness skin graft may help prevent the development of an ectropion, but the cosmetic result may not be ideal due to color and texture mismatch. A properly designed flap may provide the best functional and cosmetic outcomes.

The most suitable color and texture match in facial reconstruction is obtained when a flap is taken from the same facial aesthetic unit as the adjacent defect. Gonzalez-Ulloa first described the aesthetic facial units (Fig. 2.15).[98] Skin varies in color, texture, and appendageal characteristics, depending on the location on the face. Areas of the face that share similar skin characteristics and that are commonly bordered by visually prominent, naturally occurring anatomic landmarks are considered to be within a single aesthetic unit.[99–101] The two most complicated areas for reconstruction on the face are the nose and the lip. On the nose, there are many different small subunits divided by the skin's color, texture, and mobility.[102,103] Robinson recently published a 10-year prospective study confirming improved cosmetic results when wounds were reconstructed within aesthetic units.[104] She emphasized that when a primary defect involves multiple aesthetic units, each unit should be reconstructed individually with sutures placed in the borders between units. If a wound involves more than 50% of the subunit, then the authors often remove the unit's remaining tissue and reconstruct the unit as a whole. Although some normal tissue is sacrificed, the final cosmetic result is superior since scars are least conspicuous when they are properly placed at the junction of aesthetic units.

When designing any closure, the surgeon must identify the relaxed skin tension lines (RSTLs), which are those curvilinear lines seen at rest in elderly patients. In young patients, pinching the skin will identify these furrows. When designing a flap, it is often helpful to initially mark these RSTLs, as well as borders of cosmetic subunits, with a surgical marking pen. Tissue surrounding the wound should then be palpated, pushed, and pinched to evaluate tissue laxity and potential flap donor tissue reservoirs.[55,105] The lateral and inferior face usually has greater tissue reservoirs than the central zones of the face.[106] On the nose, the nasal sidewall and glabella are often used as tissue donor sites. Tissue may be borrowed from these areas, but incisions should be planned to be parallel to the RSTLs in order to minimize scar visibility (Fig. 2.16). When an incision is placed within an RSTL, the wound's tension vectors are parallel the lines of maximal extensibility, and there is

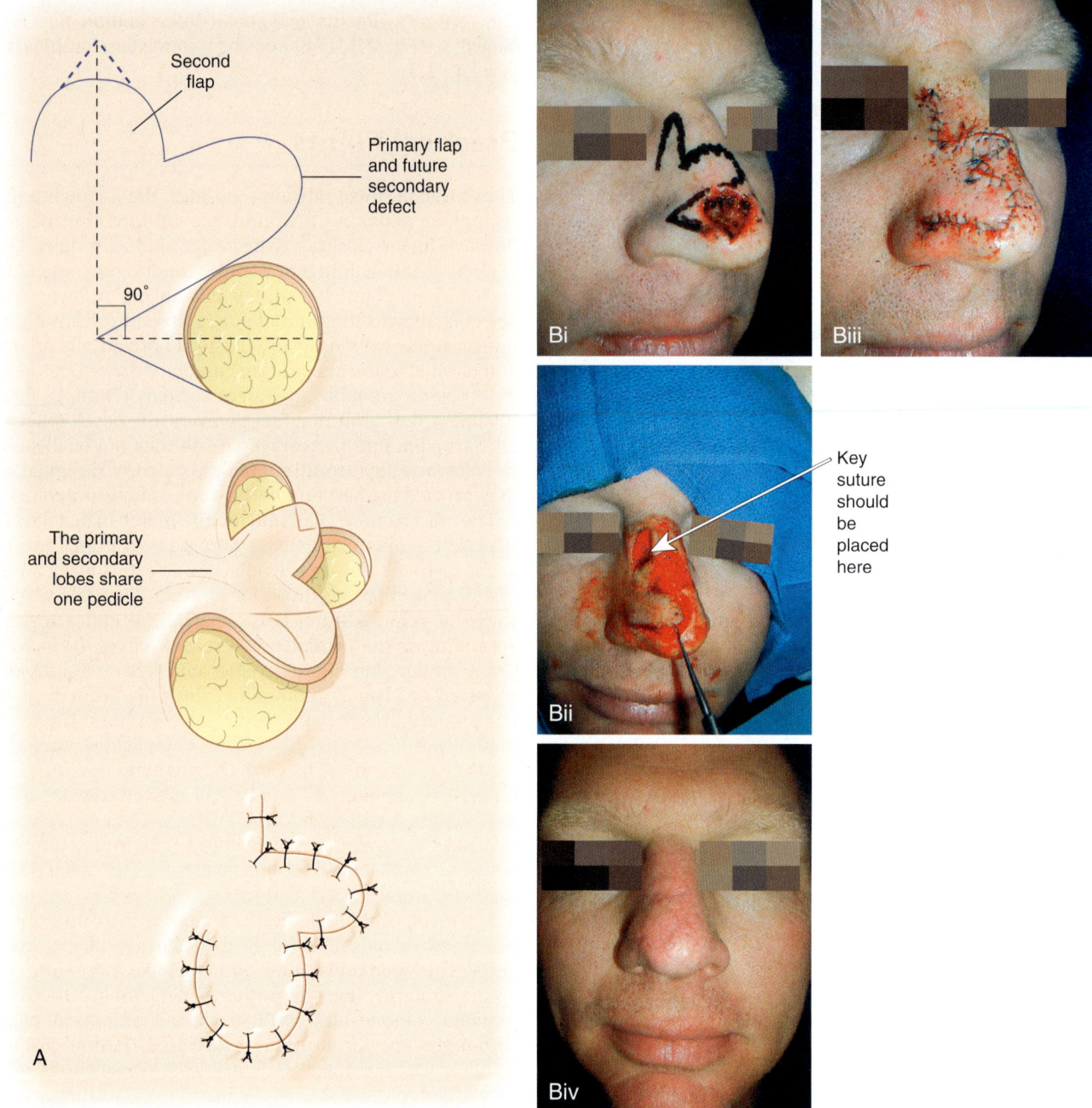

Fig. 2.13 Bilobed transposition flap. (A) In Esser's bilobed design, there are actually two flaps (lobes) raised that share a common pedicle. The primary flap is designed to close the primary defect, and the second flap fills the secondary defect. (B) In this modified bilobed flap design, the second lobe is drawn at a right angle to the first lobe and the surface area is approximately 50% of the first lobe. Since both flaps are being transposed on a single pedicle, the design must provide sufficient pedicle width to support metabolism of both lobes. The key suture is to close the tertiary defect. Panel Biv was taken at a 3-month follow-up.

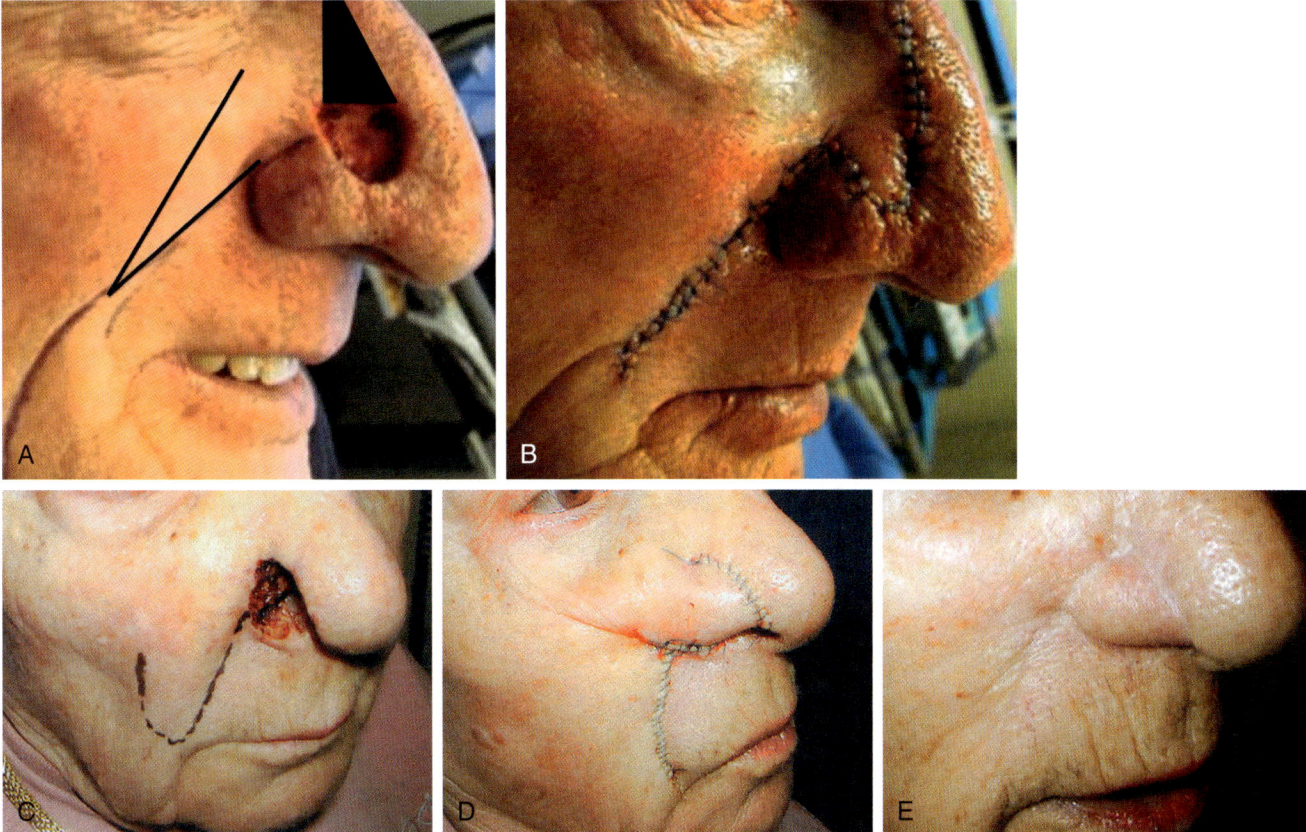

Fig. 2.14 Melolabial flaps are often used to reconstruct the nasal ala. A single staged melolabial transposition flap (A and B) is most useful for defects crossing over the alar crease into the nasal sidewall. When the defect is entirely on the nasal ala, a two-staged melolabial interpolation flap is useful such as for reconstruction of this full-thickness defect (C and D). The final result is seen at 3 months, following pedicle division (E).

less tension on the wound edge. Often it is helpful to initially design a primary closure along RSTLs. When it is obvious that the wound cannot be closed primarily, either because of the size of the wound/tension on the wound edges or if the closure would cross into a free margin or cosmetic subunit border, then use probing fingers to locate the best skin reservoir to allow wound closure with minimal tension and to produce the best functional and cosmetic results (Fig. 2.17).

Final Pearls

Prior to performing any repair, it is important to ensure complete extirpation of a malignant tumor. If a flap is placed into a wound without complete tumor removal, the tumor may grow hidden for many years before subsequent clinical detection. The tumor will not only grow beneath the flap, but also along the plane of prior tissue undermining. The result can be disastrous, with deep tumor penetration and in some cases metastasis. Using Mohs micrographic surgery/complete margin assessment or staged surgical excision to obtain negative pathologic margins is essential prior to reconstruction.

Flap success is dependent on careful patient selection. A thorough medical history must be obtained regarding factors that may affect wound healing. In addition, the patient's ability to perform ongoing wound care must be evaluated. For example, an elderly widow with poor functional status who lives alone may not be able to perform the required daily wound care. The patient may need home health arranged, frequent clinic visits for dressing changes, or an alternative reconstruction may be considered.

Follow the carpenter's motto—always measure twice and cut once. Consider all reconstructive options prior to making any incision. Wound closure should not result in unacceptable tension being placed on the wound edges or free margins. Such undue tension will lead to wound edge necrosis and/or deformity of free margins. When planning a flap, do not neglect the secondary defect. One should be able to close the secondary defect satisfactorily when placing the flap into the wound. In addition, the surgeon should always have a secondary plan to close a defect should the original idea fail.

Surgical technique and knowledge of anatomy must be refined. There is no substitution for understanding the anatomy of any area to be reconstructed. This familiarity will help one avoid transecting major cutaneous arteries and important motor nerves. Skin hooks and fine-tooth forceps should be used to avoid blunt trauma to skin edges. In addition, care should be utilized when performing undermining. Wide undermining should be used to prevent flap elevation (pin-cushioning) during healing.[53] Meticulous hemostasis must be obtained prior to final suturing.

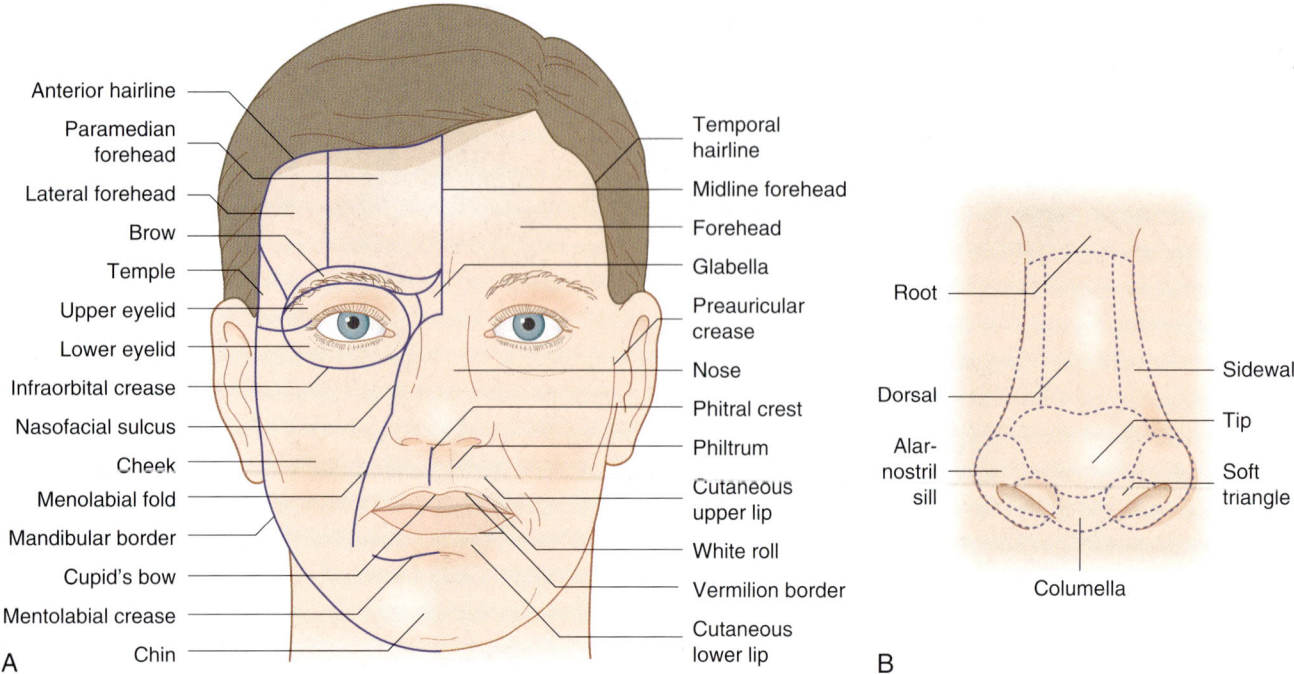

Fig. 2.15 (A) The cosmetic subunits of the face must be realized when planning a repair. The repair should be confined within the subunit when possible and incision lines may be placed within the subunit division lines for ideal hiding of scar lines. (B) The nose is divided into several cosmetic subunits including the root, dorsum, lateral sidewalls, tip, alae nasi, soft triangles, and columella. When possible, repairs should be kept within these subunits and incision scars will be best camouflaged when placed along these division lines.

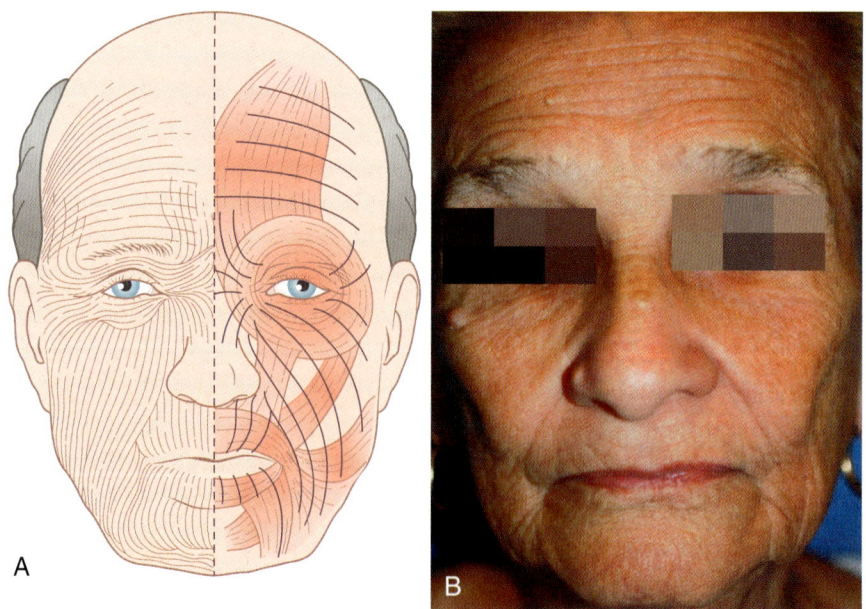

Fig. 2.16 The relaxed skin tension lines seen in a diagram (A) and in vivo (B). Incision lines should be placed within or parallel to these lines to gain an optimal final cosmetic result.

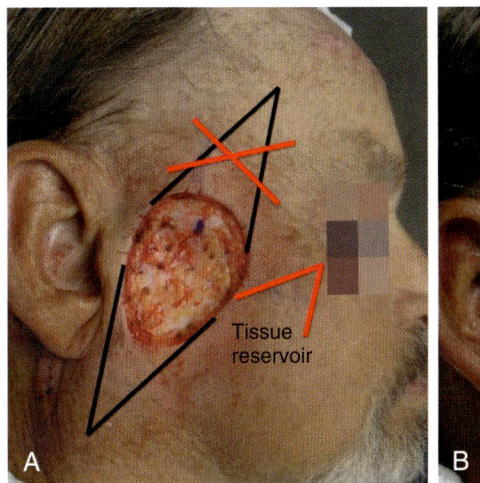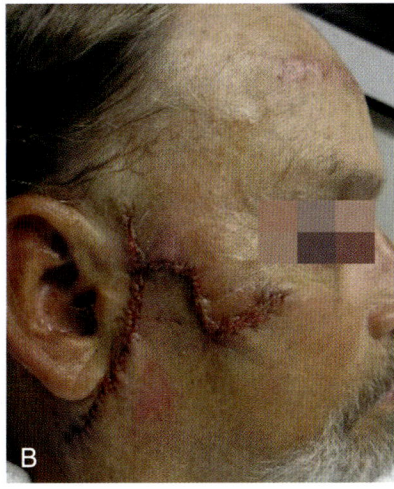

Fig. 2.17 The lateral and inferior face usually have greater tissue reservoirs than the central zones of the face. When designing a flap, it is sometimes useful to design the simple linear closure first along the relaxed skin tension lines (A). Once the tissue reservoir is identified, a flap can be designed to optimize movement of this tissue reservoir into the primary defect. In this case a modified rhombic flap is designed to utilize the tissue reservoir of the cheek while aligning the closure of the secondary defect in the periocular furrows and the primary defect in the preauricular sulcus of the face, yielding an optimal cosmetic result (B).

Moreover, any dead space beneath the flap should be eliminated, with the conservative use of tacking sutures (if you think about a drain, place one).

No wound must be reconstructed with a single modality. For example, a large defect involving the nasal sidewall and cheek may be reconstructed in units using both an advancement flap for the cheek component of the wound and a full-thickness skin graft for the nasal defect. Reconstructive surgery is a creative process, in that there are many ways to close any particular wound. Knowledge and experience lead the surgeon to pick the best solution.

References

1. Wallace AF. History of plastic surgery. *J R Soc Med.* 1978;71:834-838.
2. Cutting C, Ballantyne D, Shaw W, Converse JM. Critical closing pressure, local perfusion pressure, and the failing skin flap. *Ann Plast Surg.* 1982;8:504-509.
3. Stell PM. The pig as an experimental model for skin flap behaviour: a reappraisal of previous studies. *Br J Plast Surg.* 1977;30:1-8.
4. Daniel RK, Williams HB. The free transfer of skin flaps by microvascular anastomoses. An experimental study and a reappraisal. *Plast Reconstr Surg.* 1973;52:16-31.
5. Patterson TJ. The survival of skin flaps in the pig. *Br J Plast Surg.* 1968;21:113-117.
6. Patterson TJ. Study of the blood-supply of skin-flaps by close-up thermography. *Br J Surg.* 1969;56:381.
7. Dzubow LM. Tissue movement—a microbiomechanical approach. *J Dermatol Surg Oncol.* 1989;15:389-399.
8. Milton SH. Pedicled skin flaps: the fallacy of the length: width ratio. *Br J Surg.* 1970;57:502-508.
9. Baran NK, Horton CE. Growth of skin grafts, flaps, and scars in young minipigs. *Plast Reconstr Surg.* 1972;50:487-496.
10. Kernahan DA, Zingg W, Kay CW. The effect of hyperbaric oxygen on the survival of experimental skin flaps. *Plast Reconstr Surg.* 1965;36:19-25.
11. Donovan WE. Experimental models in skin flap research. In: Grabb WC, Myers MB, eds. *Skin Flaps.* Boston: Little, Brown; 1975:11-20.
12. Daniel RK. The anatomy and hemodynamics of the cutaneous circulation and their influence on skin flap design. In: Grabb WC, Myers MB, eds. *Skin Flaps.* Boston: Little, Brown; 1975:111-131.
13. Neligan P, Pang CY, Nakatsuka T, Lindsay WK, Thomson HG. Pharmacologic action of isoxsuprine in cutaneous and myocutaneous flaps. *Plast Reconstr Surg.* 1985;75:363-374.
14. Pearl RM. A unifying theory of the delay phenomenon—recovery from the hyperadrenergic state. *Ann Plast Surg.* 1981;7:102-112.
15. Marks NJ. Quantitative analysis of skin flap blood flow in the rat using laser Doppler velocimetry. *J R Soc Med.* 1985;78:308-314.
16. Guyton AC. *Textbook of Medical Physiology.* 6th ed. Philadelphia: WB Saunders; 1981:344-356.
17. Pearl RM, Johnson D. The vascular supply to the skin: an anatomical and physiological reappraisal—part I. *Ann Plast Surg.* 1983;11:99-105.
18. Pearl RM, Johnson D. The vascular supply to the skin: an anatomical and physiological reappraisal—part II. *Ann Plast Surg.* 1983;11:196-205.
19. Midy D, Mauruc B, Vergnes P, Caliot P. A contribution to the study of the facial artery, its branches and anastomoses: application to the anatomic vascular basis of facial flaps. *Surg Radiol Anat.* 1986;8:99-107.
20. Cutting C. Critical closing and perfusion pressures in flap survival. *Ann Plast Surg.* 1982;9:524.
21. Mathes SJ, Nahai F. The reconstructive triangle: a paradigm for surgical decision making. In: Mathes SJ, Nahai F, eds. *Reconstructive Surgery: Principles, Anatomy, and Technique.* New York: Churchill Livingston; 1997:9-36, 37-160.
22. Fazio MJ, Zitelli JA. Flaps. In: Ratz JL, Geronemus RC, Goldman MP, eds. *Textbook of Dermatologic Surgery.* Philadelphia: Lippincott-Raven; 1998:225-227.
23. Heniford BW, Bailin PL, Marsico RE Jr. Field guide to local flaps. *Dermatol Clin.* 1998;16(1):65-74.
24. Stranc MF, Sanders R. Abdominal wall skin flaps. In: Grabb WC, Myers MB, eds. *Skin Flaps.* Boston: Little, Brown; 1975:419-426.
25. Hartwell SW Jr. Local flaps of the leg and foot. In: Grabb WC, Myers MB, eds. *Skin Flaps.* Boston: Little, Brown; 1975:497-506.
26. Larrabee WF Jr. Immediate repair of facial defects. *Dermatol Clin.* 1989;7:661-676.
27. Meyers B. Understanding flap necrosis. *Plast Reconstr Surg.* 1986;78:813-814.
28. Kerrigan C, Daniel R. Critical ischemia time and the failing skin flap. *Plast Reconstr Surg.* 1982;69:986-989.
29. Zelt RG, Olding M, Kerrigan CL, Daniel RK. Primary and secondary critical ischemia times of myocutaneous flaps. *Plast Reconstr Surg.* 1986;78:498-503.
30. Guba AM, Zinner MJ, Hobson RW. Regional hemodynamics of a pedicle flap: evaluation by distribution of radioactive microspheres. *J Surg Res.* 1978;25:274-279.
31. Kerrigan CL, Zelt RG, Daniel RK. Secondary critical ischemia time of experimental skin flaps. *Plast Reconstr Surg.* 1984;74:522-526.
32. Gottrup F, Oredsson S, Price DC, Mathes SJ, Hohn DC. A comparative study of skin blood flow in musculocutaneous and random pattern flaps. *J Surg Res.* 1984;37:443-447.

33. Sasaki GH, Pang CY. Experimental evidence for involvement of prostaglandins in viability and acute skin flaps: effects on viability and mode of action. *Plast Reconstr Surg.* 1981;67:335-340.
34. Kerrigan CL, Stotland MA. Ischemia reperfusion injury: a review. *Microsurgery.* 1993;14:165-175.
35. Kay S, Green C. The effect of a novel thromboxane synthetase inhibitor dazmegrel (UK38485) on random pattern skin flaps in the rat. *Br J Plast Surg.* 1986;39:361-363.
36. Goding GS Jr, Horn DB. Skin flap physiology. In: Baker SR, Swanson NA, eds. *Local Flaps in Facial Reconstruction.* St Louis: Mosby; 1995:15-30.
37. Angel MF, Narayanan K, Swartz WM, et al. The etiologic role of free radicals in hematoma-induced flap necrosis. *Plast Reconstr Surg.* 1986;77:795-803.
38. Mellow CG, Knight KR, Angel MF, Coe SA, O'Brien BM. The biochemical basis of secondary ischemia. *J Surg Res.* 1992;52:226-232.
39. Kerrigan CL, Daniel RK. Skin flap research: a candid view. *Ann Plast Surg.* 1984;13:383-387.
40. Wang C, Kerrigan CL, Stotland MA. Kinetics of E-selectin expression in surgical flaps. *Plast Reconstr Surg.* 1997;100:1482-1488.
41. Park S, Tepper OM, Galiano RD, et al. Selective recruitment of endothelial progenitor cells to ischemic tissues with increased neovascularization. *Plast Reconstr Surg.* 2004;113:284-293.
42. Tsur H, Daniller A, Strauch B. Neovascularization of skin flaps: route and timing. *Plast Reconstr Surg.* 1980;66:85-90.
43. Pickett BP, Burgess LP, Livermore GH, Tzikas TL, Vossoughi J. Wound healing. *Arch Otolaryngol Head Neck Surg.* 1996;122:565-568.
44. Jonsson K, Hunt TK, Brennan SS, Mathes SJ. Tissue oxygen measurements in delayed skin flaps: a reconsideration of the mechanisms of the delay phenomenon. *Plast Reconstr Surg.* 1988;82:328-336.
45. Liu PY, Wang XT, Badiavas E, Rieger-Christ K, Tang JB, Summerhayes I. Enhancement of ischemic flap survival by prefabrication with transfer of exogenous PDGF gene. *J Reconstr Microsurg.* 2005;21:273-279.
46. Simman R, Craft C, McKinney B. Improved survival of ischemic random skin flaps through the use of bone marrow nonhematopoietic stem cells and angiogenic growth factors. *Ann Plast Surg.* 2005;54:546-552.
47. Gatti JE, LaRossa D, Brousseau DA, Silverman DG. Assessment of neovascularization and timing of flap division. *Plast Reconstr Surg.* 1984;73:396-402.
48. Serafin D, Shearin C, Georgiade NG. The vascularization of free flaps: a clinical and experimental correlation. *Plast Reconstr Surg.* 1977;60:233-241.
49. Klingenstrom P, Nylen B. Timing of transfer of tubed pedicles and cross flaps. *Plast Reconstr Surg.* 1966;37:1-12.
50. Cummings C, Trachy R. Measurement of alternative blood flow in the porcine panniculus carnosus myocutaneous flap. *Arch Otolaryngol.* 1985;111:598-600.
51. Demirseren ME, Yenidunya MO, Yenidunya S. Island rat groin flaps with twisted pedicles. *Plast Reconstr Surg.* 2004;114:1190-1194.
52. Leach J. Proper handling of soft tissue in the acute phase. *Facial Plast Surg.* 2001;17:227-238.
53. Summers BK, Siegle RJ. Facial cutaneous reconstructive surgery: general aesthetic principles. *J Am Acad Dermatol.* 1993;29:669-681.
54. Myers MB. Wound tension and vascularity in the etiology and prevention of skin sloughs. *Surgery.* 1964;56:945-949.
55. Myers MB, Combs B, Cohen G. Wound tension and wound sloughs—a negative correlation. *Am J Surg.* 1965;109:711-714.
56. Larrabee WF. Design of local skin flaps. *Otolaryngol Clin North Am.* 1990;23:899-923.
57. Salasche SJ. Acute surgical complications: cause, prevention, and treatment. *J Am Acad Dermatol.* 1986;15:1163-1185.
58. Myers MB. Investigation of skin flap necrosis. In: Grabb WC, Myers MB, eds. *Skin Flaps.* Boston: Little, Brown; 1975:3-10.
59. Salasche SJ, Grabski WJ. Complications of flaps. *J Dermatol Surg Oncol.* 1991;17:132-140.
60. Lanir Y. A structural theory for the homogeneous biaxial stress-strain relationships in flat collagenous tissues. *J Biomech.* 1979;12:423-436.
61. Daly CH, Odland GF. Age-related changes in the mechanical properties of human skin. *J Invest Dermatol.* 1979;73:84-87.
62. Larrabee WF Jr, Galt JA. A finite element model for the design of local skin flaps. *Otolaryngol Clin North Am.* 1986;19:807-824.
63. Lanir Y, Walsh J, Soutas-Little RW. Histological staining as a measure of stress in collagen fibers. *J Biomech Eng.* 1984;106:174-176.
64. Ridenour BD, Larrabee WF. Biomechanics of skin flaps. In: Baker SR, Swanson NA, eds. *Local Flaps in Facial Reconstruction.* St Louis: Mosby; 1995:31-38.
65. Larrabee WF, Sutton D. The biomechanics of advancement and rotation flaps. *Laryngoscope.* 1981;91:726-734.
66. Gibson T, Kenedi RM. Biomechanical properties of skin. *Surg Clin North Am.* 1967;47:279-294.
67. Swanson NA. Classifications, definitions, and concepts in flap surgery. In: Baker SR, Swanson NA, eds. *Local Flaps in Facial Reconstruction.* St Louis: Mosby; 1995:63-74.
68. Johnson TM, Swanson N, Baker SR. Concepts of sliding and lifting tissue movement in flap reconstruction. *Dermatol Surg.* 2000;26:274-278.
69. Robinson JK. Placement of the tension-bearing suture in repairing the alar facial junction. *J Am Acad Dermatol.* 1997;36:440-443.
70. Marmelzat WL. Medicine in history—Celsus (25 AD), plastic surgeon: on the repair of defects of the ears, lips, and nose. *J Dermatol Surg Oncol.* 1982;8:1012-1014.
71. Zelac NE, Swanson N, Simpson M, Greenway HT. The history of dermatologic surgical reconstruction. *Dermatol Surg.* 2000;26:983-990.
72. Hale EK. The history of flaps. *J Drugs Dermatol.* 2002;1:293-296.
73. Burow A. Beschreibung einer neuen Transplantations-methode (Methode der seitlichen Dreiecke) zum Wiederersatz verlorengegangener Teile des Gesichts. Berlin: J Nauck; 1885.
74. Gormley DE. The dog-ear: causes, prevention, and correction. *J Dermatol Surg Oncol.* 1977;3:194-198.
75. Webster RC, Davidson TM, Smith RC, et al. M-plasty techniques. *J Dermatol Surg.* 1976;2:393-396.
76. Salasche SJ, Roberts LC. Dog-ear correction by M-plasty. *J Dermatol Surg Oncol.* 1984;10:478-482.
77. Gormley DE. A brief analysis of the Burow's wedge/triangle principle. *J Dermatol Surg Oncol.* 1985;11:121-123.
78. Barron JN, Emmett AJ. Subcutaneous pedicled flaps. *Br J Plast Surg.* 1965;18:51-78.
79. Tomich JM, Wentzell JM, Grande DJ. Subcutaneous island pedicle flaps. *Arch Dermatol.* 1987;123:514-518.
80. Papadopoulous DJ, Trinei FA. Superiorly based nasalis myocutaneous island pedicle flap with bilevel undermining for nasal tip and supratip reconstruction. *Dermatol Surg.* 1999;25:530-536.
81. Krishnan R, Garman M, Nunez-Gussman J, Orengo I. Advancement flaps: a basic theme with many variations. *Dermatol Surg.* 2005;31:986-994.
82. Hairston BR, Nguyen H. Innovations in the island pedicle flap for cutaneous facial reconstruction. *Dermatol Surg.* 2003;29:378-385.
83. Vandeput J. The new bilaterally pedicled V-Y advancement flap for face reconstruction. *Plast Reconstr Surg.* 2003;111:1363-1364.
84. Skaria AM. Refinement of the island pedicle flap: parallel placed release incisions to increase translation movement. *Dermatol Surg.* 2004;30:1595-1598.
85. Pancoast J. New operation for the relief of persistent facial neuralgia. *Med Times Phila.* 1842;2:85-87.
86. Konz B. Use of skin flaps in dermatologic surgery of the face. *J Dermatol Surg.* 1975;1:25-30.
87. Dzubow LM. The dynamics of flap movement: effect of pivotal restraint on flap rotation and transposition. *J Dermatol Surg Oncol.* 1987;13:1348-1353.
88. Crow ML, Crow FJ. Resurfacing large cheek defects with rotation flaps from the neck. *Plast Reconstr Surg.* 1976;58:196-200.
89. Rieger RA. A local flap for repair of the nasal tip. *Plast Reconstr Surg.* 1967;40:147-149.
90. Marchac D, Toth B. The axial frontonasal flap revisited. *Plast Reconstr Surg.* 1985;76:686-694.
91. Deluca J, Tappeiner L, Pichler M, Eisendle K. Using the Peng flap for a wide dorsal nasal defect. *J Dtsch Dermatol Ges.* 2014;12(11):1060-1062.
92. Kaufman AJ. Bilateral vermilion rotation flap. *Dermatol Surg.* 2006;32(5):721-725, discussion 725.
93. Chase RA. Introduction: the history of vascularized composite-tissue transfers. In: Strauch B, Vasconez LO, Hall-Findlay E, eds. *Grabb's Encyclopedia of Flaps.* 2nd ed. New York: Lippincott-Raven; 1988.
94. Limberg AA. Modern trends in plastic surgery. Design of local flaps. *Mod Trends Plast Surg.* 1966;2:38-61.
95. Dufourmentel C. Closure of limited loss of cutaneous substance. So-called "LLL" diamond-shaped L rotation-flap. *Ann Chir Plast.* 1962;7:60-64.

96. Esser JFS. Gestielite lokale Nasemplastik mit zweizipfligem Lappen, Deckung des sekundaren Defektes vom ersten Zipfel durch den zweiten. *Dtsch Z Chir.* 1918;143:385-390.
97. Pharis DB, Papadopoulos DJ. Superiorly based nasolabial interpolation flap for repair of complex nasal tip defects. *Dermatol Surg.* 2000;26:19-24.
98. Gonzalez-Ulloa M. Restoration of the face covering by means of selected skin in regional aesthetic units. *Br J Plast Surg.* 1956;9:212-221.
99. Webster RC, Smith RC. Cosmetic priniciples in surgery on the face. *J Dermatol Surg Oncol.* 1978;4:397-402.
100. Dzubow LM, Zack L. The principle of cosmetic junctions as applied to reconstruction of defects following Mohs surgery. *J Dermatol Surg Oncol.* 1990;16:353-355.
101. Burget GC. Modification of the subunit principle. *Arch Facial Plast Surg.* 1999;1:16-18.
102. Burget GC, Menick FJ. The subunit principle in nasal reconstruction. *Plast Reconstr Surg.* 1985;76:239-247.
103. Burget GC. Aesthetic reconstruction of the tip of the nose. *Dermatol Surg.* 1995;21:419-429.
104. Robinson JK. Segmental reconstruction of the face. *Dermatol Surg.* 2004;30:67-74.
105. Stegman SJ. Guidelines for placement of elective incisions. *Cutis.* 1976;18:723-726.
106. Summers BK, Siegle RJ. Facial cutaneous reconstructive surgery: facial flaps. *J Am Acad Dermatol.* 1993;29:917-941.

3 Second Intention Healing and Primary Closure

MICHAEL COSULICH, MD, JEREMY ETZKORN, MD, THUZAR MYO SHIN, MD, PHD, and CHRISTOPHER J. MILLER, MD

Introduction

Second intention healing (SIH) and primary closure are the most common and basic strategies to manage wounds after skin cancer removal.[1] SIH is defined as allowing a wound to heal without suturing together the edges. Primary closure refers to direct approximation of the wound edges with sutures. For the purposes of this chapter, "primary closure" refers to a linear, or side-to-side, closure of a wound. This chapter will discuss SIH and primary closure to manage defects after removing skin cancers and other cutaneous lesions.

Second Intention Healing

PHASES OF WOUND HEALING

Healing wounds progress through a sequence of overlapping phases: inflammation, proliferation, and remodeling (Fig. 3.1). The inflammatory phase, which occurs during the first 24 to 48 hours after injury (and can last up to 2 weeks), is defined by a cellular and vascular response. This is followed by the proliferative phase, which is characterized by angiogenesis, fibroplasia, and re-epithelialization. The remodeling phase, which can last for weeks to years, is distinguished by the deposition of different matrix materials, whose composition changes over time as the scar matures.[2,3]

Healing time depends on several variables, including blood supply, wound size, and host factors. Wounds with a strong blood supply and more adnexal structures heal faster. For example, facial wounds have a robust blood supply and heal faster than wounds on the lower extremity. Deeper wounds require a longer proliferative phase for granulation tissue to fill the wound. Broader wounds take longer to heal, although healing time is not linearly proportional to wound diameter. For example, a 10-fold increase in the area of a wound may only double the healing time.[4] The health and nutritional status of the patient may also affect healing time. For example, lower extremity wounds may require excessive healing time in vasculopathic patients. Since numerous factors affect wound healing, it is not possible to generalize healing time for all wounds.

Wound contraction, which commences during the proliferative phase and extends into the remodeling phase, can account for a significant decrease in the size of the wound (Fig. 3.2).[5] The wound contracts in three phases: a plateau phase, an exponential phase, and a postexponential phase. During the exponential phase, the rate of contraction occurs in a logarithmic fashion related to the area of the wound, which explains why overall healing time is not linearly proportional to the area of the wound and why larger wounds often heal faster than expected.[5] The amount of contraction varies widely, depending on the depth and the anatomic location. Wounds on the relatively thick and inelastic tissue of the scalp may contract by 45% of their original size, whereas wounds of the medial canthus may contract by up to 78%.[5] Myofibroblasts begin to mediate wound contraction as early as 5 days after injury.[3] Partial thickness dermal wounds contract less than full-thickness wounds, and adnexal structures in the residual dermis speed re-epithelialization.[2]

APPEARANCE OF SECOND INTENTION HEALING SCARS

SIH produces scars that have a shiny texture and lack skin appendages, such as hair follicles and eccrine glands. Telangiectases usually develop on the scar's surface, especially in patients with lighter skin types. Larger wounds tend to heal with larger caliber vessels on the central surface. Smaller vessels along the periphery of the scar may fade as the scar matures and becomes relatively avascular.[4,6] A newly re-epithelialized scar is pink, but scars often become hypopigmented in lighter skin types and hyperpigmented in darker skin types.

IDEAL WOUNDS FOR SECOND INTENTION HEALING

SIH is ideal for wounds where the surrounding skin has a normally shiny texture, where wound contracture will not result in anatomic distortion, and where the blood supply at the base of the wound is robust. Many factors can influence outcomes for SIH. Certain anatomic locations are ideal for second intention healing. On the temple, forehead, bald scalp, and pretibial leg, the shiny scars formed by SIH often heal with good results and minimal morbidity (Fig. 3.3). SIH may be a good option for wounds of the hands and feet, as long as tendons are not exposed and the wound does not cross joints.[7] The pink scars from SIH mimic the natural color and texture of the vermilion lip, and the cosmetic result is often highly aesthetic.[8,9]

The contour of the anatomic site has traditionally been considered to be a good predictor of aesthetic outcome.[6,10] Wounds have been considered to heal with better aesthetic outcomes on concave versus convex surfaces. However, this dogma is an oversimplification. For example, while SIH is

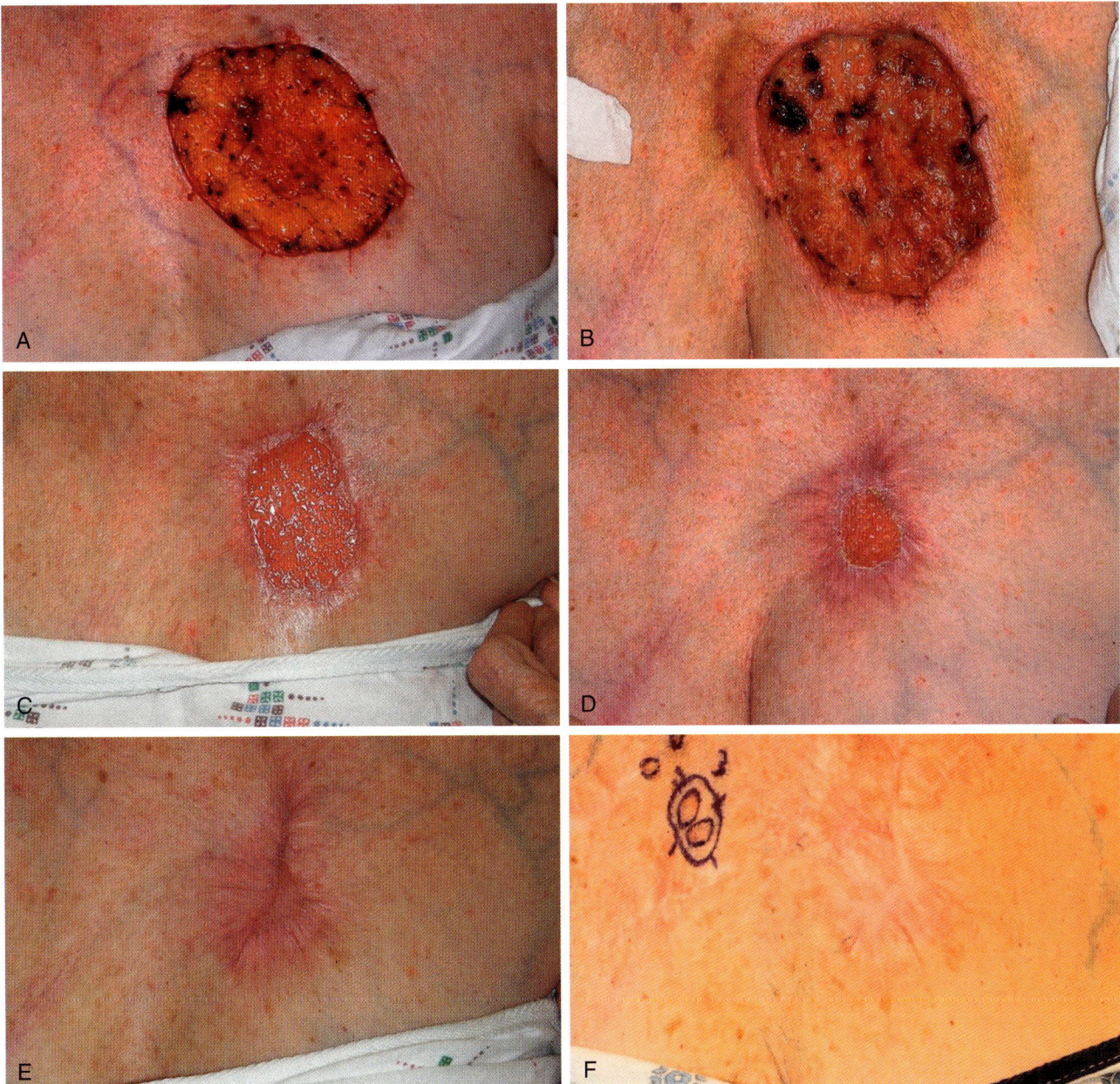

Fig. 3.1 Example of wound progressing through phases of second intention healing. (A) Wound immediately after Mohs surgery for a basal cell cancer. (B) One week after surgery, the wound remains in the inflammatory phase of healing. Note the inflammation along the wound edges and yellow fibrin at the base of the wound. The wound is relatively unchanged in size. (C) One month after surgery, the wound has fully entered the proliferative phase. The base of the wound is filled with glistening pink granulation tissue, the wound has contracted, and newly re-epithelialized skin is advancing along the periphery. (D) Two months after surgery, the wound continues to contract and the new skin continues to advance to the center of the wound. (E) Four months after the surgery, the scar has completely re-epithelialized and it has advanced to the remodeling phase. Note the central ridge along the preferred line of tension, pink color, and prominent telangiectases radiating perpendicularly to the central ridge. (F) Seven years later, the patient returns for more skin cancer treatment. The scar is now hypopigmented. Telangiectases persist.

often utilized for wounds of the concave medial canthus and can sometimes result in excellent outcomes (Fig. 3.4), SIH in this location will often create webbing from tension on the nearby eyelid skin (Fig. 3.5). SIH of the concave alar groove may result in webbing or elevation of the alar margin. By contrast, SIH can be an excellent option for wounds on convex surfaces, such as the forehead and bald scalp, which have normally shiny, taut skin.

The texture and color of the surrounding skin may influence the appearance of SIH scars. The shiny scar from SIH may contrast sharply in locations with textured skin, such as a sebaceous nasal tip (Fig. 3.6). By contrast, the shiny scar from SIH is often inconspicuous in locations with tight, shiny skin, such as the ear.[11] The surgeon must anticipate the likely result from a primary closure versus SIH. In some locations, such as the upper back and shoulders, linear

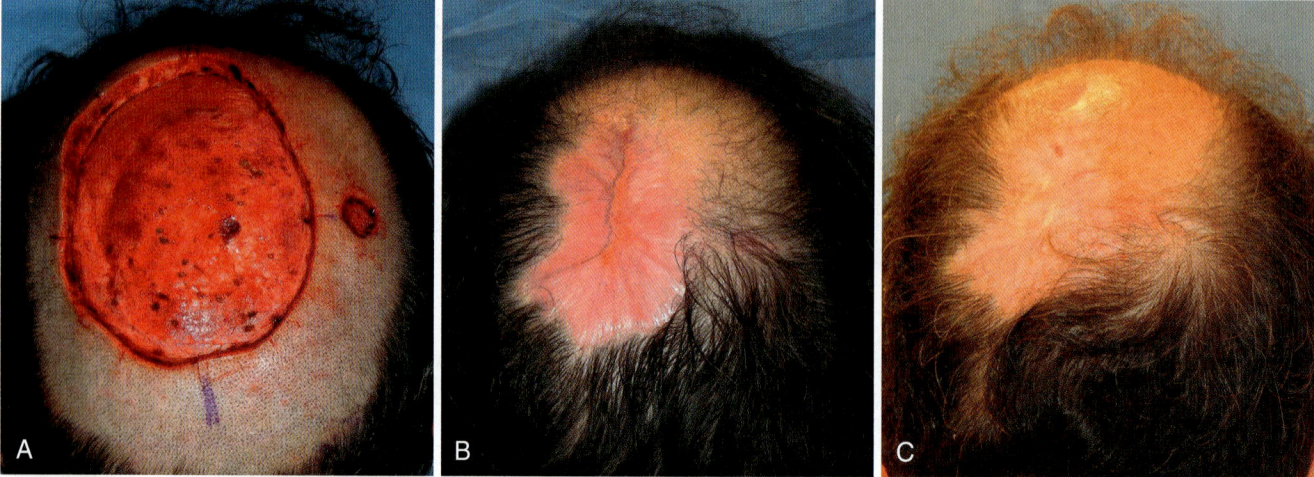

Fig. 3.2 Wounds left to heal by second intention may contract significantly. This figure demonstrates the marked contraction of a large scalp wound. (A) Wound immediately after Mohs surgery for a large basal cell cancer. (B) The wound has completely re-epithelialized 4 months after surgery. Note the pink color and telangiectases. (C) Six years later, the scar is hypopigmented.

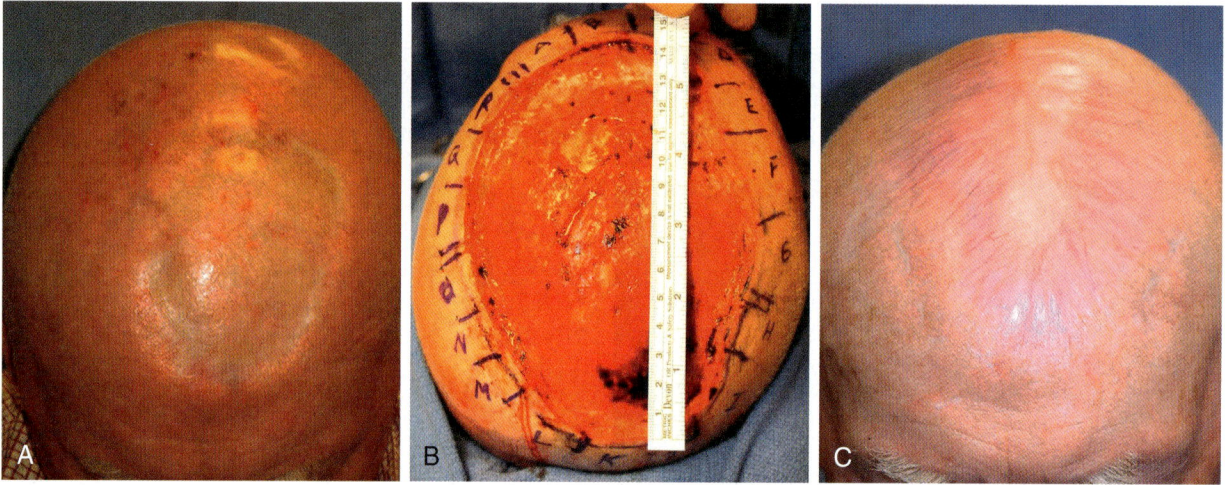

Fig. 3.3 Example of an ideal wound for second intention healing. (A) This patient presented for Mohs surgery of a desmoplastic melanoma that recurred after conventional excision. Note the conspicuous skin graft from his initial surgery. (B) Large Mohs defect. A dermal graft was placed to prevent desiccation of the periosteum, and the wound was left to heal by second intention. (C) One year after the surgery, the wound has healed with a shiny scar that simulates the tight, shiny skin of his bald scalp. Prior to this photograph, he had undergone treatment with the pulsed dye laser to reduce telangiectases.

scars have a tendency to spread and often become more noticeable than a smaller circular scar from second intention healing.

SUBOPTIMAL WOUNDS FOR SECOND INTENTION HEALING

Some wounds have predictably poor outcomes from SIH. Wounds near the eyelid, ala, and lip may contract and distort these free margins (Fig. 3.7). SIH of wounds with exposed "white structures," such as bone, cartilage, and tendons, may result in desiccation and prolonged healing. If soft tissue coverage of exposed bone and cartilage is not possible, fenestration of exposed cartilage and burring of exposed bone may improve the blood supply and promote healing (Fig. 3.8).[12] Finally, SIH may distort contours when wound contraction places tension on nearby loose skin.

PATIENT FACTORS AFFECTING DECISIONS ABOUT SECOND INTENTION HEALING

Patient-specific factors may influence decisions about SIH. Patients must be willing and able to care for the wound until healing is complete. Patients with poor dexterity and vision may not be capable of independent wound care. A caretaker may be necessary for wounds in difficult-to-reach anatomic locations. Patients who are active or have wounds in visible areas may prefer reconstruction to speed healing. Finally, patients with limited income may not be able to afford expensive wound care supplies.

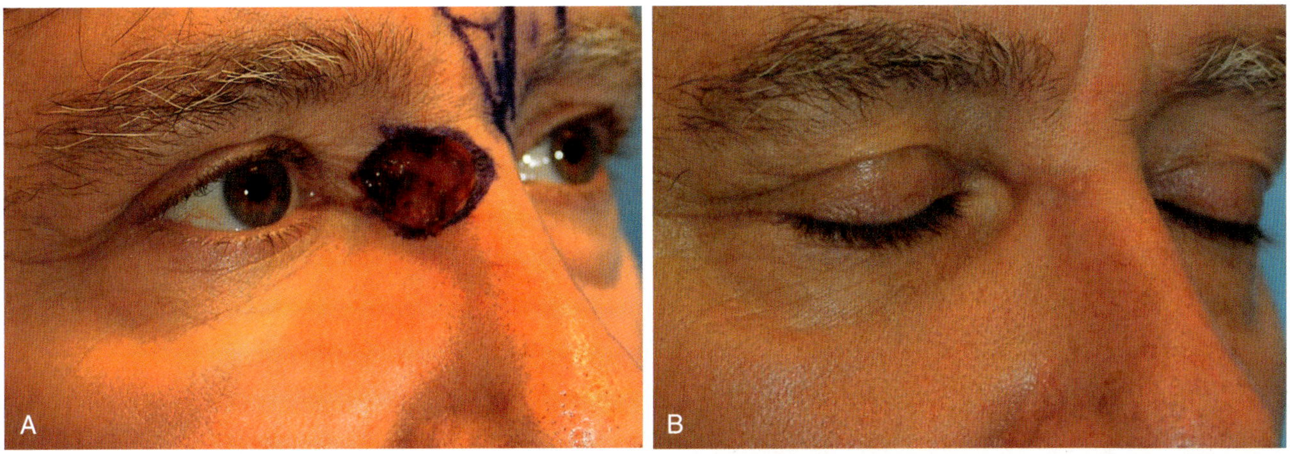

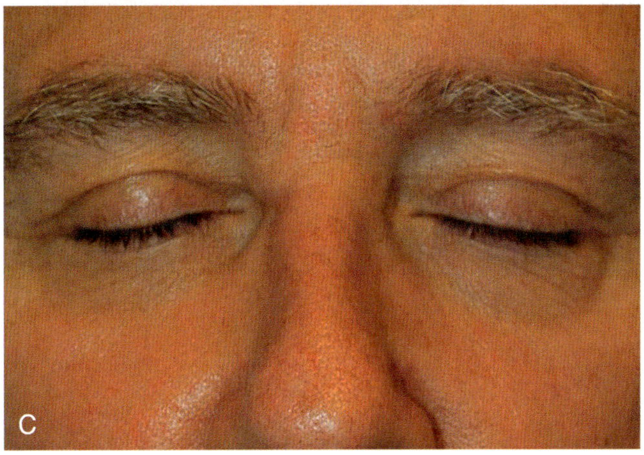

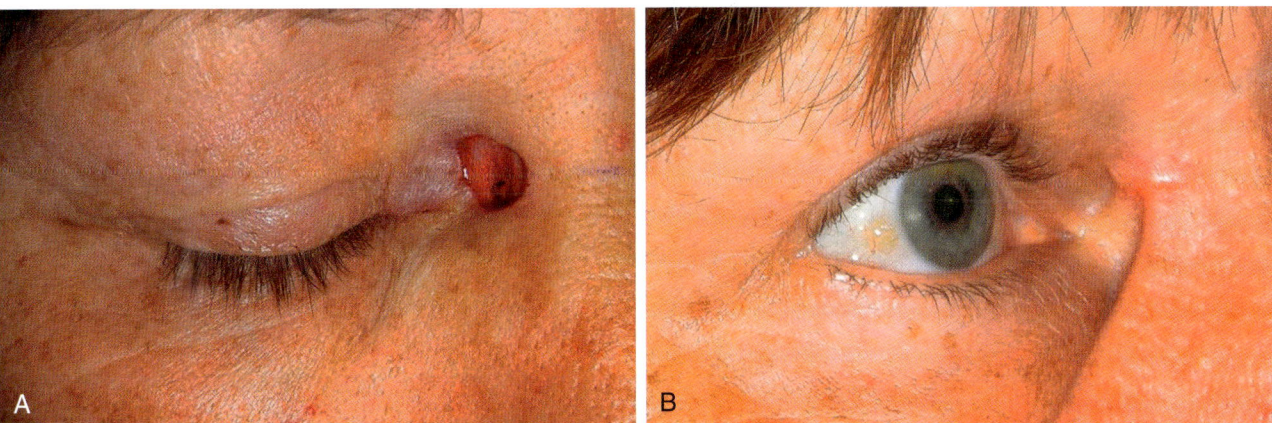

Fig. 3.4 Wounds of the medial canthus can sometimes heal by second intention with excellent cosmetic results. (A) Wound from Mohs surgery in the right medial canthus. The wound was left to heal by second intention. (B) Three months after surgery, the wound has healed with a highly aesthetic result. (C) Frontal view of the wound after 3 months.

Fig. 3.5 Wounds in concave areas may heal with noticeable scars, especially if scar contraction places tension on nearby loose skin. (A) Small wound from Mohs surgery in the concave medial canthus. The wound was left to heal by second intention. (B) Two months after the surgery, her wound has healed with a hypertrophic scar, and she has prominent webbing from tension on the loose skin of the adjacent lower eyelid.

SECOND INTENTION HEALING AS AN ADJUNCT TO RECONSTRUCTIVE SURGERY

SIH may supplement reconstructive surgery. SIH may prepare some wounds for better outcomes after skin grafting. If immediate skin grafting will not restore contour of deep wounds, grafting may be delayed until granulation tissue has filled the wound bed (Fig. 3.9). Wounds that cross concavities, such as the alar groove, may benefit from partial reconstruction with a local skin flap and SIH of the portion of the wound at the alar groove. To avoid retraction after SIH of wounds near the alar margin, free cartilage grafts may first be placed at the base of the wound.[13] To speed healing, purse-string closures may shrink the wound size prior to SIH.[4]

WOUND CARE DURING SECOND INTENTION HEALING

Two Cochrane reviews of dressings, topical agents, and antibiotics for use during SIH both concluded that there is a lack of high-quality studies showing superiority of any particular regimen.[14,15] A relatively basic regimen is usually sufficient. The wound is initially covered with petrolatum and a nonadherent, absorbent pressure dressing that remains in place for 24 to 48 hours. After this period, the wound may be cleansed with a mild soap and water once or twice daily, and kept moist with petrolatum and a bandage until re-epithelization is complete.[4] The moist environment prevents crust formation, decreases pain, and accelerates healing.[6] When crusting or scabbing occurs, manual or enzymatic debridement may be necessary to reduce delays in the healing process. SIH has consistently been associated with less postoperative pain than other reconstructions[16,17] and has a low incidence of infection with proper wound care.[4]

COMPLICATIONS

Failure to account for contraction can lead to anatomic distortion after SIH of wound near free margins, such as the nasal ala and eyelid.[6] Formation of excess granulation tissue can delay healing (Fig. 3.10).[6] High potency topical steroids reduce granulation tissue and speed healing. Erosive pustular dermatosis is thought to be associated with trauma,[18] and can occur with SIH. As it is easily confused with infection, the surgeon must be aware of this potential complication. It is commonly treated with topical corticosteroids.[19] Newly re-epithelialized wounds tend to be more fragile and can be easily sheared with incidental trauma. Contour of the healing wound is unpredictable, so wounds may heal with either hypotrophic or hypertrophic scars.

CONCLUSION

SIH can be an excellent choice and lead to highly aesthetic outcomes for appropriate wounds. While patients may initially be wary of SIH, and surgeons often feel compelled to attempt a sutured closure, a recent study demonstrated that patient satisfaction for SIH is equivalent to that of primary closure in appropriately selected wounds.[20,21] If SIH results in an unsatisfactory scar, surgical reconstruction can be performed at a later date. Judicious use of SIH avoids complications and enhances outcomes.

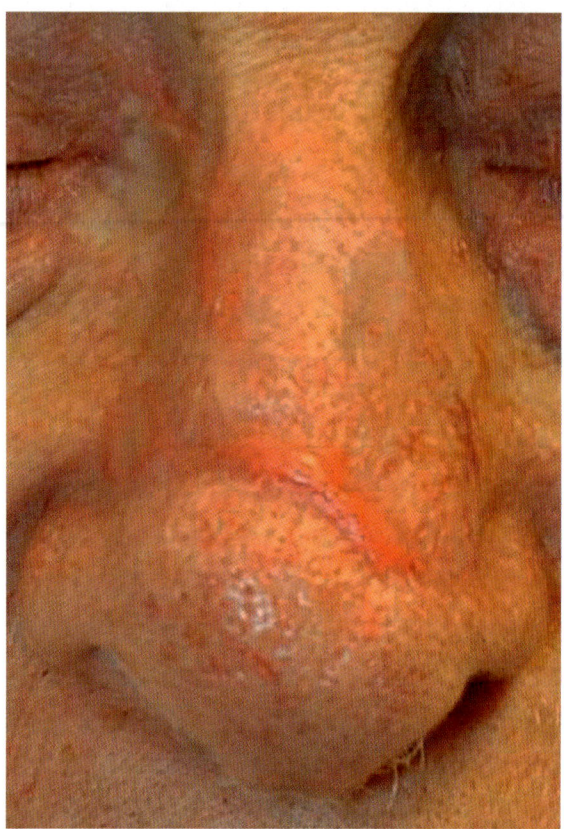

Fig. 3.6 The shiny scars from second intention healing may be conspicuous in areas where the skin is normally textured. This patient's shiny scar on the nasal supratip contrasts sharply with the sebaceous skin of his nasal tip.

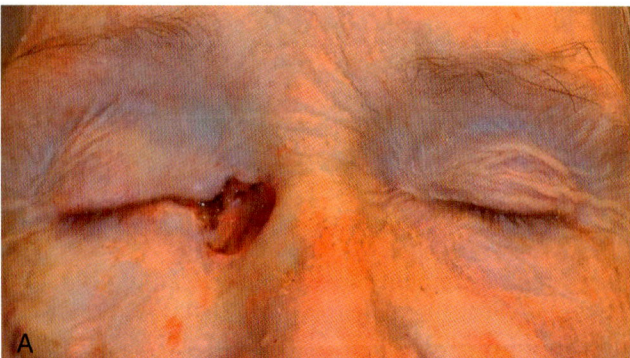 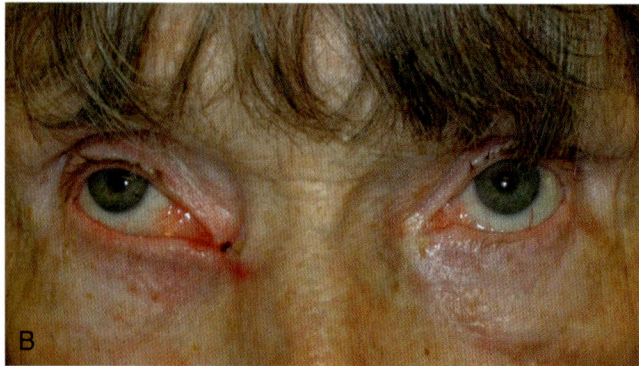

Fig. 3.7 Wound contraction may distort adjacent free margins. (A) Mohs surgery defect in the right medial canthus. The patient had dementia and declined reconstruction. (B) Two months after the surgery, wound contraction has resulted in ectropion of her medial lower eyelid.

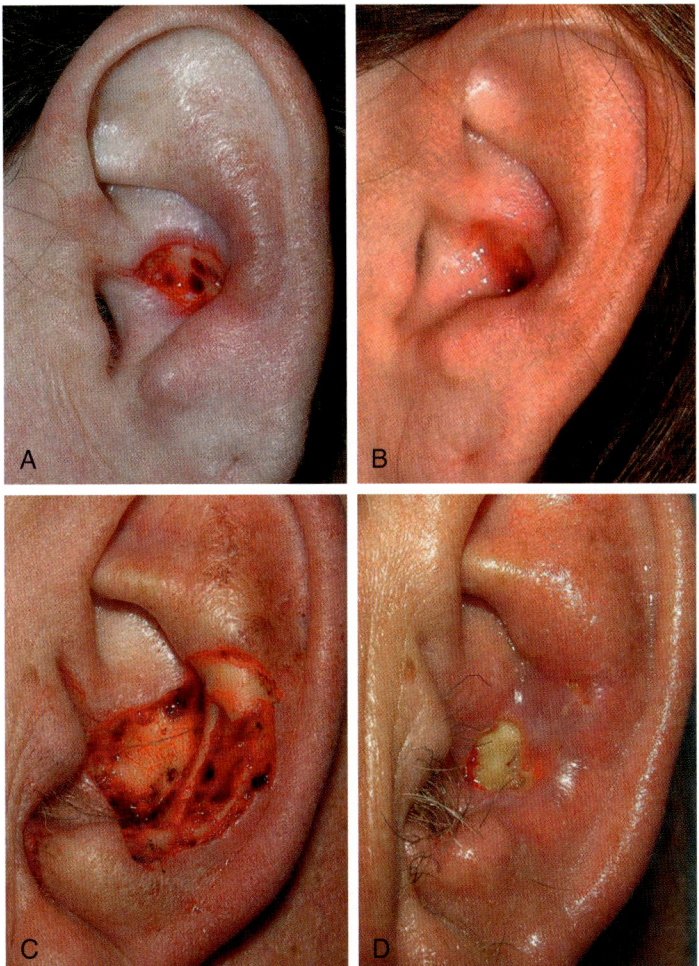

Fig. 3.8 Fenestration of exposed cartilage can prevent desiccation of cartilage and speed healing. (A) Wound of cymba concha with exposed cartilage. Note the windows made with punch incisions through the cartilage. (B) Fourteen days after the surgery, granulation tissue covers the entire wound, and she has no chondritis. (C) Wound of antihelix and cavum concha. Note that the cartilage is intact and perichondrium has been removed from the portion of the wound in the cavum concha, but there is a window through the cartilage along the antihelix. (D) One month after the surgery, approximately 75% of the wound has re-epithelialized. The portion of the wound with the cartilage window has healed fastest.

Primary Closure

Primary closure refers to a linear, or side-to-side, closure of a wound with sutures. An elliptical or fusiform closure is the most common method of repairing wounds after excision of cutaneous lesions. Although the term "elliptical" is commonly used, the term "fusiform" more accurately describes the spindle-shaped design of a primary closure. Whereas an ellipse has a curved shape along its entire boundary, a fusiform design has two sides that taper to a sharp point at each end. For the purposes of this chapter, the terms "elliptical" and "fusiform" will be used interchangeably to describe the linear closure of a wound with a layer of dermal sutures and cutaneous sutures.

PHASES OF WOUND HEALING

Compared to SIH, primary closure speeds the progression of wounds through the inflammatory, proliferative, and remodeling phases of healing.[2] The tensile strength of the sutured wound increases over time. Relative to normal skin, the tensile strength of a sutured wound is estimated to be about 20% after 3 weeks, 40% at 1 month, and 80% at 12 months, which is the maximum level it will achieve.[2,3]

PRINCIPLES OF RECONSTRUCTION

The following principles guide the design of a fusiform excision. First, preserve or restore the position of free margins, such as the eyelid, distal nose, lips, and helical rim. Second, preserve and restore the normal contour of the skin. Third, align the linear closure in cosmetic subunit junction lines, if possible. Fourth, orient the fusiform excision along relaxed skin tension lines, if possible. Preserving and restoring free margins and contour trump all other design considerations. Even if the scar line itself is minimally apparent, onlookers will readily note distorted free margins and contour.

Preserve and Restore the Position of Free Margins

Fusiform excisions can either pull or push the position of free margins, such as the eyelids, distal nose, lips, and helical rim. The pushing and pulling effects on free margins depend

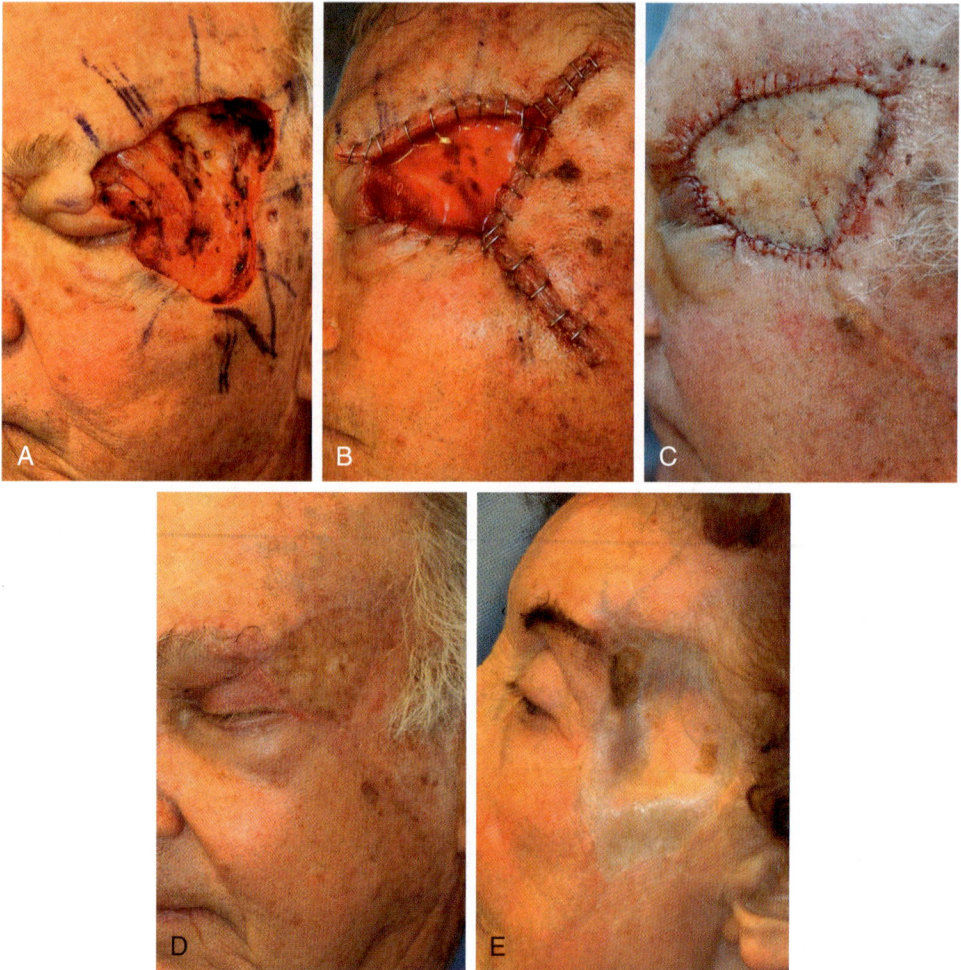

Fig. 3.9 Second intention healing is a good strategy to build volume in a wound before grafting. (A) This patient had a deep defect extending to the lateral orbital rim and temporal fossa. (B) The wound was partially closed and a dermal graft was placed to prevent desiccation of the exposed orbital rim. (C) After granulation tissue grew flush with the skin surface, a full-thickness skin graft was placed. (D) Two months after the graft, he has healed with good contour. (E) A different patient demonstrates how the volume of a skin graft cannot restore contour when placed immediately on a deep wound. She would have benefited from delaying the graft until second intention healing had developed granulation tissue to the surface of the wound.

on the orientation of the ellipse. The tension vectors of the closure are perpendicular to the long axis of the ellipse (Fig. 3.11). Tension is greatest at the center of the ellipse, where the gap between the two sides is greatest, and it progressively decreases toward the apices of the ellipse. Closure of fusiform excisions oriented parallel to free margins will pull them away from their natural position (Fig. 3.12). Orienting the fusiform excision with the long axis perpendicular to free margins prevents pulling from tension during the closure. For example, to prevent ectropion, orient the fusiform excision perpendicular to the lower eyelid.

While orienting a fusiform excision with its long axis perpendicular to free margins may prevent "pulling," this proper design predictably "pushes" free margins. The long axis of a fusiform excision elongates as the curved lines are pulled to form a single straight line (Fig. 3.13). The amount of elongation increases as the angles at the apices of fusiform excision increase.[22] As the axis lengthens, it pushes the nearby tissue, an effect most notable at free margins. Pushing up the lower eyelid or lower lip is usually inconsequential, because gravity usually restores the free margins to their original position (Fig. 3.14). However, pushing down on the upper lip is more likely to persist and may require revision at a later date. Increasing the length:width ratio of the fusiform excision decreases the angles at the apices and minimizes this "pushing" effect. An alternative reconstruction, such as an M-plasty, or an advancement or transposition flap, should be considered if there is not adequate space to lengthen the fusiform design and decrease the apical angles.[22]

Preserve and Restore Normal Contour

Preserving and restoring contour is essential to disguise a scar. Elevated contours unnaturally reflect light, and depressed contours cast noticeable shadows. The most common reason for elevated contours after primary closure is standing cone deformities, a term describing redundant tissue that puckers at the apices of a primary closure. The formation of standing cones depends primarily on the angle of the apex of the fusiform excision. Apical angles greater than 30 degrees usually create standing cone deformities.

The apical angles correlate with the length:width ratio of the fusiform excision. As the length:width ratio increases, the angles at the apices decrease. A length:width ratio of

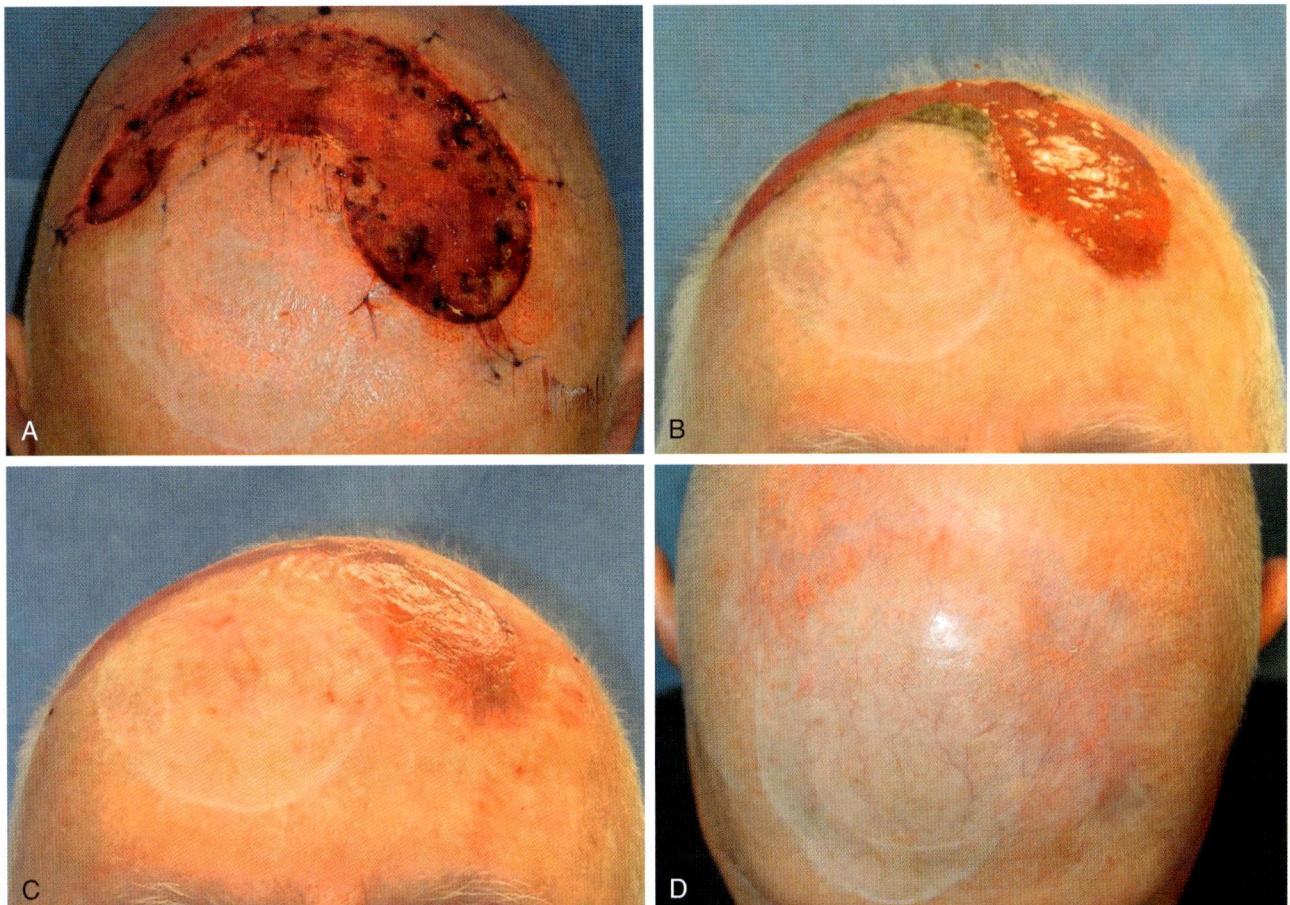

Fig. 3.10 (A) Mohs surgery defect after removal of a melanoma in situ that recurred after conventional excision. Note the hypopigmented skin graft from the initial surgery. The Mohs defect was allowed to heal by second intention. (B) Two months after the surgery, the patient has excessive granulation tissue. High potency topical steroids were prescribed twice daily. (C) Two weeks later, the granulation tissue has receded flush with the skin. He went on to heal uneventfully. (D) Twenty-two months after the surgery, his scar from second intention healing is less conspicuous than the initial skin graft. Prior to this photograph, telangiectases of the scar were treated with pulsed dye laser.

3:1, which is often proposed as the ideal ratio,[23] results in apical angles closer to 70 degrees and a high likelihood for standing cone deformities.[24] The length:width ratio must be increased to 4:1 or 5:1 to create apical angles of less than 30 degrees.

The need to elongate fusiform excisions varies with tissue elasticity. In areas where the skin is bound down and inelastic, such as the pretibial lower extremity and nasal tip, redundant tissue cones will often form despite a 30-degree apical angle. Increasing the length:width ratio to 4:1 or 5:1 to create apical angles of 15 to 20 degrees may be necessary to avoid standing cones in these locations.[25] By contrast, a shorter length to width ratio and apical angles slightly greater than 30 degrees may have little risk of contour deformity on elastic skin, such as the scrotum.

Depressed contours usually result from poor surgical technique or excessive tension on the wound. Suboptimal surgical technique may result in inverted scars and misaligned wound edges. Details of surgical technique are beyond the scope of this chapter, and readers are referred to more comprehensive references.[26,27]

Excessive wound tension also creates depressed contours. Tension is greatest at the center of the ellipse, where the gap between the two sides is greatest, and it progressively decreases toward the apices. Primary closure of tight wounds in anatomic locations with compressible deep tissue, such as the calf or deltoid, may heal a bowed scar that has a depressed central contour. Wounds that cross convexities, such as the jawline, may heal with depressed central contour as the wound contracts along the long axis of the closure. Failure to close all anatomic layers of a wound may also result in inverted scars. For example, closure of the dermis and epidermis but not the galea aponeurotica may heal with inverted scars on the scalp.

Orient Scars Along Cosmetic Subunit Junction Lines

Cosmetic subunit junction lines are natural boundaries with lines, shadows, and reflections that distinguish different anatomic areas on the body. They are relevant for surgical design on the face and relatively unimportant everywhere else on the body. Prominent examples on the face are the nasolabial fold, philtral columns, alar grooves, naso-facial sulcus, and eyebrow. Because the observer expects to see shadows or reflections in these areas, scars oriented along these cosmetic subunit junction lines are less perceptible. Scars should not be oriented in cosmetic subunit junction

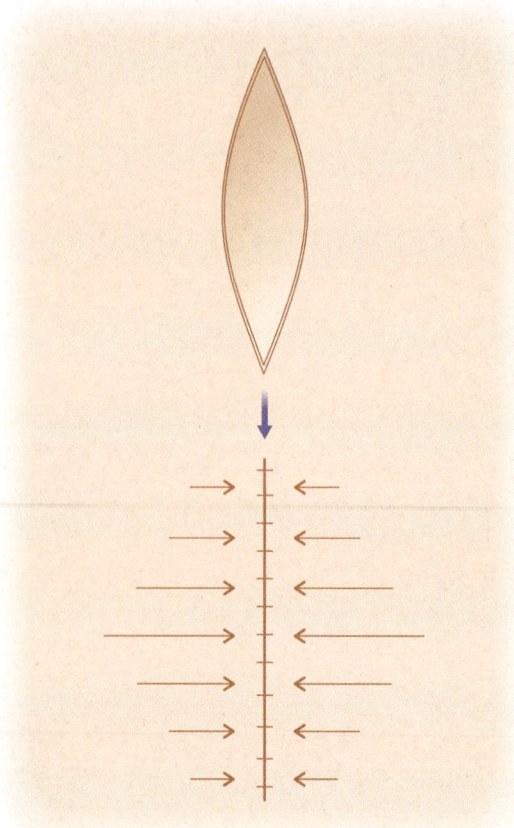

Fig. 3.11 Parallel tension vectors are present along the entire sutured wound. Tension is greatest at the center of the sutured wound and progressively decreases towards the apices.

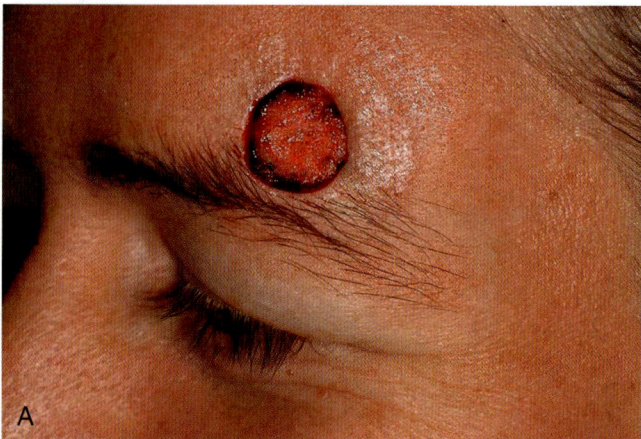

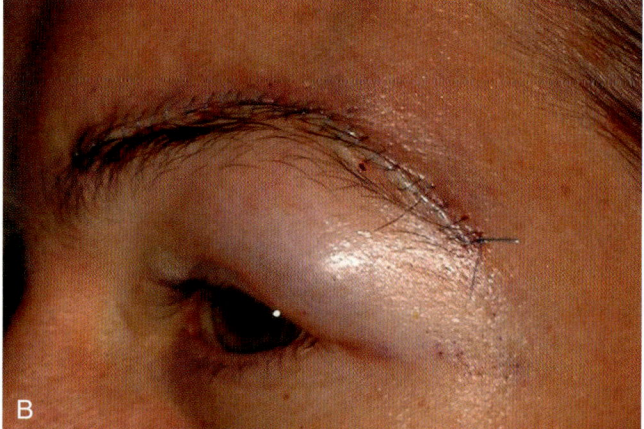

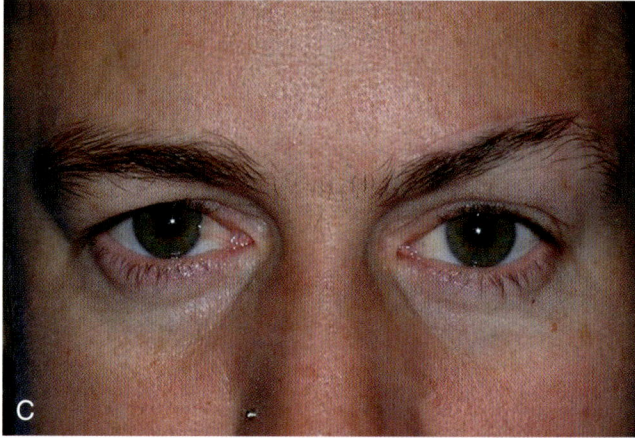

Fig. 3.12 (A) The patient has a small wound above her eyebrow. (B) A linear closure was used to hide the scar along the cosmetic subunit junction line of the eyebrow and forehead. (C) The faulty design of the excision predictably pulled up on her eyebrow and created markedly asymmetrical eyebrow position. An alternative reconstruction, such as an advancement flap, would have kept tension vectors parallel to her eyebrow and preserved its position.

lines if they distort free margins or contour. For example, avoid closing wounds along the alar groove or suprabrow if it elevates the free alar margin or brow position (see Fig. 3.12).

Orient Scars Along Relaxed Skin Tension Lines

Orienting fusiform excisions with the long axis along relaxed skin tension lines can decrease wound tension. Relaxed skin tension lines roughly correspond to the wrinkles on the body. On the face, contracting the muscles of facial expression, which insert directly to the dermis, accentuates the wrinkles perpendicular to the muscular contraction. On the trunk and extremities, skeletal muscles do not insert into the skin, and the relaxed skin tension lines must be assessed by pinching the skin. Increased numbers of parallel lines will form when the skin is pinched in one direction versus the other. It is important to assess for relaxed skin tension lines on the trunk and extremities in the neutral anatomic position: the patient is upright with arms by the sides and palms facing forward. Note that perceived lines of tension can change based on the patient's position.

Of all the principles for design of primary closures, orienting scars along relaxed skin tension lines is least important. With precise surgical technique, scars will heal well even if they cross relaxed skin tension lines. For example, vertically oriented scars on the forehead are usually preferable to placing scars in the horizontal wrinkles, because they preserve the position of the eyebrow.

VARIATIONS OF THE FUSIFORM EXCISION

This section provides an overview of the modifications to the standard fusiform design.

Crescentic Excision

Whereas the standard fusiform closure joins two sides of equal length to produce a straight scar, the crescentic excision joins two sides of unequal length to produce a curvilinear scar. This variation may be desirable in locations, such as the buccal cheek, where relaxed skin tension lines have a gentle curve (Fig. 3.15). One limb of the crescent is straight, and the second limb is curved. Closure of the unequal limbs bows the scar toward to the side of the longer, curved limb. A greater discrepancy in the lengths of the limbs results in greater curvature of the scar.

The crescentic excision may increase the risk for a contour deformity from a standing cone along the longer limb. A greater difference in length between the two limbs increases the size of the standing cones. Meticulous suture technique is necessary for precise wound edge alignment.

S-Plasty

Whereas the standard fusiform excision has a straight long axis, the S-plasty has a longer curving, "lazy-S" long axis (Fig. 3.16). As noted previously, primary closures can develop depressed and inverted scars over convex surfaces as contraction shortens the scar. This inversion can be prevented through a "lazy-S design" that increases the total length of the design but keeps the linear distance between the two ends constant.[28,29] Scar contraction will usually cause the final shape to straighten out, but the degree of inversion is decreased because of the extra length gained by the design. The S-plasty is especially useful to decrease inversion over the chin, mandible, and dorsal forearms (Fig. 3.17).

The S-plasty also reorients tension vectors. Whereas the standard fusiform excision has tension along a single vector, the curvy design of the S-plasty creates nonparallel tension vectors. The design is particularly useful for defects with a

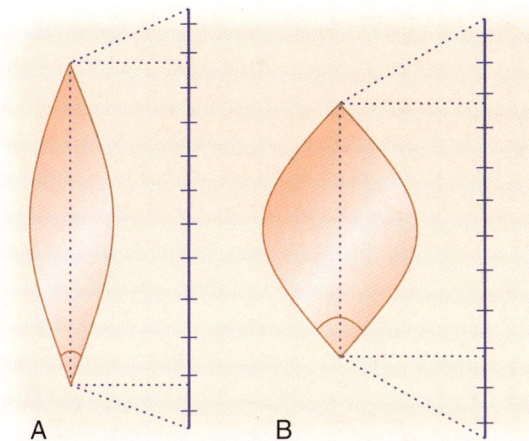

Fig. 3.13 (A) The long axis of a fusiform excision elongates as the curved lines are stretched to form a straight, sutured wound. (B) The amount of elongation increases as the angle at the apices of the wound increases.

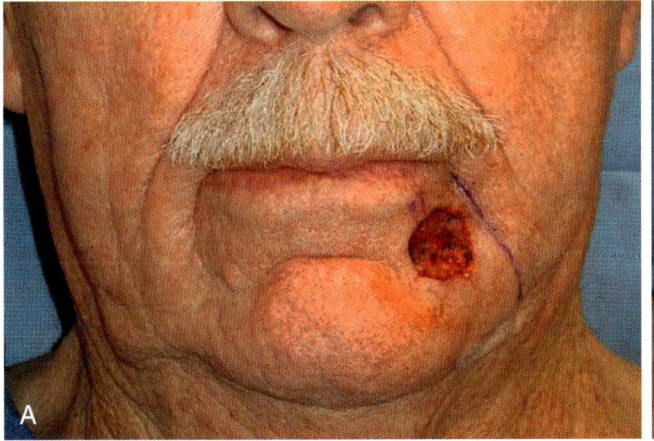

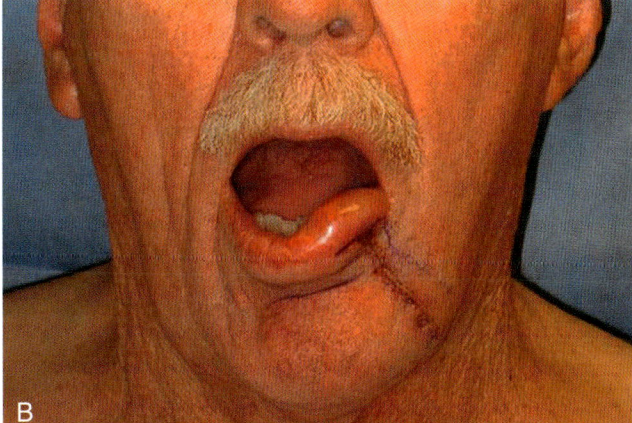

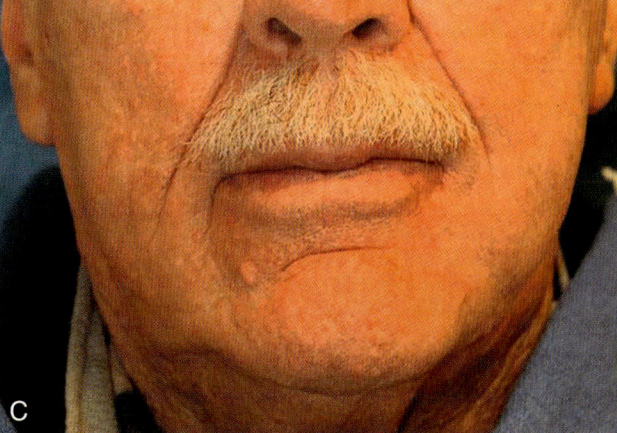

Fig. 3.14 (A) Defect after Mohs surgery for a skin cancer of the lower cutaneous lip. (B) The wound was reconstructed with a primary closure oriented perpendicularly to the free margin of the lip. Note how elongation of the wound has pushed up on the lower lip. (C) Three months after the surgery, gravity has restored the normal position of the lip.

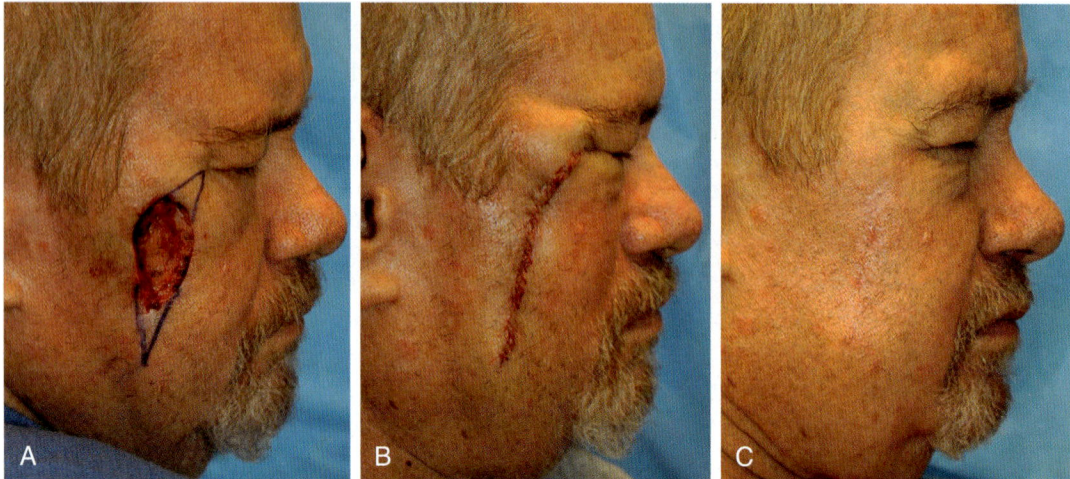

Fig. 3.15 Crescentic excision. (A) Design of a crescentic excision to close a defect of the zygomatic cheek. Note that the posterior limb of the design is curved, and the anterior limb is relatively straight. (B) Appearance immediately after suturing the wound. The scar has bowed with a gentle curve toward the longer, posterior limb. (C) Three months after the surgery, the scar is minimally apparent.

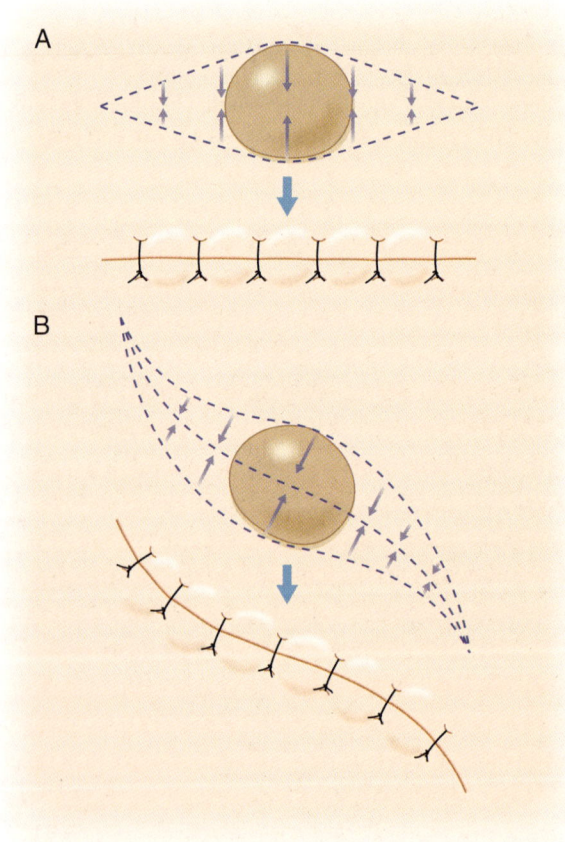

Fig. 3.16 (A) Classic ellipse with horizontal vectors of tension and straight line closure. (B) Classic S-plasty allowing for more diagonal vectors of tension and curved S-shaped suture line.

horizontal long axis on the preseptal lower eyelid and infraorbital cheek. By designing a "lazy-S" shape so that the superior and inferior standing cones at each end of the wound are perpendicular to the free margin, the tension vectors are reoriented to be parallel to the free margin which avoids a downward pull on the eyelid.

Order and placement of sutures are critical for an S-plasty. After excising of the specimen with the proper "S" shape, it is imperative that the surgeon take horizontal bites between the opposing edges and not diagonal bites. Diagonal bites will result in a linear scar that is inadvertently greater in length than the initial design. Inexperienced surgeons also often create unnecessarily long scars by "chasing" redundant tissue cones. Precise placement of the initial buried suture is essential to avoiding both of these results. If placed properly, the first suture will form crescent-shaped defects on both sides of the suture. These crescents will be oriented in different directions from each other. Meticulous placement of subsequent buried sutures will produce the desired S-shape.

M-Plasty

The M-plasty reduces the total length of a scar to avoid encroaching upon important neighboring structures such as the eyelid or lip,[30,31] or to reduce the risk of webbing by keeping the scar from crossing a concavity (Figs. 3.18 and 3.19). The M-plasty may also be useful for primary closure of a wound with asymmetric widths (Fig. 3.20). One or both sides of the standard fusiform design may be modified, depending on where the reduction in length is needed. The triangle at the apex of the wound is converted to two adjacent triangles that form an "M" shape. The new triangles that are formed should also have apical angles of 30 degrees and should be half the length of the initial triangle. The triangle may be advanced into the linear part of the closure to decrease the pushing motion created by the unavoidable lengthening that occurs with a standard linear closure. This can be especially useful to minimize downward push from vertical closures near the free margin of the upper lip.

3 • Second Intention Healing and Primary Closure   45

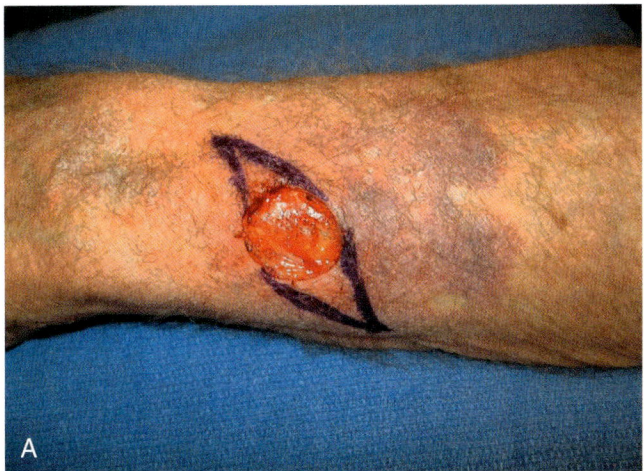
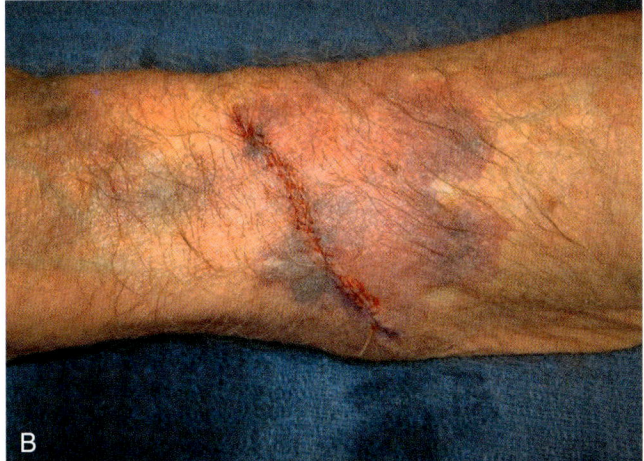
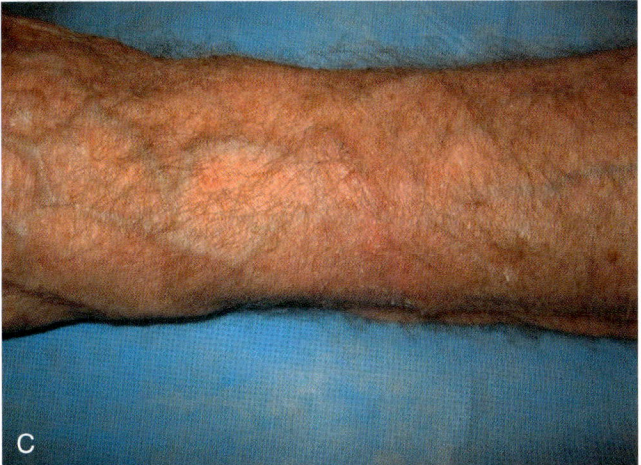

Fig. 3.17 S-plasty. (A) S-plasty design for a Mohs defect over the convex, dorsal ulnar forearm. (B) Immediately after primary closure, the suture line retains its "lazy-S" shape. (C) One month after the surgery, the wound has healed with excellent contour and no inversion.

If an even shorter scar is necessary, the process can be repeated on each of the two newly formed triangles, which will result in four adjacent triangles. Previously termed a "nested" M-plasty, this variation is helpful for lesions on flat or concave surfaces.[32] Some have argued that the M-plasty is better conceptualized as a modified V-Y plasty, and have proposed widening the shoulders of the adjacent triangles to avoid compression-derived tissue protrusion.[31]

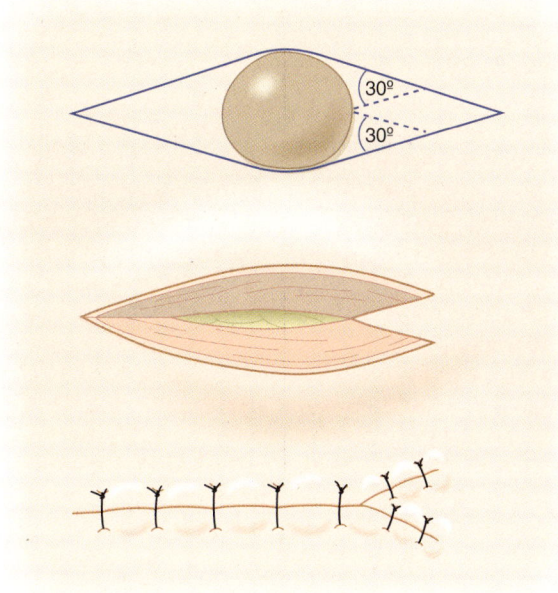

Fig. 3.18 M-plasty. Instead of completing the ellipse, the dashed lines are incised as shown, reducing the length of the scar.

Serial Elliptical Excisions

Some lesions, such as congenital melanocytic nevi, can be so large that complete excision in a single stage is not possible or desirable, due to the amount of tension required for closure. In these situations, serial excision of the lesion is often utilized to prevent a potentially disfiguring scar (Fig. 3.21). Serial excision takes advantage of the skin's inherent tissue creep and allows a lesion to be removed in numerous stages. The number of required stages is dictated by the size of the lesion relative to the lesion's specific anatomic location. When performing serial excisions, the normal design principles of elliptical excision do not all apply. The initial elliptical excision should be designed to be the length of the lesion and should have apical angles of less than 30 degrees. It takes roughly 8–12 weeks for the skin to heal and relax before another excision can be performed. The process is repeated until the lesion is completely excised. The final scar is usually shorter and finer than the anticipated scar from a single, large excision.

STANDING CONE DEFORMITIES: CAUSES AND CORRECTIONS

Standing cone deformities, often referred to as "dog ears," are protrusions of redundant tissue that form near the apices of primary closures and alter the normal contour of the skin. Standing cone deformities most commonly form due to angles wider than 30 degrees at the apices of a fusiform excision, suturing wounds of unequal length (e.g., crescentic excision), primary closures with insufficient length:width ratio, especially on convex surfaces, and excessive deep tissue near the apices of a wound after excision of an ellipse.[33]

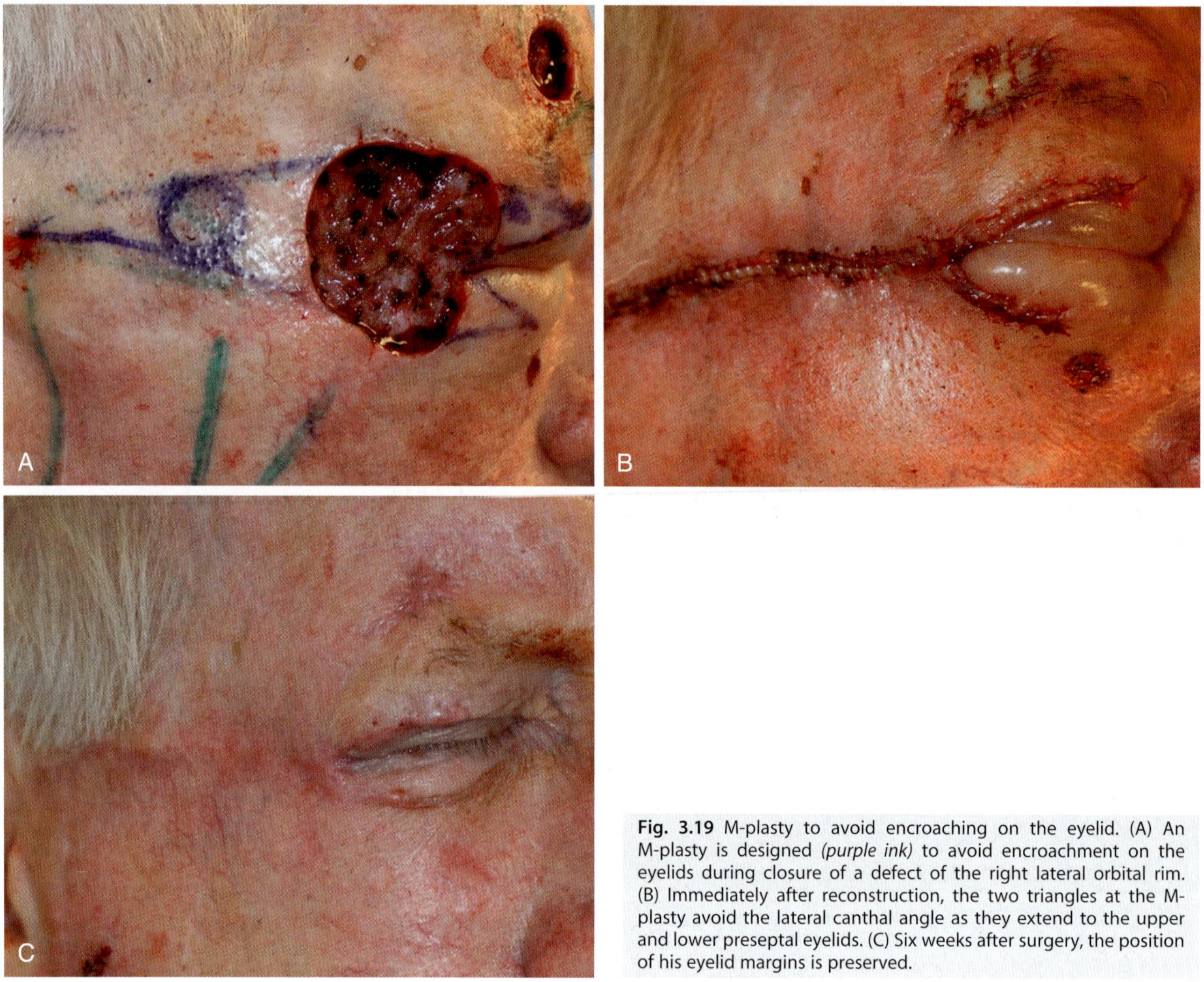

Fig. 3.19 M-plasty to avoid encroaching on the eyelid. (A) An M-plasty is designed *(purple ink)* to avoid encroachment on the eyelids during closure of a defect of the right lateral orbital rim. (B) Immediately after reconstruction, the two triangles at the M-plasty avoid the lateral canthal angle as they extend to the upper and lower preseptal eyelids. (C) Six weeks after surgery, the position of his eyelid margins is preserved.

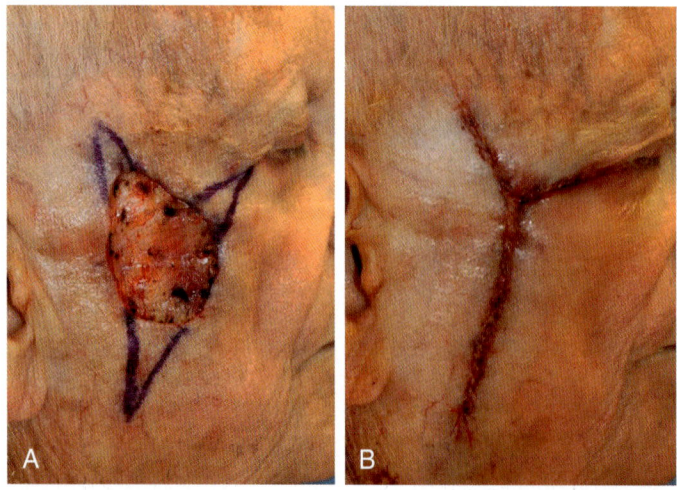

Fig. 3.20 (A) A modified M-plasty is designed to reconstruct an asymmetric wound. (B) Immediately after reconstruction.

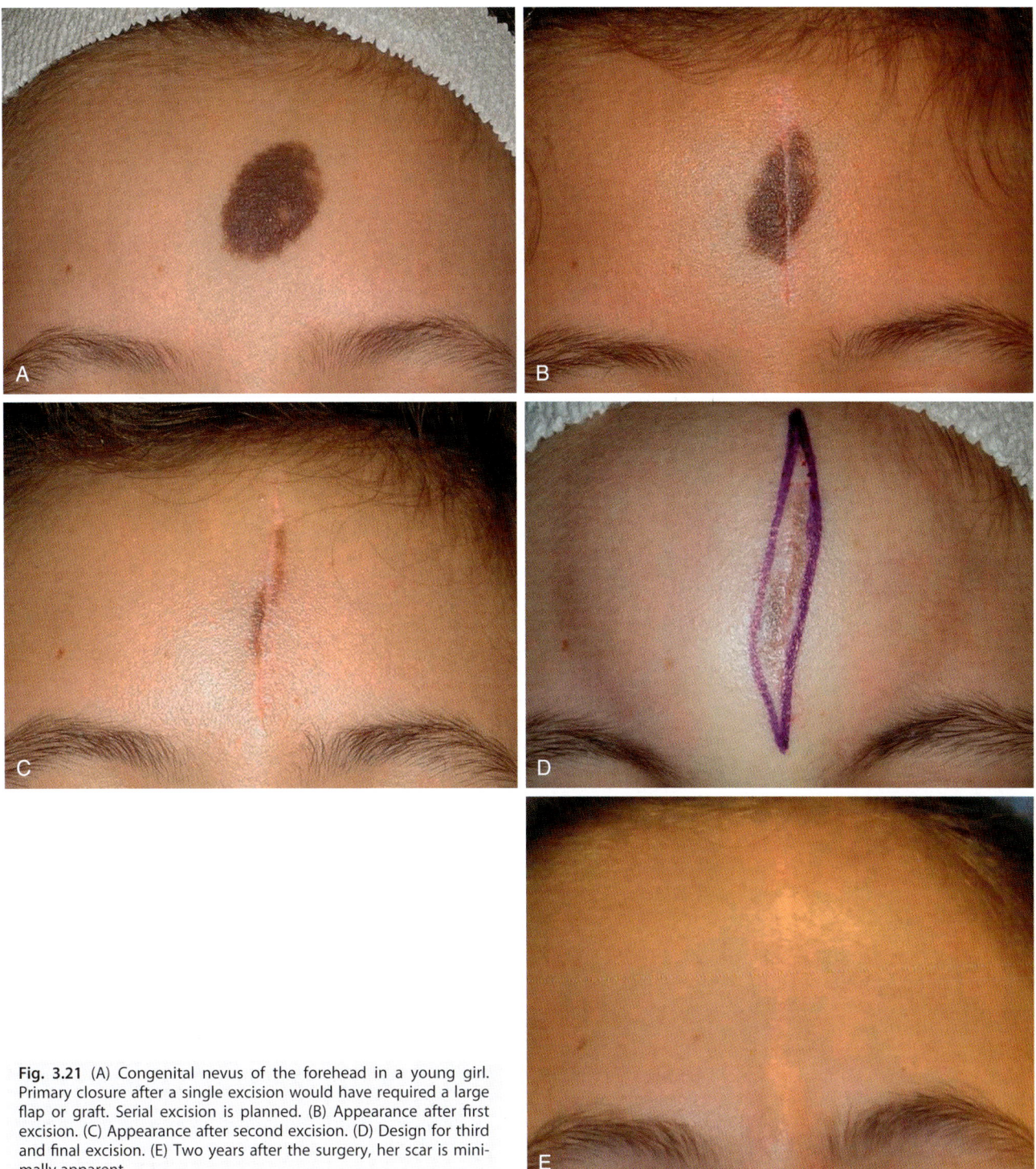

Fig. 3.21 (A) Congenital nevus of the forehead in a young girl. Primary closure after a single excision would have required a large flap or graft. Serial excision is planned. (B) Appearance after first excision. (C) Appearance after second excision. (D) Design for third and final excision. (E) Two years after the surgery, her scar is minimally apparent.

The following design principles minimize the formation of standing cones:

- design fusiform excisions with apical angles of 30 degrees or less;
- increase the length:width ratio and decrease the apical angles for fusiform excisions on tight, convex surfaces or compressible deep tissue;
- suture wound edges of unequal length with meticulous technique and the rule of halves;
- use careful surgical technique, including incising with sharply vertical edges to a uniform depth, excising the tissue with a uniform plane at the base of the wound and undermining around the entire wound.[26,28]

To correct a standing cone deformity, first define the size of the cone by pulling up on the peak of the redundant tissue up with a forceps or skin hook (Fig. 3.22). Note that the tissue can be manipulated to point the cone in different directions. If desired, use a marking pen to define the base

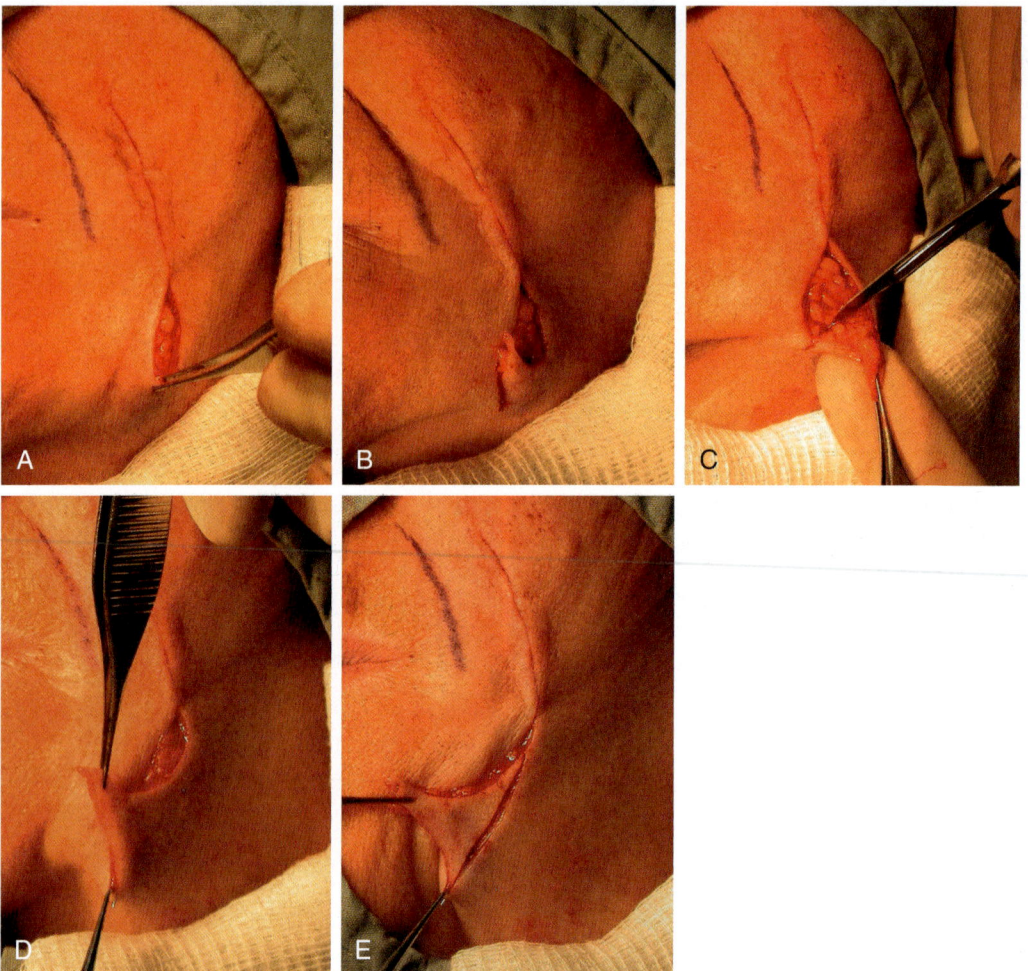

Fig. 3.22 Technique to remove standing cone deformities. (A) A forceps is used to pull up on the peak of the redundant tissue and to define the base of the standing cone. (B) An incision has been made through the dermis along the base of one side of the cone. Note that the skin does not drape freely, since it has yet to be undermined. (C) A scalpel is used to undermine the redundant skin. (D) The undermined skin drapes freely over the wound. (E) A second incision has been made to match the location of the first incision. The cone is removed and the edges are sutured in a layered fashion.

of the standing cone. Still pulling up on the peak of the redundant skin, incise through the dermis along the base of one side of the cone. Be careful to keep the scalpel perpendicular to the plane of the retracted skin as it is altered when being pulled up by the forceps or skin hook. Undermine the redundant skin and drape it flat over the initial excision. Make a second incision along draped flap to match the first incision and remove the tissue. The edges of the wound should align precisely for closure with sutures.

COMPLICATIONS OF PRIMARY CLOSURE

Many of the complications arising from primary closure result from an unsound design that violates the principles of reconstruction. If the excision is designed so that tension vectors are oriented parallel rather than perpendicular to a free margin, there is risk of distortion if the wound is close enough to the margin. Consequent ectropion, eclabium, or elevation of the eyebrow will noticeably distort a patient's appearance. When designs fail to maintain a sufficient length to width ratio or have apical angles that are excessively obtuse, redundant tissue cones will cause obvious contour deformities. Standing cones may form if there is a discrepancy in the length of opposing wound edges, such as an aggressively designed crescentic excision. Webbing is a complication commonly seen when a primary closure crosses a concave surface, such as the medial canthus or root of the nose. A Z-plasty is often necessary to correct the deformity.

Complications are sometimes a consequence of flawed surgical technique. Hematomas or seromas may form if there is failure to properly close the dead space for deeper wounds. Spitting sutures, which most often occur around 6 weeks postoperatively, can result from the placement of buried sutures too superficially or poor knot cutting technique.[34] This reaction can be delayed up to 5 to 6 months for some sutures such as polytrimethylene carbonate (Maxon). If the superficial sutures bear too much tension, spread scars and track marks often result. While some amount of spreading may be inevitable in certain locations or young, elastic skin, it can be lessened by longer-acting buried dermal absorbable sutures.[35]

Some complications are unavoidable and specific to the patient. Some patients will be prone to hypertrophic scarring and keloid formation due to a genetic predisposition.[36] A history of hypertrophic scarring and keloid formation should be queried prior to surgery. The areas of the upper trunk (chest, shoulders, upper back) as well as the periauricular skin are particularly susceptible. This possibility should be discussed with the patient at the time of surgery. Likewise, younger patients with elastic skin should be forewarned about the likelihood of a spread scar.

CONCLUSION

SIH and primary closure are workhorse options to manage cutaneous wounds. Basic principles guide wound selection and help achieve predictable outcomes. Variations of the traditional elliptical excision can reduce complications and improve results.

References

1. Alam M, Helenowksi IB, Cohen JL, et al. Association between type of reconstruction after Mohs micrographic surgery and surgeon-, patient-, and tumor-specific features: a cross-sectional study. *Dermatol Surg.* 2013;39:51-55.
2. Lamel S, Li J, Kirsner RS. Wound healing. In: Robinson J, Hanke CW, Siegal DM, Fratila A, eds. *Surgery of the Skin: Procedural Dermatology.* 3rd ed. Philadelphia: Elsevier Saunders; 2015:95-113.
3. Morton LM, Phillips TJ. Wound healing and treating wounds: differential diagnosis and evaluation of chronic wounds. *J Am Acad Dermatol.* 2016;74:589-605.
4. Lam TK, Lowe C, Johnson R, Marquart JD. Secondary intention healing and purse-string closures. *Dermatol Surg.* 2015;41(suppl 10):S178-S186.
5. Mott KJ, Clark DP, Stelljes LS. Regional variation in wound contraction of Mohs surgery defects allowed to heal by second intention. *Dermatol Surg.* 2003;29:712-722.
6. Zitelli JA. Secondary intention healing: an alternative to surgical repair. *Clin Dermatol.* 1984;2:92-106.
7. Bosley R, Leithauser L, Turner M, Gloster HM Jr. The efficacy of second-intention healing in the management of defects on the dorsal surface of the hands and fingers after Mohs micrographic surgery. *Dermatol Surg.* 2012;38:647-653.
8. Gloster HM Jr. The use of second-intention healing for partial-thickness Mohs defects involving the vermilion and/or mucosal surfaces of the lip. *J Am Acad Dermatol.* 2002;47:893-897.
9. Leonard AL, Hanke CW. Second intention healing for intermediate and large postsurgical defects of the lip. *J Am Acad Dermatol.* 2007;57:832-835.
10. Zitelli JA. Wound healing by secondary intention: a cosmetic appraisal. *J Am Acad Dermatol.* 1983;9:407-415.
11. Hochwalt PC, Christensen KN, Cantwell SR, et al. Comparison of full-thickness skin grafts versus second-intention healing for Mohs defects of the helix. *Dermatol Surg.* 2015;41:69-77.
12. Drosou A, Trieu D, Goldberg LH. Scalpel-made holes on exposed scalp bone to promote second intention healing. *J Am Acad Dermatol.* 2014;71:387-388.
13. Campbell T, Eisen DB. Free cartilage grafts for alar defects coupled with secondary-intention healing. *Dermatol Surg.* 2011;37:510-513.
14. Norman G, Dumville JC, Mohapatra DP, Owens GL, Crosbie EJ. Antibiotics and antiseptics for surgical wounds healing by secondary intention. *Cochrane Database Syst Rev.* 2016;(3):CD011712.
15. Vermeulen H, Ubbink D, Goossens A, de Vos R, Legemate D. Dressings and topical agents for surgical wounds healing by secondary intention. *Cochrane Database Syst Rev.* 2004;(2):CD003554.
16. Firoz BF, Goldberg LH, Arnon O, Mamelak AJ. An analysis of pain and analgesia after Mohs micrographic surgery. *J Am Acad Dermatol.* 2010;63:79-86.
17. Chen AF, Landy DC, Kumetz E, et al. Prediction of postoperative pain after Mohs micrographic surgery with 2 validated pain anxiety scales. *Dermatol Surg.* 2015;41:40-47.
18. Allevato M, Clerc C, del Sel JM, et al. Erosive pustular dermatosis of the scalp. *Int J Dermatol.* 2009;48:1213-1216.
19. Patton D, Lynch PJ, Fung MA, Fazel N. Chronic atrophic erosive dermatosis of the scalp and extremities: a recharacterization of erosive pustular dermatosis. *J Am Acad Dermatol.* 2007;57:421-427.
20. Stebbins WG, Gusev J, Higgins HW II, Nelson A, Govindarajulu U, Neel V. Evaluation of patient satisfaction with second intention healing versus primary surgical closure. *J Am Acad Dermatol.* 2015;73:865-867.
21. Kantor J. Primary surgical closure versus second intention healing after Mohs micrographic surgery: patient satisfaction and clinical implications. *J Am Acad Dermatol.* 2016;75:e35.
22. Etzkorn JR, Sobanko JF, Miller CJ. Free margin distortion with fusiform closures: the apical angle relationship. *Dermatol Surg.* 2014;40:1428-1432.
23. Hussain W, Mortimer NJ, Salmon PJ. Optimizing technique in elliptical excisional surgery: some pearls for practice. *Br J Dermatol.* 2009;161:697-698.
24. Moody BR, McCarthy JE, Sengelmann RD. The apical angle: a mathematical analysis of the ellipse. *Dermatol Surg.* 2001;27:61-63.
25. Cook J, Zitelli JA. Primary closure for midline defects of the nose: a simple approach for reconstruction. *J Am Acad Dermatol.* 2000;43:508-510.
26. Miller CJ, Antunes MB, Sobanko JF. Surgical technique for optimal outcomes: part I. Cutting tissue: incising, excising, and undermining. *J Am Acad Dermatol.* 2015;72:377-387.
27. Miller CJ, Antunes MB, Sobanko JF. Surgical technique for optimal outcomes: part II. Repairing tissue: suturing. *J Am Acad Dermatol.* 2015;72:389-402.
28. Zitelli JA. TIPS for a better ellipse. *J Am Acad Dermatol.* 1990;22:101-103.
29. Sebastian S, Bang RH, Padilla RS. A simple approach to the S-plasty in cutaneous surgery. *Dermatol Surg.* 2009;35:1277-1279.
30. Salasche SJ, Roberts LC. Dog-ear correction by M-plasty. *J Dermatol Surg Oncol.* 1984;10:478-482.
31. Wisco OJ, Wentzell JM. When an M is a V: vector analysis calls for redesign of the M-plasty. *Dermatol Surg.* 2009;35:1271-1276.
32. Krishnan RS, Donnelly HB. The nested M-plasty for scar length shortening. *Dermatol Surg.* 2008;34:1236-1238.
33. Weisberg NK, Nehal KS, Zide BM. Dog-ears: a review. *Dermatol Surg.* 2000;26:363-370.
34. Clayton AS, Stasko T. Surgical complications and optimizing outcomes. In: Bolognia JL, Jorizzo JL, Schaffer JV, eds. *Dermatology.* 3rd ed. Philadelphia: Elsevier Saunders; 2012:2459-2472.
35. Kia KF, Burns MV, Vandergriff T, Weitzul S. Prevention of scar spread on trunk excisions: a rater-blinded randomized controlled trial. *JAMA Dermatol.* 2013;149:687-691.
36. Trace AP, Enos CW, Mantel A, Harvey VM. Keloids and hypertrophic scars: a spectrum of clinical challenges. *Am J Clin Dermatol.* 2016;17:201-223.

Videos for this chapter can be found online by accessing the accompanying Expert Consult website.

4 Advancement Flaps

CHRISTIE R. TRAVELUTE, MD, and ROBERTA SENGELMANN, MD

Flap Design and Considerations

Advancement flaps are the oldest and most basic methods of adjacent tissue transfer in cutaneous surgery.[1] They can be thought of as sliding flaps that move along a single vector directly into the surgical defect (Figs. 4.1 and 4.2). After the defect is closed, the surrounding tissue provides the secondary movement or opposing force.[2] The flap is designed by extending two parallel incisions (not necessarily of the same length) from one side of a surgical defect (Fig. 4.3). Because the flap is created from adjacent skin, one edge of the defect becomes the advancing tip of the flap. This basic design has also been called a U-plasty or rectangular flap. The prominent horizontal lines make the advancement flap particularly useful in the reconstruction of the eyebrow and forehead areas. It can also be effective for reconstruction of defects on the upper lip, dorsal nose, and helical rim.

The primary advantage of an advancement flap lies in its ability to redistribute standing cones (dog-ears) to a more favorable location that is not necessarily contiguous with the defect. When a circular wound is closed with a linear side-to-side closure, standing cones develop adjacent to the apices. In both rotation and transposition flaps, a standing cone develops at the pivotal base, where it must be excised to allow for full movement of the flap.[3] The geometry of an advancement flap allows for excision of tissue redundancy anywhere along the length of the flap. In this way the incisions can be hidden within relaxed skin tension lines (RSTLs) or cosmetic unit junction lines.

There are several factors that must be taken into account when designing an advancement flap. The most important consideration is the amount of tissue laxity available for closure of the defect. An advancement flap does not lower the tension of closure much beyond that which can be achieved with a side-to-side closure, and it is not a good choice for large defects without surrounding laxity. With experience, the surgeon can estimate the degree of tissue mobility and identify tissue reservoirs by pinching and stretching the defect and surrounding skin. The importance of physical manipulation of tissue to estimate mobility cannot be stressed enough. After the flap is incised from the surrounding tissue, it relies on the blood supply within its pedicle to maintain viability. The flap's perfusion is determined largely by its dimensions, its thickness, the quality of the vasculature within its pedicle, and the tension placed upon it during closure.[4] Blood flow to the tip of the flap is inversely related to the tension of wound closure, and even a wide, well-perfused flap is at risk for necrosis if placed under too much strain.[5]

Any form of wound closure has the potential to distort a free margin, but advancement flaps, which are strictly linear, carry a significant risk if not oriented correctly. The surgeon can estimate the potential for asymmetry by pinching the defect closed in the direction of the flap's movement. If this maneuver distorts a free margin, then the flap should be reoriented or another form of reconstruction considered. Other important considerations in flap design include determining the best location for incision lines and where to displace standing cones.[6]

Flap Mobilization and Key Sutures

After the flap design has been determined, the proposed incision lines should be marked on the skin prior to infiltrating additional local anesthesia. This allows for more accurate placement without distortion by tumescence. To ensure symmetry, these markings should be confirmed with the patient in the upright position. After local anesthesia is achieved, the surgical defect may be undermined in all directions prior to incising the flap. This allows the surgeon to assess the degree of tissue laxity and to reconfirm the surgical plan. It is wise to approach each reconstruction with several alternatives in mind, recognizing that intraoperative adjustments in the surgical plan may be necessary. For example, there are times when unexpected laxity may allow for a less complex closure with comparable cosmesis and lower morbidity. Conversely, situations can arise in which there is less movement than expected, requiring flap modification. The potential for either scenario always exists, and it is best to have considered all potential outcomes before starting any surgical procedure. It is usually helpful to make incisions that keep the most options available first and save those that lock into a particular closure for last.

The classic advancement flap is designed for a rectangular defect, but it is not always necessary to square the edges of a circular defect prior to incising the flap.[7] In fact, it may be prudent to wait until the flap has been mobilized to evaluate whether the recipient defect should be modified or the flap tip rounded. Because flap viability is directly related to the length and thickness of the pedicle and not the shape of the flap distal to it, the surgeon is free to choose the option that achieves the best aesthetic result.[4] In fact, there may be times when it is deemed wise to enlarge the defect to allow the suture lines to fall within RSTLs (Fig. 4.4).

In general, the maximum length for a random pattern flap on the face is limited to three to four times the width of the pedicle.[8] The surgeon may consider making the initial incisions slightly shorter than were originally designed to accommodate unexpected laxity discovered

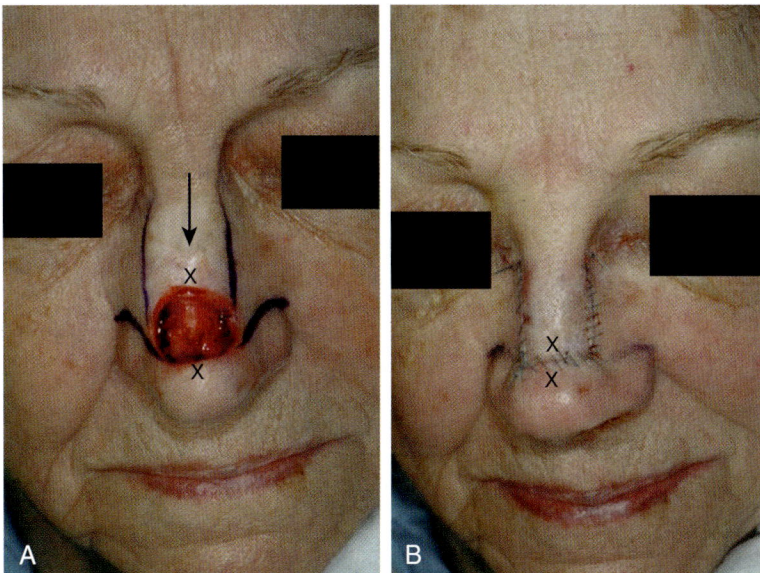

Fig. 4.1 Rintala flap. (A) Single rectangular advancement flap with tissue reservoir located in the glabella and incision lines along the cosmetic junction lines of the nasal dorsum. In this case, Burow triangles are placed at the base of the flap within relaxed skin tension lines. The *arrow* indicates the primary motion of the flap. (B) Immediate postoperative appearance.

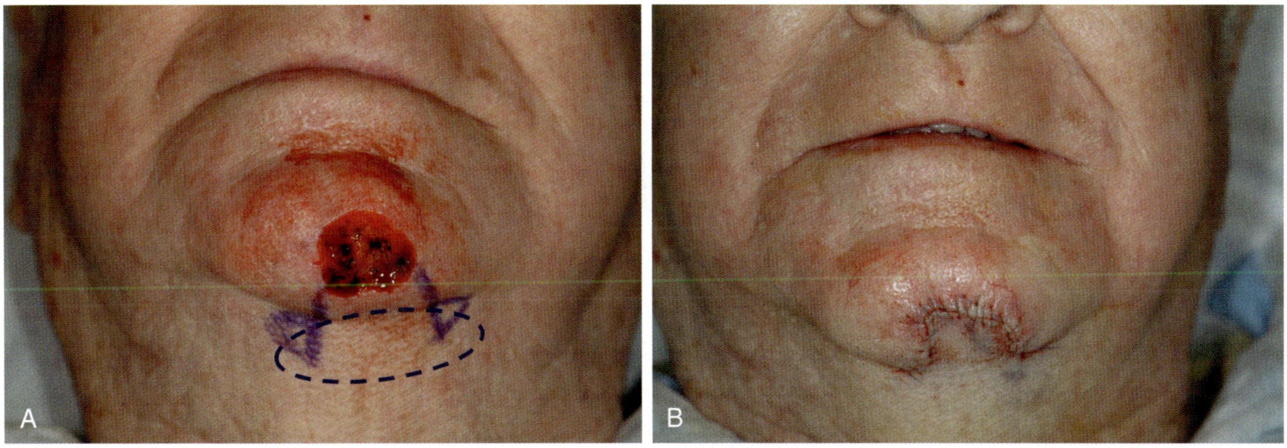

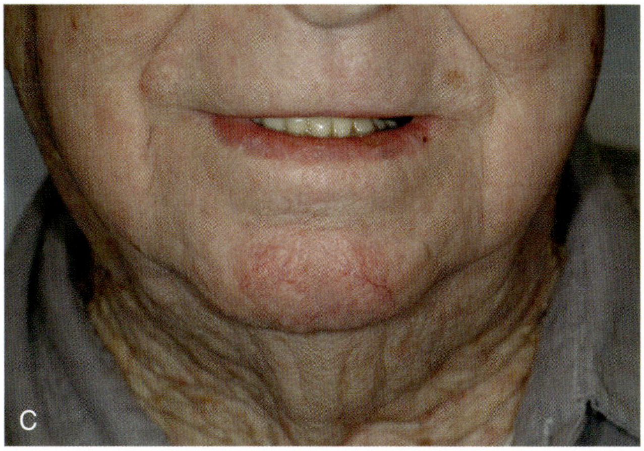

Fig. 4.2 Rectangular advancement flap. (A) Surgical defect, which does not have sufficient immediate surrounding tissue laxity to allow primary closure. *Blue oval* identifies the submental tissue reservoir the flap will rely upon. (B) Immediate postoperative appearance. (C) Appearance 6 weeks after surgery.

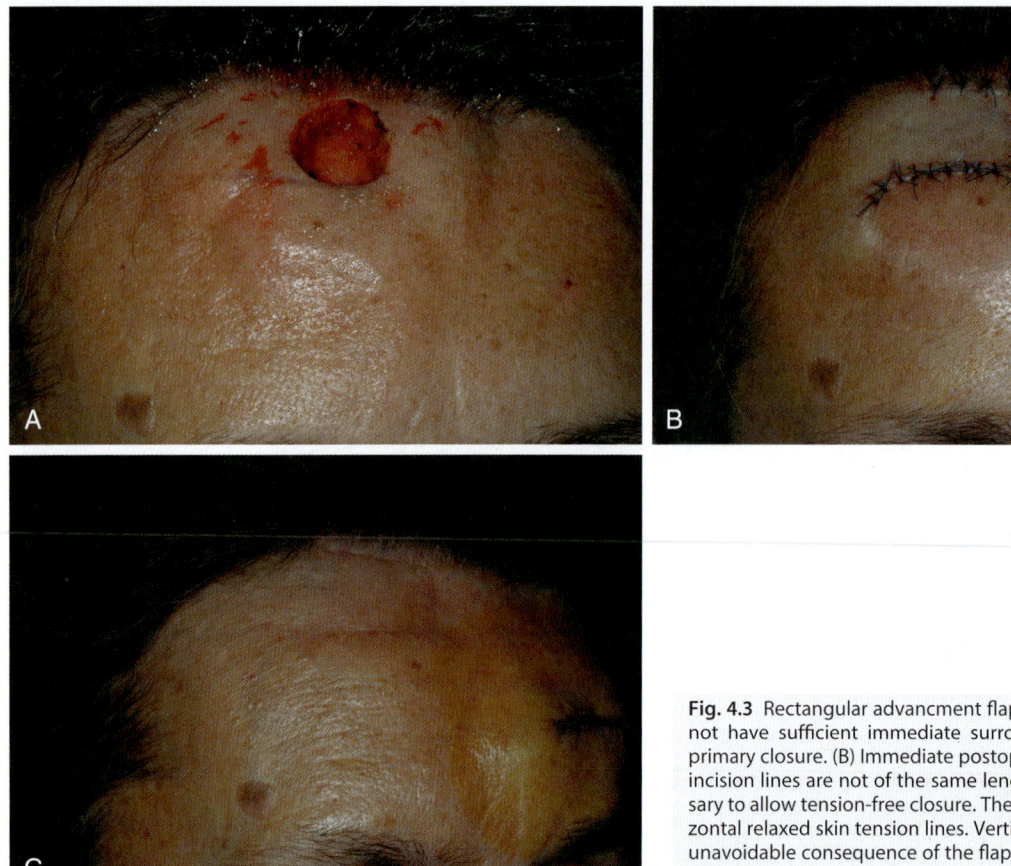

Fig. 4.3 Rectangular advancment flap. (A) Surgical defect that does not have sufficient immediate surrounding tissue laxity to allow primary closure. (B) Immediate postoperative appearance. Note flap incision lines are not of the same length and only as long as necessary to allow tension-free closure. They are designed to fall into horizontal relaxed skin tension lines. Vertical line is more noticeable but unavoidable consequence of the flap. (C) Appearance 3 weeks after surgery.

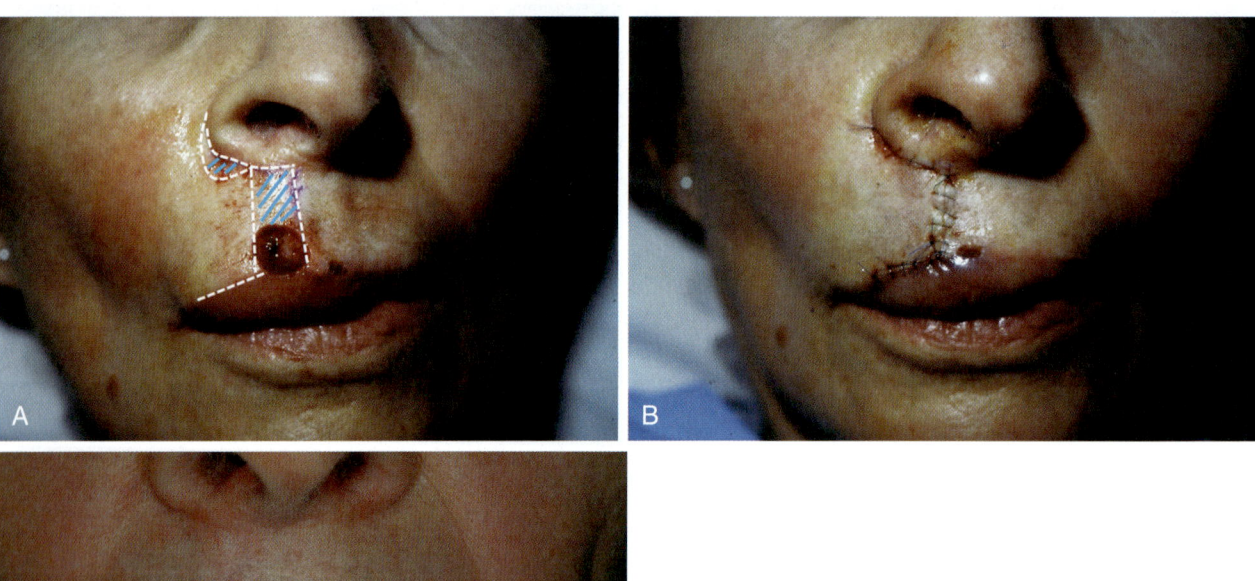

Fig. 4.4 Webster perialar crescentic advancement flap. (A) Flap design marked with *dotted lines*. Tissue that will be sacrificed to allow suture lines to fall within relaxed skin tension lines is marked with *blue shading*. (B) Immediate postoperative appearance. Tissue redundancy at inferior edge sewn out by the rule of halves. (C) Appearance 4 months after surgery.

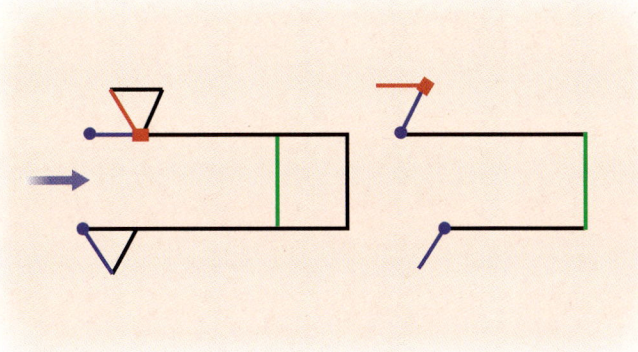

Fig. 4.5 Diagram of Burow triangle excision. Inverted Burow triangle is placed at the superior edge and traditional Burow triangle is placed at the inferior edge.

after undermining. These incisions can always be extended if additional length is needed. The flap should be thick enough to fill the defect and include the subdermal vascular plexus with at least a portion of the upper subcutaneous fat. In the absence of vital anatomic structures, the flap should become progressively thicker as it extends towards the base of the pedicle. This allows for larger-caliber vessels to be recruited and increase the likelihood of flap survival. If there is a question of sufficient blood supply, studies have shown it may be appropriate to deepen the defect to accommodate a thicker flap with more robust perfusion.[4]

In an advancement flap, the entire flap and surrounding skin should be undermined in all directions. This increases mobility, distributes tension more evenly, and, by spreading out the forces of contracture that will occur during wound healing, may limit the development of pin-cushioning.[9] The exact undermining depth will vary with the location of the defect.[10] In anatomic danger zones, such as over the zygoma and mandible and within the posterior triangle of the neck, the dissection must remain in the upper subcutaneous fat and above motor nerves, or permanent functional loss may result. Small defects on the forehead can be undermined in the subcutaneous fat above the frontalis fascia. However, large forehead defects are best dissected in the subgaleal plane. In hair-bearing locations such as the eyebrow, the undermining should be well into the subcutis and deep to the hair papillae. The nose should be undermined in the submuscular plane and the ears above the perichondrium. After undermining has been performed, the flap is pulled gently into the defect to test its mobility. If this maneuver produces excessive tension, the most common cause is insufficient undermining. If tension remains despite wide undermining, the surgeon may consider lengthening the flap or converting it into a bilateral advancement flap to obtain additional tissue movement.[11]

If the surgical defect is secondary to Mohs micrographic surgery, it is likely that the wound edges are beveled. Prior to insetting the flap, the beveled tissue should be excised flush with the epidermis to create a crisp 90-degree vertical edge. After the recipient site has been prepared and undermining completed, judicious hemostasis should be achieved. There is a delicate balance between inadequate hemostasis, which increases the risk for hematoma, and excessive thermal injury that induces inflammation and increases the potential for infection. Small vessels in the skin edge will tamponade with closure and usually do not require electrocoagulation. Large vessels should be clamped and individually spot-electrocoagulated or suture-ligated. After the flap is able to slide into the defect with minimal tension and hemostasis has been obtained, the key suture is placed in the advancing edge to close the wound. In an advancement flap, the key suture closes the primary defect and serves to align the flap.

By design, an advancement flap has skin edges of unequal lengths, and closure of the primary defect almost always creates tissue redundancies along the outer edges of the surrounding skin. In most cases it is best to wait until the flap has been undermined and the primary defect closed before excising the standing cones, because tissue stretch and accommodation often leave them smaller than were expected preoperatively. Not infrequently, the redundant tissue may be distributed itself by the "rule of halves" and will not require excision at all.[12]

If excision is necessary, one common method is to remove the standing cones as Burow triangles. These triangular cones can be excised at the base of the flap to create a flared or "hockey stick–shaped" suture line. Alternatively, in advancement flaps, they may be placed at any point along the skin edge. The traditional Burow triangle is oriented with its base placed along the wound edge and apex pointing away from the flap, but the apex may be inverted if a zigzag suture line is desired (Fig. 4.5). This maneuver lengthens the overall suture line but may decrease the extent of contraction and in certain instances be more inconspicuous than a linear scar.[13]

Flap Modifications and Applications

H-PLASTY OR BILATERAL ADVANCEMENT FLAP

In the H-plasty or bilateral advancement flap, parallel incisions are created on opposite sides of the defect. The two limbs of the flap are then advanced centrally to form an H-shaped suture line (Fig. 4.6). This flap is most useful for

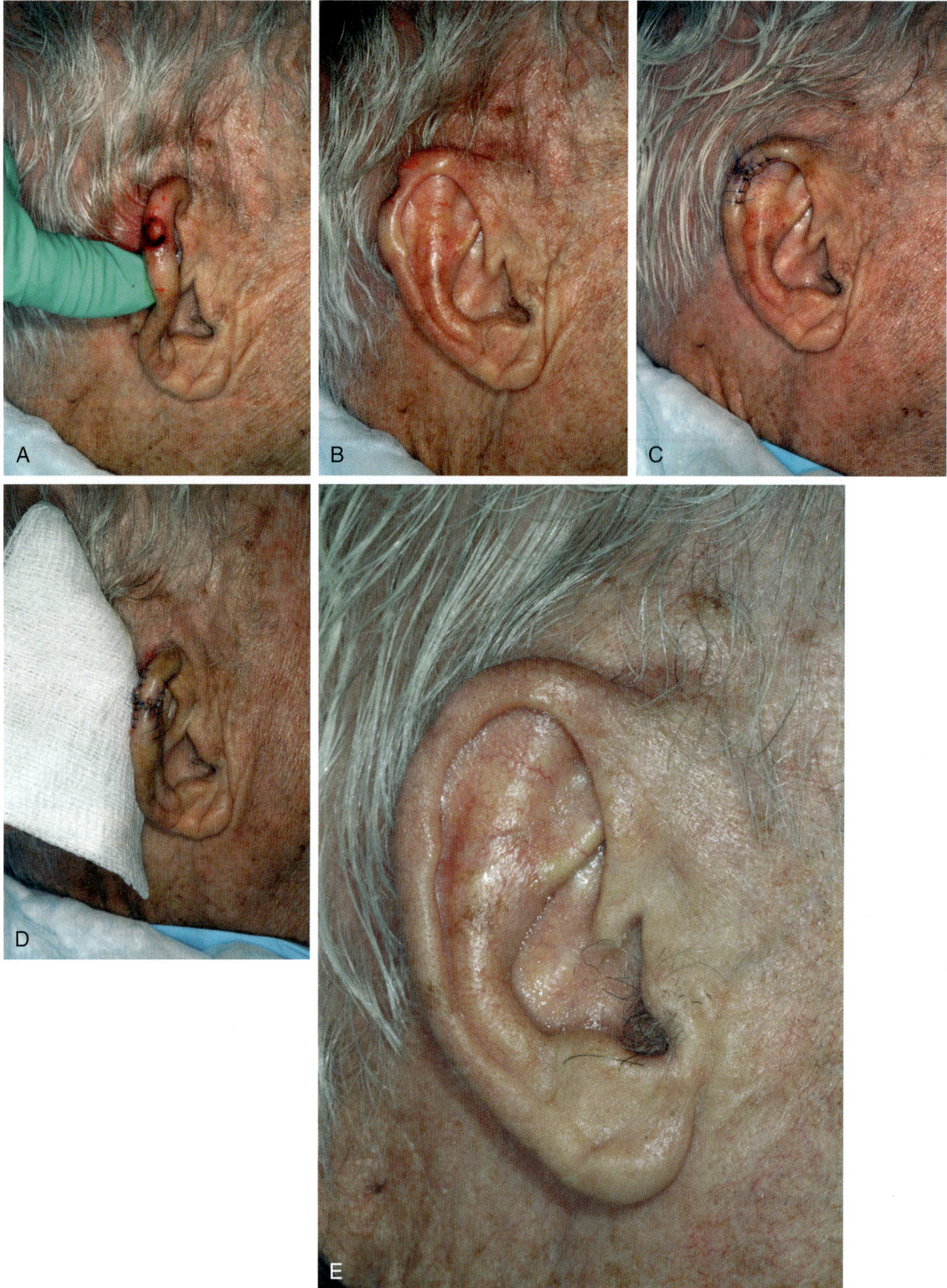

Fig. 4.6 H-plasty. (A) and (B) Surgical defect. (C) and (D) Immediate postoperative appearance. Tissue redundancy sewn out by the rule of halves. (E) Appearance 3 months after surgery.

locations with prominent horizontal lines, such as the forehead, eyebrow, or helical rim. The incision lines do not need to be exactly parallel and may be curved to conform to RSTLs (Fig. 4.7). The advantage of an H-plasty is that each flap must advance only half as far as the single flap design. It is used in situations in which a unilateral flap will not provide adequate tissue for tension-free wound closure.[14] A significant drawback to the H-plasty is the multiple linear incisions required for its execution (Fig. 4.8). Depending on the anatomic location, it may be prudent to incise and elevate one of the flaps on the least conspicuous side to see whether this achieves sufficient movement to close the

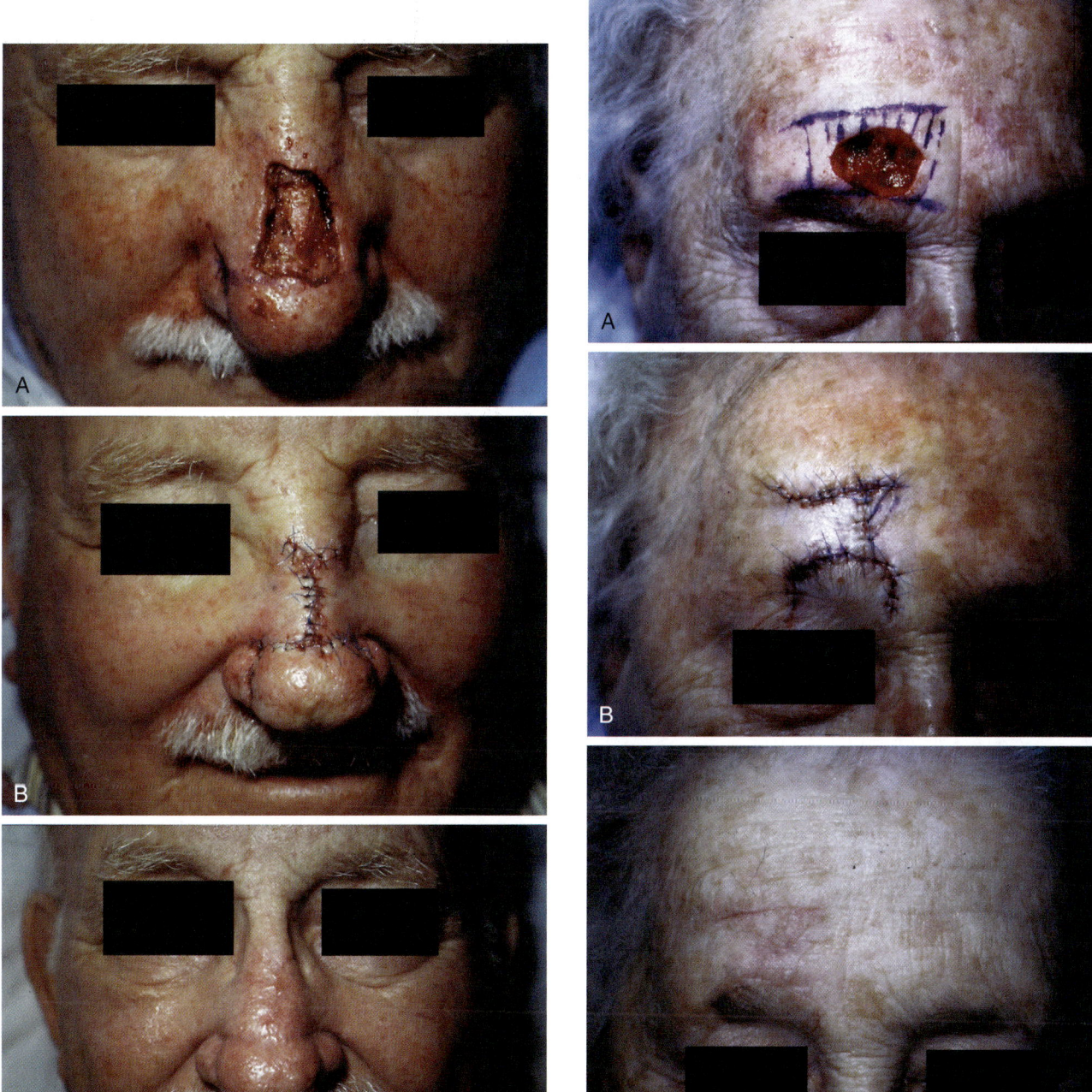

Fig. 4.7 H-plasty. (A) Surgical defect. (B) Immediate postoperative appearance. Not flap edges are angled to fall into relaxed skin tension line rather than being strictly geometric. (C) Appearance 8 weeks after surgery.

Fig. 4.8 H-plasty. (A) Surgical defect with relaxed skin tension line marked to aid in flap design. (B) Immediate postoperative appearance. Note variations in management of Burow triangles. On the inferior edge they are excised at 90 degrees to minimize transection of eyebrows. At the patient's upper right, the Burow triangle is excised at a 30-degree angle to be less angular and visible. It is sewn out by the rule of halves at the patient's upper left. (C) Appearance 8 weeks after surgery.

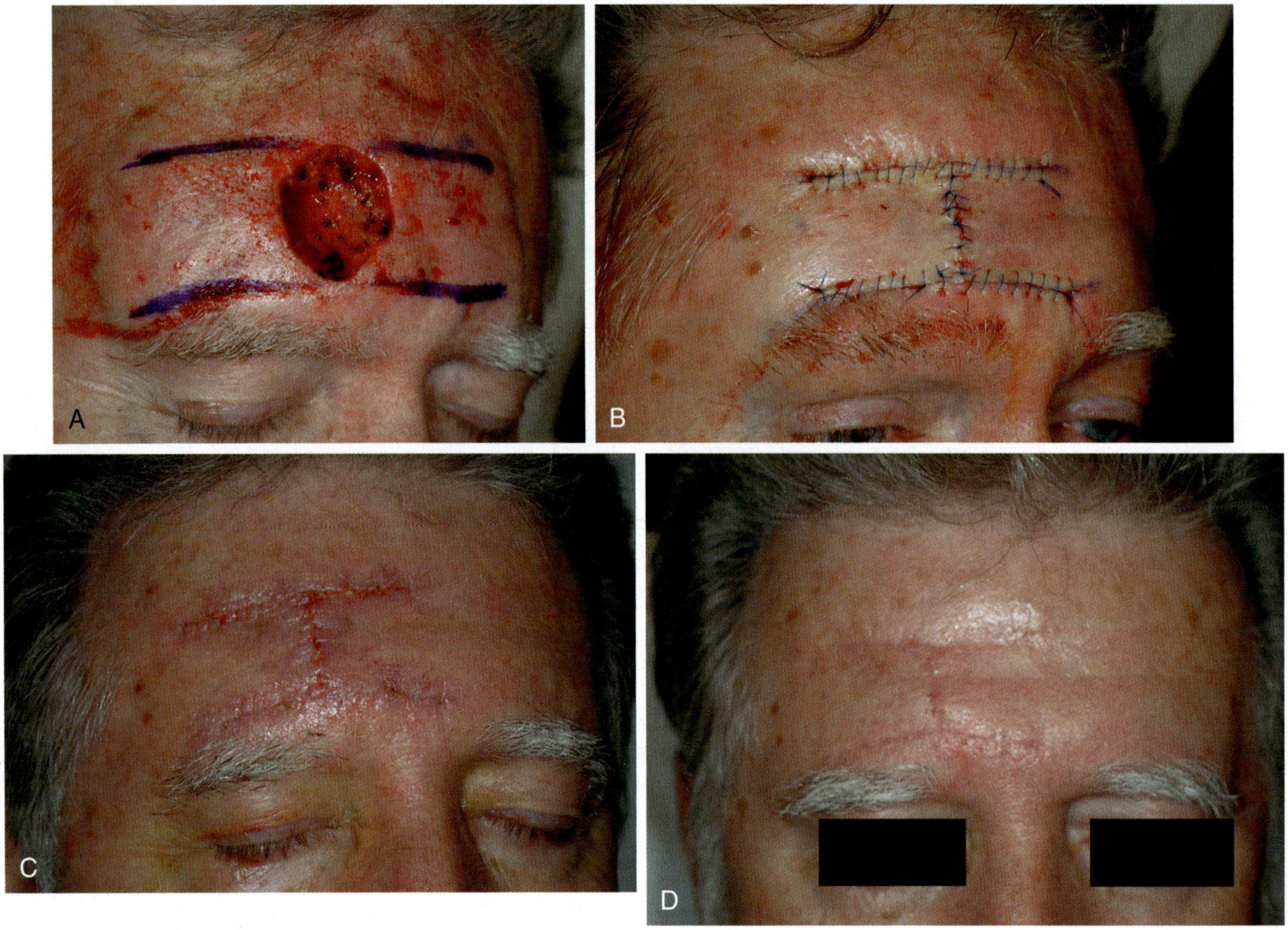

Fig. 4.9 H-plasty. (A) Surgical defect with relaxed skin tension line marked to aid in flap design. (B) Immediate postoperative appearance. Tissue redundancy sewn out by the rule of halves. (C) Appearance at 1 week suture removal. (D) Appearance at 8 weeks. Not visible contracture of vertical suture line. Horizontal lines may have contracted to the same degree but are not visible. This can be avoided by placing a Z-plasty in the advancing edge of the flap.

defect. If there is excessive tension despite wide undermining, the second flap can be incised. However, keep in mind that both of the flaps do not need to be the same size. After hemostasis has been achieved, the key suture is placed in the advancing edges of both flaps and closes the primary defect. Similar to the single advancement flap or U-plasty, tissue redundancies will occur along the edges of each flap that will need to be excised as Burow triangles or redistributed by the rule of halves. Another drawback to the H-plasty is scar contraction. This can be much more evident when adjacent to a free margin (Fig. 4.9). Placing a Z-plasty in the advancing edge of the flap can serve to widen it and offset this effect (Fig. 4.10).

T-PLASTY

The T-plasty is a bilateral advancement flap that is also known as an A to T (when the defect is triangular), V to T (an inverted A to T), and O to T (when the defect is oval). The T-plasty is simple in its design, with the vertical height of the flap approximately twice the height of the defect and the base incisions extending one defect diameter in each direction (Fig. 4.11).[15] The incision lines do not need to be exactly linear and may be adjusted to conform to RSTLs (Fig. 4.12). If desired, an M-plasty can be placed in the apex of the triangle to decrease the vertical length of closure.[16] Both flaps must be undermined widely to allow full mobility and tension-free closure.

After hemostasis has been achieved, the key suture closes the primary defect and creates tissue redundancy along the

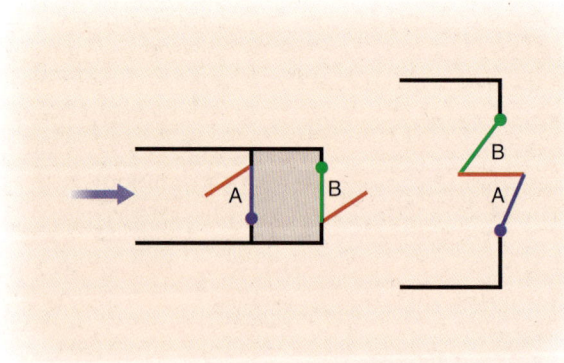

Fig. 4.10 Diagram of Z-plasty at flap's edge to widen the tip. (A) Advancing flap edge portion of Z-plasty. (B) Surrounding tissue edge portion of Z-plasty.

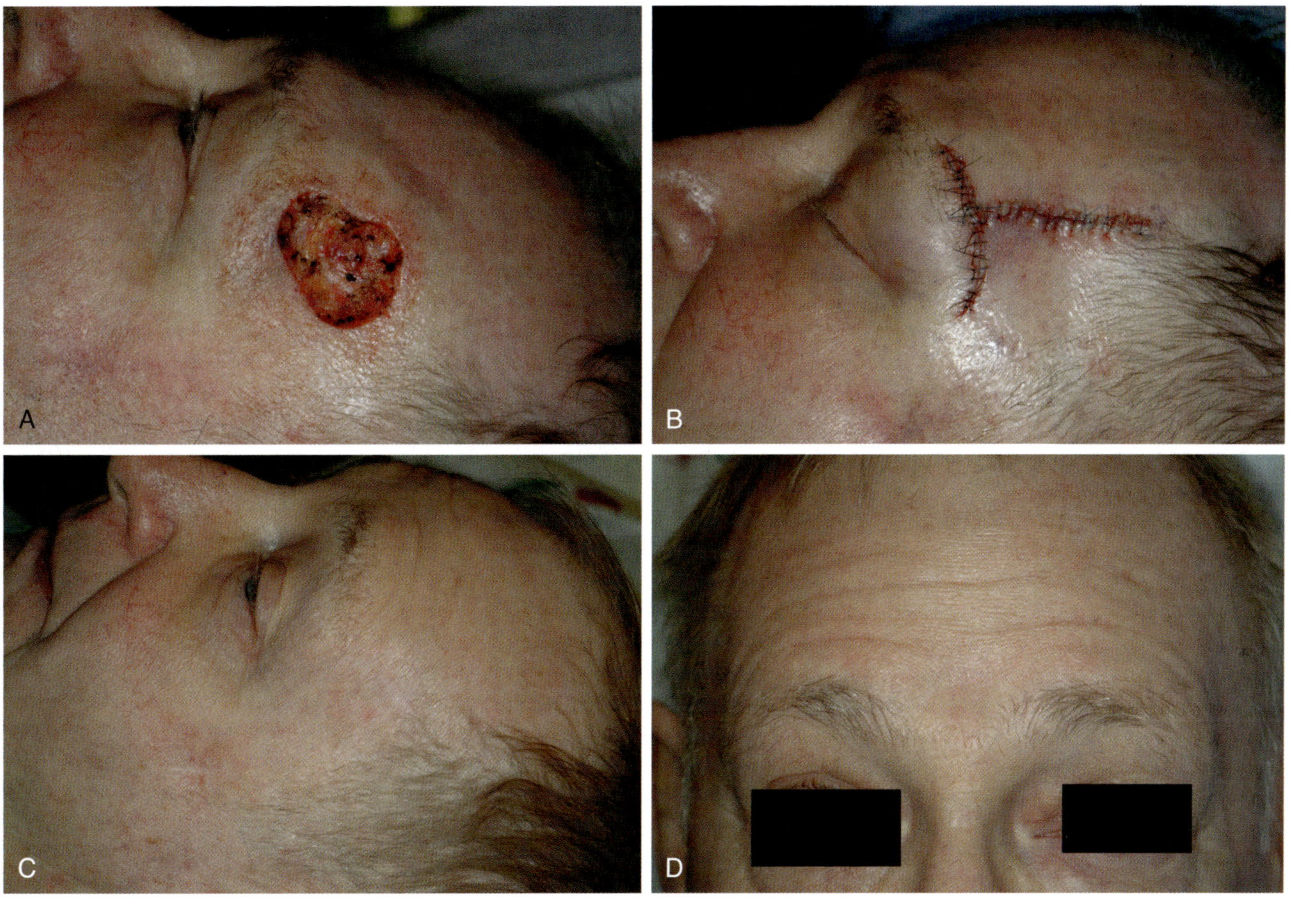

Fig. 4.11 T-plasty. (A) Flap designed by converting the circular defect to a triangle and placing the base along the ridge of the orbital frontal bone. (B) Immediate postoperative appearance. (C) Appearance 6 months after surgery. (D) Frontal view demonstrating symmetry and full function of temporal branch of facial nerve.

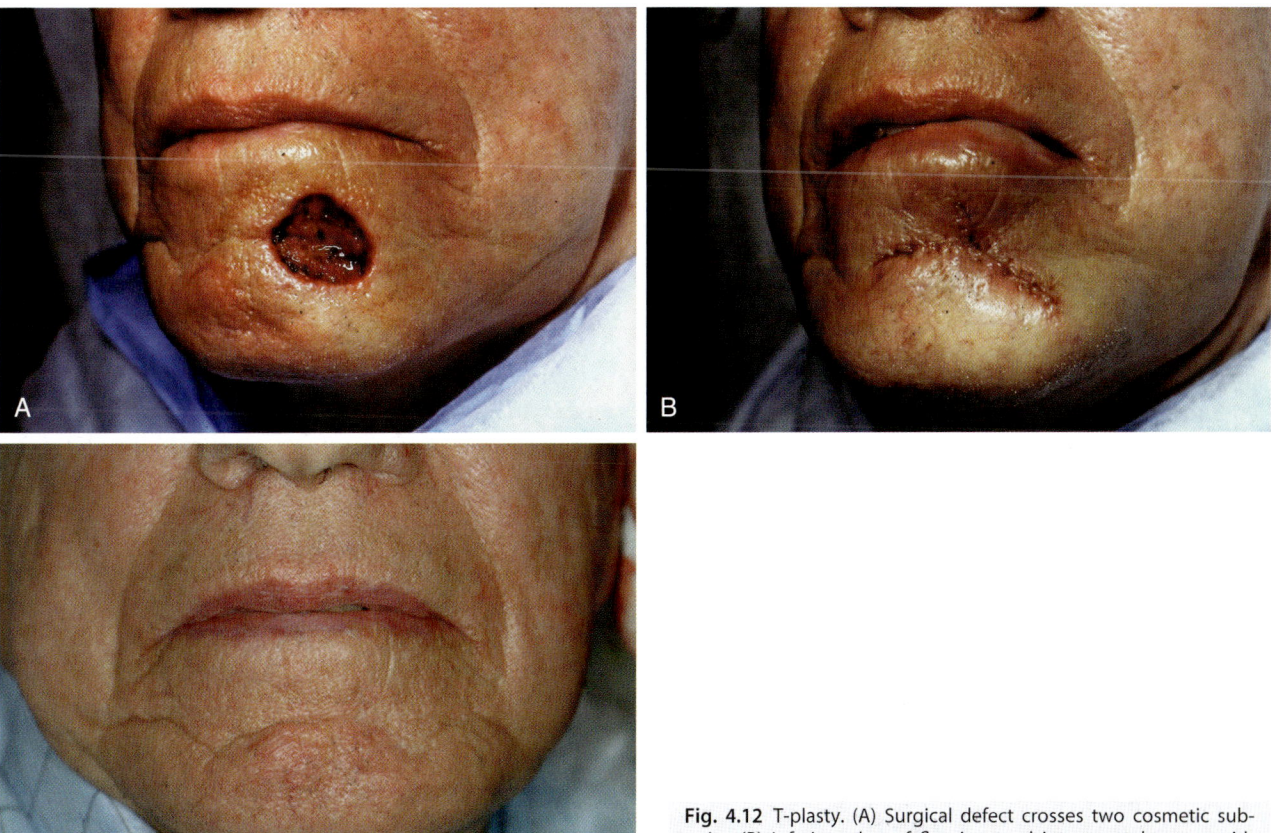

Fig. 4.12 T-plasty. (A) Surgical defect crosses two cosmetic subunits. (B) Inferior edge of flap is pexed into mental crease with periosteal suspension sutures. (C) Appearance at 6 months.

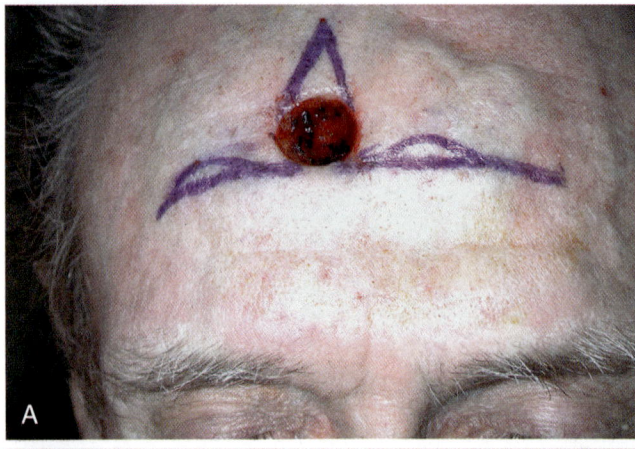
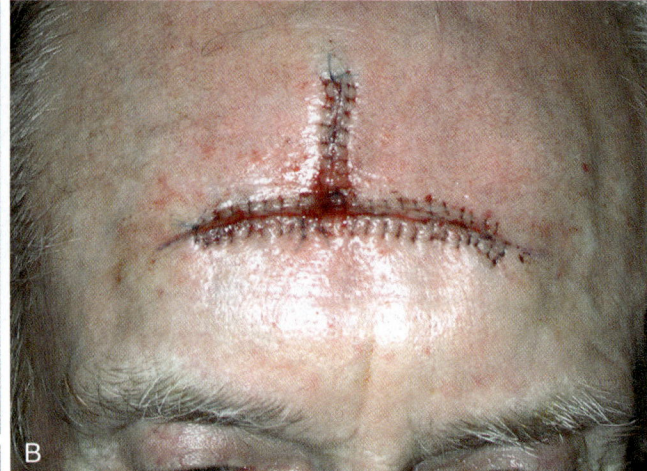
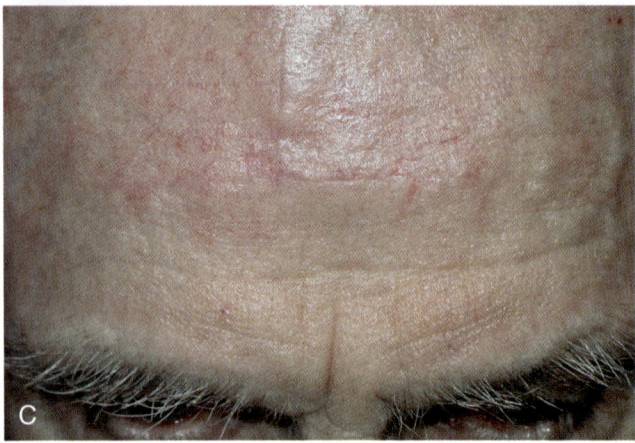

Fig. 4.13 T-plasty. (A) Flap demonstrates excision of tissue redundancy by the crescentic technique. (B) Immediate postoperative appearance. (C) Appearance 2 months after surgery.

base of the flap. These standing cones can be redistributed by the rule of halves, or excised. An alternative to the Burow triangle method is to excise the standing cones with curvilinear or crescentic incisions that redistribute the redundancy along the length of closure (Fig. 4.13).[17] This crescentic technique serves to lengthen the shorter advancing flap edge so that it more closely matches the length of the outer skin edge and thus mitigates the need for standing cone repair. It has the benefit of not creating additional incision lines and seems to be best suited when tissue is being moved over bony convexities. Because the vector of closure for the secondary defect changes with this maneuver and may become somewhat vertical, care must be taken not to elevate an adjacent free margin. This technique should not be used with an H- or a U-plasty because the crescents would be excised from both edges of a flap that was relatively a narrow flap to begin, thereby possibly increasing the risk for ischemia. The key advantages of the T-plasty are that the T portion of the flap can be placed along anatomic boundaries, which hides a large portion of the scar within a cosmetic junction line, and its broad pedicles provide a reliable vascular supply (Fig. 4.14).[18]

L-PLASTY

For defects with sufficient laxity, an O to L or L-plasty may be performed. This is an extremely useful flap in facial reconstruction and takes advantage of tissue laxity that is displaced to one side of the defect. The vertical limb is designed similarly to a T-plasty, and the advancing limb should extend to the tissue reservoir along RSTLs. Tissue redundancy is either redistributed by the rule of halves or lengthened with the crescentic technique (Figs. 4.15 and 4.16). If excision of a Burow triangle is necessary, the suture line is no longer L-shaped and it is best referred to as a Burow triangle flap (see next section).

BUROW TRIANGLE FLAP

In 1855 the German surgeon Karl August von Burow described a method for excision of the standing cones created by flap closure that bears his name, the Burow triangle. An advancement flap based on the excision of this redundant tissue is also named in his honor, the Burow triangle flap or Burow wedge flap. This flap moves in a single direction and is most effective for defects in which tissue laxity is limited to one side of the defect (Fig. 4.17). It is also useful for repair of defects in close proximity for which advancement of the flap closes both defects with one movement (Fig. 4.18).[19]

For a single defect, a linear incision is extended from the defect along a cosmetic junction or RSTL. This incision is usually two to three times as long as the width of the surgical defect but will vary with anatomic location and laxity. The incision may be extended to take advantage of a tissue reservoir or to allow better camouflage of the Burow

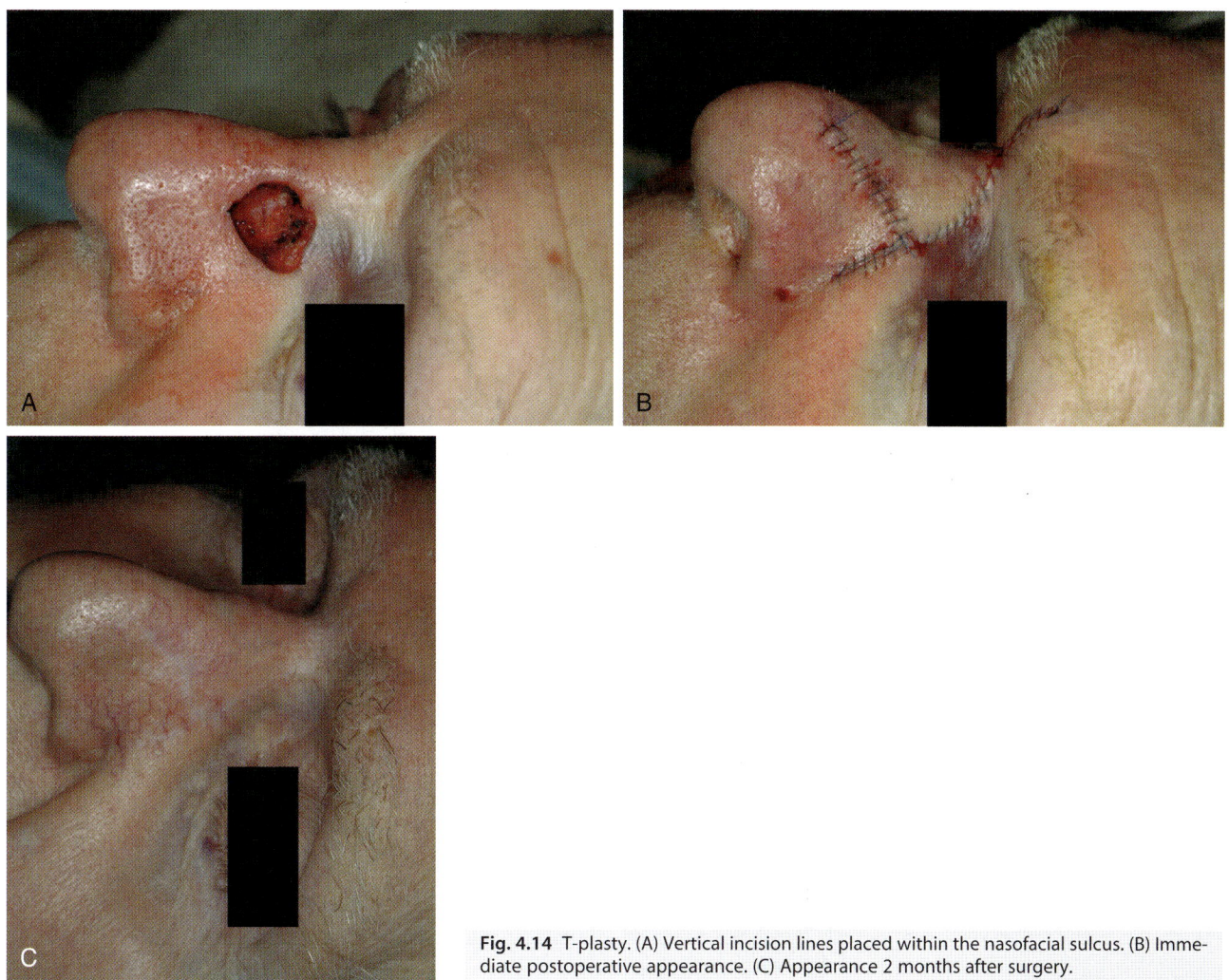

Fig. 4.14 T-plasty. (A) Vertical incision lines placed within the nasofacial sulcus. (B) Immediate postoperative appearance. (C) Appearance 2 months after surgery.

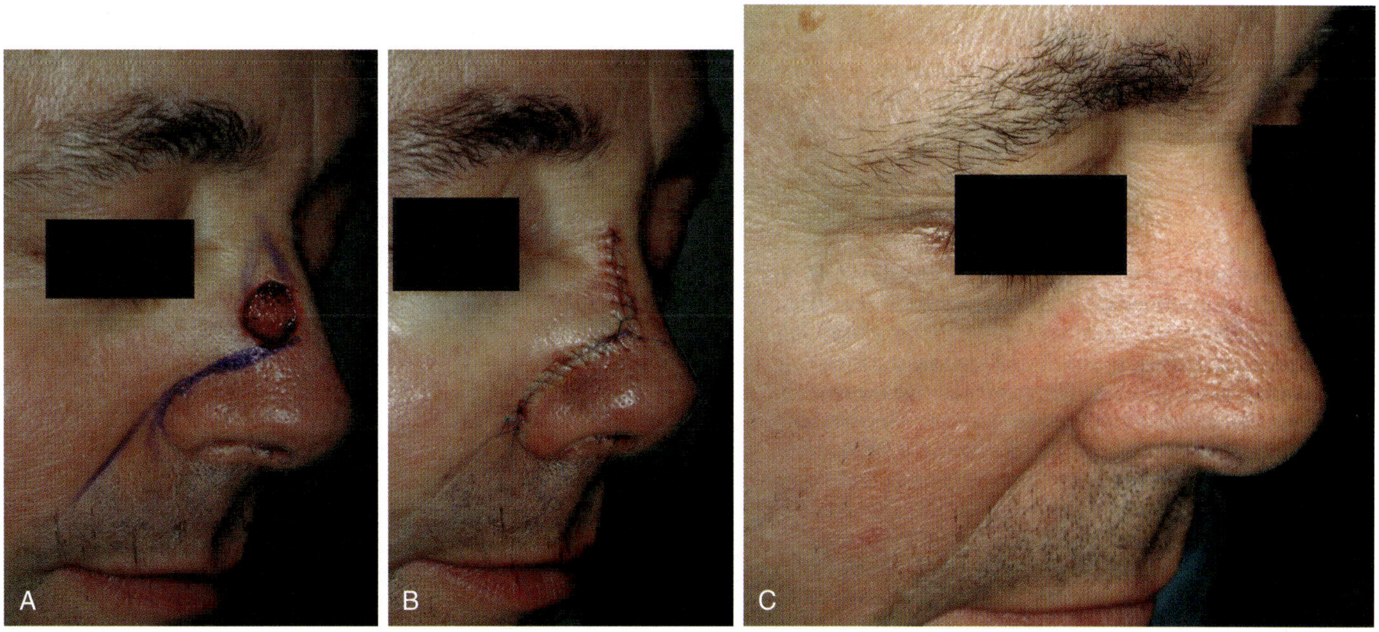

Fig. 4.15 L-plasty. (A) Flap designed with suture lines placed within the alar crease and nasal dorsum. (B) Immediate postoperative appearance. (C) Appearance 1 year after surgery.

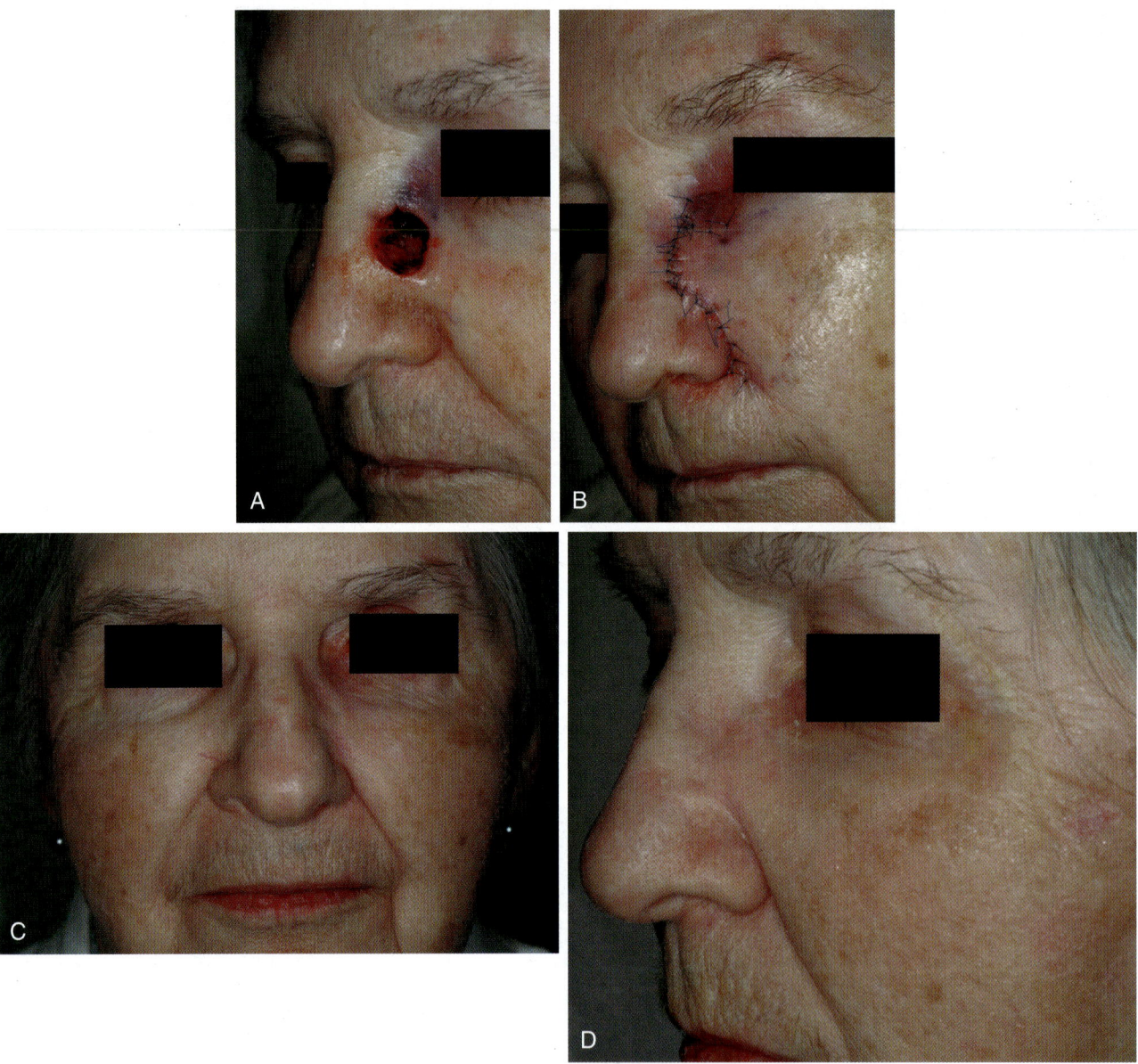

Fig. 4.16 L-plasty. (A) Flap designed with suture lines placed within the alar crease and nasal dorsum. (B) Immediate postoperative appearance. Note M-plasty placed at superior pole of suture line to shorten overall length and extension toward medial canthus. (C) and (D) Appearance 6 months after surgery.

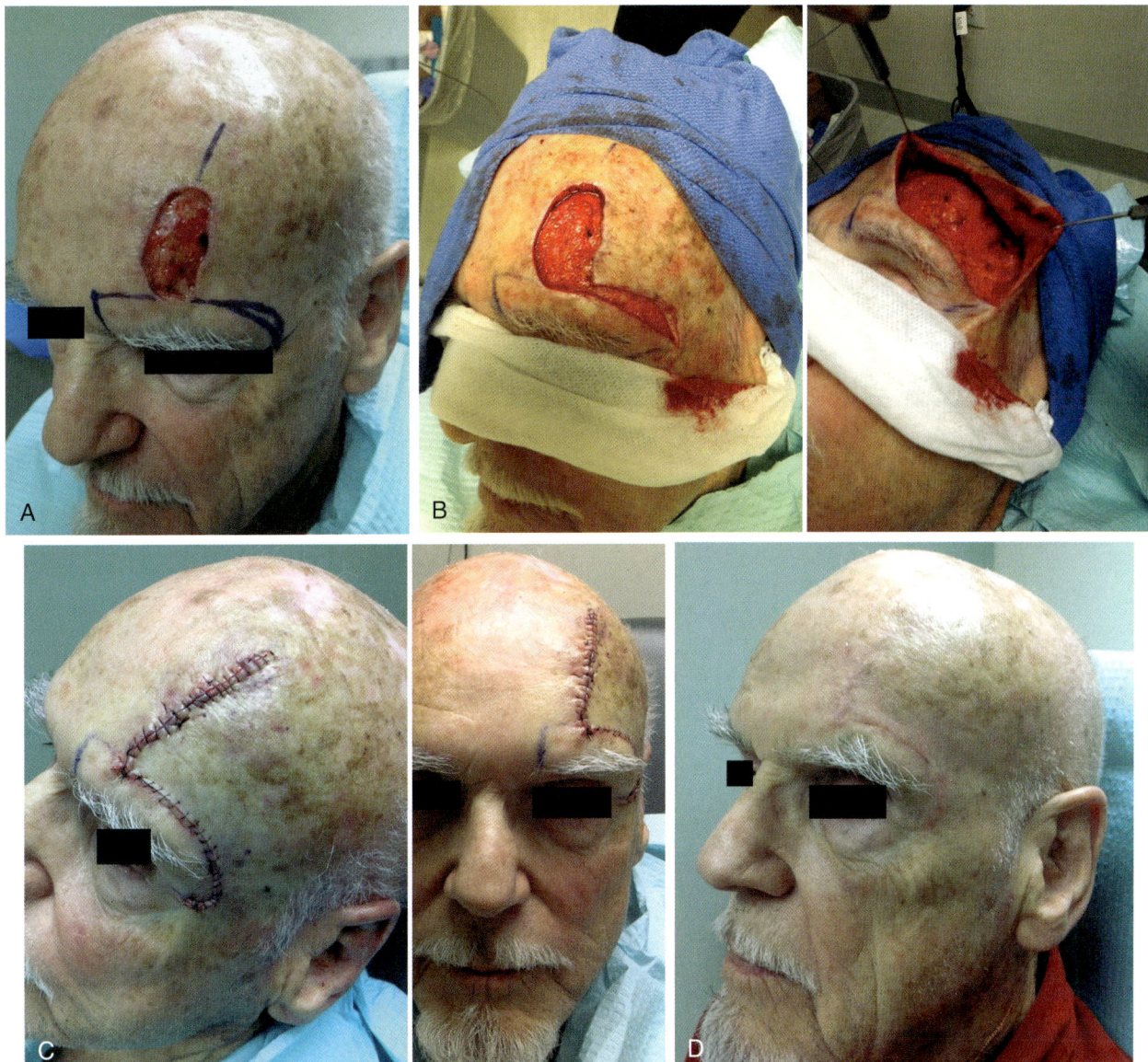

Fig. 4.17 Burow triangle flap. (A) Preoperative planning anticipates the possible need to convert this flap into a T-plasty. (B) A single slap is incised, elevated, and widely undermined. This allows for a tension-free closure eliminates the need for extending the flap bilaterally. (C) Immediate postoperative appearance (D) Appearance 2 months after surgery.

triangle. Classically the Burow triangle is excised at the base of the flap but may be excised at any point that provides for maximal cosmesis (Figs. 4.19 to 4.21). For two defects in close proximity, the incision is placed along the bridge of tissue, connecting them in such a way that the Burow triangles are displaced over both defects (see Fig. 4.18). This conserves tissue and closes both defects with one single motion.

CHEEK ADVANCEMENT

The cheek advancement flap is a widely based unilateral flap used to close medium- to large-sized defects of the medial cheek, nasofacial sulcus, and lateral nose. The primary movement is from lateral to medial. The inferior incision is frequently hidden within the melolabial fold or along RSTLs that run parallel to it. Depending on the location of the defect, the superior incision can be hidden along the nasofacial crease (see Fig. 4.16) or within the junction of the lower eyelid and cheek (Fig. 4.22). One drawback to using an infraorbital incision is the potential for edema due to disruption of lymphatics, which usually lasts weeks to months and in some cases may be permanent.

In this flap, similar to other advancement flaps, the key suture closes the primary defect and creates standing cones that must be redistributed or excised. Suspension or tacking sutures that extend from the dermal portion of the flap to the periosteum of the underlying bone are used to decrease any downward pull on the eyelid or blunting of the nasofacial sulcus.[20] Suspension sutures have the potential to

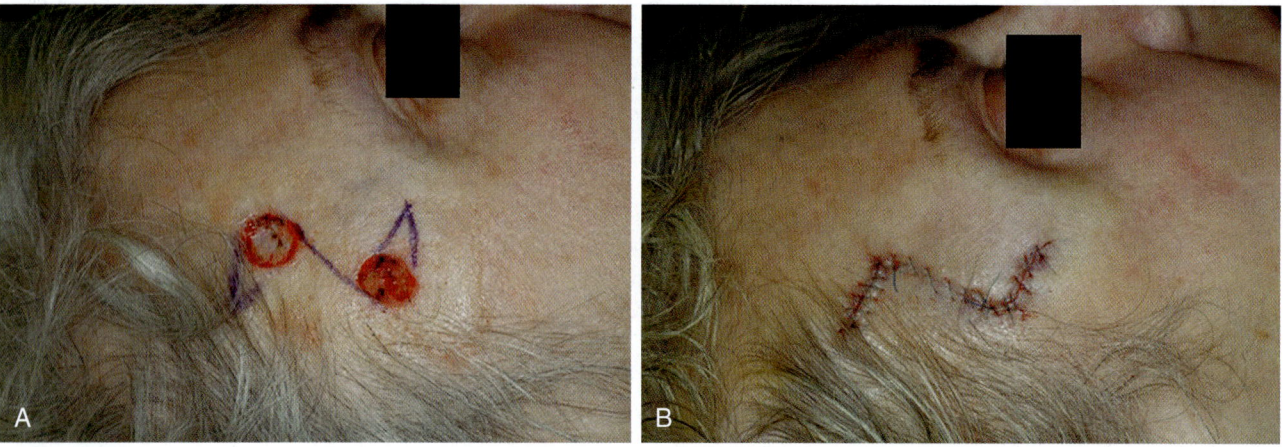

Fig. 4.18 Burow triangle flap. (A) Two defects in close proximity closed with a single flap. (B) Immediate postoperative appearance.

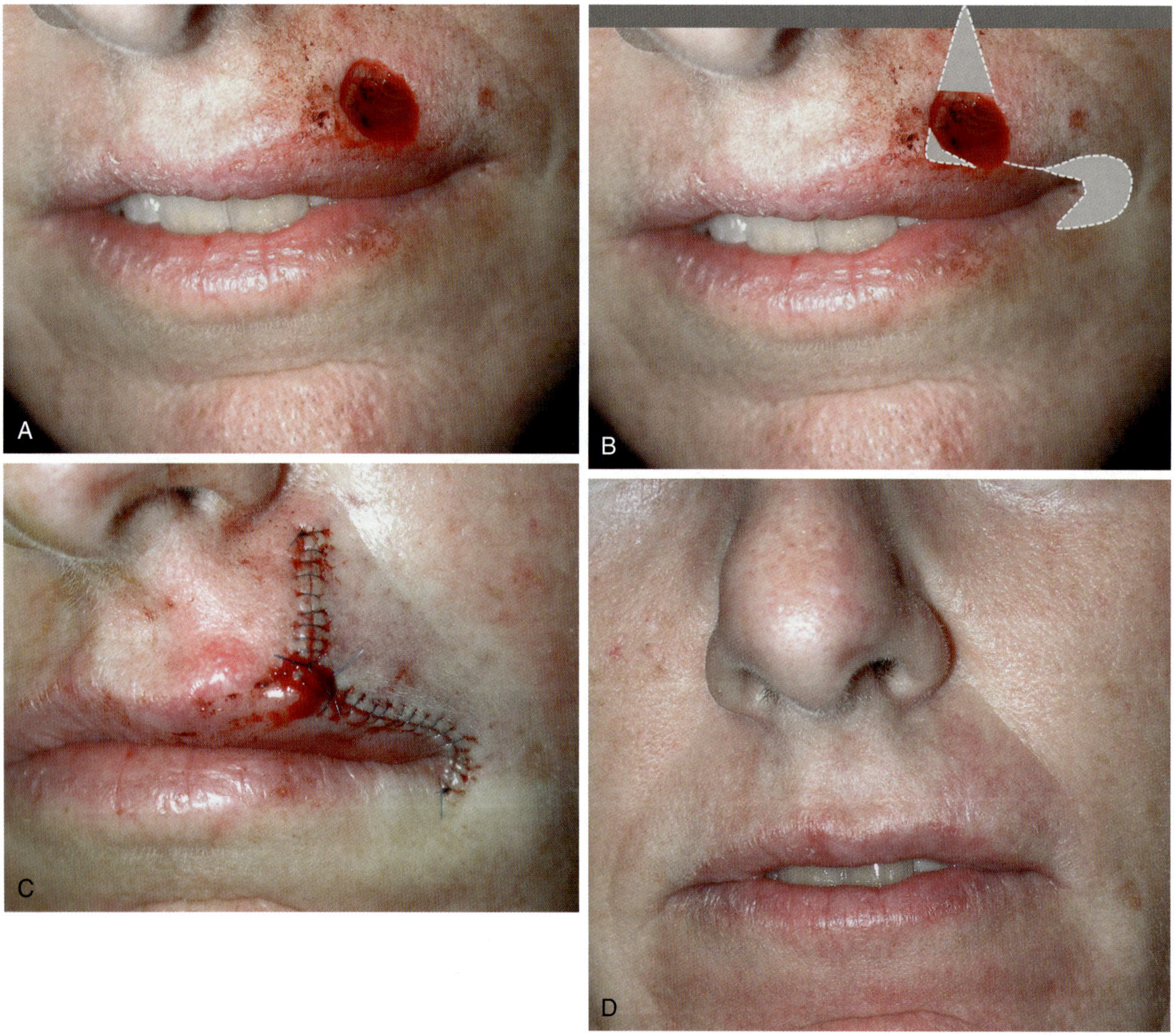

Fig. 4.19 Burow triangle flap. (A) Immediate postoperative appearance. (B) Flap design with anticipated sacrifice of tissue to allow flap to fall into relaxed skin tension lines. Burow triangle will be excised at oral commissure. (C) Immediate postoperative appearance. (D) Appearance 3 months after surgery.

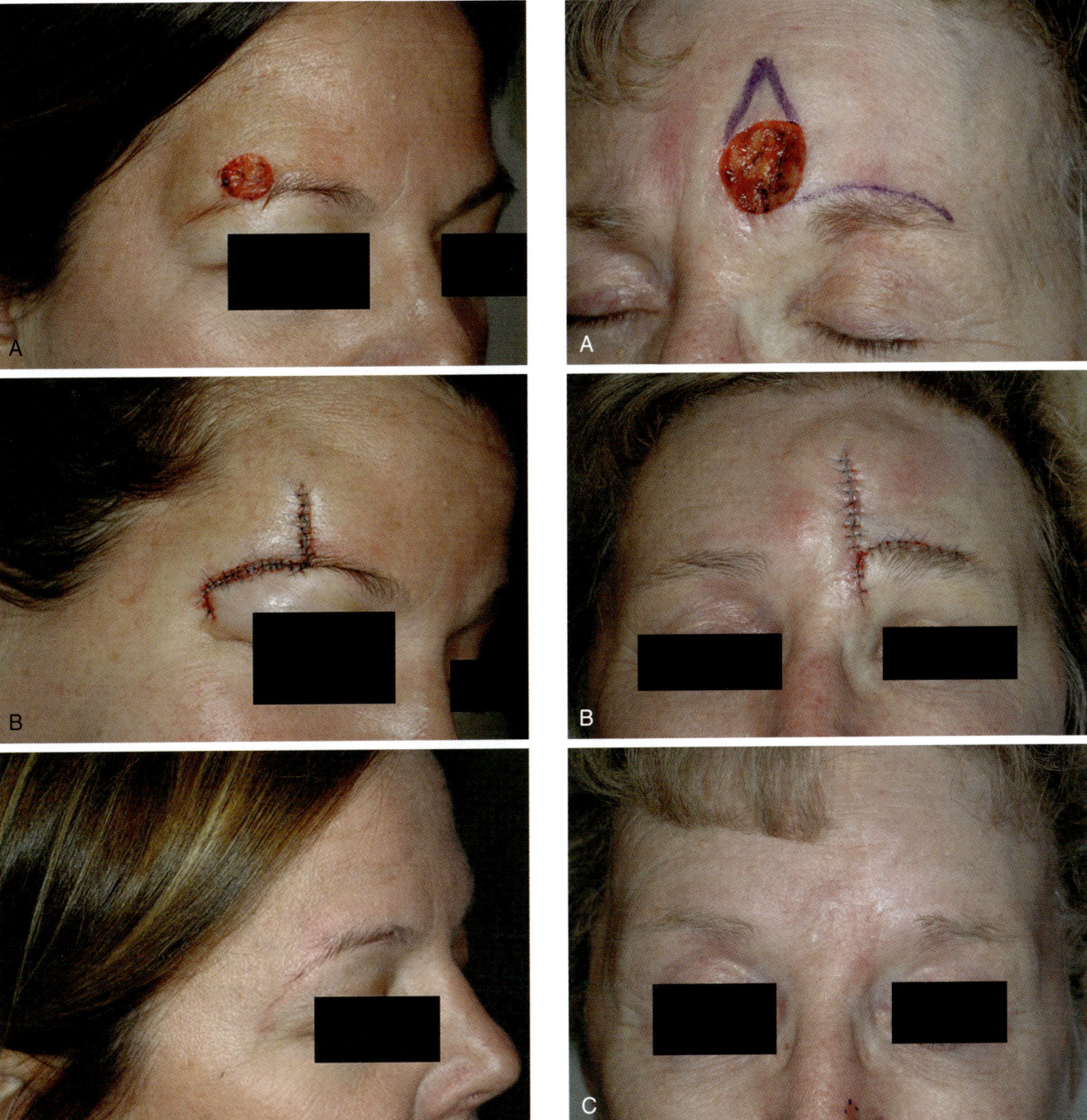

Fig. 4.20 Burow triangle flap. (A) Immediate postoperative appearance. (B) Suture lines placed in relaxed skin tension lines and cosmetic subunit junction lines for maximum cosmesis. (C) Appearance 3 months after surgery.

Fig. 4.21 Burow triangle flap. (A) Immediate postoperative appearance. (B) Burow triangle excised at the proximal edge of the flap into the glabella. (C) Appearance 4 months after surgery.

impinge on blood flow and should be placed parallel to the blood vessels supplying the flap and not used if there is concern for ischemia. An alternative approach for reconstruction across a concavity is to advance the flap just up to the sulcus and suture it in place. The perpendicular surface is either allowed to heal by second intention or repaired with a full-thickness skin graft harvested from a Burow triangle.

HELICAL RIM ADVANCEMENT FLAP

The helical rim advancement flap can be an extremely useful method for repairing defects on the helix. As with other advancement flaps, sufficient tissue laxity must be present and the length-to-width ratio should not exceed 3:1 or 4:1. In the classic version, a full-thickness incision is placed through the cartilage and auricular skin and extended inferiorly from the defect along the scaphoid fossa

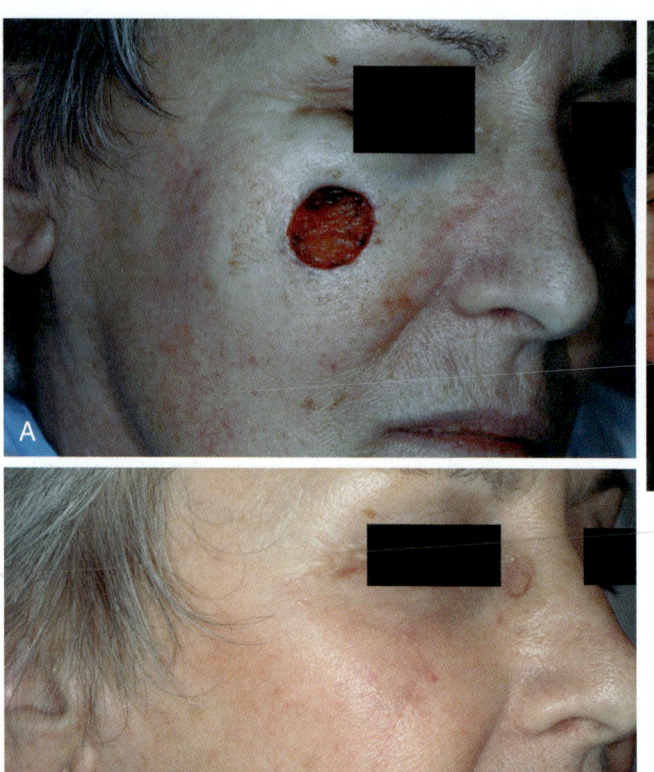
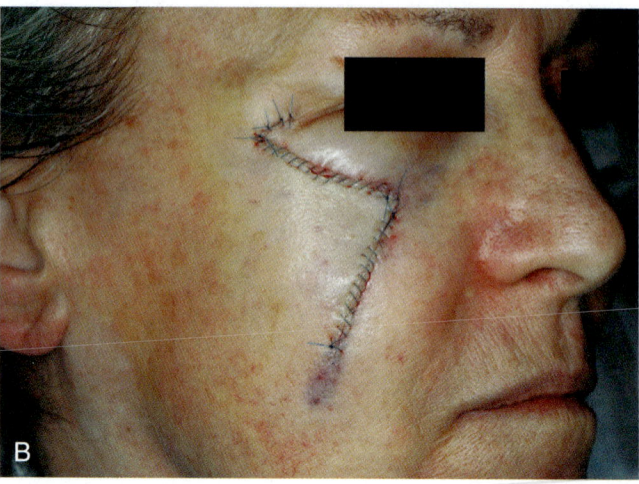

Fig. 4.22 Cheek advancement flap. (A) Horizontal incision placed along the orbital cheek junction. Primary movement is horizontal and limits any downward pull on the eyelid. (B) Immediate postoperative appearance. (C) Appearance 2 months after surgery.

to the lobule, which provides the tissue reservoir. For defects of the mid to superior helix, this creates a long, narrow pedicle that is at risk for ischemia.

In 1967 Antia and Buch described a modified chondrocutaneous advancement flap in which the incision, instead of being through and through, is limited to the anterior auricular skin and cartilage.[21] The postauricular skin is left intact and dissected above the perichondrium to the postauricular sulcus. This modification allows for the same mobility as the classical version but with a more reliable blood supply (Fig. 4.23). In both flaps, after wide undermining is performed and hemostasis is achieved, the flap is advanced along the curvature of the helical rim to close the defect. If there is too much tension or the movement produces cupping of the ear, a Burow triangle can be placed in the lobule to lengthen the flap. Alternatively the rotational arc can be shortened by shaving the scaphal cartilage (Fig. 4.24).[22] For additional movement, a second flap can be incised superior to the helical crus, which is then detached and repositioned posteriorly toward the defect in a V-to-Y fashion or a full-thickness wedge can be excised.

A significant disadvantage to both versions of the helical rim advancement flap is that they may cause ear asymmetry by shortening the overall height of the ear and/ or by cupping.[22] This is particularly true for large defects, and if marked asymmetry is anticipated, another form of reconstruction should be considered. For unexpected asymmetry, the contralateral ear can be shortened with a wedge excision for a better match. A second concern is that any inversion of the suture line results in a highly visible notch along the curve of the helical rim. There are several methods for limiting this risk, which include careful wound edge eversion with vertical mattress sutures, modification of the flap tips with Z-plasties, and full-thickness interlocking step-cuts.[23,24]

CRESCENTIC ADVANCEMENT FLAP

Webster Perialar Crescentic Flap

Webster published his experience with the crescentic perialar cheek advancement flap for upper lip repair in 1955.[25] He described a method for lengthening the flap's superior skin edge by excising a crescentic-shaped piece of tissue from the perialar cheek. This maneuver removes intervening redundant skin and facilitates the flap's advancement into the upper lip defect (Fig. 4.25; see also Fig. 4.4). The superior standing cone is displaced laterally to the perialar sulcus instead of into the nostril.

Modifications of the Crescentic Advancement Flap

The perialar sulcus is an ideal location to hide an incision line and many variations from Webster's classic design are possible. For example, defects up to a centimeter in diameter

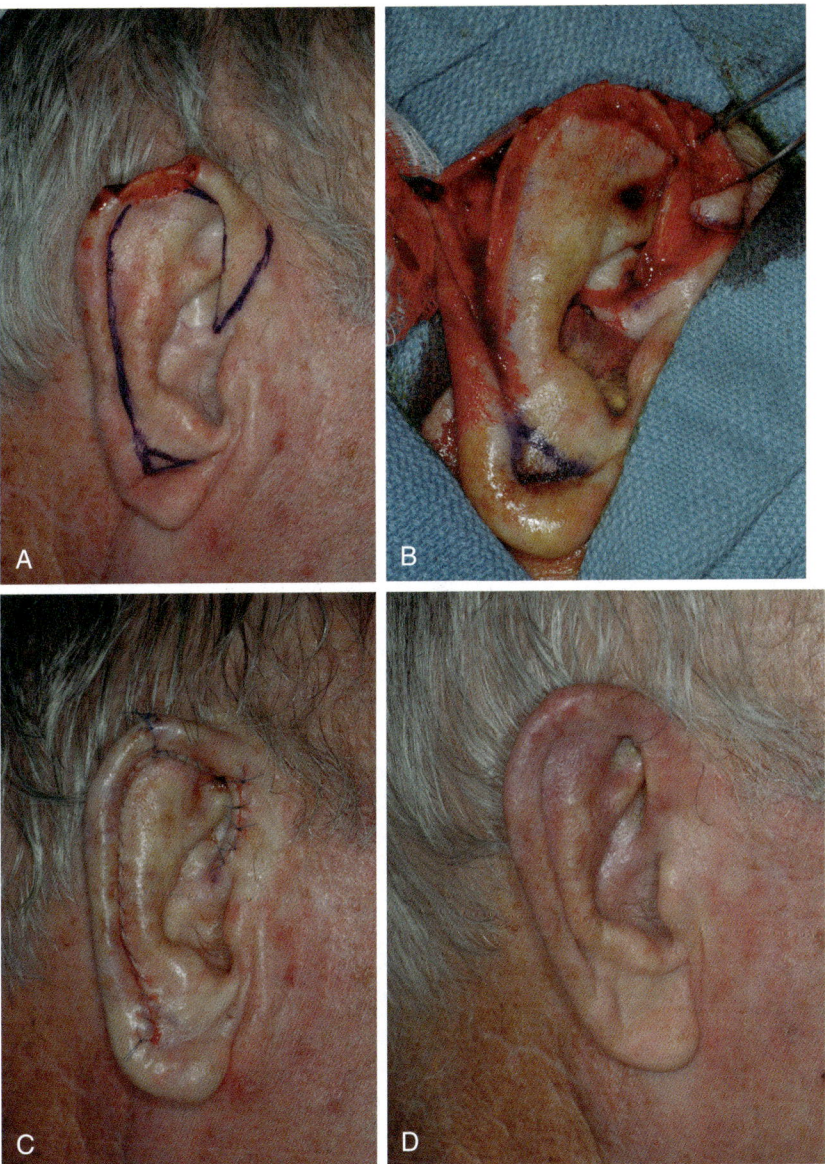

Fig. 4.23 Helical rim advancement flap. (A) Flap design. (B) Flap dissected widely to the postauricular sulcus. No need to extend incision into lobule, which can shorten the vertical height of the ear. (C) Flap sutured into place for a tension-free closure. (D) Appearance 3 months after surgery. Mild blunting of the helical roll, which could have been avoided by keeping the suture line within the scaphoid fossa.

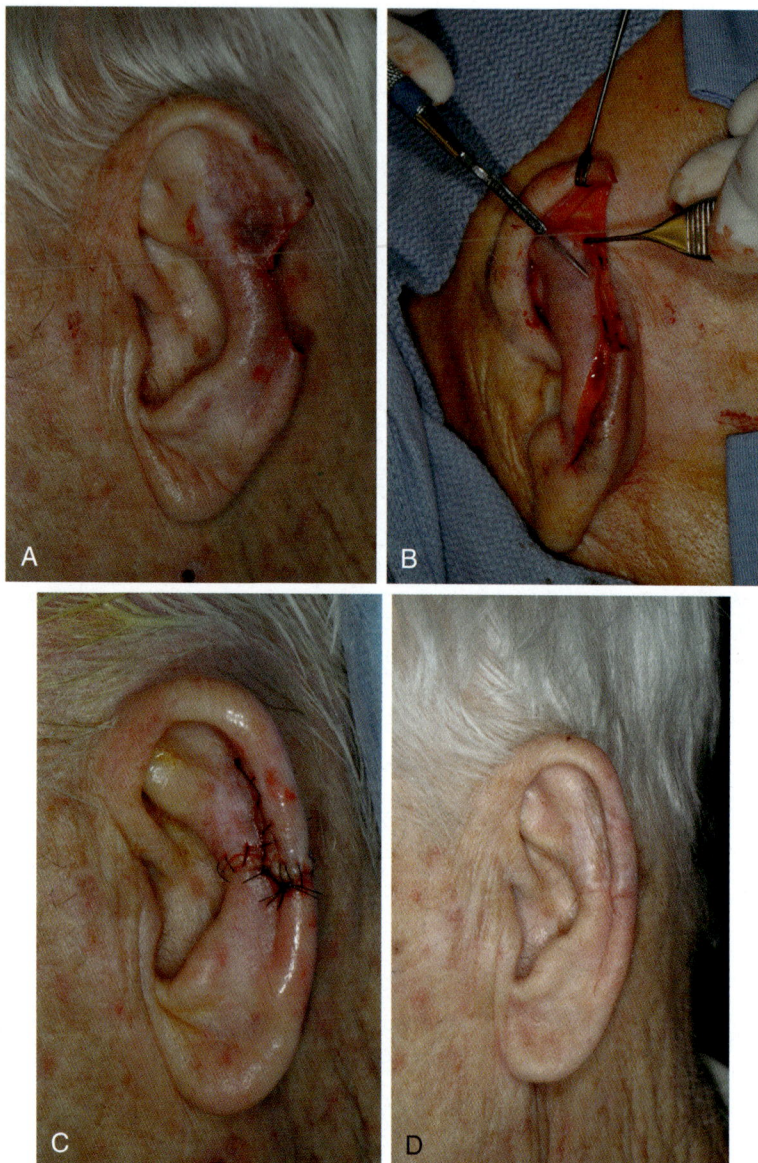

Fig. 4.24 Combination wedge and helical rim advancement flap. (A) Preoperative appearance. (B) Flap elevated but still restricted. Excision of scaphoid cartilage decreases the arc of rotation necessary to suture the flap into place and decreases cupping of the ear. (C) Completed repair. (D) Appearance 2 months after surgery.

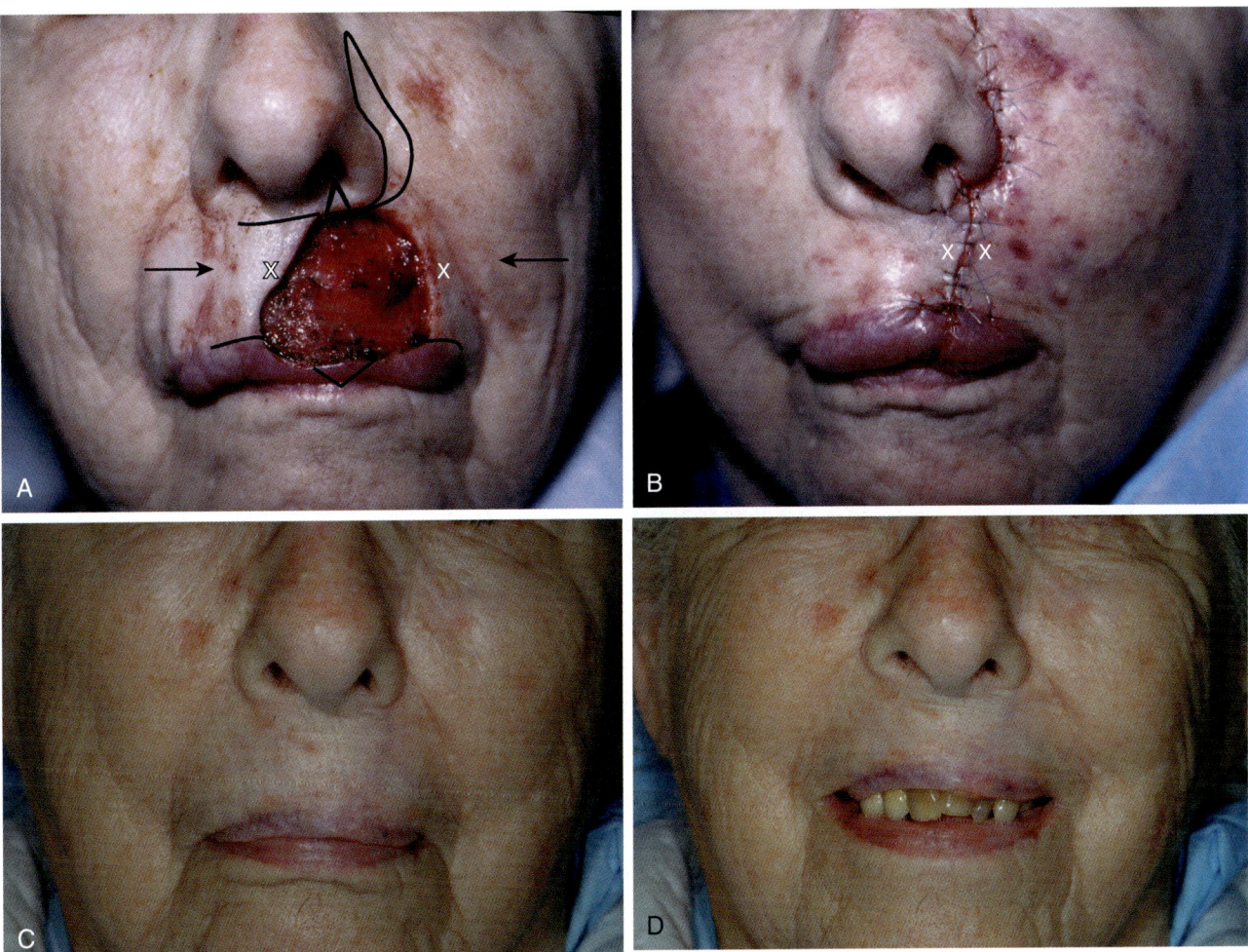

Fig. 4.25 (A) Perialar crescentic flap for large surgical defect after excision of deeply infiltrative basal cell carcinoma. Defect extends through orbicularis oris muscle with intact mucosa. Flap design and complex repair requiring reapproximation of the orbicularis oris muscle to maintain oral function and patency. (B) Immediate postoperative appearance. (C) and (D) Appearance 1 year after surgery.

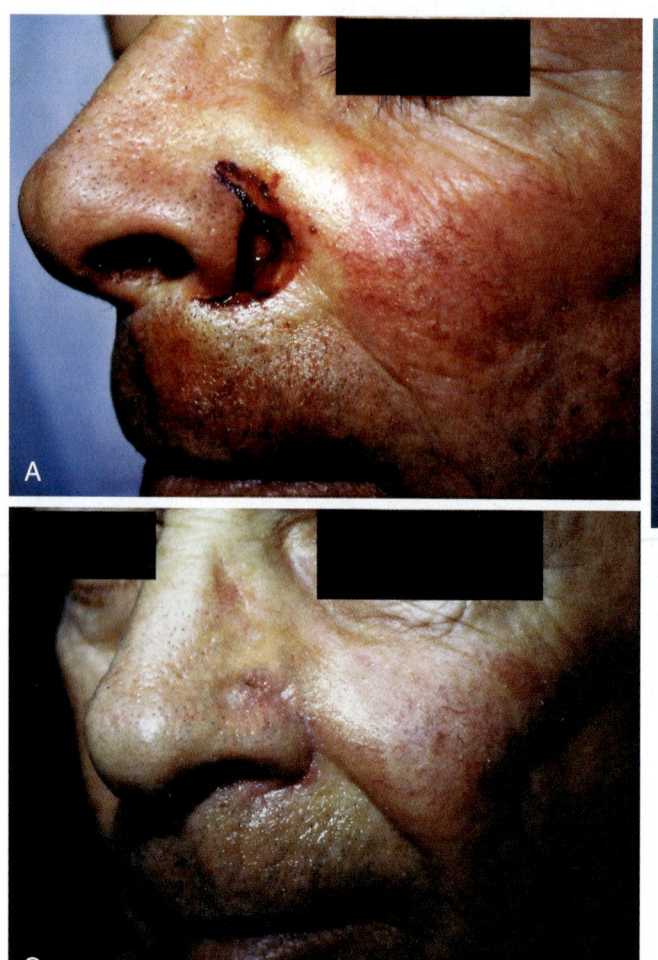
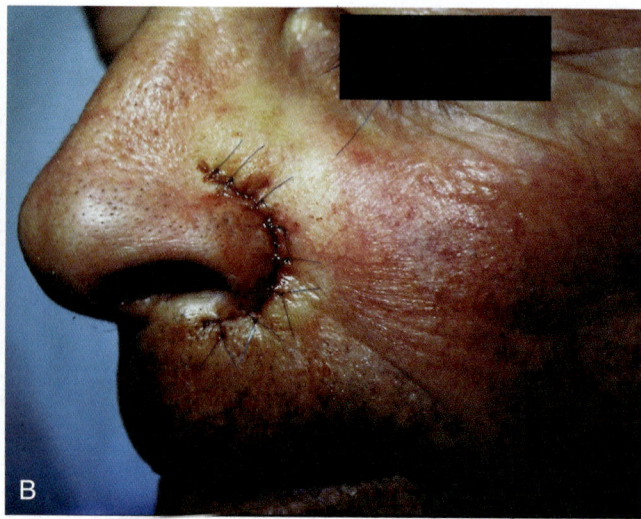

Fig. 4.26 (A) Modification of the crescentic advancement flap with incisions placed within the alar sulcus. (B) Immediate postoperative appearance. (C) Appearance 2 months after surgery, full-face view.

on the perialar lip and cheek can be advanced into the sulcus, where the standing cones are excised as a continuation of the crescent and the suture line is hidden entirely within this natural curve (Fig. 4.26).

PENG FLAP

For repair of central nasal tip defects, Peng et al. suggested a "pinch" modification to the Rintala flap that shortens the vertical incision lines and widens the pedicle.[26] The geometry of placing a Rintala flap into a circular defect necessitates that healthy tissue must be sacrificed, by either trimming the flap tips or squaring the defect. In the Peng modification, instead of vertical incisions, the flap limbs are extended laterally from the middle of the wound along the alar groove and then superiorly in a linear fashion along the nasofacial sulcus. The flap is advanced inferiorly, and the tips are rotated medially to form a rounded and slightly convex tip. This maneuver shortens the overall flap length to 1.5 to 1.8 times the vertical height of the defect and does not affect flap survival. However, it does elevate the ala slightly. Rowe et al. suggested starting the incision for the rotating arms of the flap as far distal as possible and not mid-defect as described by Peng et al. (Fig. 4.27).[27] This modification decreases the amount of vertical advancement involved in the flap and increases the amount of rotation into the defect. This will serve to shorten the length of the lateral vertical incisions and help facilitate closure, given there is some laxity lateral to the defect. Careful attention must be paid to the position of the nasal ala during this closure. Any significant distortion may be cosmetically unacceptable.

Disadvantages

The two major drawbacks of an advancement flap are that in most circumstances it does not recruit tissue for closure and, unless diligently designed and executed, has a propensity to distort free margins. It is not the repair of choice for large defects without surrounding laxity or nearby tissue reservoirs. Another disadvantage is that most advancement flaps are designed with straight lines and thus, if not appropriately placed, may be highly visible.

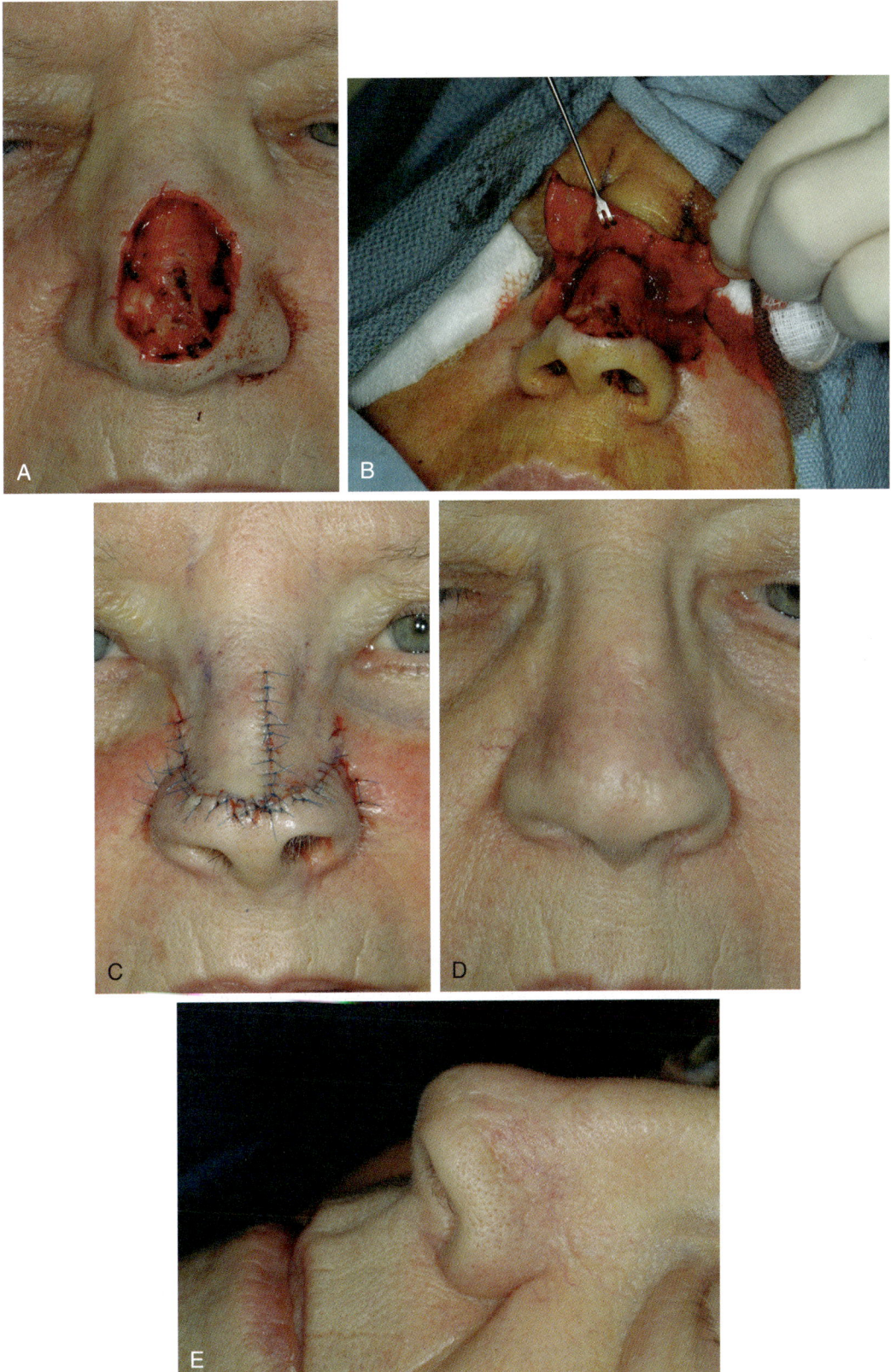

Fig. 4.27 Peng or "pinch" modification of the linear advancement flap. (A) Surgical defect with denuded and partially resected cartilage. (B) Elevation of the flap in the submuscular plane. (C) Burow triangles excised along alar cheek sulcus. Moderate tip elevation is expected and usually temporary. (D) and (E) Appearance 6 months after surgery. Note resolution of tip elevation and good side contour.

References

1. Spencer WG. *Celsus on Medicine: Books VII–VIII Volume VII*. Cambridge: Harvard University Press; 1994.
2. Larrabee WF Jr. A finite element model of skin deformation. I. Biomechanics of skin and soft tissue: a review. *Laryngoscope*. 1986;96:399-405.
3. Dzubow LM. The dynamics of flap movement: effect of pivotal restraint on flap rotation and transposition. *J Dermatol Surg Oncol*. 1987;13:1348-1353.
4. Memarzadeh K, Sheikh R, Blohme J, Torbrand C, Malmsjo M. Perfusion and oxygenation of random advancement skin flaps depend more on the leng than thickness of the flap than on the width to length ratio. *Eplasty*. 2016;16:e12.
5. Larrabee WF Jr, Holloway GA Jr, Sutton D. Wound tension and blood flow in skin flaps. *Ann Otol Rhinol Laryngol*. 1984;93:112-115.
6. Burget GC, Menick FJ. Aesthetic restoration of one-half of the upper lip. *Plast Reconstr Surg*. 1986;78:583-593.
7. Dzubow LM. Chemosurgical report: indications for a geometric approach to wound closure following Mohs surgery. *J Dermatol Surg Oncol*. 1987;13:480-486.
8. Brodland DG. Advancement flaps. In: Roenigk RK, Roenigk HK, eds. *Roenigk & Roenigk's Dermatologic Surgery: Principles and Practice*. New York: Marcel Dekker; 1996:825-834.
9. Kaufman AJ, Kiene KL, Moy RL. Role of tissue undermining in the trapdoor effect of transposition flaps. *J Dermatol Surg Oncol*. 1993;19:128-132.
10. Boyer JD, Zitelli JA, Brodland DG. Undermining in cutaneous surgery. *Dermatol Surg*. 2001;27:75-78.
11. Larrabee WF Jr, Sutton D. The biomechanics of advancement and rotation flaps. *Laryngoscope*. 1981;91:726-734.
12. Weisberg NK, Nehal KS, Zide BM. Dog-ears: a review. *Dermatol Surg*. 2000;26:363-370.
13. Suzuki S, Matsuda K, Nishimura Y. Proposal for a new comprehensive classification of V-Y plasty and its analogues: the pros and cons of inverted versus ordinary Burow's triangle excision. *Plast Reconstr Surg*. 1996;98:1016-1022.
14. Brown MD. Advancement flaps. In: Baker SR, Swanson NA, eds. *Local Flaps in Facial Reconstruction*. St. Louis: Mosby; 1995:91-107.
15. Stevens CR, Tan L, Kassir R, Calhoun K. Biomechanics of A-to-T flap design. *Laryngoscope*. 1999;109:113-117.
16. Webster RC, Davidson TM, Smith RC, et al. M-plasty techniques. *J Dermatol Surg*. 1976;2:393-396.
17. Moody BR, Sengelmann RD. Standing cone avoidance via advancement flap modification. *Dermatol Surg*. 2002;28:632-634, discussion 635.
18. Hirshowitz B, Mahler D. T-plasty technique for excisions in the face. *Plast Reconstr Surg*. 1966;37:453-458.
19. Boggio P, Gattoni M, Zanetta R, Leigheb G. Burow's triangle advancement flaps for excision of two closely approximated skin lesions. *Dermatol Surg*. 1999;25:622-625.
20. Robinson JK. Placement of the tension-bearing suture in repairing the alar facial junction. *J Am Acad Dermatol*. 1997;36:440-443.
21. Antia NH, Buch VI. Chondrocutaneous advancement flap for the marginal defect of the ear. *Plast Reconstr Surg*. 1967;39:472-477.
22. Calhoun KH, Slaughter D, Kassir R, Seikaly H, Hokanson JA. Biomechanics of the helical rim advancement flap. *Arch Otolaryngol Head Neck Surg*. 1996;122:1119-1123.
23. Ramsey ML, Marks VJ, Klingensmith MR. The chondrocutaneous helical rim advancement flap of Antia and Buch. *Dermatol Surg*. 1995;21:970-974.
24. Butler CE. Reconstruction of marginal ear defects with modified chondrocutaneous helical rim advancement flaps. *Plast Reconstr Surg*. 2003;111:2009-2013.
25. Webster JP. Crescentic peri-alar cheek excision for upper lip flap advancement with a short history of upper lip repair. *Plast Reconstr Surg*. 1955;16:434-464.
26. Peng VT, Sturm RL, Marsh TW. Pinch modification" of the linear advancement flap. *J Dermatol Surg Oncol*. 1987;13:251-253.
27. Rowe D, Warshawski L, Carruthers A. The Peng flap: the flap of choice for the convex curve of the central nasal tip. *Dermatol Surg*. 1995;21:149-152.

Videos for this chapter can be found online by accessing the accompanying Expert Consult website.

5 Rotation Flaps

GLENN D. GOLDMAN, MD

A rotation flap employs an arciform incision adjacent to an operative wound in order to recruit laxity from multiple directions and redirect flap closure tension.[1] Adjacent tissue laxity assists flap rotation into the primary defect, and the tension vector is redirected in part to the secondary defect/motion of the flap. Rotation flaps recruit laxity by lysing deep restraint and by widely severing and redirecting dermal restraint. Rotation flaps may also displace dog-ears to more favorable locations.

Well-designed rotation flaps create scar lines that are hidden along facial boundaries or within relaxed skin tension lines. There are few repairs as elegant and seemingly simple as a well-designed and well-executed rotation flap. In practice, flaps that utilize only rotational motion are uncommon. Most rotation flaps combine several different types of motion, and most incorporate a significant degree of tissue advancement. Rotation flaps have long been utilized in plastic and general surgery for the reconstruction of larger truncal wounds including pilonidal excisions. In the last three decades, rotation flaps have found a greater use for the reconstruction of facial wounds.

Rotation Flap Design: Basic Principles

The classic rotation flap incorporates a triangulated defect and a smooth curvilinear arc. The long arciform dermal incision achieves substantial reduction in tension in the primary motion of the repair. Rotation flaps are sometimes hindered in their movements by the inherent stiffness of the tissue at the point of pivotal restraint along the lagging edge of the rotation arc. Such restraint may cause the tip of a properly designed flap to fall short of its destination at the apex of the primary operative wound (Fig. 5.1). In many cases, the tip is simply advanced under some tension to close the wound, but this may impair distal flap viability. To overcome this issue, the arc of the flap may be extended and the leading edge of the flap lengthened. When the elongated rotation is executed, the extended tip of the flap drapes without tension where it meets the distant point of the primary defect (Fig. 5.2).[2,3] This concept has been demonstrated in vivo in a porcine model.[4]

A rotation flap can frequently be closed without undermining beneath the point of pivotal restraint; however, for optimal flap motion, this area of restraint should be undermined (Fig. 5.3). This is particularly important with the dorsal nasal flap, where maximal rotation is required to close a defect located in the inelastic skin of the distal nose. Proper undermining of the pivot point accomplishes the release of deep restraint and usually allows substantial motion of the flap. This undermining is not without some risk, as too much undermining may interfere with deep vascular perforators. However, the reduction in tension on the flap tip usually more than compensates for any diminishment in pedicle vascularity.

A back cut into the rotation flap's body can improve flap mobility, particularly on relatively immobile skin such as on the scalp.[5] A back cut frees both deep and lateral restraint and can prove valuable in reducing closure tension, but a back cut also has the potential to compromise the vascular supply of the flap's pedicle. The more ample the residual vascular input, the more extensive of a back cut may be created. If, as in the case of the dorsal nasal flap, the remaining pedicle contains large-caliber axial vessels, the width of the pedicle may be safely narrowed and a substantial back cut will be tolerated. The defect from a back cut is usually closed with a V-to-Y repair, trimming excess tissue from the apex of the flap as indicated. Alternately, the apex may be closed with a Z-plasty.

FLAP LENGTH

Rotation flaps create long incision lines. A longer arc of flap rotation facilitates closure of the narrowed secondary defect and minimizes wound closure tensions, both in the primary and secondary motions of the repair.[6] In addition, a longer rotation flap allows for easier redistribution of tissue redundancy along the longer outer arc of rotation. Thus the incision lines for rotation flaps typically need to be longer than one would initially expect if the flap is to be placed under minimal tension and if the unwanted displacement of structures surrounding the primary defect is to be avoided. A common error in scalp reconstruction is to undersize a rotation flap with the resultant inability to close the operative wound.

FLAP CURVATURE

Most rotation flaps are designed with an arc that transects about one-quarter of a circle. Such a flap design reliably redistributes tension vectors along the secondary operative defect. Rotation is limited by the surface restraint of the pivot point. The greater the curvature of a flap, the greater degree of rotation can be accomplished. Similar to a back cut, a greater curvature actually cuts into the pedicle and permits greater freedom of movement by freeing pivotal restraint. However, too great of an arc of rotation will actually redirect tension "backward" and may negate the decrease in tension that the rotation flap was supposed to accomplish (Fig. 5.4).

Because rotation flaps require long incision lines to achieve appropriate flap motion, in many facial locations other flap options may be preferable. Rotation flaps have

5 • Rotation Flaps

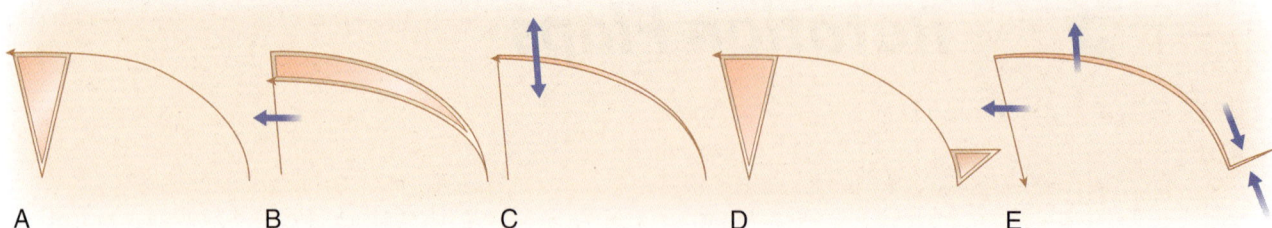

Fig. 5.1 Classic rotation flap. As primary defect is closed, a secondary defect develops. Secondary flap movement closes this defect. When the tip of a rotation flap is created as a simple arc taken off of a round defect (A), the flap will "fall short" and fail to meet the superior edge of the primary defect (B). The flap's leading edge will only meet the far edge of an operative wound if the flap tip is also advanced in a secondary motion (C). Note also that flap rotation typically produces a dog-ear redundancy at the flap's pivot point (D). The dog-ear must be excised to achieve proper flap contour (E).

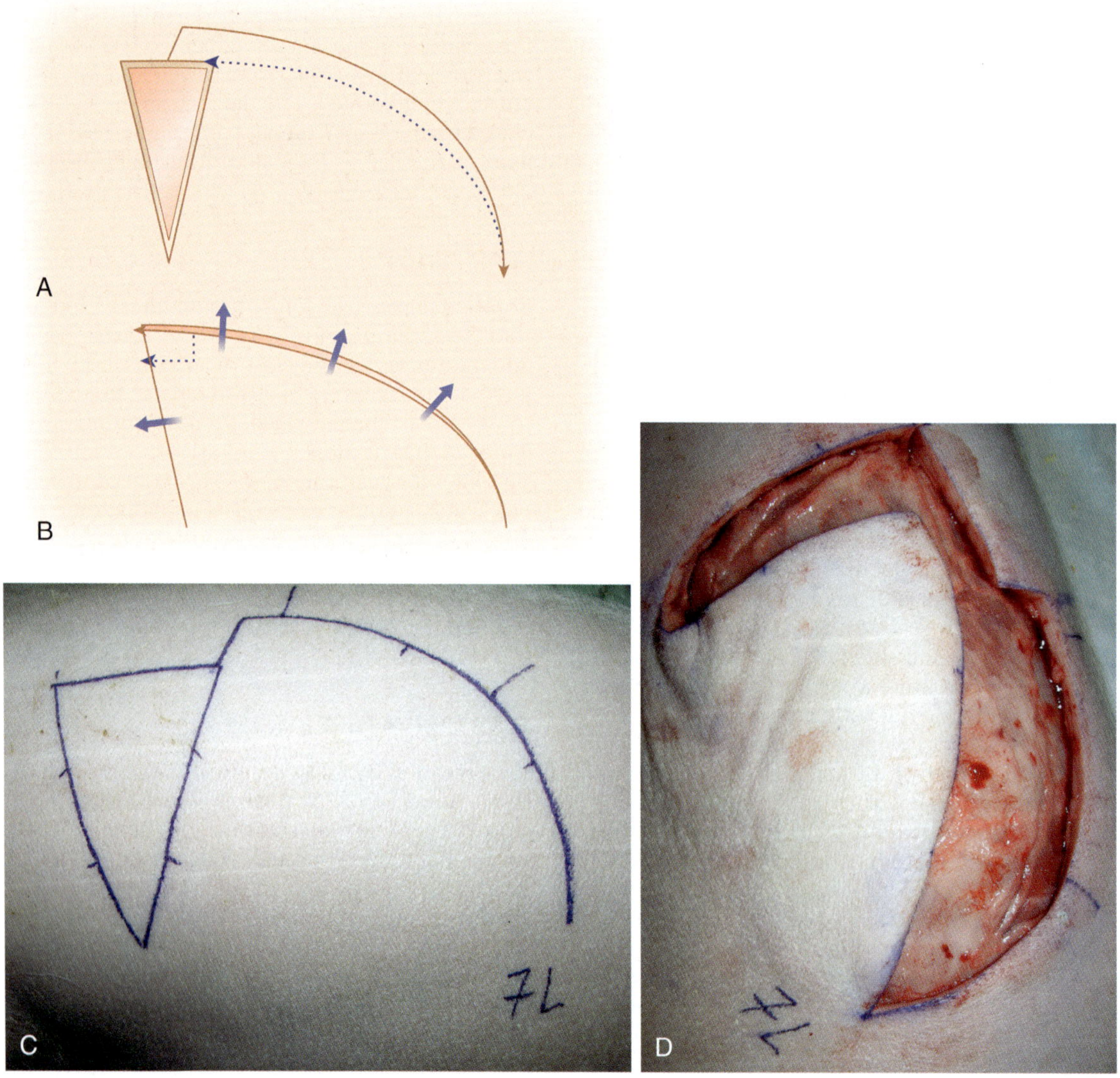

Fig. 5.2 Lengthening the leading edge of the rotation arc (A) overcomes pivotal restraint and minimizes secondary flap motion. Note the lack of need to rely on tissue advancement around the primary defect with the extended leading edge design of this rotation flap (B). This is demonstrated in vivo in a porcine model. The leading edge of the flap is elongated (C). Following incision and undermining the flap easily rotates into place and the leading edge of the flap will close under minimal tension (D).

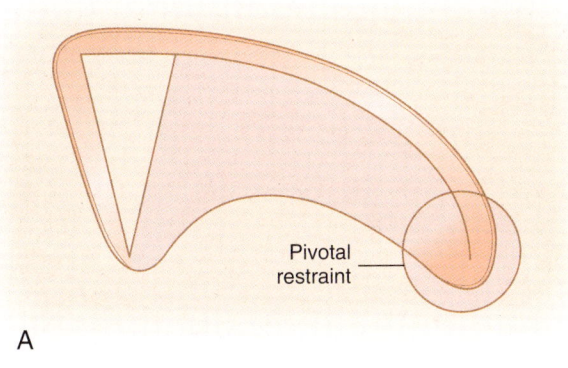
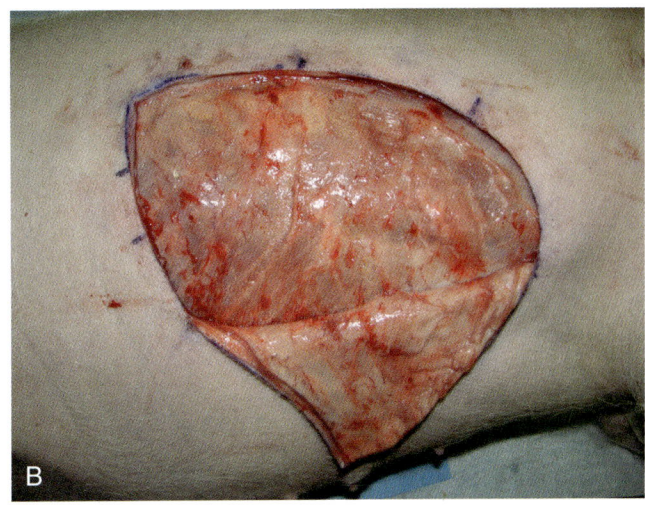

Fig. 5.3 For optimal flap mobilization the base of a rotation flap is undermined (shaded areas) to eliminate pivotal restraint (A). The appropriate extent of flap undermining is demonstrated in a porcine model (B).

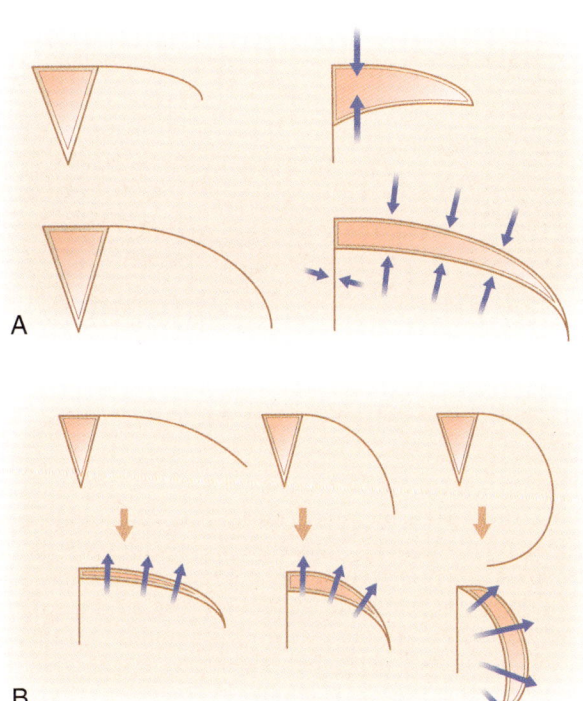

Fig. 5.4 A greater arc of rotation narrows the rotation flap's pedicle and increases mobility (A). Note also that greater flap length minimizes the relative width of the secondary defect at any point along the flap's arc. Rotation arcs greater than 90 degrees redirect tension in unwanted "backward" directions (B).

their greatest utility in the closure of scalp, temple, and cheek defects. In select cases, rotation flaps are also quite valuable on the nose. On the scalp, a lack of adjacent skin mobility requires rotation flaps to be especially long in order to close even small to moderate-sized operative wounds. On the cheek, rotation flaps are particularly useful for the repair of medially located wounds, because the rotation flap can effectively mobilize the large reservoir of loose skin in the entire area of the lateral cheek.[7] Infraorbital wounds can be closed with rotation flaps that recruit substantial laxity from the temple. Because rotation flaps tend to be rather "short" flaps when the distance from the flap base to the tip is considered, their vascular supply is quite predictable, and ischemic failures of the flaps are very uncommon if the flaps are closed under low tension.

Bilateral Rotation Flaps

Bilateral or dual rotation flaps utilize rotation from two sides of an operative defect to allow for wound closure where motion from one side would either be inadequate to close the wound or where symmetry of the repair is desired for enhanced cosmesis. Bilateral rotation flaps are most useful for large forehead wounds where a bicoronal incision is utilized (Fig. 5.5), for chin defects where the arc of the bilateral rotation lies within the mental crease, and lip defects where it is preferable to spread the tension out evenly over the entire lip.

O–Z ROTATION FLAP

The construction of an O–Z flap involves the creation of opposing rotation flaps, one of which takes origin from one side of the operative wound and the other as a mirror image from the opposing side of the defect. In the design of the O–Z flap, however, there is great flexibility. The paired flaps can be designed to rely upon pure rotational movement, or there can be varying amounts of flap advancement introduced into the operative design. As with traditional rotation flaps, the movement of O–Z flaps produces paired standing cone redundancies near the flaps' pivot points, and these redundancies are either excised or sewn out by the rule of halves. The O–Z repair has its greatest application on the scalp,[8] where the flap's prominent incision lines are typically hidden beneath a blanket of hair (Fig. 5.6).

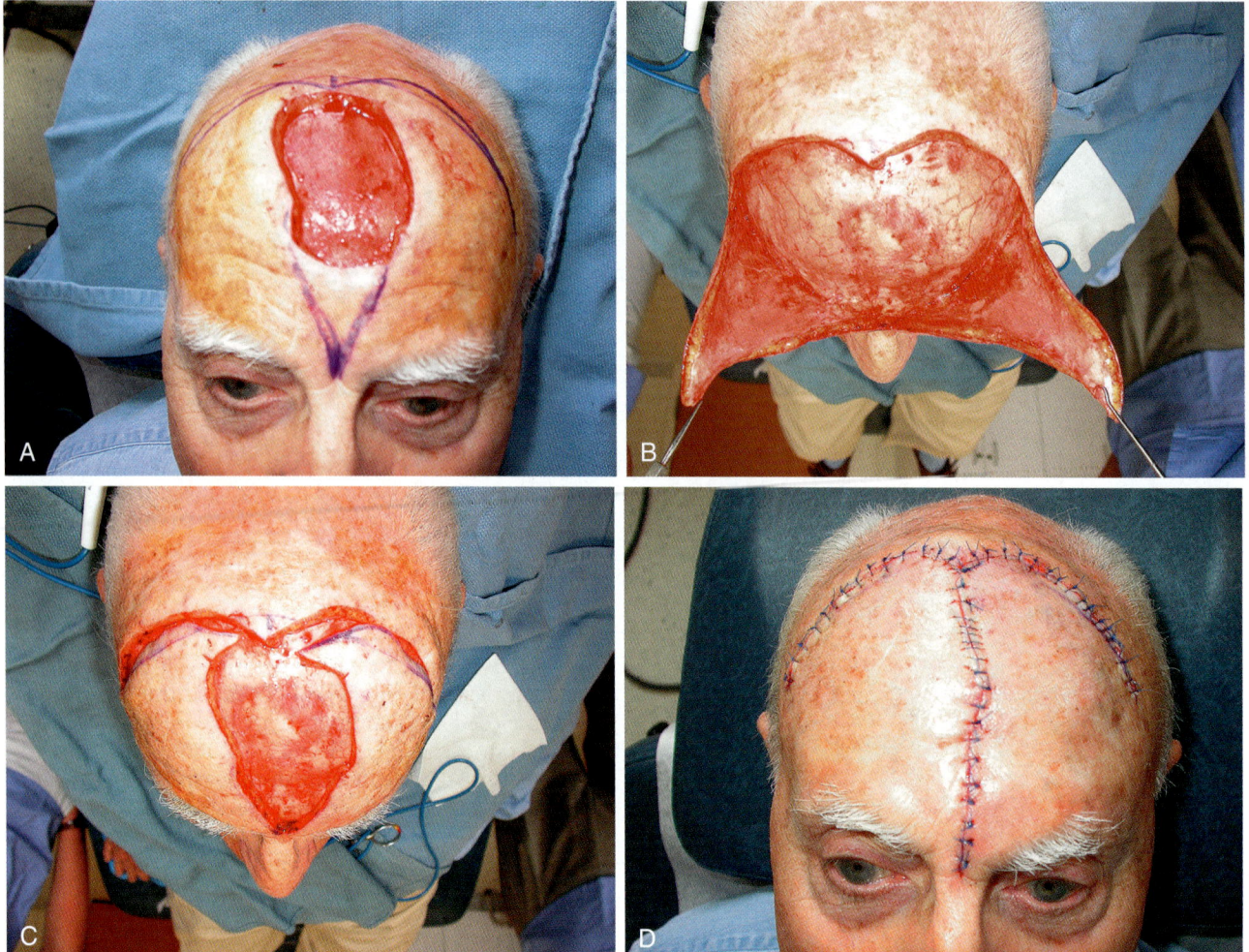

Fig. 5.5 Bilateral forehead/scalp rotation flaps for a large operative wound resulting from Mohs surgery for advanced basal cell carcinoma (A). Note that the flaps' rotation arcs extend beyond the upper pole of the operative wound (B). The flaps are widely undermined (C), and a dog-ear redundancy is removed inferiorly (D).

Selected Rotation Flaps

DORSAL NASAL ROTATION FLAP

Surgical defects of the distal third of the nose present unique reconstructive challenges. The skin of this area is stiff, sebaceous, and inflexible. Although some broad distal nasal wounds may be appropriately repaired with skin grafts, grafts often result in texture and color disparities, and grafts will not reliably survive over exposed cartilage. Many local nasal flaps do not allow adequate tissue movement for larger defects and can produce alar asymmetry and tip elevation. Distant pedicled flaps provide superior outcomes but require multiple surgical procedures.

In 1967 Rieger introduced the dorsal nasal rotation flap for the reconstruction of distal nasal wounds (Fig. 5.7).[9] The Rieger flap is a random pattern rotation flap that pivots on a muscular pedicle from the medial canthus and nasofacial sulcus. The flap described by Rieger is a full-thickness rotation of the entire nasal dorsum with a glabellar back cut to improve flap mobility. The flap is designed with a long sweeping arc that extends from the superior aspect of the defect to the nasofacial sulcus, past the contralateral medial canthus to a midpoint just superior to the glabella. In order to include the abundantly perfused underlying nasal musculature, the flap is elevated at the level of the underlying perichondrium or periosteum. Although not originally described by Rieger, it is often beneficial to change undermining planes at the glabella and elevate the flap above the procerus and medial inferior corrugators in this area. This avoids the transfer of thick glabellar skin to the thin skin of the contralateral medial canthus. The point of pivotal restraint with the dorsal nasal flap is located in the areas of the ipsilateral medial canthal tendon and the attachment of the nasal musculature to the nasofacial sulcus. As with all rotation flaps, undermining in the area of pivotal restraint can improve flap mobility, but this undermining should be performed under direct visualization in order to protect the flap's vascular pedicle. Properly executed, the dorsal nasal flap can be used to repair distal nasal defects up to 2 cm in diameter and is most useful for medium-sized distal nasal defects too large to be repaired with bilobed transposition flaps and too small to warrant the use of two-staged pedicled flaps (Fig. 5.8A).

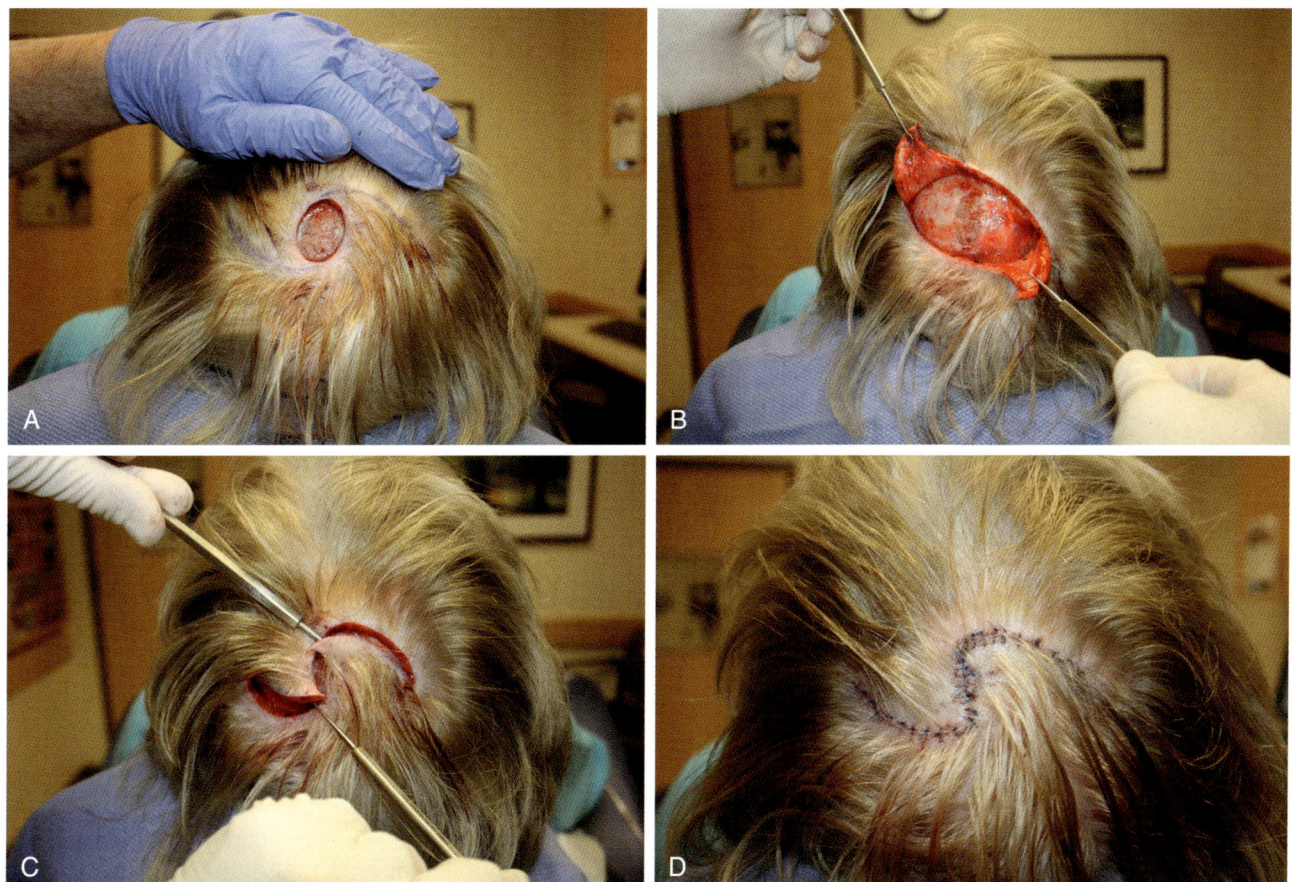

Fig. 5.6 A moderate but tight wound of the scalp with a depth to bone is best closed directly. Bilateral rotation flaps allow for recruitment of laxity from multiple directions and lyse dermal restraint along two long arcs (A). The flaps are elevated and undermined (B) and the wound closes under minimal tension (C). The completed repair (D) will be hidden by scalp hair.

The dorsal nasal flap, the variations of which have been eloquently reviewed by Dzubow,[10] has several advantages. Local nasal skin is used to repair a nasal wound, and in general, a good texture and color match along with a minimally visible scar are achieved. The scars of the dorsal nasal flap are hidden in the cosmetic junctions of the alar crease and the nasofacial sulcus and within the glabellar frown lines. The dorsal nasal flap has a predictable blood supply and rarely suffers from vascular compromise. The main disadvantages of the dorsal nasal flap are its size and its generous undermining requirements. If pivotal restraint is inadequately freed, rotation is limited, and closing the wound may place undesirable tension on the free margin of the nose. If the defect is on the central nasal tip, insufficient flap rotation will cause the tip to elevate. Whereas in older patients this elevation, if symmetric, may not be a concern and may actually be beneficial because of correction of age-related nasal tip ptosis,[11] in younger patients tip elevation produces a "pig nose" deformity. Flaps used to repair lateral wounds may produce to alar elevation and asymmetry. By lengthening the flap and extending the leading edge beyond the defect, the surgeon can achieve sufficient flap rotation to prevent free margin elevation. Not all noses are alike. Elongate noses with relatively thin, nonsebaceous skin are readily repaired with the dorsal nasal flap, whereas shorter noses and those with thicker sebaceous tissue prove more challenging. Although longer incision lines may create aesthetic concerns in the early postoperative period, a longer arc of flap rotation will reduce the likelihood of the alar tip distortion that can result from a smaller flap.

VARIANTS OF THE DORSAL NASAL FLAP

Axial Dorsal Nasal Rotation Flap

Marchac based his dorsal nasal flap variant on an axial pedicle of vessels that emerge near the medial canthus.[12,13] Based on reliable perforators emanating from the angular artery, the pedicle could be safely narrowed, allowing for removal of a long vertical triangular dog-ear along the ipsilateral nasal sidewall. Removal of this standing cone allowed for optimal rotation and also diminished the fullness of the ipsilateral sidewall that resulted from rotation of the flap into the operative wound. To ensure flap viability—especially adequate venous drainage—not only the arterial perforators but also a sling of nasalis muscle should be preserved in the vascular pedicle.

Heminasal Rotation Flap

In 1973 Rigg modified the dorsal nasal flap by designing a repair that utilized only a portion of the skin of the dorsal nose.[14] The incision of the heminasal flap he described

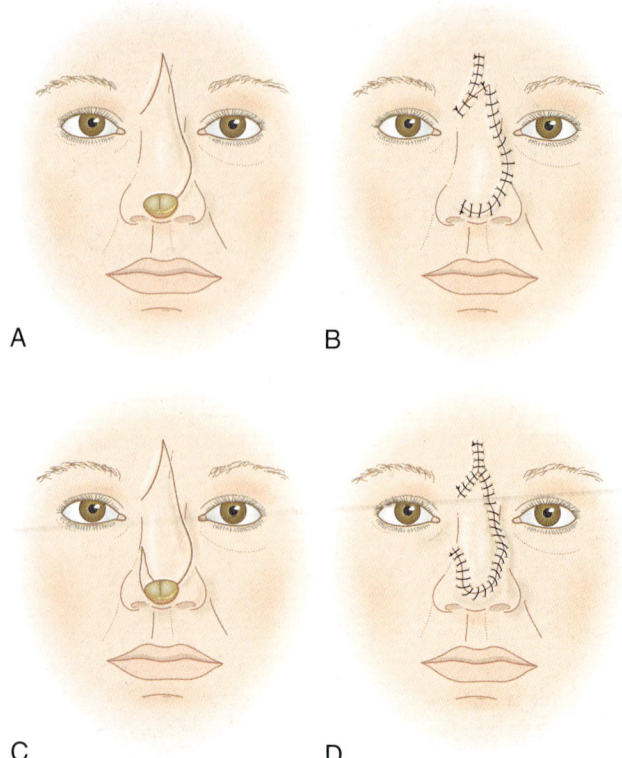

Fig. 5.7 (A) The classic dorsal nasal flap as designed by Rieger. Back-cut into glabella is closed with a Z-plasty. (B) A broad lateral pedicle is elevated above periosteum. The long sweeping circumference along the contralateral nasofacial sulcus allows for ample flap rotation and closure without tip elevation. (C) The modifications made by Marchac and Toth include basing the flap on an axial pedicle near the medial canthus and removing a vertical standing cone on the ipsilateral side. (D) Greater rotation may be achieved with this variation, and there is less tendency for dog-ear formation along the ipsilateral sidewall. The flap does require more incisions and has a greater potential for edema because of the limited pedicle size.

always necessary to extend the back cut superiorly onto the glabella or to extend the flap's curvilinear excision far laterally onto the contralateral nasal sidewall. Small lateral and inferior wounds that are repairable with bilobed or nasalis sling island flaps may also be suitably repaired with small rotation flaps carefully elevated above the nasalis musculature (Fig. 5.9). Such "distal nasal" rotation flaps are more sparsely reported in the medical literature, but they are useful in select cases.

THE SPIRAL FLAP

A common operative wound from a basal cell carcinoma is a defect of the medial to mid alar crease. Such wounds encompass both loss of nasal tissue and tissue from the adjacent cheek. Reconstruction of this area has been fraught with the creation of bridging between the cheek and nose. A novel solution developed by Cook creates a spiral or pinwheel flap to close the wound while recreating the alar crease.[16] The flap is a laterally based rotation that originates at the distal operative wound and spirals superiorly and then laterally, with an increasing radius. The flap is elevated either above or below nasalis. As it is rotated into place, the tip is folded back to the base. The tip of the flap replaces the ala, and the base of the flap advances in to the medial cheek. Due to the induced kinking of the flap, there is a natural tendency to invert and recreate the alar crease. The authors of the original paper leave the flap attached to the underlying nasalis, but the flap may be elevated just above the muscle out to the nasofacial sulcus in order to achieve greater mobility (Fig. 5.10).

TENZEL AND MUSTARDE ROTATION FLAPS

In 1966 Mustarde described a cheek rotation flap for lower eyelid reconstruction.[17] In 1975 Tenzel and Stewart described a similar rotation flap from the temple for repair of full-thickness lower eyelid defects.[18] The classic Mustarde flap is a large rotation of cheek and temple skin with extension of the flap's incisions into the distant preauricular cheek. The Tenzel semicircular flap is a similarly designed rotation of a skin and orbicularis muscular flap from the temple and lateral canthal areas, combined with a cantholysis of one crus of the lateral canthal tendon in order to facilitate flap rotation. Originally described by the author as an advancement flap, the Tenzel flap actually constitutes a combination of advancement and rotation about a pivot point on the zygoma. A superiorly arcing semicircular incision lateral to the canthus allows for the recruitment of adjacent tissue for reconstruction of the lower lid. Both the Mustarde and Tenzel flaps utilize the primary motion of the flap to support the eyelid, and both flaps direct wound closure tensions toward the temple superolaterally and toward the cheek medially. Because the flaps disperse tensions in these directions and are tacked down to the periosteum of the lateral orbital rim, unwanted vertically directed tension along the eyelid margin is avoided, and the appropriate position of the lower lid can be maintained. Similar to the design of the rotating dorsal nasal flap, the Mustarde and Tenzel flaps' long arcs of rotation allow the redistribution of the volume of the primary defect along a narrowed secondary defect. Because the secondary defect with both

places the free edge of the flap directly on the midline dorsum of the nose to the glabella, and then back cuts to the ipsilateral inner canthus. This repair is most useful for relatively small lateral nasal wounds, where it provides a suitable alternative to the bilobed transposition flap. Similarly, defects of the lateral inferior nasal sidewall can sometimes be readily repaired with a mirror image heminasal rotation flap where the free margin of the flap rotates along the nasofacial sulcus. This repair requires that the flap rotate freely enough to avoid elevation of the ipsilateral nasal ala.

Other Variants

For supratip and tip wounds, the optimal nasal rotation flap usually has a pedicle based on the opposite side of the nasal bridge. More lateral defects are often best repaired either via a transposition flap or via a heminasal rotation flap with the pedicle based on the same side of the defect. In many cases, a flap that utilizes only the nasal skin and avoids the glabella will suffice to close even a substantial distal operative wound (see Fig. 5.8B).[15] The dorsal nasal flap can be suitably modified for smaller defects. With such smaller flaps, it is not

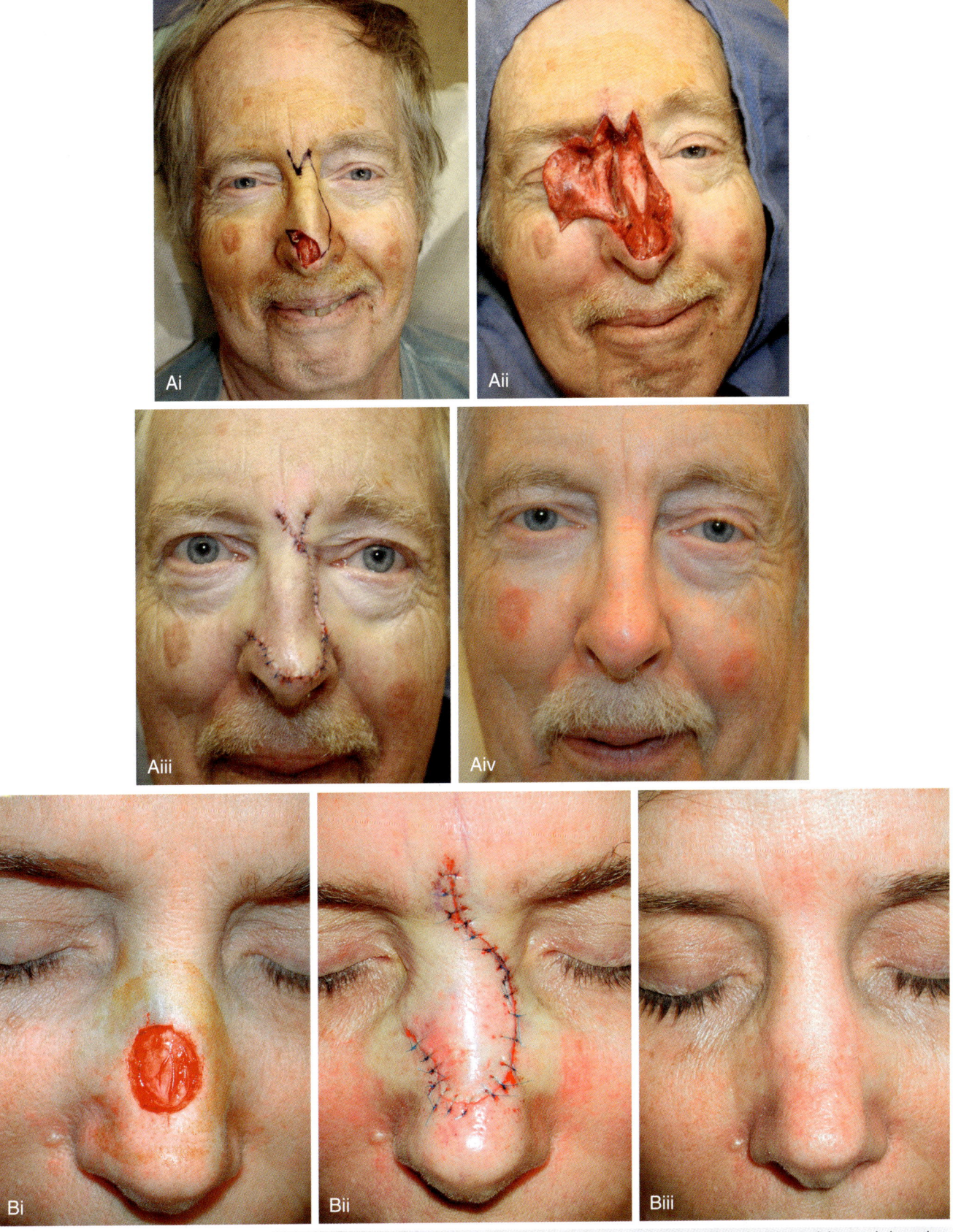

Fig. 5.8 (A) Dorsal nasal flap. (Ai) A surgical defect following Mohs surgery for a basal cell carcinoma. A large arciform incision is delineated along the tip and sidewall, extending to the glabella. A standing tissue cone will be removed above the wound. (Aii) The flap is elevated. The distal flap is elevated above the contralateral nasalis. The main bulk and base of the flap is elevated at perichondrium/periosteum. (Aiii) The flap drapes into place under little tension to repair the operative wound. (B) Modified dorsal nasal flap. A defect on the nasal dorsum (Bi) is repaired with a more proximal dorsal heminasal rotation flap (Bii). The flap allows for repair of a defect on the nasal bridge that is too large for primary side-to-side closure, and the aesthetic results of the flap are ideal, despite the complexity of the flap's incision lines (Biii).

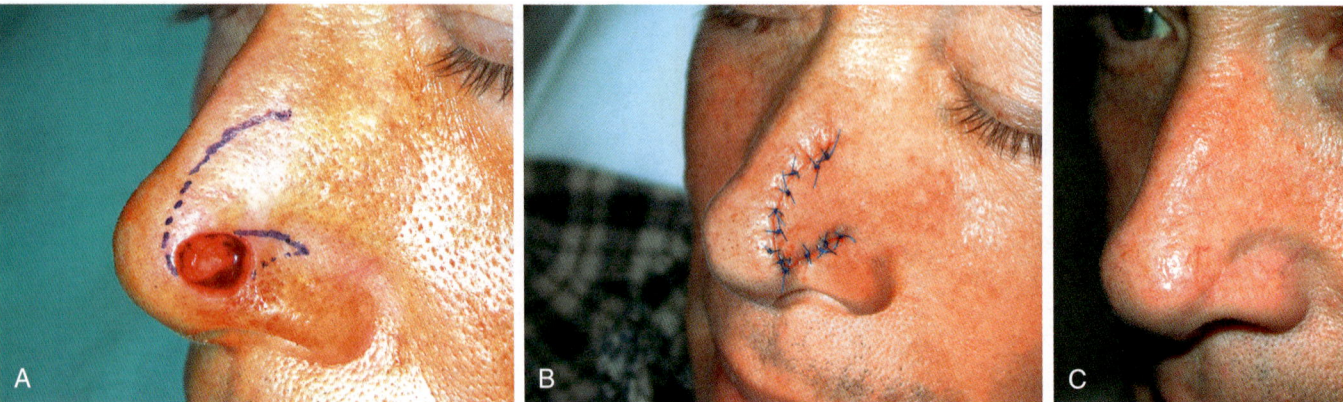

Fig. 5.9 Surgical wound of the distal nose may be repaired with relatively small superiorly based rotation flaps (A). Unlike the standard dorsal nasal flap, these small flaps are elevated above the nasal musculature. Flap rotation is accomplished without distortion of the alar margin (B), promoting acceptable cosmetic results (C).

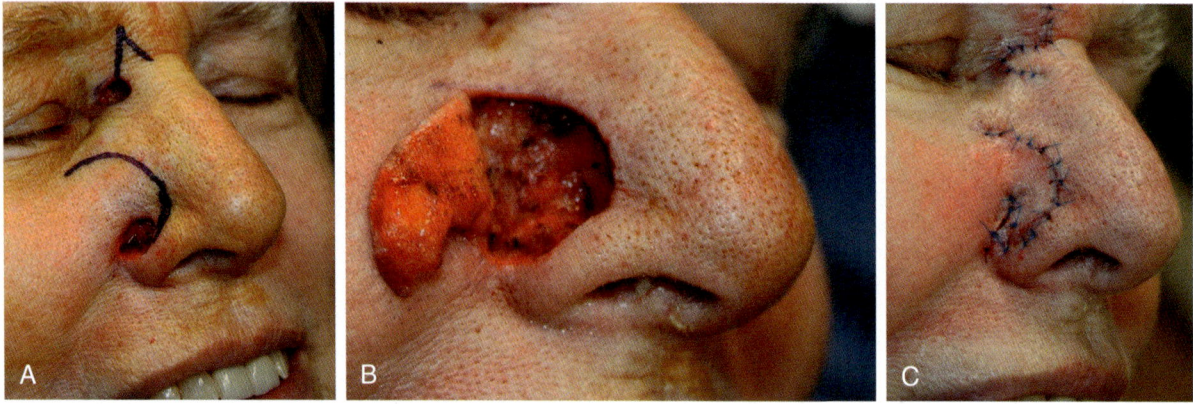

Fig. 5.10 Spiral rotation flap. This flap is most useful for defects which span the alar crease. The rotation is designed to arc from the medial aspect of the wound superiorly and laterally (A). The flap is elevated (B) and rotated onto itself to recreate the alar crease (C).

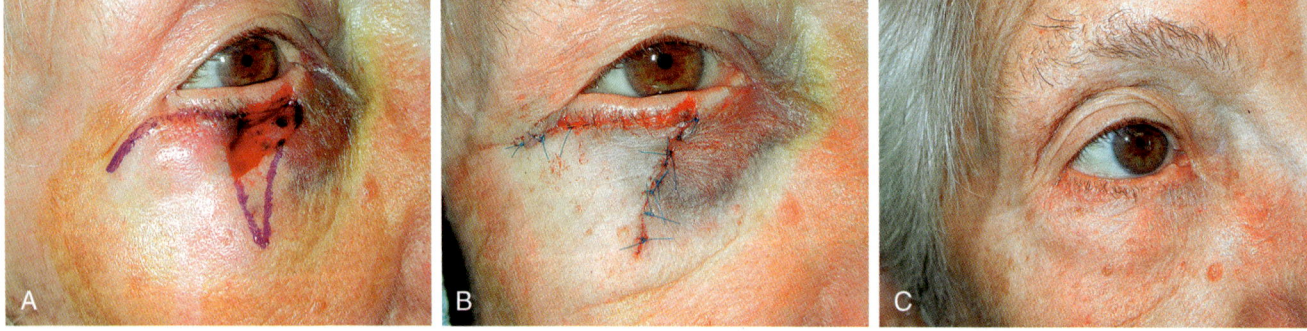

Fig. 5.11 For a wound near the eyelid's margin, a modified Tenzel flap (A) combines features of rotation and advancement. The flap is elevated just above the orbicularis oculi musculature. This flap combines elements of rotation and advancement (B), and recruitment of loose tissue near the lateral canthus prevents the development of an ectropion (C).

of these flaps is located within the compliant and mobile skin of the temple and cheek, distortion of the surrounding structures is minimized.

These useful rotation flaps have been commonly modified,[19,20] and they are reliable for the repair of defects of the lower eyelid and defects that span the lower lid and adjacent cheek or zygoma. The most commonly employed flap variant is a modified Tenzel flap used to repair partial-thickness defects of the mid to lateral lower eyelid (Fig. 5.11). From the superior extent of the surgical defect, a curvilinear rotation is extended laterally and superiorly past the lateral canthus and onto the temple. If the arc of rotation is not extended superiorly, an ectropion may develop. The flap is elevated just above the orbicularis oculi superomedially, above the medial insertions of the superficial musculoaponeurotic system (SMAS) inferiorly, and over the superficial temporal fascia superolaterally. Tension is directed horizontally along the vector of the primary motion. As the wound

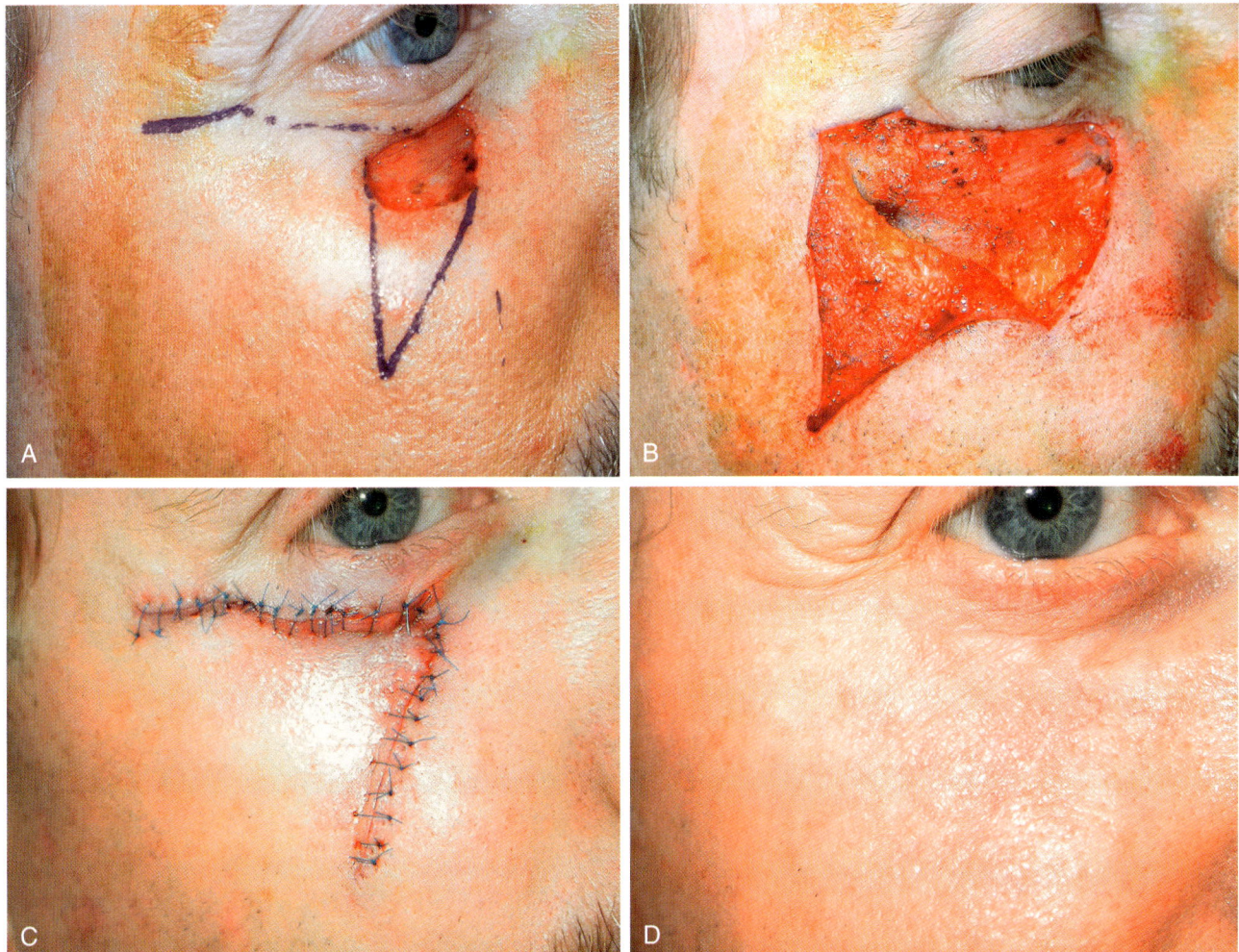

Fig. 5.12 With infraorbital rotation flaps, extending the flap's incision superior and lateral to the lateral canthus (A) oversizes the flap and supports the eyelid upon flap motion, thus preventing a tendency to produce an ectropion. The flap is undermined just above orbicularis superiorly and above superficial musculoaponeurotic system (SMAS) inferiorly (B). With appropriate flap undermining and suturing (C), the aesthetic results are ideal (D).

is closed, the temporal arc of the rotation/advancement supports the lower lid and prevents ectropion. This is one type of rotation flap where the maximum tension vector remains mainly in the direction of the primary motion. By having an oversized arc of rotation, the flap places essentially no tension on the medial portion of the secondary defect, thus avoiding tension on the lower lid margin. The modified Tenzel flap often produces temporary edema of the lower lid due to the obstruction of the laterally draining lymphatic channels, and this may persist for several months. As noted earlier, the modified Tenzel flap is also useful for sizeable defects that involve not only the lid but also the area just below the infraorbital crease over the zygoma or more medial cheek (Fig. 5.12).

MEDIAL CHEEK ROTATION FLAP

Defects of the medial cheek near the junction of the lower lid and nasal sidewall can often be repaired linearly or with local tissue advancement. It is common, however, to be presented with a postoperative wound that is inferior and lateral to the medial canthus, oval in shape, and oriented along the lower lid crease. Such elongate wounds are often due to the tendency of basal cell carcinomas in this region to extend along the infraorbital crease as a path of lower resistance. Similarly, sizeable defects including portions of lateral nose, medial cheek, and inferomedial lower lid are common. Advancement in this location can be difficult because of the relatively minimal horizontal laxity of the medial cheek. Linear repair places tension on the medial lower lid margin and can produce either a "pulled lid" appearance or a medial ectropion. For these reasons, very large defects in this area can be repaired with large sweeping rotation/advancement flaps that extend to the temple, but for smaller wounds, elegant and smaller medial cheek rotation flaps are often suitable. In such repairs, curvilinear dog-ear incisions are designed along the lower lid crease to triangulate the primary defect. The arc of this rotation flap extends down along the nasofacial sulcus and nasolabial fold, where a dog-ear excision at the inferior extent may be required. The flap is elevated just above the orbicularis oculi superiorly, at the level of the nasalis medially, and just above the levator labii superioris inferiorly. When this flap is elevated just above the facial musculature and within the loose fat of the medial cheek, it is usually a very easy flap elevation with minimal bleeding. Once the deep and lateral

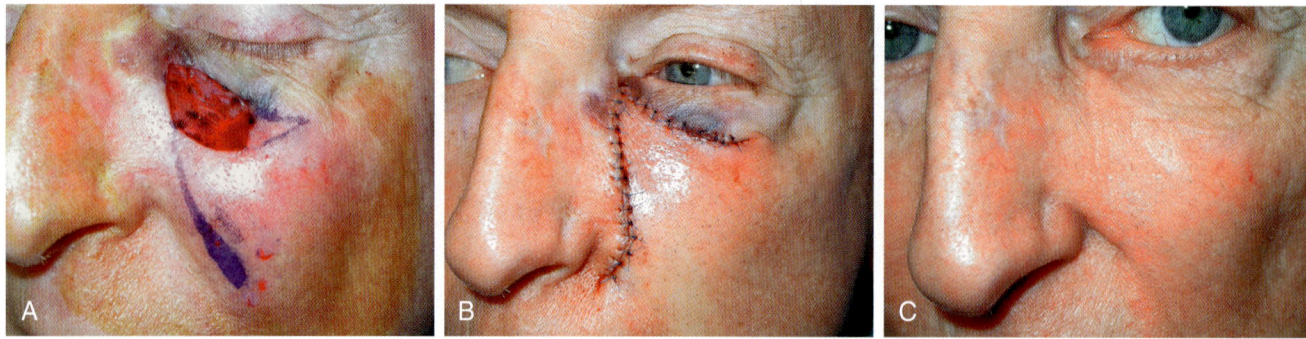

Fig. 5.13 The medial rotation of a cheek flap (A) directs all wound closure tension along the area of secondary motion and toward the tip of flap repair (B). By tacking the rotating tip to the underlying nasal periosteum, there is essentially no tension on the primary operative wound. This supports the medial lower lid and prevents ectropion (C).

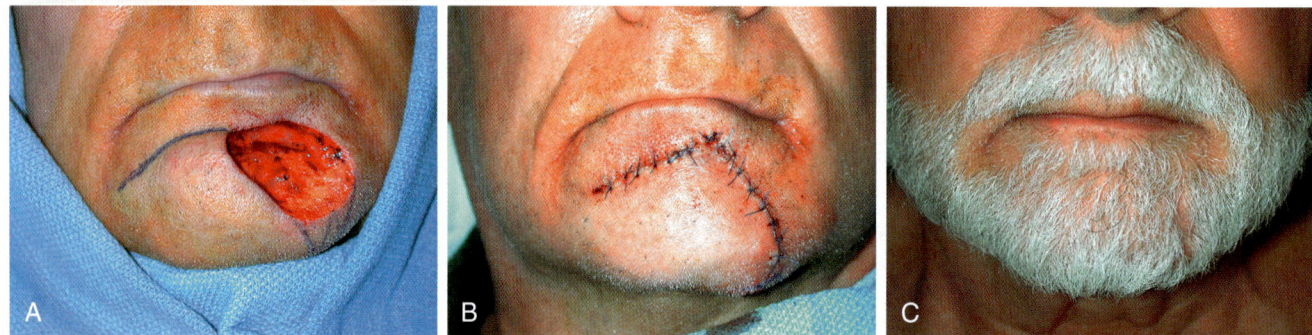

Fig. 5.14 Large chin defects (A) are readily repaired by rotation (B) with the arc of the rotation flap hidden within the mental crease (C).

restraints have been freed, the flap will rotate superomedially under minimal tension. In order to support the lower lid and prevent ectropion, the dermis of the center of the tip of the flap is tacked carefully to the periosteum of the nasal bone or medial maxilla (Fig. 5.13). This critical single stitch, which can be a 4-0 Vicryl suture, supports the weight of the flap and closes the primary defect along the lid crease. The nasofacial sulcus is then repaired with a bilayered closure. Only one or two deep sutures are usually required along the cheek–lid junction.

Although this flap may seem quite large for the repair of a small wound, there are few complications more problematic than cicatricial ectropion, and this rotation reliably prevents tension on the eyelid. It is common to have substantial lid edema for a week or two following surgery, but this does not typically persist.

CERVICOFACIAL ROTATION FLAPS

Cheek defects of up to 5 to 10 cm diameter may be repaired with long sweeping cervicofacial rotation flaps. The cervicofacial rotation is drawn as an arc from the superior aspect of the operative wound superolaterally arcing past the zygoma, in front of the ear, and far down onto the neck. The flap is elevated within the loose, deep facial adipose superiorly and laterally and then just above the platysma inferiorly on the neck. The flap must be thoroughly undermined under the medial and inferior pedicle to free the flap's rotation over the jaw. If the rotation is extended inferiorly to the clavicle, enormous facial operative wounds can be suitably repaired.[21,22]

ROTATION FLAPS ON THE CHIN AND LIP

Rotation flaps may be utilized to repair large chin defects. The arc or rotation is placed along the mental crease, and a triangular dog-ear is removed beneath the primary operative wound. Elevated just above the mentalis muscle and undermined over the mandible, chin rotation flaps can move a great distance and reliably close large wounds (Fig. 5.14). Defects of the lateral portion of the upper lip adjacent to the ala are readily repaired with small rotation flaps in which the arc of the rotation starts at the alar crease and extends inferolaterally along the nasolabial fold. As the flap rotates into the primary defect, the nasolabial fold is pulled slightly medially, but this is not usually noticed by the casual observer. The small standing or redundant cone that results from flap rotation into the primary defect is removed inferior to the primary operative defect. This flap works best in patients who have a substantial apical triangle of lip between the lateral alar crease and the nasolabial fold.

Plane of Flap Elevation and Surgical Undermining

Rotation flaps must be liberated from attachments to the deeper subcutaneous tissues before they can properly move. Undermining is very effective at reducing wound closure tension, and a properly designed and undermined flap repair is ideally draped over the operative wound under minimal tension. Sharp undermining with a scalpel or

Shea undermining scissors under direct visualization is preferred by many surgeons, since the flap can be elevated within a uniform and predictable plane.[23] When a fascial plane such as the SMAS or muscular plane is encountered, undermining can often be accomplished with great precision using electrosection.

Rotation flaps are elevated and undermined in defined planes based on anatomic location. Cheek flaps are usually elevated within the subcutaneous fat in the larger, looser fat lobules near the depth of the subcutis. Flaps on the forehead are typically elevated just above the frontalis musculature. Although this plane of elevation requires careful separation of the subcutis from the underlying skeletal muscle, it prevents the numbness and arterial transection that can occur with deeper flap elevation. Scalp rotation flaps are most appropriately elevated beneath the galea in the bloodless tissue plane immediately above the periosteum. Some small distal nasal rotations are elevated above the nasal musculature, but in general, most nasal rotation flaps are elevated just above the perichondrium. This deeper plane of undermining on the nose is associated with far less bleeding, and the inclusion of richly perfused skeletal muscle with the bases of these flaps makes the flaps nearly immune to ischemic insult.

Suspension (or tacking) sutures are sutures that anchor a portion of a flap repair to underlying immobile structures such as the periosteum. Suspension sutures are used to shift tension away from the edges of a flap, to reorient the tension vector of a flap, or to tack down a flap at a point of facial concavity where the flap would otherwise tent and create a potential dead space.[24] Tacking is usually performed with a nonabsorbable suture such as 4-0 Vicryl. A classic example of how a tacking suture may be utilized to redirect tension is a medial cheek rotation flap used to close an infraorbital wound. The dermis of the advancing edge/tip of the flap is tacked to the nasal sidewall at the superior and medial extent of the rotation. This single suture effectively closes the primary defect and takes all tension off of the leading edge of the flap, thus preventing ectropion formation. Similarly, tacking sutures are often used to tack large cheek and temple rotation flaps to the zygoma or to the lateral orbital rim or temple.

Conclusion

Rotation flaps allow for the redirection of tension vectors and for the mobilization of tissue utilizing laxity that lies at a distance from the operative wound. The arc and size of a rotation flap must be properly designed to minimize unwanted secondary motions. Rotation flaps are versatile because wound closure tensions may be redirected by simply altering suture placement. In some cases, the tensions may be equally shared between the primary and secondary motions, whereas in other cases, almost all tension may be directed along one vector, thus preventing pull in the direction where the result would be adverse (pull on a free margin, ectropion, for example). Rotation flaps should be elevated within the loose deeper subcutis or within a deeper plane in order to preserve needed vascular supply.

The flap's pedicle or its arc of rotation must be undermined beneath the point of pivotal restraint in order to allow for appropriate flap motion. The most aesthetic rotation flaps incorporate designs that place suture lines along natural cosmetic junctions. The concepts of rotation flaps are defining aspects of reconstructive surgery, and rotation flaps are reliable reconstructions for the repair of challenging operative wounds.

References

1. Dzubow LM. Rotation flaps. In: Dzubow LM, ed. *Facial Flaps. Biomechanics and Regional Application.* Norwalk, CT: Appleton and Lange; 1990:31-41.
2. Ahuja RB. Geometric considerations in the design of rotation flaps in the scalp and forehead region. *Plast Reconstr Surg.* 1988;8:900-906.
3. Dzubow LM. The dynamics of flap movement: effect of pivotal restraint on flap rotation and transposition. *J Dermatol Surg Oncol.* 1987;13:1348-1353.
4. Lichon V, Barbosa N, Gomez D, Goldman G. An elongated leading edge facilitates rotation flap closure: an in vivo demonstration. *Dermatol Surg.* 2016;42:100-104.
5. Kroll S, Margolis R. Scalp flap rotation with primary donor site closure. *Ann Plast Surg.* 1993;30:452-455.
6. Larrabee WF, Sutton D. The biomechanics of advancement and rotation flaps. *Laryngoscope.* 1981;91:726-734.
7. McGregor IA. Local skin flaps in facial reconstruction. *Otolaryngol Clin North Am.* 1982;15:77-98.
8. Albom MJ. Repair of large scalp defects by bilateral rotation flaps. *J Dermatol Surg Oncol.* 1978;4:906-907.
9. Rieger RA. A local flap for repair of the nasal tip. *Plast Reconstr Surg.* 1967;40:147-149.
10. Dzubow LM. Dorsal nasal flaps. In: Baker SR, Swanson NA, eds. *Local Flaps in Facial Reconstruction.* St Louis, MO: Mosby; 1995:225-246.
11. Preaux J. Le lambeau nasal de Rieger. Histoire, raffinements techniques et indications. *Ann Chir Plast Esthet.* 2000;45:9-16.
12. Marchac D. Lambeau de rotation frontonasal. *Ann Chir Plast Esthet.* 1970;15:44-49.
13. Marchac D, Toth B. The axial frontonasal flap revisited. *Plast Reconstr Surg.* 1985;76:686-694.
14. Rigg BM. The dorsal nasal flap. *Plast Reconstr Surg.* 1973;52:361-364.
15. Greeen RK, Angeles J. A full skin rotation flap for closure of soft tissue defects in the lower one-third of the nose. *Plast Reconstr Surg.* 1996;98:163-166.
16. Mahlberg MJ, Leach BC, Cook J. The spiral flap for nasal alar reconstruction: our experience with 63 patients. *Dermatol Surg.* 2012;38:373-380.
17. Mustarde JC. The use of flaps in the orbital region. *Plast Reconstr Surg.* 1970;45:146-150.
18. Tenzel RR, Stewart WB. Eyelid reconstruction by the semicircle flap technique. *Ophthalmology.* 1978;85:1164-1169.
19. Rao GP, Frank HJ. Surgical management of lower-lid basal cell carcinoma involving the medial canthus: a modification of the Mustarde cheek rotation flap. *Ophthal Plast Reconstr Surg.* 1998;14:367-369.
20. McGregor IA. Eyelid reconstruction following subtotal resection of upper or lower lid. *Br J Plast Surg.* 1973;26:346-354.
21. Shestak KC, Roth AG, Jones NF, Myers EN. The cervicopectoral rotation flap—a valuable technique for facial reconstruction. *Br J Plast Surg.* 1993;46:375-377.
22. Katz AE, Grande DJ. Cheek-neck advancement-rotation flaps following Mohs excision of skin malignancies. *J Dermatol Surg Oncol.* 1986;12:949-955.
23. Boyer JD, Zitelli JA, Brodland DG. Undermining in cutaneous surgery. *Dermatol Surg.* 2001;27:75-78.
24. Salache SJ, Jarchow R, Feldman BD, Devine-Rust MJ, Adnot J. The suspension suture. *J Dermatol Surg Oncol.* 1987;13:973-978.

Videos for this chapter can be found online by accessing the accompanying Expert Consult website.

6 V-Y Flaps and Island Flaps

JOEL COOK, MD

Many variables must be considered when examining a surgical defect and considering reconstructive options. The effective restoration of soft tissue contours improves results by reducing the visual impact of the reconstructive scars. Closure options for soft tissue defects include primary closure (side-to-side repair), split- or full-thickness skin grafts, and local or distant skin flaps. For smaller and less complex defects in areas with adequate regional tissue laxity, primary closure may often be a suitable repair choice. To achieve good cosmetic results with primary closure, the surgeon must recognize the limitations of adjacent tissue reservoirs. The mobility of nearby facial structures and their tolerance for movement must be determined prior to initiating the surgical repair. When the defect is too large to rely on local tissue laxity to close the wound in a side-by-side fashion, a skin graft or flap may be considered. Both full- and split-thickness skin grafts may be used to repair cutaneous wounds in a wide variety of locations; the uses of skin grafts are discussed elsewhere in this text. Although skin grafts may sometimes provide excellent final cosmetic results, they suffer from several limitations. To achieve excellence in cutaneous reconstruction, the surgeon must replace the missing tissue with tissue of identical or nearly identical character. When compared with the recipient site skin, the donor site skin should have a similar amount of sun damage, sebaceous glands, terminal hair, etc. Because skin grafts are usually harvested from sites not adjacent to the surgical defect, the harvested skin's character is often unlike that of the missing skin. Moreover, to ensure the survival of a full-thickness skin graft, all of the subcutaneous fat and portions of the dermis must be removed from the graft prior to its placement. The graft, therefore, may lack sufficient volume to adequately fill the surgical wound or avoid the forces of postoperative wound contraction. For these reasons, flap repairs may be better suited for many wounds.

The flap repair of soft tissue defects is unsurpassed in its ability to provide functional preservation, contour restoration, and overall cosmetically appropriate reconstruction. A cutaneous flap is defined as a mobile attached unit of skin and soft tissue with its associated blood supply. Flaps are used extensively to repair a wide variety of soft tissue defects following skin cancer surgery in all anatomic locations. Flaps are widely used because they can often overcome many of the pitfalls seen with alternative repair options. Cutaneous flap surgery is safe and reproducible.[1] Although cutaneous flaps may yield excellent results, they are not without the potential for some surgical risks and operative complications. It is important that the cutaneous surgeon have a firm knowledge of relevant anatomy, flap physiology, and flap design to maximize the opportunity for success. The nuances of proper surgical technique prove to influence operative outcomes significantly. Care must be extended to flap choice, flap design, incision and flap harvesting, and suture technique.

Cutaneous flaps are typically classified based on one of two systems: either the type of principal movement (rotation, transposition, advancement, or interpolation) or blood supply (random or axial patterned).[2] Because the majority of flaps performed by dermatologists are random-pattern cutaneous flaps, skin flaps are more commonly classified on the basis of movement. Random-pattern flaps of varied design are supplied by the richly anastomotic dermal vasculature; they lack the axial-pattern flaps' larger-caliber, named vessels in their bases. When these flaps are properly designed and executed, the abundant vascular supply of the dermis affords random-patterned flaps optimal chances for survival.

Advancement flaps are technically straightforward flaps; they are important in cutaneous reconstruction. The classical advancement flap is a sliding flap formed by a U-shaped incision. While this flap design has some reconstructive utility, it is prone to distal flap necrosis if the length is excessive or the flap is inset under excessive closure tensions. There are several modifications of the classical advancement flap that have expanded the flap's utility. These include, among others, the O-T, A-T, Burow advancement, and V-Y flaps. All of these rely on the linear advancement of adjacent skin and soft tissue to allow surgical repair.

The V-Y advancement flap is a random-pattern cutaneous flap that is useful in repairing small- to medium-sized facial wounds.[3-19] The classical advancement flap recruits contiguous tissue to repair an adjacent defect by creating a flap elevated to its base after two parallel incisions are made (Fig. 6.1). The traditional advancement flap, in this regard, is limited by the mechanics of the flap's design. With the simple advancement flap, a length:width ratio of less than 3:1 must usually be maintained to ensure perfusion of the distal portion of the elevated flap. The highest-tension portion of the flap is most distal to the flap's vascular input. Advancement flaps designed with length:width ratios exceeding 3:1 or flaps inserted under significantly elevated wound closure tensions may be subject to an inordinately high risk of distal ischemic necrosis. The V-Y flap has surmounted this pitfall, which has sometimes limited the usefulness and success of the classical advancement flap. The V-Y flap is designed with the nutrient vascular pedicle closer to the flap's leading edge so as to provide a greater and more predictable vascular supply (Fig. 6.2). The preserved central vascular pedicle significantly improves the perfusion of the

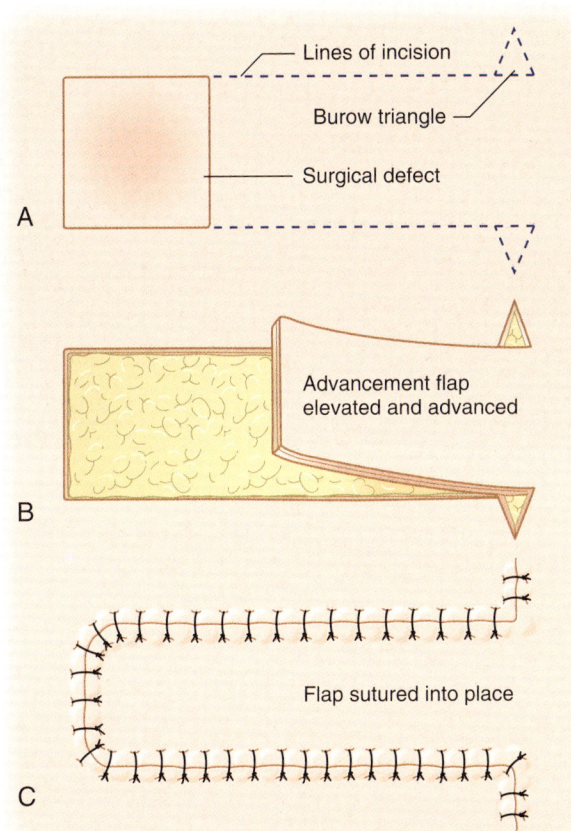

Fig. 6.1 (A–C) The classic advancement flap is created by two parallel incisions. The flap is then elevated and advanced to close the surgical defect.

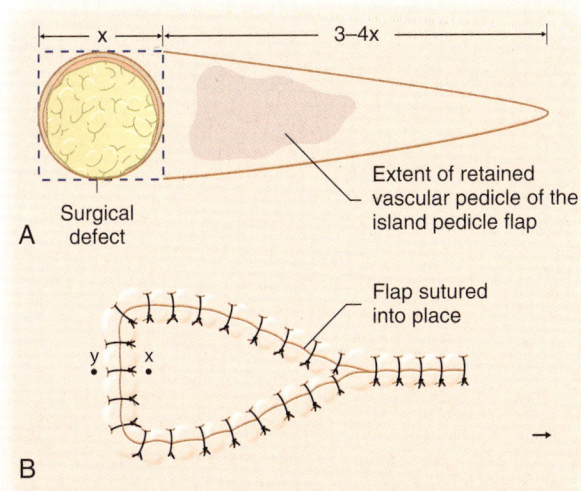

Fig. 6.2 (A, B) Design of the traditional V-Y flap.

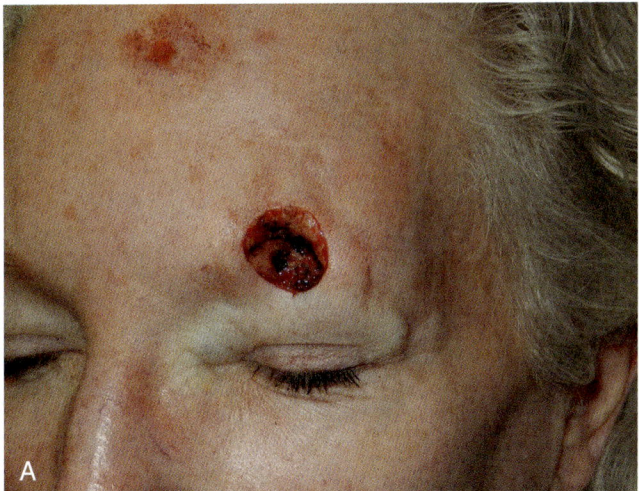
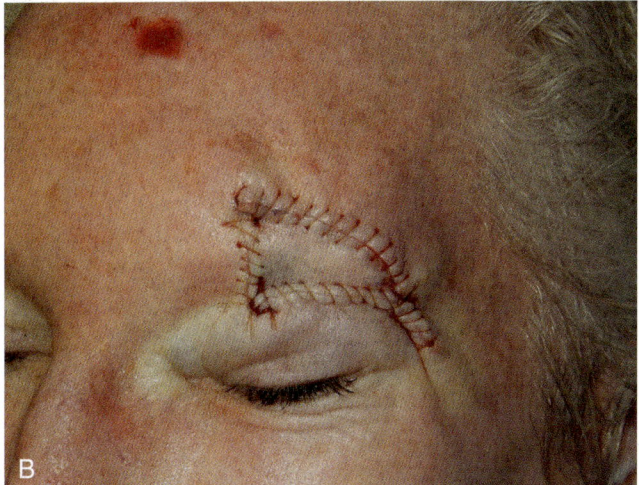
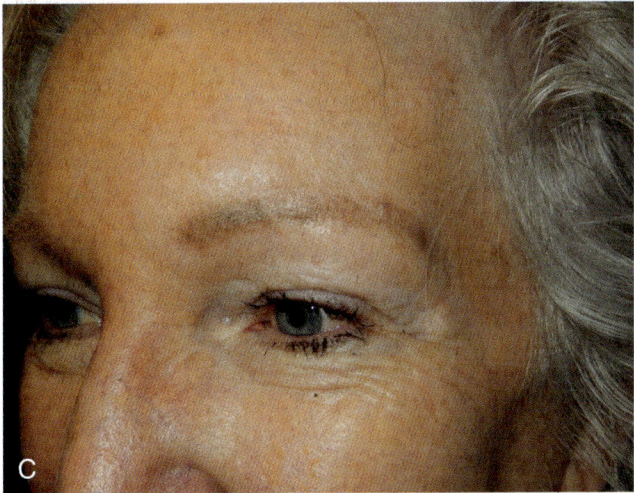

Fig. 6.3 (A–C) A traditional V-Y flap is used to advance the lateral brow and create a normal-appearing brow postoperatively.

flap's anterior margin and eliminates the relative ischemia at the leading edge of the longer traditional advancement flap. Because it has an abundantly perfused central pedicle, the flap can tolerate longer incisions and greater closure tensions than the classical advancement flap. The careful identification and preservation of a nutrient vascular pedicle in the V-Y flap is therefore critical for the success of the flap. The classic design of the V-Y flap is best used to repair defects where the long incisions may be camouflaged (e.g., upper cutaneous lip, cheek near anatomic borders, and brow) (Figs. 6.3–6.5).[3,7,10,11,13,17] The flap may also be used to effectively repair defects of the nasal dorsum, nasal

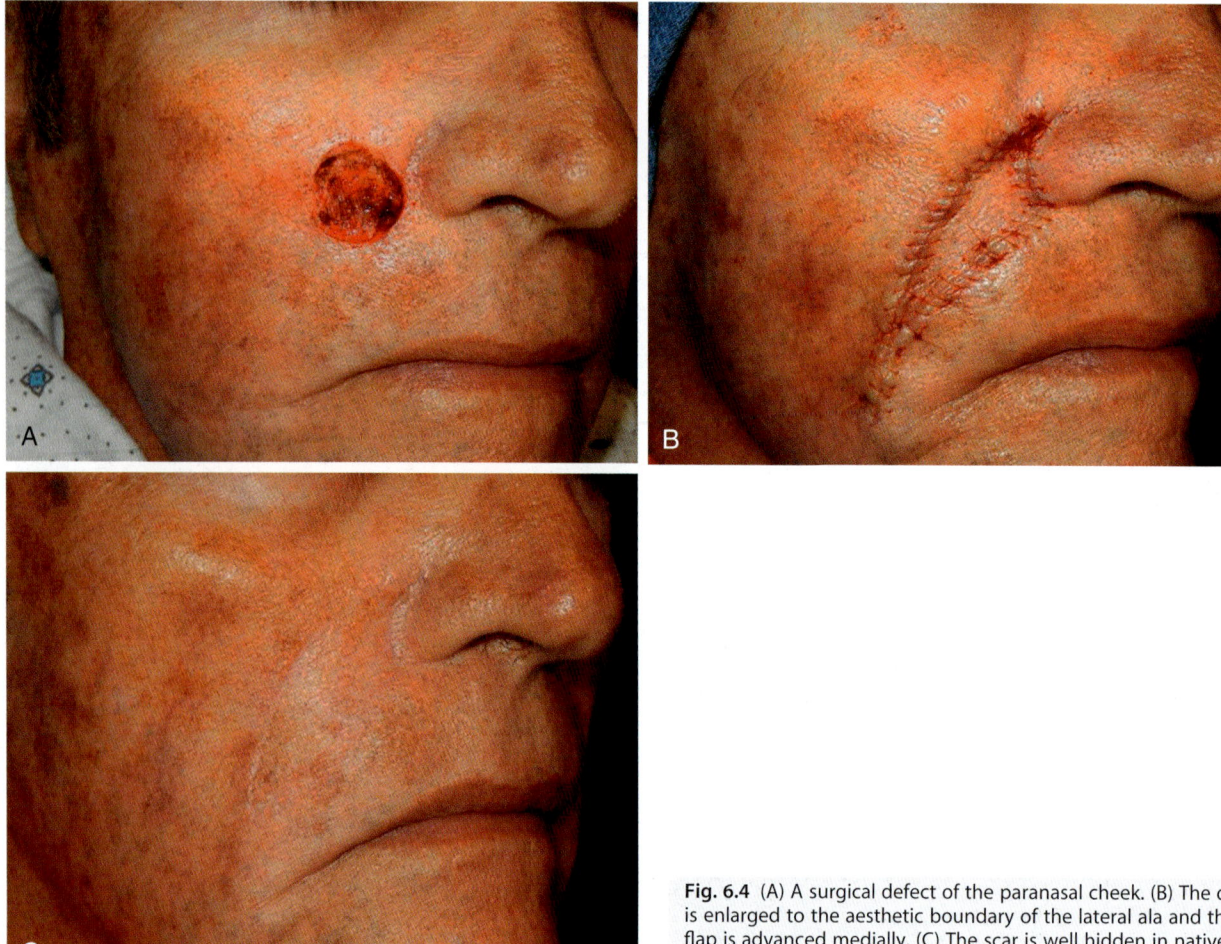

Fig. 6.4 (A) A surgical defect of the paranasal cheek. (B) The defect is enlarged to the aesthetic boundary of the lateral ala and the V-Y flap is advanced medially. (C) The scar is well hidden in native anatomic boundaries.

ala, forehead, and nonfacial locations.[15,16,18,19] In the classic design of the V-Y flap, the preserved nutrient vascular pedicle is directly underneath the central portion of the mobile flap. Variations of the flap with the vascular pedicle relocated to a lateral margin, a de-epithelialized distal flap, and a flap with bilevel muscular pedicles have been described previously (Fig. 6.6).[3,6,12,15,20] At times, opposing V-Y flaps may be used (Figs. 6.7 and 6.8). However, in the author's opinion, none of these modifications can surpass the predictably reproducible results seen with the classic design of the flap with a central vascular pedicle.

The V-Y advancement flap has been commonly referred to (and billed) as an island pedicle flap. Centers for Medicare and Medicaid Services (CMS) has recently redefined and restricted the use of the term *island pedicle flap* to those flaps requiring identification and dissection of an anatomically named axial vessel. Since the majority of the flaps used in dermatologic surgery are local flaps not based on named vessels, they should be referred to and billed as V-Y advancement flaps.

Technique

The proper design and execution of the V-Y flap is obviously critical to achieving reproducible aesthetic results with minimal operative risk. Once a defect has been selected for repair with a V-Y flap, operative consent is obtained from the patient. Routine prepping, draping, and infiltration with a local anesthetic then follow. The flap is designed as a V-Y tissue advancement. Although usually depicted as an isosceles triangle with straight edges, the flap's long axes may be curved so as to place the resultant incision lines along the borders of the facial cosmetic units (e.g., curvilinear incisions in the melo-labial fold and along the vermilion border for a flap used in upper lip reconstruction). The flap may also be designed with the initial lines coming off the defect running straight for a short distance before tapering into the V shape. This displaces the area of tension farther away from the defect and may be useful in areas where there is no tissue laxity in the immediate area of the defect.

The flap has a robust central vascular pedicle that consists of dermis, subcutaneous tissue, and underlying facial musculature. This pedicle nourishes the flap with a predictable vascular support available in few other random-pattern cutaneous flaps. Although categorically a random-pattern cutaneous flap, the V-Y flap has a more abundant and predictable blood supply than that of many other alternative flap reconstructive options. This improved vascular support may be beneficial in patients with increased risks of tissue ischemia (smokers, patients with prior exposure to radiation therapy, etc.). Moreover, the limited amount of required

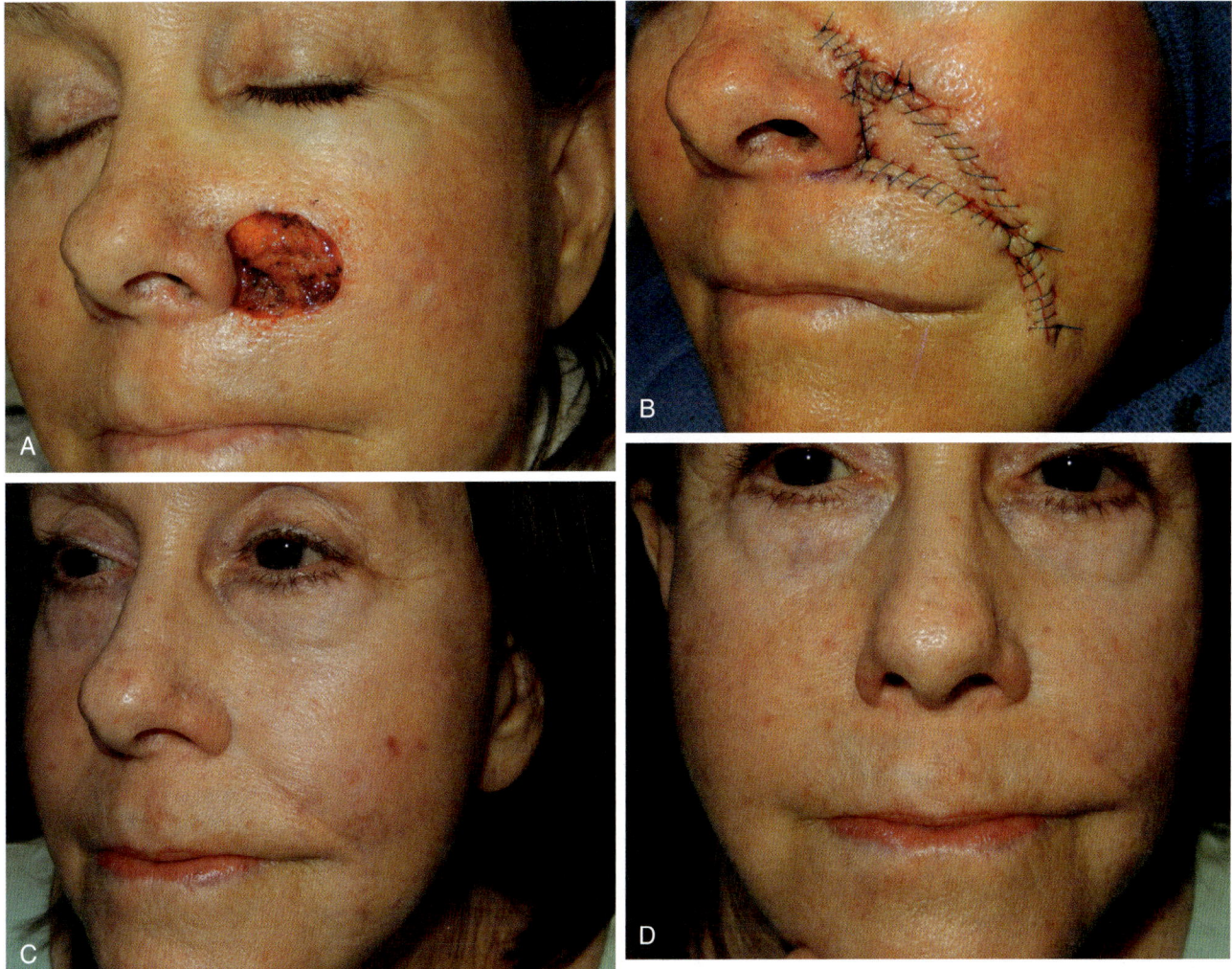

Fig. 6.5 (A) A surgical defect of the medial cheek and upper lip. (B) A V-Y flap is advanced medially to fill the surgical defect. (C, D) Postoperative result. Because the central portion of the flap is not undermined, the native melo-labial fold is preserved.

undermining and tissue mobilization associated with the execution of the V-Y flap may make this flap an excellent choice in patients taking anticoagulants or those with bleeding diatheses. As compared with a rotation or advancement flap used to repair similarly sized defects, the V-Y flap typically requires less undermining, which may lead to a lower risk of postoperative bleeding complications.[21,22]

Following adequate tumor extirpation, the defect to be repaired with the island pedicle flap is thoroughly analyzed. The flap produces the best results when it is harvested from within the same cosmetic unit as the surgical wound. This, however, is not an absolute requirement for flap success. The flap is classically designed as an isosceles triangle adjacent to the primary defect. The length of the triangle is typically 3 to 4 times the width of the surgical defect. The apex of the triangle's long sides is an angle of approximately 30 degrees. After the flap is designed, if the wound has resulted from a Mohs extirpation, the circular surgical defect is converted to a square and the beveled dermis removed.[23] It is the opinion of the author that a squared-off island flap inserted into a squared-off surgical defect has less chance of elevation (trap-dooring) and resultant failure of contour restoration than a rounded flap placed into a rounded defect. The phenomenon of trap-dooring is poorly understood. As a flap contracts in the postoperative period, circumferential movement of incipient scar tissue may force the flap to become elevated above the surrounding skin. Although this elevation may prove aesthetically displeasing, it can usually be corrected with massage, intralesional corticosteroids, and simple observation, thereby avoiding the need for additional operative procedures. Despite previously published recommendations to oversize the flap, the best surgical results are obtained when the flap is slightly undersized.[23,24] For that reason the width of the properly designed V-Y flap should be slightly smaller than the width of the primary surgical defect. Although this minimal undersizing requires some degree of secondary tissue movement from around the borders of the primary surgical defect, it reduces the risk of postoperative flap protuberance. Oversizing or equivalent sizing the V-Y flap to the defect simply stuffs too much flap

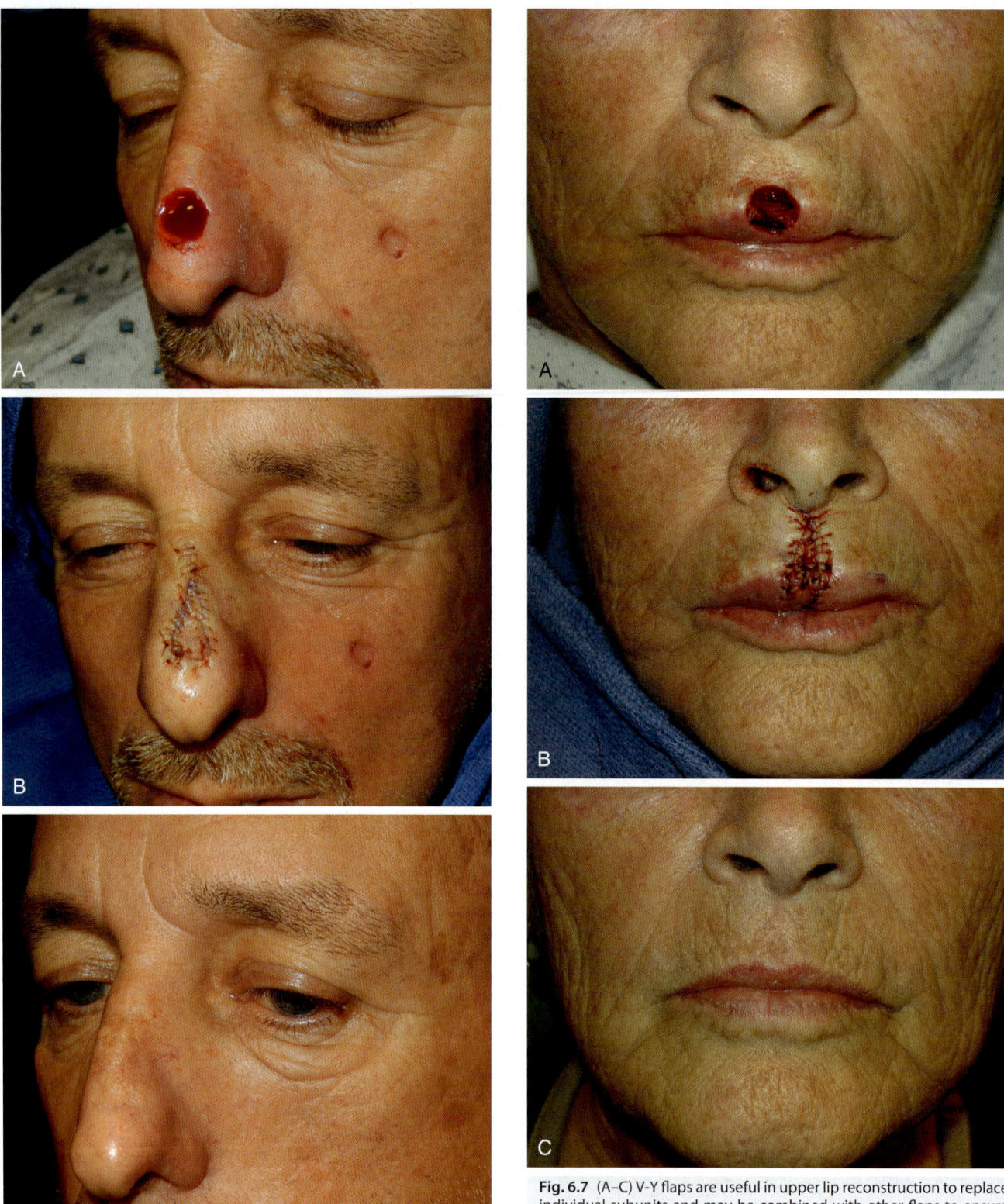

Fig. 6.6 (A) Surgical defect of the supratip. (B) A V-Y flap based on a lateral pedicle with bilevel undermining is advanced into the defect and sutured in place. (C) Postoperative result with no additional procedures.

Fig. 6.7 (A–C) V-Y flaps are useful in upper lip reconstruction to replace individual subunits and may be combined with other flaps to ensure neutral wound position upon healing.

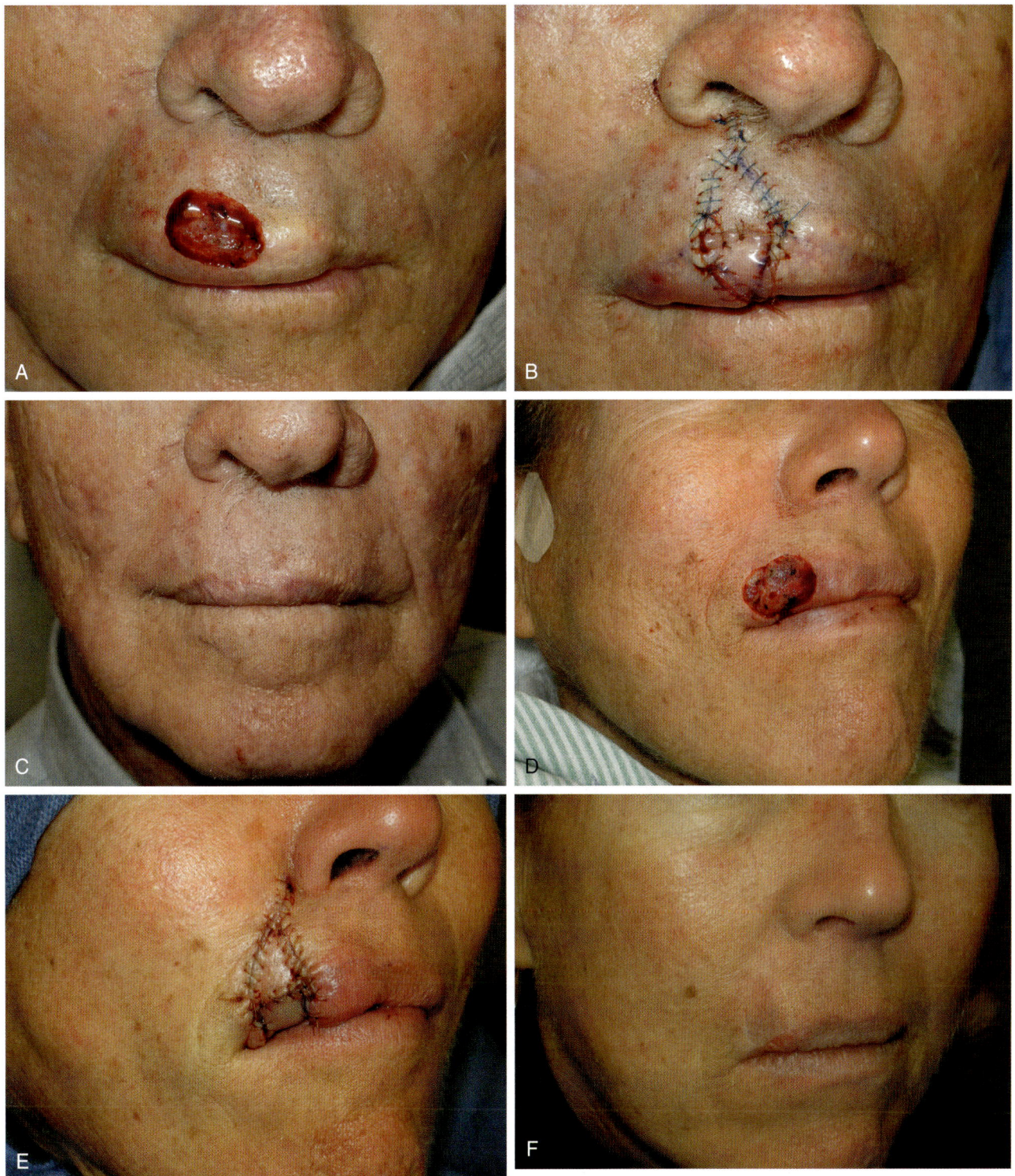

Fig. 6.8 (A–C) A mid-upper lip defect repaired with opposing V-Y flaps (one for the cutaneous lip and one for the vermilion lip). (D–F) A lateral upper lip defect repaired with a cutaneous V-Y flap and mucosal advancement flap.

into the surgical defect, and the flap, when cicatricial forces begin to contract, decompresses anteriorly, producing an unsightly, redundant flap that will detract from the typical aesthetic success seen with the smaller flap's design.

After the flap has been designed with attention to anatomic boundaries and flap geometry, the flap is sharply incised. The margins of the flap's donor area are then undermined to facilitate flap advancement and donor-site closure. It is important to recognize the degree of secondary tissue movement that will be required in all cases in order to avoid unwanted anatomic distortion. The primary defect's peripheral margins are also undermined at an identical depth. Undermining the pedicle of the V-Y flap itself presents the most risky portion of the reconstruction. If undermining is inadequate, the flap will prove difficult to mobilize and thus excessive tensions may be required for closure. These inappropriately elevated tensions increase the risk of flap ischemia and may produce associated anatomic distortion. Conversely, if the flap is undermined without careful attention to the preservation of the central vascular pedicle, insufficient vascular supply may fail to nourish the nascent flap. Although facial flaps may have a greater and more predictable vascularity than similarly designed flaps in other locations, the V-Y flap may be used in nonfacial reconstruction with identical design. A central pedicle of 40% to 50% of the flap's area is typically adequate to ensure the flap's survival. A significant restriction to the linear advancement of the flap may originate at the narrow apex (tail) of the flap. The apex of the flap may be incised and elevated to increase the forward sliding motion of the flap. This undermining and elevation of the flap's tail greatly improve the flap's mobility, but it should be limited to the exact extent necessary to advance the flap. Increasing the extent of undermining reduces the size of the nutrient vascular pedicle and therefore increases the risk of ischemic flap necrosis. The advancing margin of the flap is also undermined for several millimeters, principally to assist with accurate reapproximation of the wound edges. This small amount of undermining also significantly improves flap movement, particularly when the tail of the flap has also been liberated from its underlying attachments.

After undermining of the recipient site, the donor site, and the anterior and posterior margins of the flap, the flap and surrounding skin are elevated and hemostasis is achieved. After the achievement of adequate hemostasis, the flap is advanced in a V-Y manner to fill the surgical defect. The initial suture (the key stitch) is placed at the midpoint of the flap's anterior margin to a corresponding point along the opposite margin of the primary surgical defect. This suture is placed with particular care to make sure that the flap is carefully aligned and thus to minimize the risk of subsequent anatomic distortion. Suture technique is critical to achieve operative success. To compensate for the inevitable wound contraction seen in the postoperative period, the flap must be sutured into place with care. Buried vertical mattress sutures of absorbable material are placed in the mid-dermis. If placed correctly, each successively placed buried suture will lower the central portion of the slightly undersized island pedicle flap. Once the buried sutures have been placed, the center of the flap should be depressed 2 to 3 mm below the surrounding skin. This slight flap recession is important to provide a well-contoured flap after wound healing has been completed, since the flap will inevitably rise to a small extent as wound contraction occurs at the flap's bed in the early postoperative period.[24] The author has never observed a recessed flap that failed to eventually elevate to a proper position.

After the flap has been secured with properly placed buried sutures, the epidermis is reapproximated with a running cuticular suture. Drains are rarely used, even with larger flap procedures. Tip stitches at the apex of the flap are not typically required. The wound is bandaged and wound care instructions are given to the patient. Oral antibiotics may be prescribed as needed. The sutures are removed at an appropriate postoperative interval, typically at 5 to 7 days for facial flaps. The V-Y flap repair rarely needs any postoperative refinement such as scar revision, debulking, or dermabrasion.

The classically designed V-Y flap is a hearty flap that may be used to repair a wide variety of facial defects with elegance and minimal procedural morbidity. The flap repairs wounds with skin of excellent color and textural match. The advancement V-Y flap should be viewed as an ideal reconstructive choice for soft tissue defects of the cutaneous lip, eyebrow, and medial cheek. Although previous authors have championed the flap as a viable reconstruction choice for distal nasal defects, the flap may prove problematic on the lower nose if the mobility of the nasal skin is limited or misjudged.[6] In such a case, prominent nasal distortion may result after inadequate flap advancement because a reliance on secondary tissue movement to close the primary surgical defect is required. For small- to medium-sized distal nasal wounds, alternative reconstructive choices (the bilobed and other flaps) may prove to be superior selections.

Modifications

When preoperative assessment predicates that a central pedicle may limit the flap's movement, lateral pedicles may be used to increase flap movement and maintain adequate flap perfusion. This design modification may prove to be important in certain anatomic areas (the temple, for example). Alternative modifications may also increase the usefulness of the V-Y flap. The advancing margin of the flap may be de-epithelialized and buried in yet another variation of the flap (Fig. 6.9).[15] This removal of the distal flap's epidermis may provide a soft tissue platform upon which to reconstruct a nasal sill or medial canthus. The anterior limb of the created V-Y flap may be folded upon itself rather than amputated to replace disparate aesthetic subunits (Fig. 6.10). Modifications of the V-Y flap's design may improve the versatility of the flap and allow the flap to be used with larger facial wounds and in less traditional locations such as the upper nose and lateral ala Fig. 6.11. With large facial and nonfacial wounds, dual island pedicle flaps may be useful. These double V-Y flaps may be of equal or unequal size. The dual flaps are designed, elevated, and mobilized with the identical techniques previously described for the single V-Y flap.

When immediately adjacent tissue is not suitable for advancement, a donor site removed and not contiguous to the surgical defect may be utilized (the transposition island pedicle flap).[12] With this design, the flap is modified to

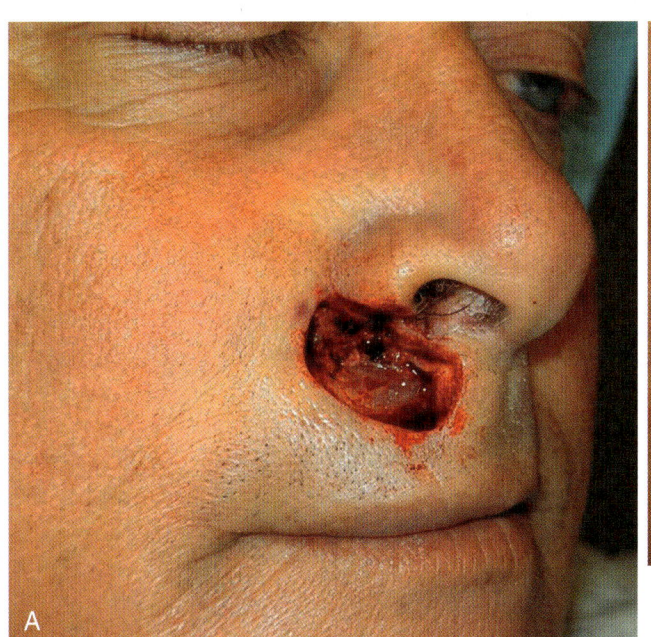
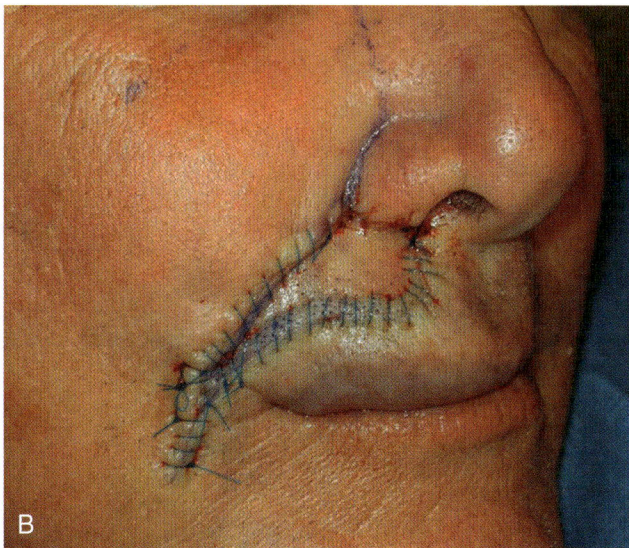
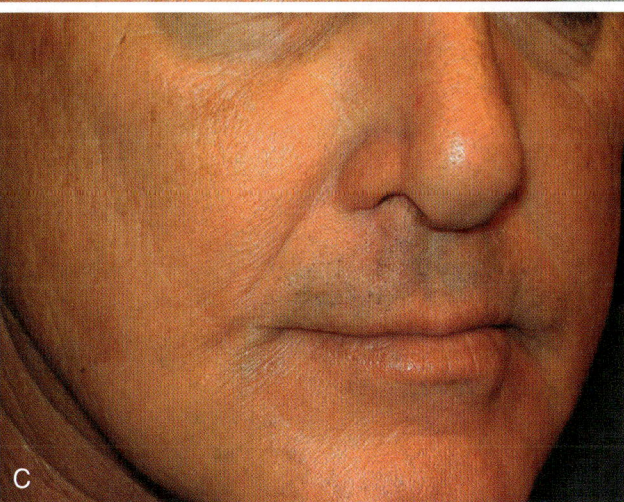

Fig. 6.9 The distal end of the flap may be de-epithelialized to create a base for lateral alar repair. (A) A defect of the upper lip and lateral ala with a significant portion of the ala having been surgically removed. (B) The distal flap's epidermis has been removed and the nasal ala inserted into the portion of the flap that is devoid of epithelium. (C) Postoperative result with no additional procedures.

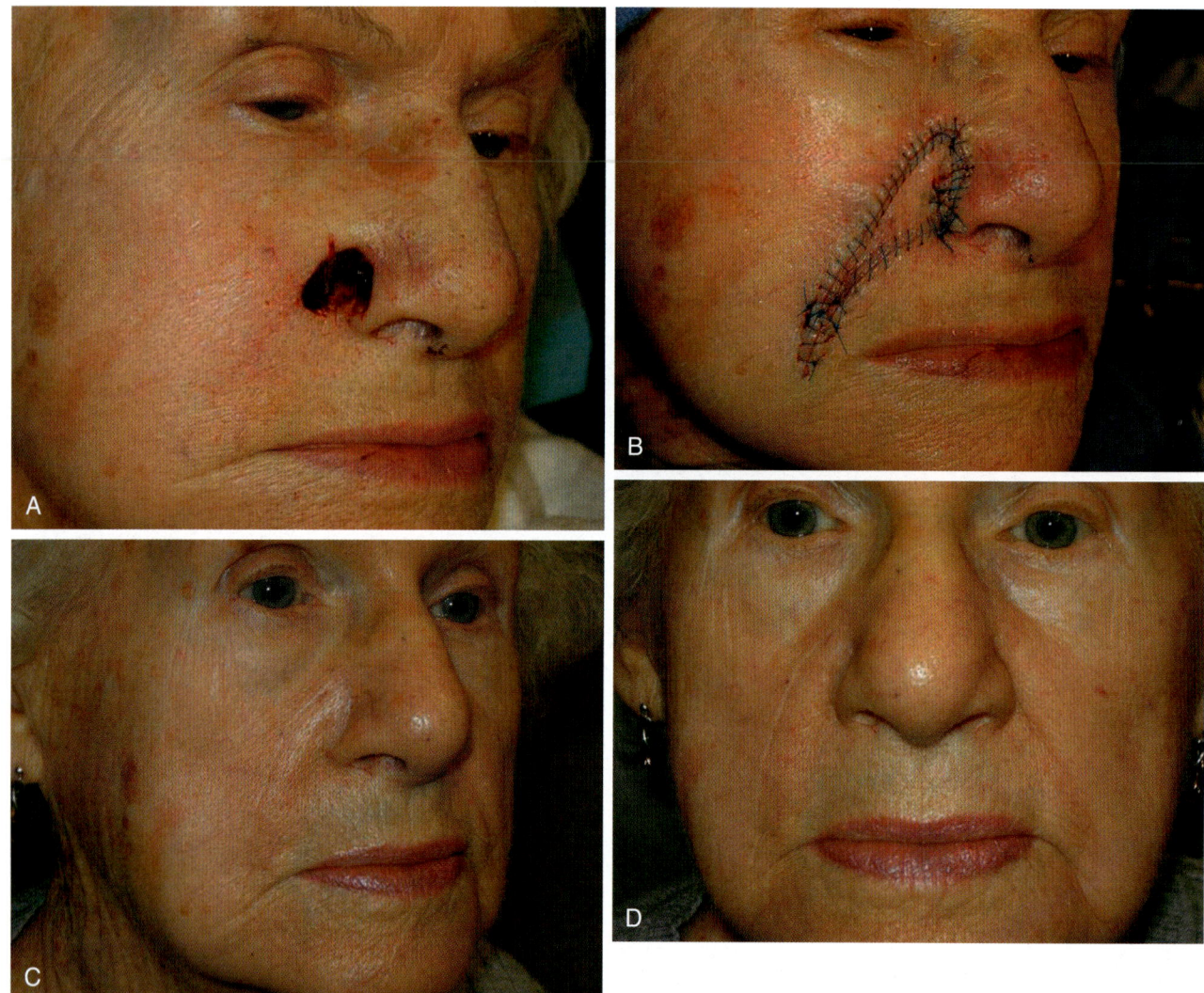

Fig. 6.10 When surgical defects involve more than one cosmetic unit, the V-Y flap may be advanced and folded upon itself to recreate individual aesthetic units. (A) A defect of the upper lip and lateral ala with a significant portion of the ala having been surgically removed. (B) The advancing arm of the flap is retained and rotated upon itself to resurface the nasal subunit. (C, D) Postoperative result with no additional procedures.

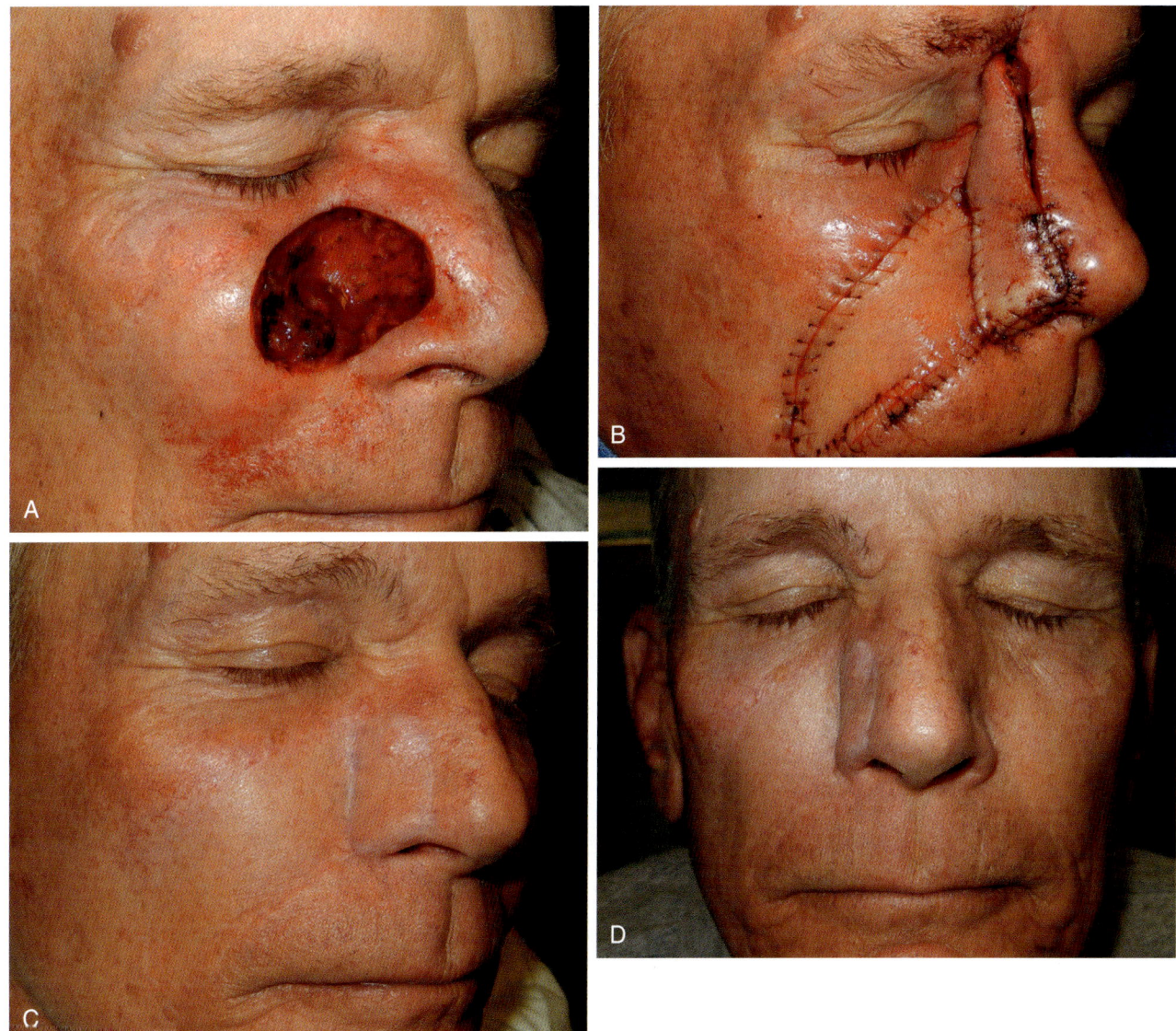

Fig. 6.11 The V-Y flap may be used with other flaps for larger or more complex surgical wounds. (A) A moderate-sized deep defect of the nose and medial cheek. (B) The nasal portion is repaired with a paramedian forehead flap and cartilage graft. The cheek portion of the defect is repaired with a V-Y advancement flap. (C, D) The surgical site seen 1 year postoperatively and prior to tertiary procedures to refine the nasal contour. The V-Y flap has replaced the cheek portion of the defect, with minimal visible scarring.

recruit tissue from a donor site near to but not contiguous with the primary defect. The island flap is thus an interpolated flap much like the paramedian forehead flap or the cheek interpolation flap. This modification of the flap's design may prove to be an ideal solution to the reconstruction of lateral nasal ala or upper nasal dorsum wounds. In both areas, the design of the transposition island flap is similar. The wound's template is transferred to a nearby reservoir of matching skin (usually located at a distance two or more times the diameter of the surgical defect from the wound) (Fig. 6.12). The template is then placed over the proposed donor site and it is confirmed that there is enough tissue laxity to allow interpolation of the flap. The design of the flap can be conceptually compared to the design of the melo-labial interpolation or paramedian forehead flap. However, the epidermis from the proximal portion of the flap (from the flap's origin to the margin of the placed template) is removed, with particular attention to ensure that the subcutaneous tissue with its vascular supply is preserved.[25] The standing cutaneous deformity distal to the template is then removed. The island flap is then elevated with care to protect the deep, proximal vascular pedicle. The flap is then transposed, tunneled, and inset into the primary surgical defect. The proximal portion of the pedicle, lacking an overlying epidermis, is buried and covered with the repair. The donor site of the flap is then repaired. This one-stage repair of defects that have been traditionally repaired with two-stage flaps may prove useful in certain clinical circumstances, such as that of a poor candidate for staged reconstructive efforts or a patient who lives a long distance from the treating physician. However, because the burying of this flap's pedicle can occasionally cause a significant

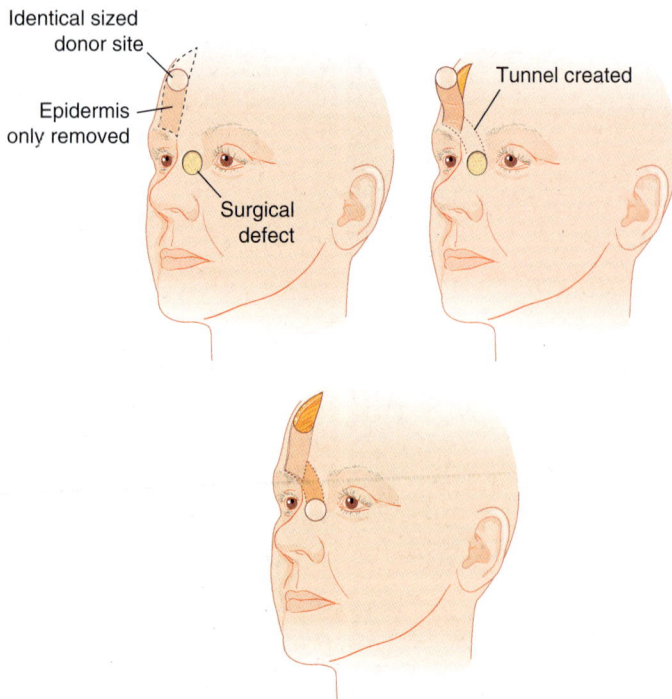

Fig. 6.12 An interpolated flap can be de-epithelialized and tunneled as a single-stage procedure.

elevation/deformity near the flap's pivot point, this modification of the island pedicle flap is unlikely to entirely replace the more classically designed interpolation flaps, since the latter retain a vascular pedicle that is removed in a second surgical procedure performed several weeks after the initial creation of the flap (Figs. 6.13–6.15). This fullness near the flap's pivot point typically subsides with time and with the use of intralesional corticosteroids, but the shadowing and elevation near the flap's donor site may prove persistently troubling to the aesthetically demanding patient. By de-epithelializing the proximal pedicle of this transposition-type island flap, the operative risk of necrosis to the distal portion of the flap may be increased. However, with appropriate flap design and execution, this one-stage repair of defects traditionally repaired with staged interpolation flaps may provide reproducible functional and aesthetic success.

Auricular defects may also represent significant operative challenges. The three-dimensional complexity of the ear and its aesthetic prominence may obviate simpler repair options such as primary closure. Although healing by second intention and skin grafting may afford good postoperative results, larger and more significant surgical wounds may require flap closures to achieve aesthetic and functional success. The V-Y advancement flap has been previously described as a reconstructive method for conchal or scaphoid fossa defects (Figs. 6.16 and 6.17).[18,19] In such a situation, an appropriate donor site overlying the mastoid is selected. A template of the wound is transferred to this mastoid skin and a V-Y flap is incised and elevated as previously described. The flap, with its preserved vascular pedicle, is then passed through a full-thickness defect in the ear. The flap is then inserted into the wound located on the anterior aspect of the ear (the flip-flop flap). The inclusion of musculature in the flap's base significantly improves the flap's vascularity. The flap's donor site can be allowed to granulate or can be repaired with a full-thickness skin graft. This one-stage repair offers excellent postoperative results when used for appropriate surgical defects.

Complications

The vascular support of the V-Y flap and its modified versions is superior to that of more traditional advancement flaps, making necrosis very uncommon with proper surgical technique. The suture lines are relatively long for the size of the repaired surgical defect and may prove visually distracting in selected patients. Proper surgical technique minimizes this risk. If placed at anatomic boundaries or cosmetic subunits borders, this visual impact is lessened significantly.

Both the V-Y flap and the island flap are circumferential flaps that may prove prone to trap-dooring. Fortunately this may be lessened with proper surgical technique, as described previously. If present, a trap-door elevation typically responds well to conservative measures such as massage and intralesional corticosteroids and/or 5-fluorouracil.

In summary, these details regarding the variations of the advancement flap may improve operative success. The well-preserved vascular pedicle provides durability and predictability to the flap. The classically designed V-Y flap with a central pedicle provides unsurpassed results for reconstructing different-sized defects in a variety of anatomic

Text continued on p. 98

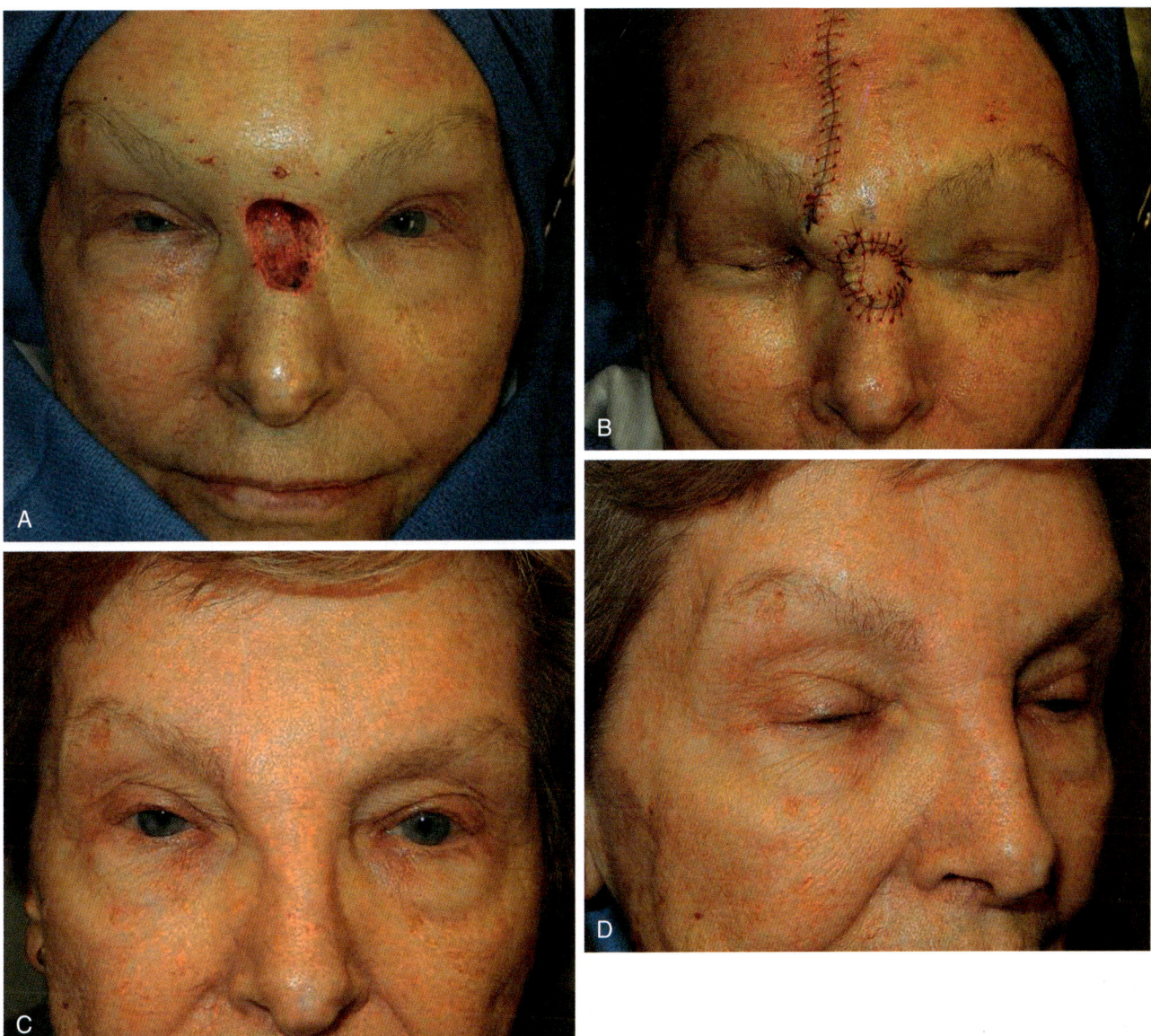

Fig. 6.13 Interpolated island flaps may be useful in situations where conventional interpolated (paramedian forehead or cheek interpolation) flaps may be less than ideal. (A) A deep defect of the nasal root with the nasal bone exposed, devoid of periosteum. (B) A paramedian forehead flap is designed with the proximal portion of the flap's epidermis removed; the flap is then further incised and elevated. The flap is tunneled; it exits the superior border of the surgical defect and is sutured into place. The flap's donor site on the forehead is repaired. (C, D) The postoperative result with no additional procedures shows minimal fullness of the nasion at the site of the retained and buried proximal flap pedicle.

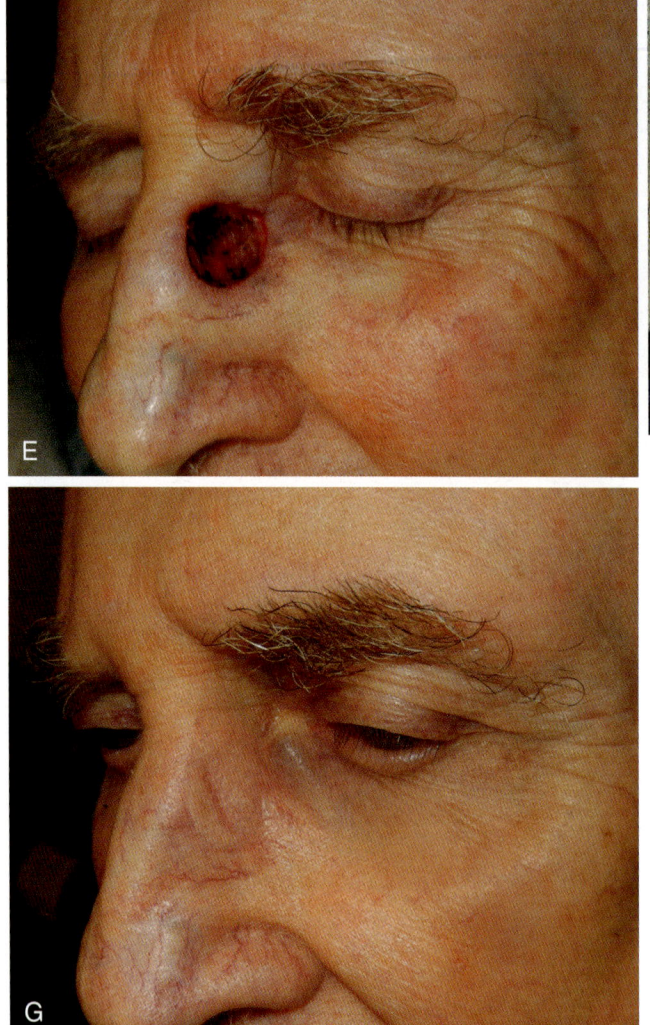
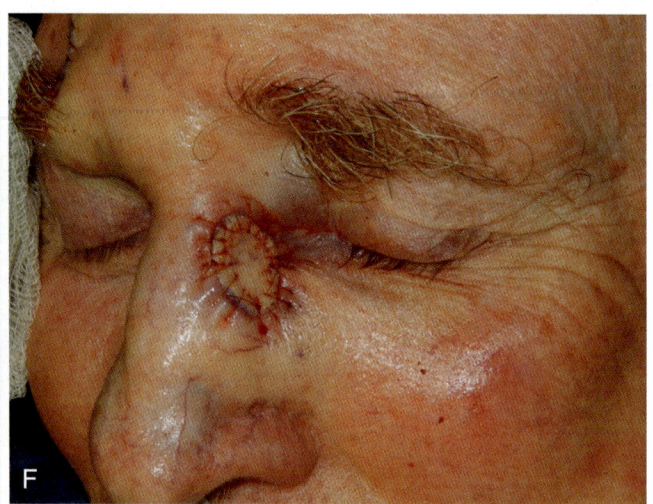

Fig. 6.13, cont'd (E–G) A medial canthal defect repaired with the identical technique.

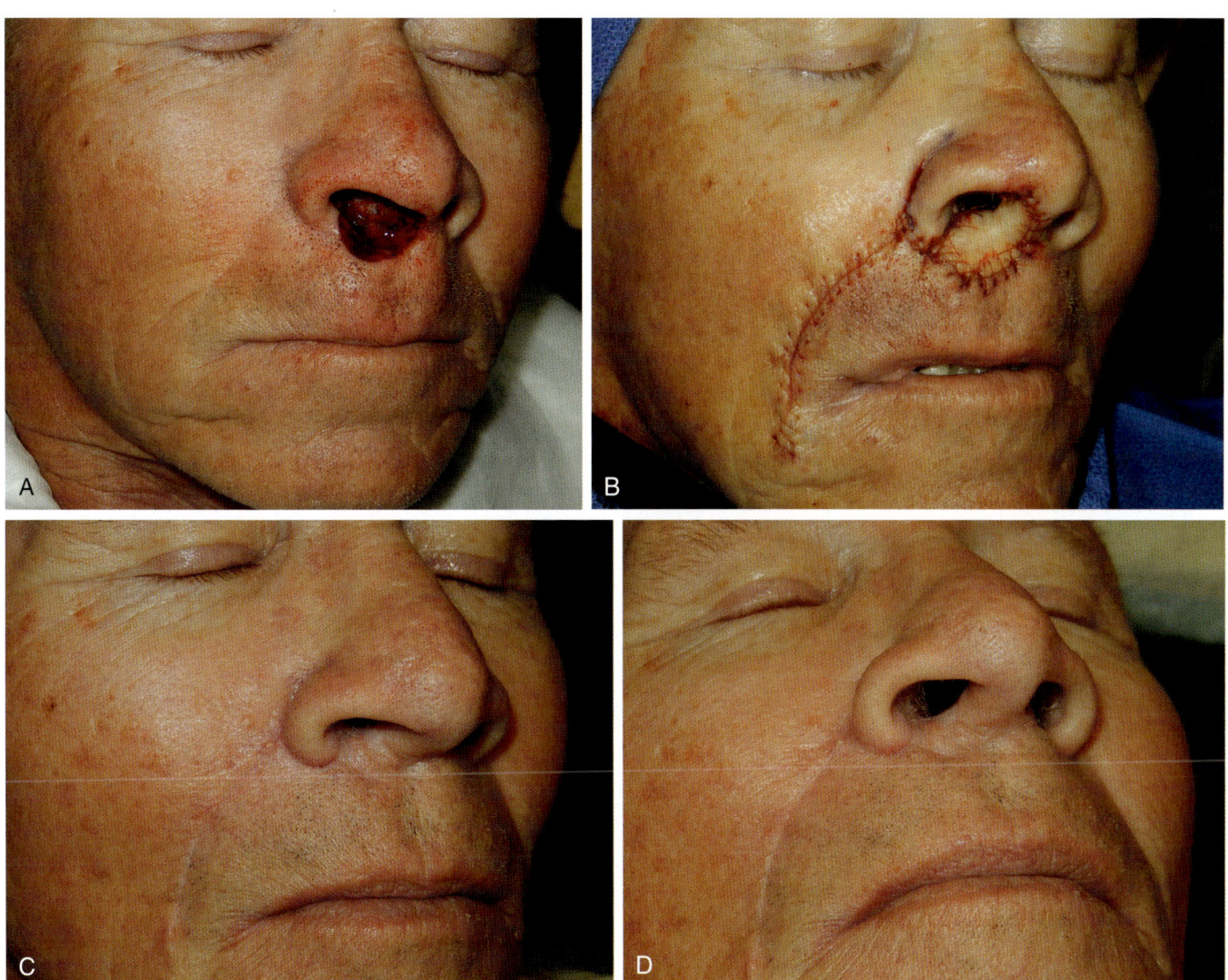

Fig. 6.14 (A, B) A defect of the nasal sill repaired with a tunneled island flap designed in the same way as a cheek interpolation flap, except that the proximal portion of the flap's epidermis is removed and the flap is tunneled into place. (C, D) The postoperative result with no additional procedures.

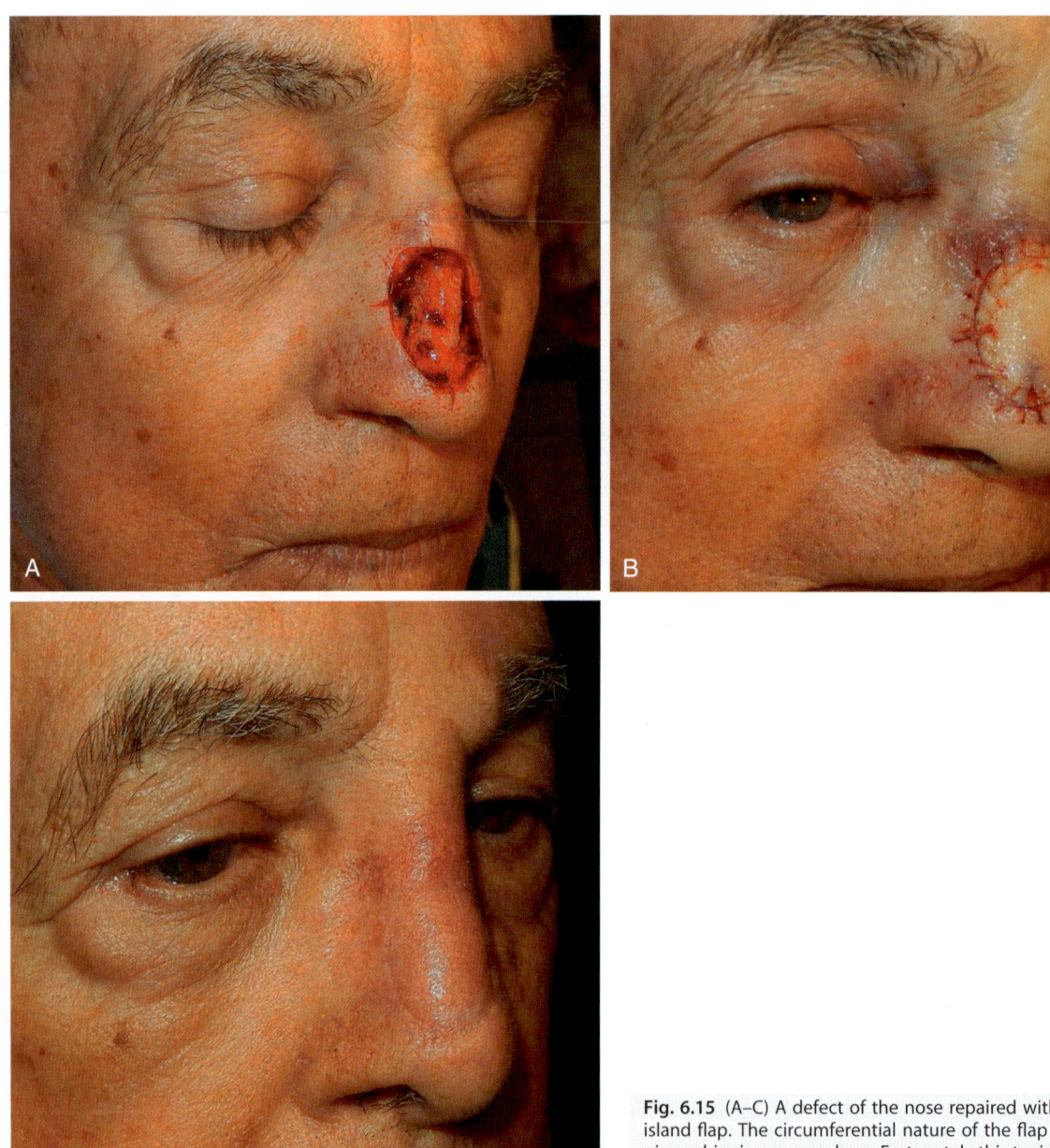

Fig. 6.15 (A–C) A defect of the nose repaired with an interpolated island flap. The circumferential nature of the flap predisposes it to pin-cushioning as seen here. Fortunately this typically resolves with massage, intralesional corticosteroid, and time.

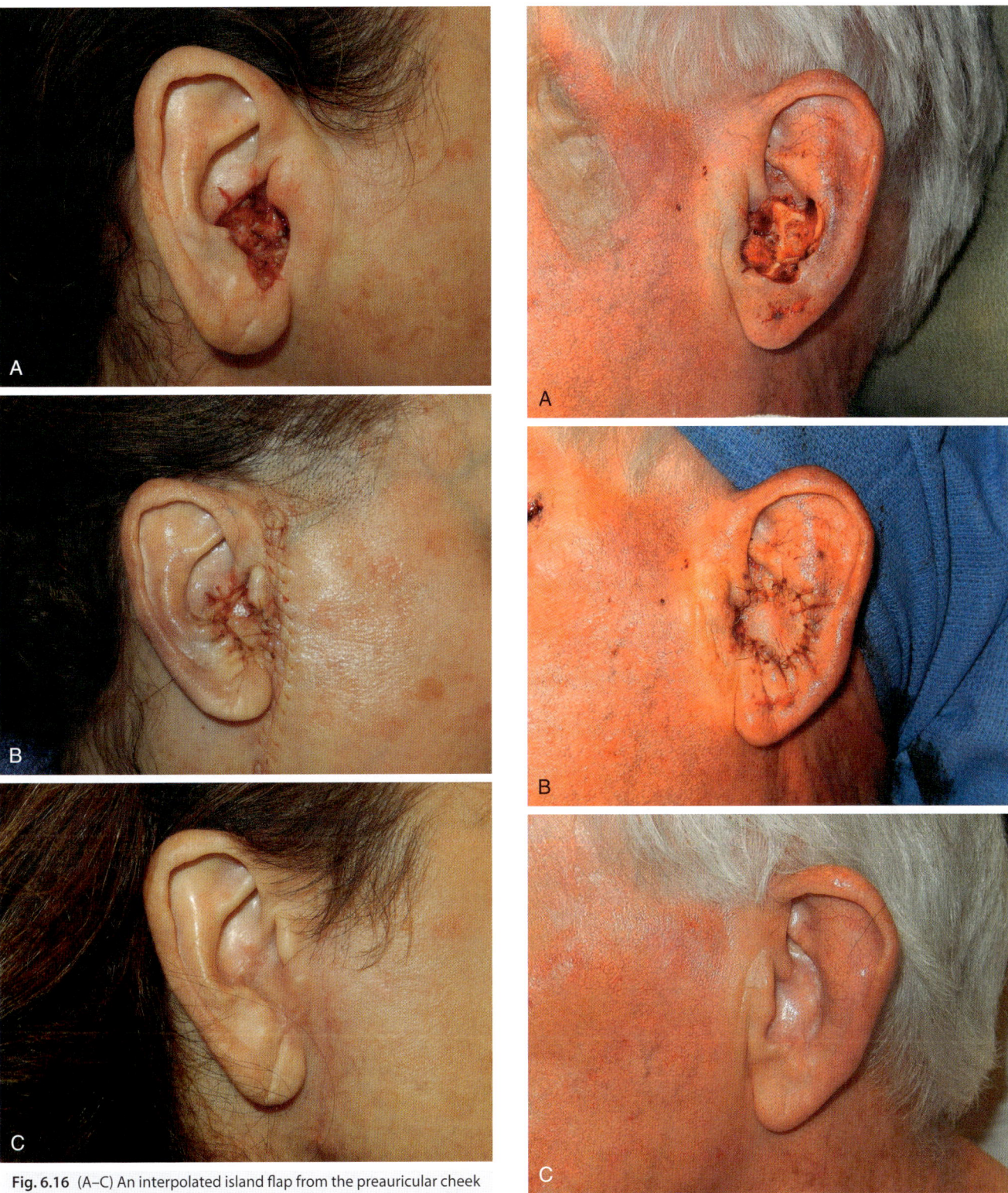

Fig. 6.16 (A–C) An interpolated island flap from the preauricular cheek used to repair a defect of the concha, antitragus, and outer auditory canal. The flap has healed with no stenosis of the canal and minimal donor scarring.

Fig. 6.17 (A–C) Mastoid pull-through flap (flip-flop flap) is useful for repairing defects of the concha, where skin grafting or healing by second intention are not options. The flap is incised, centered about the retroauricular sulcus, and advanced through a created full-thickness incision in the conchal cartilage; it is then sutured into place.

locations. Modifications of the flap's design may expand the flap's usefulness in repairing defects of the nose, ear, and other locations. With proper design and execution, the flap rewards the reconstructive surgeon with excellent cosmesis. The flap's carefully identified and dissected vascular supply makes flap necrosis unlikely. If the flap is bulky, it may be subject to pin-cushioning. If the flap is designed and executed with care, this is a very uncommon problem. If the skin's mobility near the flap's origination or insertion points is misjudged, excessive secondary tissue movement may result in anatomic distortion and aesthetically inferior results. These variations of the advancement flap (V-Y flap and transposed island flap) should occupy a significant place in the reconstructive surgeon's armamentarium.

References

1. Cook JL, Perone JB. A prospective evaluation of the incidence of complications associated with Mohs micrographic surgery. *Arch Dermatol.* 2003;139:143-152.
2. Goding GS, Hom DB. Skin flap physiology. In: Baker SR, Swanson NA, eds. *Local Flaps in Facial Reconstruction.* St. Louis: Mosby; 1995:15-30.
3. Zitelli JA, Brodland DG. A regional approach to reconstruction of the upper lip. *J Dermatol Surg Oncol.* 1991;17:143-148.
4. Field L. The subcutaneously bipedicled island flap. *J Dermatol Surg Oncol.* 1980;6:454-460.
5. Ono I, Gunji H, Sato M, Kaneko F. Use of the oblique island flap in excision of small facial tumors. *Plast Reconst Surg.* 1993;91:1245-1251.
6. Papadopoulos DJ, Trinei FA. Superiorly based nasalis myocutaneous island pedicle flap with bilevel undermining for nasal tip and supratip reconstruction. *Dermatol Surg.* 1999;25:530-536.
7. Narsete TA. V-Y advancement flap in upper lip reconstruction. *Plast Reconstr Surg.* 2000;105:2464-2466.
8. Davis WH. Sideburn reconstruction with an arterial V-Y hair bearing scalp flap after excision of basal cell carcinoma. *Plast Reconst Surg.* 2000;106:94-97.
9. Hatoko M, Kunahara M, Shiba A, et al. Earlobe reconstruction using a subcutaneous island pedicle flap after resection of earlobe keloid. *Dermatol Surg.* 1998;24:257-261.
10. Kaufman AJ, Grekin RC. Repair of central upper lip (philtral) surgical defects with island pedicle flaps. *Dermatol Surg.* 1996;22:1003-1007.
11. Gardner ES, Goldberg LH. Eyebrow reconstruction with the subcutaneous island pedicle flap. *Dermatol Surg.* 2002;28:921-925.
12. Hairston BR, Nguyen TH. Innovations in the island pedicle flap for cutaneous facial reconstruction. *Dermatol Surg.* 2003;29:378-385.
13. Carvalho LM, Ramos RR, Santos ID, et al. V-Y advancement flap for the reconstruction of partial and full thickness defects of the upper lip. *Scand J Plast Reconst Surg Hand Surg.* 2002;36:28-33.
14. Yiomaz M, Menders A, Barutcu A. Submental artery island flap for reconstruction of the lower and mid-face. *Ann Surg.* 1997;39:30-35.
15. Yildirim S, Aköz T, Akan M, Avci G. Nasolabial V-Y advancement for closures of the midface defects. *Dermatol Surg.* 2001;27:656-658.
16. Guerrerosantos J. Frontalis musculocutaneous island flap for coverage of forehead of defect. *Plast Reconst Surg.* 2000;105:18-22.
17. Kim KS, Huang JH, Kim DY, et al. Eyebrow island flap for reconstruction of a partial eyebrow defect. *Ann Plast Surg.* 2002;48:315-317.
18. Humpreys TR, Goldberg LA, Niemer DR. The postauricular (revolving door) island pedicle flap revisited. *Dermatol Surg.* 1996;22:148-150.
19. Fader DJ, Johnson TM. Ear reconstruction utilizing the subcutaneous island pedicle (flip flop) flap. *Dermatol Surg.* 1999;25:94-96.
20. Pontes L, Ribeiro M, Vrancks JS. Guimadaes J. The new bilaterally pedicled V-Y advancement flap for facial reconstruction. *Plast Reconst Surg.* 2002;109:1870-1874.
21. Field LM. Undermining subcutaneous island flaps. *Arch Dermatol.* 1988;124:20-27.
22. Chan ST. A technique of undermining a V-Y subcutaneous island flap to maximize advancement. *Br J Plast Surg.* 1988;41:62-67.
23. Otley CC, Roenigk RK. Surgical pearl: preparing the defect for an island pedicle flap. *J Am Acad Dermatol.* 1997;2:257-258.
24. Cook JL. Commentary on: Yildirim S, Akoz T, Akan M, Avci G. Nasolabial V-Y advancement for closures of the midface defects. *Dermatol Surg.* 2001;27:656-658, 658–660.
25. Park SS. The single-stage forehead flap in nasal reconstruction. *Arch Facial Plast Surg.* 2002;4:32-36.

Videos for this chapter can be found online by accessing the accompanying Expert Consult website.

7 Transposition Flaps

ASHISH C. BHATIA, MD, JOE OVERMAN, MD, and THOMAS E. ROHRER, MD

Flap Design and Considerations

A transposition flap is a random-pattern flap that borrows skin laxity from an adjacent area to fill a defect in an area with little or no skin laxity and redirects the tension vectors of the closure. This technique is especially valuable in preventing the distortion of free margins. The flap gains its name from the "transposition" or movement of a flap of donor tissue up and over normal/uninvolved tissue to its resting place within the surgical defect. The flap movement is rotational in nature from its pedicle base to the surgical defect. The flap is tethered to a pedicle and rotates into position. Care must be taken in the design of the flap as to not overrotate or put excessive tension on the flap such that the vascular pedicle is compromised.

Transposition flaps have several advantages over other types of flaps. They redistribute and redirect tension, assisting in the closure of defects that would otherwise be closed under unacceptably high tension or distort a nearby free margin, creating functional or aesthetic impairment. Transposition flaps are generally smaller than comparable repairs using advancement or rotational flaps. Because transposition flaps, like all local flaps, use adjacent tissue, they generally offer an excellent color and textural match to the recipient site. The geometric design used in transposition flaps eliminates long suture lines, which can otherwise distort the natural curvature and appearance of the repair region. The geometric broken line scar may also be thought of as a disadvantage of transposition flaps because all of the flaps' lines cannot be placed directly in relaxed skin tension lines or cosmetic unit junctions.

The most common transposition flaps in cutaneous surgery include rhombic flaps (single-lobed flaps), bilobed and trilobed flaps, and banner flaps. Knowledge of the tissue dynamics used in these three basic transposition flaps can be carried over to the planning and execution of numerous flap variations, including note flaps, trilobed flaps, and tetralobed flaps.[1] Although technically complex in their design and execution, in the hands of a skilled surgeon, transposition flaps can produce excellent aesthetic and functional surgical outcomes.

Rhombic and Single-Lobed Transposition Flaps

DESIGN

The classic rhombic flap, first described by Limberg in 1963,[2] is a single-lobed transposition flap that creates a secondary defect perpendicular to the primary defect that, when closed, provides tissue to close the primary defect and redirects the tension vector 90 degrees.[3] This design greatly decreases the wound tension on the primary defect.[4] Subsequent design modifications by DuFourmentel[5] and Webster[6] enabled more tension sharing between the primary and secondary defects by reducing the angles and sizes of the flaps' primary lobes.[7]

In planning a classic rhombic flap, the surgeon converts the primary defect, which in practice is usually round or oval, into a four-sided parallelogram centered on the middle of a round defect or on the midline of the short axis of an oval defect,[8–12] with each side of equal length and tip angles equal to 60 and 120 degrees. (Fig. 7.1).[13] It is important to take the convexities and concavities of the face into account when making measurements.[8] Note[14] and banner flaps[15] follow the same principle; however, they arise tangentially off a round or oval defect (Fig. 7.2).[16]

This rhombic shape forms the recipient site for the flap, as well as the template upon which the required incisions are planned. In the classic design (see Fig. 7.1), the flap's incision lines are drawn by extending a line (line AB) outward from one of the obtuse tips for a length equal to that of one side of the rhombus. From the free end of the extending line (line AB), a second line (line BC) is drawn parallel to and equal in length to one of the near sides of the rhombus. The tip angle of the flap's primary lobe in this configuration is 60 degrees. The incised flap is then lifted and transposed into place. The vector of maximal wound closure tension is thus redirected from that of closing the primary defect to that of closing the new secondary defect created in the execution of the flap. This allows for an effective 90-degree redirection of the tension vector.

Although the classic rhombic transposition flap can be designed and executed off of the long axis of the rhombus, there are two advantages to designing it off of the short axis of the defect.[17] First, this design keeps the flap as small as possible while filling the primary defect completely. Second, the design minimizes the arc through which the flap must rotate to reach the defect.[18,19] There are four possible flap designs off of the short axis for any rhombic defect (Fig. 7.2). The best choice among the four flap configurations depends on the adjacent anatomic structures, the adjacent skin type, and where the resulting scar line will be best hidden. The optimal placement of the flap's closure lines are planned according to the adjacent relaxed skin tension and/or cosmetic unit junction lines. Because the majority of the wound closure tension is placed on the closure of the secondary defect, the secondary defect's closure is usually designed to be aligned with the relaxed skin tension lines. The tissue redundancy at the base of the primary defect created by the rotation of the transposition flap is removed

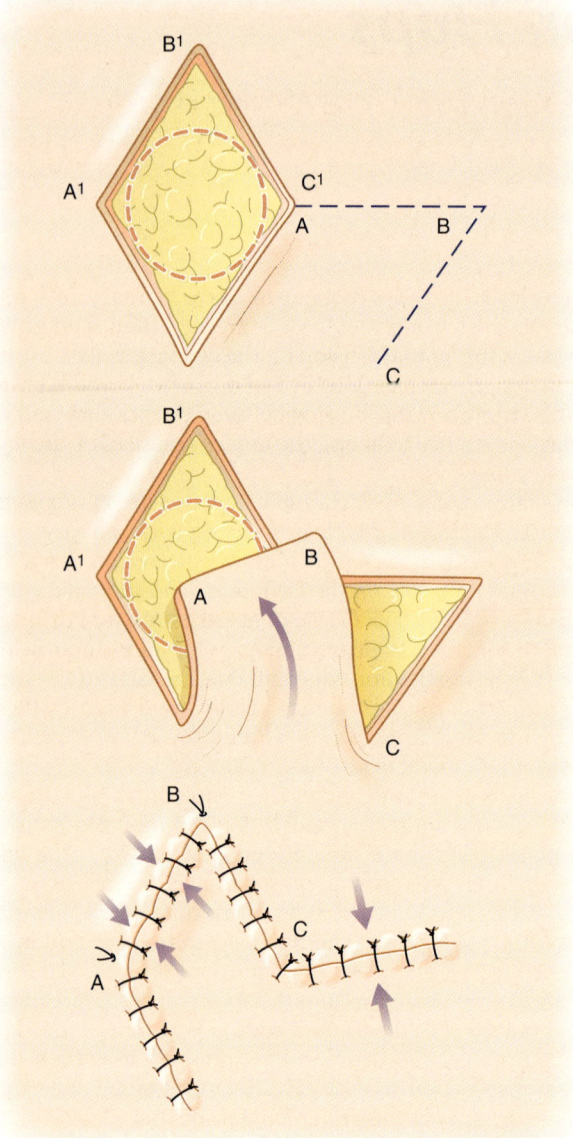

Fig. 7.1 The classic rhombic flap.

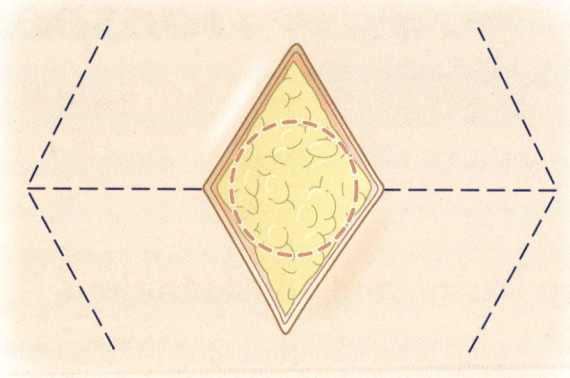

Fig. 7.2 Four possible configurations of rhombic flaps drawn off of the short axis of the rhombus-shaped defect.

with trimming of a triangle in the area of the flap's pivot point. This area is known as Burow triangle. As a common alternative approach the tip of the transposed tissue is rounded to fit a circular defect, or the defect may be squared off to accommodate the angular flap. This choice can be made based upon which option is likely to yield the optimal aesthetic result (Fig. 7.3).

A thorough understanding of wound closure tension vectors is essential to the planning, execution, and outcome of any closure. The primary tension component of a classic rhombic flap occurs with the closure of the secondary defect. A second set of tension forces is generated at the tip of the flap when it is moved into the primary defect. These forces are due to resistance to movement at the flap pedicle and effective shortening of the length of the flap during the rotation into the recipient site. Dzubow has described these forces as pivotal restraint.[20] The thicker/stiffer the skin and the greater the angle of rotation, the greater the pivotal restraint. Securing the flap tip to the far end of the recipient site under great tension can lead to tip ischemia and necrosis. Therefore rhombic flaps, as with all single-lobed transposition flaps, should be designed such that their angle of rotation is 90 degrees or less.[16]

There are two modifications of flap design that can be used in certain situations to minimize the shortening of the flap and reduce the tension at the flap tip. When the leading edge and the secondary limb of the flap's primary lobe are extended/lengthened, the flap is slightly enlarged (Fig. 7.4). This lengthening can compensate for the inevitable shortening that results from pivotal restraint at the flap's base. Lengthening the flap by this method will help to ensure the flap rests in the primary defect without undue tension at its tip. An alternate method to lengthen the flap and minimize tip tension at closure is to design the flap with a slightly more obtuse angle (greater than 120 degrees) at the flap's origination point (Fig. 7.5). This design decreases the degree of rotation necessary during flap execution and subsequently reduces pivotal restraint. Wide undermining around the flap also assists in the redistribution of tension vectors and contractile forces during the healing phase.

Z-PLASTY EFFECT OF TRANSPOSITION FLAPS

All transposition flaps have the ability to induce vertical Z-plasty-like lengthening of the repair area; this lengthening can be decreased by the addition of additional lobes.[21] In other words, the radius of the arc of rotation is greater with fewer lobes. By going from a single lobe to bilobed repair, an additional Z-plasty is effectively added. The result of this is the central limbs of the Z-plasty and the radius (or vertical height) of the repair are shortened as compared with a single-lobe repair. Likewise, in the same fashion the trilobed further shortens the surgical repair relative to the bilobed flap with the addition of another Z-plasty.[22] The Z-plasties are easier to visualize if one imagines the lobes of the flap as triangles. The secondary lobe width is often reduced as much as 10% to 15% because this Z-plasty–lengthening effect reduces the size of the secondary defect.[8]

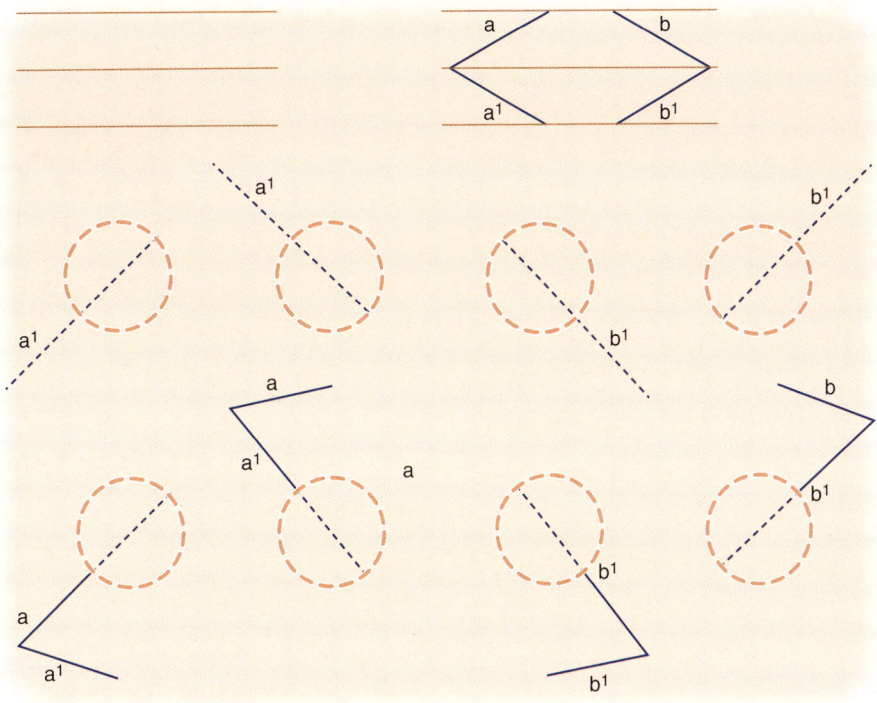

Fig. 7.3 Options for optimal placement of rhombic flaps.

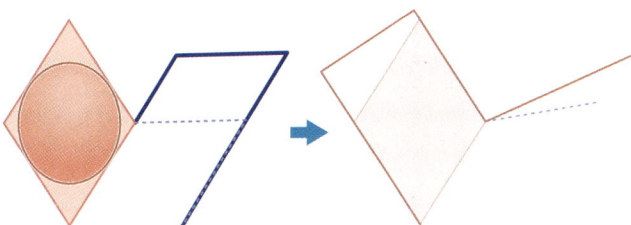

Fig. 7.4 Lengthening the flap is one option for planning a closure with minimal tip tension.

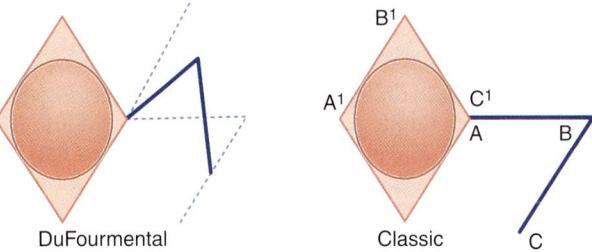

Fig. 7.6 The DuFourmentel flap. Note the narrowed tip angle and more obtuse leading edge angle compared with the classic rhombic flap.

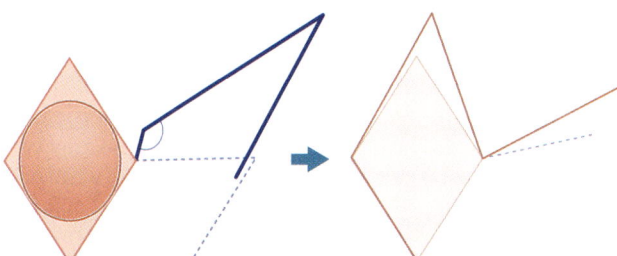

Fig. 7.5 Increasing the angle of the flap also acts to minimize tension and lengthen the flap.

Modified Rhombic Flaps

DUFOURMENTEL FLAP

This modification of the classic rhombic transposition flap narrows the angle of the tip of the secondary defect and creates a shorter arc of rotation for the flap. This allows easier closure of the secondary defect and some sharing of the tension between the primary and secondary defects. As in the classic rhombic flap, the DuFourmentel variant of the rhombic flap is designed by extending the first line from the short axis of the rhombic defect (Fig. 7.6). However, the angle at which the first line is extended from the rhombus differs from the classic rhombic flap in that it bisects the angle formed by the first line of the classic rhombic flap (which extends straight from the short axis of the rhomboid defect) and the line formed by extending one of the sides of the rhomboid from the same corner. The length of the first line is equal to that of a side length of the rhomboid. The second line originates from the free end of the first line and is drawn parallel to the long axis of the rhomboid. This second line's orientation results in a slightly widened pedicle base, a decrease in the tip volume of the flap, a decrease in the amount of movement necessary to execute the flap, and the introduction of some degree of tissue advancement

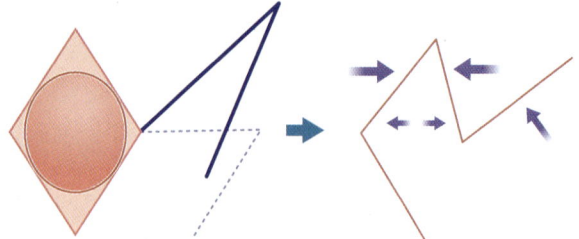

Fig. 7.7 The Webster modification to the rhombic flap.

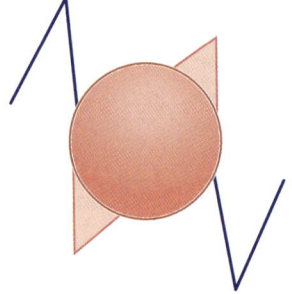

Fig. 7.8 Note the two flaps designed to fill the single defect, thus effectively sharing the tension.

along the long axis of the rhomboid defect. In most cases a tissue redundancy at the base of the leading edge of the flap is generated; this should be removed by excising a slightly larger "dog-ear" at the base of the flap.

The oblique orientation of the leading edge of the DuFourmentel flap relieves some of the pivotal restraint at the flap's base, resulting in additional lateral tip tension instead of vertical tip tension seen with the classic rhombic flap design. This allows use of the DuFourmentel flap in situations where lateral tension is more acceptable than vertical tension.

WEBSTER 30-DEGREE ANGLE FLAP

The Webster modification of the rhombic transposition flap makes the angle of the flap even more acute than the DuFourmentel variant and allows for even greater tension sharing between the primary and secondary defects.[23] A Webster 30-degree angle flap is planned similarly to the DuFourmentel flap, with the exception that the distal tip of the flap is designed to have an angle of 30 degrees (Fig. 7.7). This more acute angle produces a slimmer design and narrower pedicle. The Webster design of the rhombic flap also frequently incorporates an M-plasty in the closure of the Burow triangle excision at the flap's base. The flap width is approximately 50% of that of the defect; thus the flap relieves only approximately half of the tension from the primary defect. Closure of the flap is therefore partially dependent upon secondary motion at the site of the surgical defect. This design modification is used in situations in which some laxity exists in the horizontal axis of the rhombus-shaped defect. Given that more tension is placed on the primary defect with this design, care must be taken not to distort adjacent anatomic structures.

DOUBLE 30-DEGREE ANGLE FLAP

Another variation of the rhombic transposition flap uses two flaps to borrow laxity from either side of a defect. Essentially resembling a series of Z-plasties, the double 30-degree angle flap is planned by drawing two 30-degree angle flaps, one from each short axis of the rhombus and in opposite directions (Fig. 7.8).

RHOMBIC FLAP EXECUTION: FLAP MOBILIZATION AND KEY SUTURES

As with all reconstructive procedures, transposition flaps should be designed while patients are in upright (or near upright) positions. This places the forces of gravity on the face in the typical resting position, allowing more appropriate flap planning. In addition, the defect should not be overly distorted with local anesthetic before designing the flap. The tissue surrounding the defect is then manipulated with a probing hand, and a determination of the local tissue laxity and the adjacent anatomic structure mobility is made. The most appropriate flap is drawn out on the skin with a sterile surgical marker. Even the most experienced surgeons typically mark their lines of incision before reconstruction. The old carpentry adage holds true in reconstructive surgery: "measure twice, cut once." After designing the flap, anesthetizing the area, and prepping and draping, skin incisions oriented directly perpendicular to the surface of the skin are made along the flap's proposed lines to the depth of the subcutaneous tissue.

It is very important to make certain that all skin edges are squared off prior to closure. Leaving beveled tissue at the corners or edges places unnecessary force on the tissue edges during closure and prevents proper wound edge eversion. In most cases, it is preferable to remove the redundant Burow triangle at the pivot point of the flap before insetting the flap. Although there are certain cases in which the exact position of the redundant triangle is not as important, this triangle is usually designed to lie in a predetermined location to optimize the final aesthetic result.

The flap is raised at the desired plane with sharp dissection. The plane of dissection is based upon both the anatomic location and the depth of the primary defect. The defect, flap, and undermined tissue should all be of the same relative thickness. The proper undermining plane may vary from the superficial subcutaneous fat to just above the periosteum, depending on the anatomic location and depth of defect. The entire area surrounding the flap and the primary defect is undermined widely to fully mobilize the borrowed tissue and to dissipate contractile forces over a wider area during the healing phase. Failing to sufficiently undermine concentrates the forces of contracture during wound healing on the scar itself, and this may result in depressed wound edges and/or pin-cushioning of the flap.

After undermining, the entire defect, the adjacent undermined zone, and the underside of the flap should be visually inspected for hemorrhage. This may be facilitated with the use of a skin hook, which assists in reflecting the flap and free edges without introducing unnecessary trauma to the epidermis. To better visualize bleeding at the recesses of the

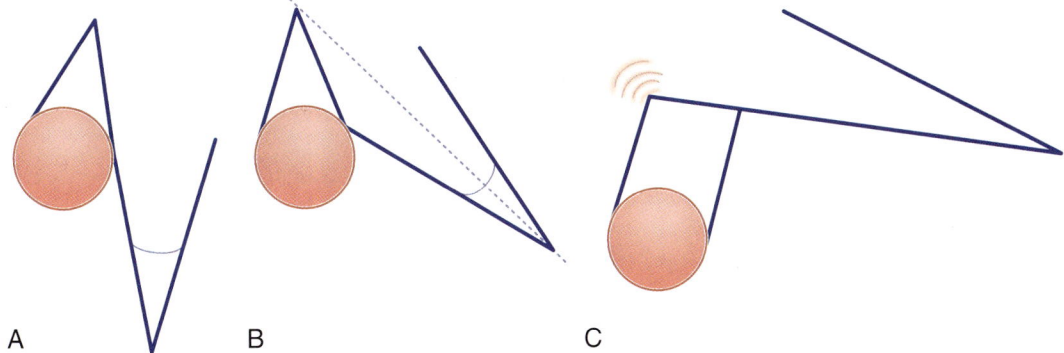

Fig. 7.9 Examples of banner flaps with increasing angles from A to C. Note the greater redundancy at the pivot point of the flap with the largest angle (C).

undermined tissue, the surgeon should push the skin beyond the wound's edge back toward the defect, with the fourth finger of the hand holding the skin hook. It is important to get sufficient and precise hemostasis. Postoperative bleeding and hematoma formation can often result in an unfavorable aesthetic result. Similarly, excessive use of tissue cautery, especially at the wound edges, may necrose tissue and produce widened scars. A fine Bishop-Harmon forceps may be used to grasp any visualized bleeding vessel and serve as an appropriate conductor for a very short burst of electrocautery current. This maneuver helps minimize necrosis of the surrounding area by eliminating widespread, indiscriminate use of electrocautery. Charred tissue needlessly increases healing time and may serve as a nidus for infection.

After hemostasis has been achieved, the flap is lifted and transposed over the intervening skin into the primary defect. At this point, the secondary defect can be closed by approximating the dermal edges with a tension-bearing stitch. This stitch is executed by placing a buried vertical mattress suture using a slowly dissolving suture material, such as Vicryl. Proper suturing technique cannot be stressed enough. Undyed suture material is usually selected to minimize visibility in the event that the suture is placed too superficially or is brought to the surface during the healing phase as a "spitting suture."

Obtaining good wound eversion and wound edge approximation is absolutely critical in achieving aesthetic results. Without these, closures have little chance of being relatively imperceptible after healing has been completed. The optimal time to obtain proper wound eversion is during the placement of the subcutaneous sutures. A properly placed buried vertical mattress suture is one of the skilled reconstructive surgeon's best tools. It everts the closure line and takes the pressure off the healing wound edge, placing it in the dermis slightly distant to the edge. This allows the wound to heal under little tension and leaves the thinnest possible scar line. After the wound has been everted and closed under minimal tension, cutaneous sutures are meticulously placed to keep the wound edges fully approximated during the initial healing phase. These cutaneous sutures may be fast-absorbing or nonabsorbable materials. If nonabsorbable suture material is used, the sutures, when used in areas of the head and neck, should be examined and removed at 5 to 7 days following the procedure.

Other Transposition Flaps

BANNER-TYPE FLAPS

Banner-type flaps are random-pattern, finger-shaped flaps that, like other transposition flaps, tap into adjacent skin to borrow laxity and cover a defect. Banner transposition flaps produce longer, linear secondary scars typically placed at the junction of two cosmetic units, allowing the surgeon to optimally camouflage a long scar.[24]

The fundamental design of the banner flap consists of a finger-shaped flap drawn with a width equal to the width of the defect and a length equal to the distance from the pivot point to the far edge of the defect (Fig. 7.9). The flap is transposed and rotated in an arc around the pivot point to fill the defect. Because the banner flap is a long random pattern flap with a narrow pedicle, the risk of vascular compromise may be high if the flap is too long or if it is harvested from an area of minimal vascularity. Unless the flap is based on a larger-caliber artery, the flap is typically designed to rotate through an angle of 60 degrees to 120 degrees instead of the originally described 180 degrees. In either scenario, a tissue redundancy is generated by the rotational motion of the flap. When removing this redundancy, the excision should be designed in a direction away from the pedicle of the flap to avoid narrowing the pedicle of the flap even further. This will minimize the risk of compromising the blood flow to the flap and maximize its viability.

BANNER TRANSPOSITION FLAP MOBILIZATION AND APPLICATION

Although not commonly used, typical locations for use of the banner flap include the nasal ala, the superior helix of the ear, and the medial anterior ear. At the nasal ala and inferior lateral side wall, a classic nasolabial transposition flap, a variant of a banner flap, can be designed, with the resulting scar hidden within the nasolabial fold (Fig. 7.10). Although this flap has been maligned for blunting the nasofacial groove, when used properly in the appropriate patient, it offers an excellent reconstructive option for some nasal defects. The flap should be designed so the closure of the secondary defect is hidden in the nasolabial fold but does not come too close to the inferior lateral ala, where blunting

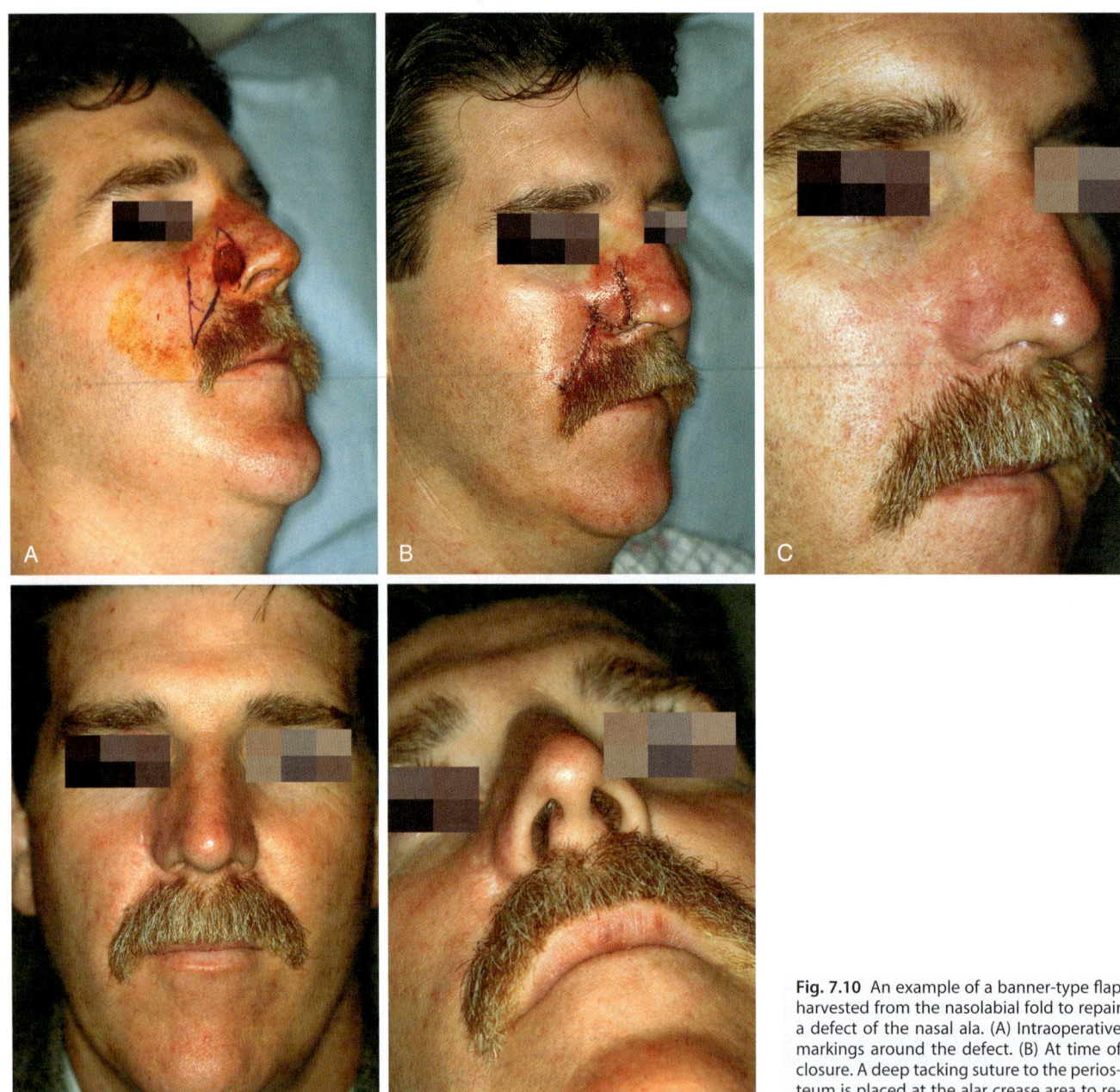

Fig. 7.10 An example of a banner-type flap harvested from the nasolabial fold to repair a defect of the nasal ala. (A) Intraoperative markings around the defect. (B) At time of closure. A deep tacking suture to the periosteum is placed at the alar crease area to re-create the alar groove. (C–E) Appearance 3 months after closure.

of the isthmus (the triangle of flat skin where the upper lip, ala, and nasolabial fold meet) could occur. The redundant Burow triangle superior to the primary defect should be designed to leave the resultant scar on the lateral nasal sidewall.

When the flap is raised, the cheek donor site should be widely undermined. Care should be taken not to harvest more adipose tissue than necessary. If too much adipose is taken while harvesting the flap, the nasolabial fold will be flattened, resulting in cheek asymmetry. When the flap is transposed into place, it should be anchored to the nasal sidewall with a periosteal suture. This reduces tension on the flap. In addition, a tacking suture from the underside of the flap to the area where the alar crease is located on the recipient bed helps re-create the alar groove. This is critical in achieving an aesthetic result with this flap.

The flap is then appropriately trimmed and thinned to match the defect. If this is done before the tacking sutures, it is easy to trim too much off the end, not taking into account the extra length required to re-create the alar crease. Conversely, not trimming and thinning the flap enough may lead to pin-cushioning.

To repair defects of the superior helix, a banner flap can be taken from behind the superior aspect of the ear. The secondary defect is closed along the postauricular sulcus, and the flap is transposed into place along the helix. As with any repair of the helix, it is important to remember the convex nature of the area and to allot enough tissue to

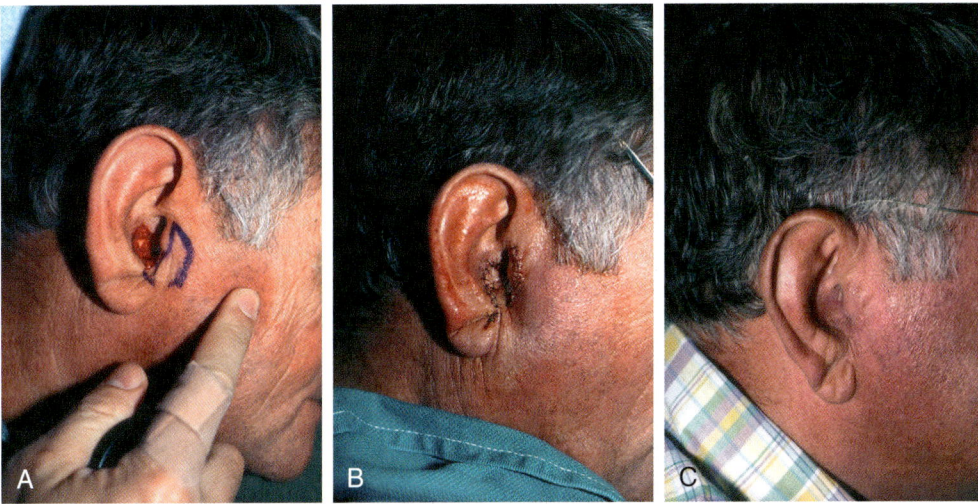

Fig. 7.11 Repair of a conchal bowl ear lesion with a banner-type transposition flap. (A) Defect with banner flap drawn. (B) Banner flap inset and sutured. (C) Flap at 3-month follow-up.

re-create this. A simple flat measurement across the defect will not give the true volume of tissue required for reconstruction. By using a slightly wider (not thicker) flap, the forces of contraction during healing will usually elevate the flap slightly in the middle and re-create the convex nature of the helix. Attaining proper wound edge eversion with well-placed buried subcutaneous mattress sutures is critical at the distal aspect of the flap where it joins the helix. If this edge is not everted properly, it will usually contract and appear as a noticeable notch on the helix.

A banner flap may also be used to correct defects of the medial anterior ear, such as the concha, tragus, or crus of the helix (Fig. 7.11). Tissue is harvested from the preauricular area and transposed into the defect. This donor area typically provides ample tissue laxity. Because it is a cosmetic unit junction area (like the melolabial fold and postauricular sulcus), the preauricular area offers an excellent location for placing a minimally visible linear or curvilinear scar. Defects in concha may also be allowed to heal by secondary intention with excellent results.

MULTILOBE TRANSPOSITION FLAPS

In a single-lobe transposition flap such as the rhombic flap, there is considerable tension across the tip of the flap, which creates pull on the original defect. If there is not sufficient tissue laxity to accommodate this, undesirable distortion can occur. The multiple-lobe flap that uses the lengthening dynamics of the Z-plasty preventing that pull and at the same time recruits tissue from more distant sites with greater laxity to donate to the repair. Therefore these flaps are particularly useful around free margins or critical structures, such as wounds on the alar margin, lips, eyelids, and eyebrows.[25] The addition of multiple lobes also widens the pedicle base, decreasing the likelihood of vascular compromise.

BILOBED FLAP

The bilobed flap commonly used nowadays is a highly evolved transposition flap. Its design actually consists of two transposition flaps, used in succession, which follow the same direction of rotation over intervening tissues.[26,27] The flap allows the surgeon to extend the reach of the transposition flap and borrow laxity from donor sites at a greater distance from the defect. The second lobe also decreases the degree of the arc through which the pedicle moves to borrow from the distal site.

The bilobed flap was first described for use in nasal reconstruction by Esser in 1918,[28] where he designed a flap with each lobe traveling 90 degrees, resulting in a significant dog-ear at the proximal advancing border of the primary lobe. When this type of closure is attempted in the highly sebaceous, thick zones of the lower nose, distortion of the alar rim is inevitable. The bilobed flap became a workhorse flap in nasal reconstruction only after Zitelli published several design modifications to it in 1989.[23] His modifications corrected the original flap's two major drawbacks: large angles of flap transposition and the production of a dog-ear deformity that typically needed an additional revision procedure. This produced an excellent reconstructive option for the very unforgiving, sebaceous terrain of the lower nose. Zitelli's modifications are illustrated in Fig. 7.12. Cook also contributed to modifications of the design with several reviews of the design and application.[29,30]

When executed, a bilobed flap resembles the motion of a rotation flap. The modified bilobed flap is designed by drawing the two lobes along a 90-degree arc off of the tip of the center of the primary defect. Unlike the original bilobed flap, the pivot point of this arc extends beyond the width of the defect, incorporating the dog-ear at one side of the circular defect. This is essential to avoid a large, tissue-distorting standing cone. With the larger radius of the arc, the individual lobes travel through fewer degrees of rotation, minimizing the amount of pivotal restraint seen in the original bilobed design. The standing cone should be oriented in an attempt to place this scar in a well-hidden location, such as the alar crease.[30]

The modified bilobed flap calls for the primary lobe to have a width equal to the width of the primary defect (Fig. 7.13). In cases in which there is some degree of laxity in the skin surrounding the primary defect, the primary lobe can be designed up to 10% narrower than the width of the

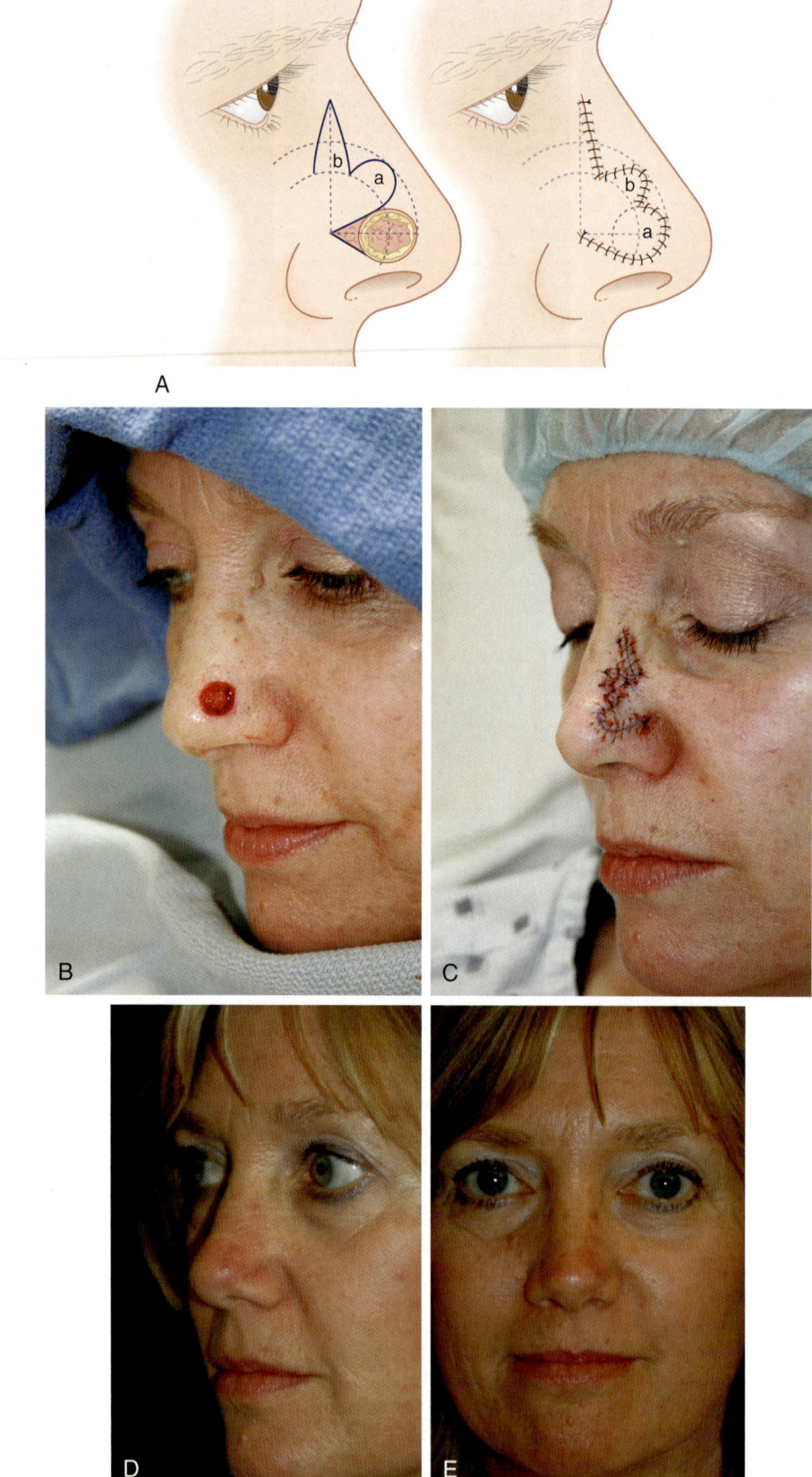

Fig. 7.12 The bilobed flap. (A) Design of Zitelli bilobed flap. (B) 0.8 cm defect on the left nasal supratip. (C) Inset and sutured bilobed flap. (D) 3-month postoperative follow-up oblique angle. (E) 3-month postoperative follow-up frontal view.

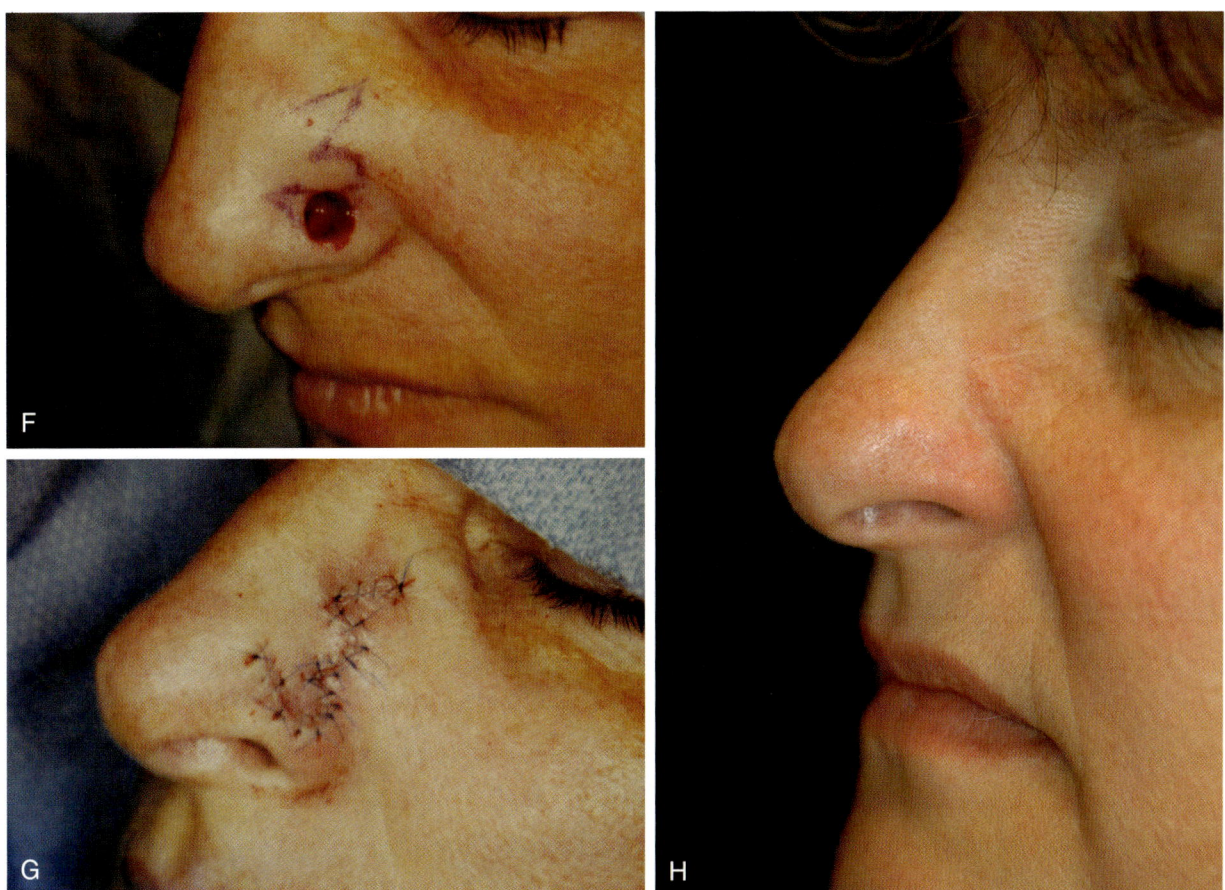

Fig. 7.12, cont'd (F) 0.7 cm defect in the mid ala. (G) Medially based bilobed flap at inset. (H) 3-month postoperative follow-up.

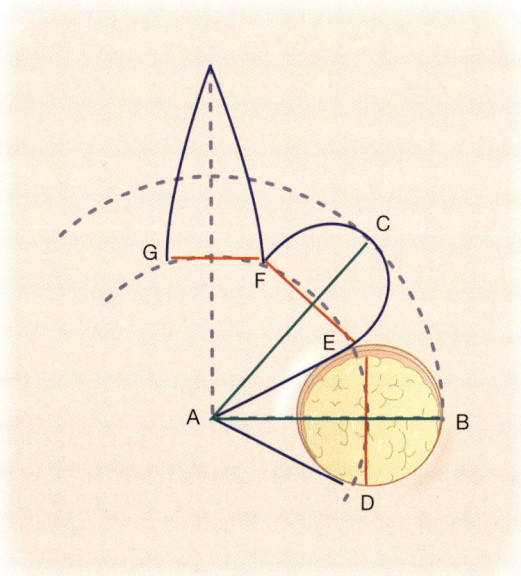

Fig. 7.13 The bilobed flap. Note the angle between line AB and AC should be roughly 45 degrees. The width of the secondary lobe E–F should be the same as the width of the defect D–E to avoid any tension on the primary defect. The tertiary lobe may be designed slightly smaller than the primary and secondary if there is some redundancy in the secondary defect area.

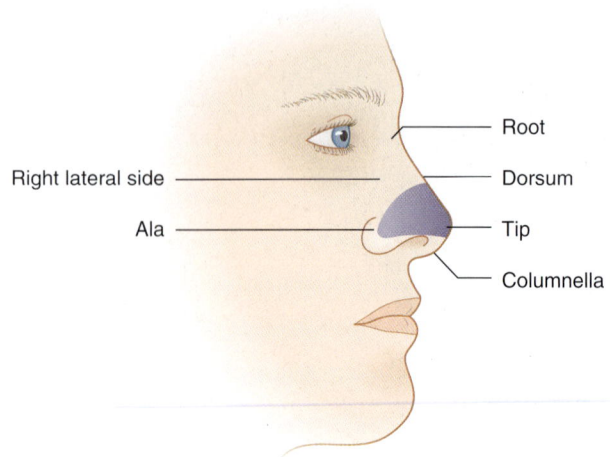

Fig. 7.14 Optimal zone for bilobed flaps on the nose.

primary defect. Subsequently, the second lobe can also be designed with a smaller width if there is sufficient tissue laxity in the areas of the secondary and tertiary defects. The second lobe, which creates the tertiary defect, should be designed at a 90-degree angle to the midline of the redundant Burow triangle at the pivot point of the flap. Because the majority of the tension is in the closure of the tertiary defect, it should be oriented in such a manner as to not distort any nearby free margins. For example, it is typically oriented perpendicular to the nasal ala when the bilobed flap is used in distal nasal reconstruction.

Some shortening of the lobes of the flap should still be anticipated because of the pivotal restraint through the arc of flap rotation. To compensate for this, the first lobe may be drawn to extend slightly beyond the edge of the primary defect. The angle of separation between the midline that bisects the defect and primary lobe should ideally be 45 degrees. This minimizes both the surgical effort needed to execute the flap and the tension on the edges of the flap after it is in place. A less acute takeoff angle, such as 30 degrees decreases the arc of rotation and decreases the Z-plasty advantage of the double transposition.[8] Using a greater takeoff angle, such as 60 degrees, increases the arc of rotation but narrows the flap pedicle.

The bilobed flap may be designed in several different directions on the nose. In general, however, more medial defects are usually closed with laterally based bilobed flaps, whereas more lateral defects are closed with medially based bilobed flaps. The bilobed flap is most often selected for reconstruction of defects located over the nasal tip and supratip, the distal nasal sidewall, the medial nasal ala, the auricular helix, and the posterior ear (Fig. 7.14).

These are areas with little local tissue laxity and high potential for distortion with side-to-side closure. The bilobed flap is often described as the flap of choice for repair of defects of the lower one-third of the nose. Familiarity with the bilobed flap and its modifications is essential for surgeons treating nonmelanoma skin cancers.

Bilobed Flap: Mobilization and Key Sutures

Bilobed flaps are usually incised down to the periosteum and undermined and mobilized out to the nasofacial groove in a submuscular (nasalis) plane. This maximizes both flap mobility and vascularity. Wide undermining of the entire area, including the flap and recipient bed, will help distribute the tension vectors of closure throughout the flap and surrounding tissue and minimize the risk of pin-cushioning.[29] As with other flaps, the bilobed flap should not be oversized, and it should rest flush or slightly below the level of the surrounding tissue. The height of the flap is usually best adjusted by trimming the depth of the recipient bed rather than trimming the underside of the flap. This will minimize the chance of vascular compromise of the flap by excess thinning.

The standing cone deformity (SCD) is the center point of the arc of rotation in a bilobed flap, and therefore it is generally advisable to remove it before rotation.[29,30] The angle of the SCD should be chosen with regard to effects closure tension will have on the neighboring free margins. The SCD should be designed to be 0.75 to 1.5 times the primary defect diameter.[29,30,31] The first key suture closes the tertiary defect and pushes the flap toward the primary defect. The second key suture secures the primary lobe into the surgical defect. The exact location of the second key suture must be skillfully chosen by the surgeon such that it avoids dynamic distortion within the repair, correctly aligns the standing cone, and adequately accounts for the size of the primary lobe relative to the surgical defect.[8] Once in place it is important to ensure the SCD preserves contour and the primary lobe is in place before doing any trimming to the flap.

TRILOBED FLAP

An additional lobe can be added on to a bilobed flap to create a trilobed flap. The primary advantages of the trilobed flap are the ability to recruit tissue from areas of laxity even more distant and/or to rotate tension vectors to a greater degree than possible with a single or bilobed transposition flap. For example, when repairing inferior-malar defects, bilobed flaps have a tendency to cause either ipsilateral alar elevation because of secondary tension vectors, ipsilateral alar depression because of "bulldozing" and Z-plasty lengthening, or contralateral alar elevation if tension vectors on the secondary lobe are oblique rather than vertical.[16,29,30] The design, mechanics, and principles of trilobed flaps are essentially the same as bilobed flaps (Fig. 7.15). In trilobed flaps, the third lobe extends the arc of rotation to angles of 120 degrees to 150 degrees allowing for a change in the tension vectors of the donor site as compared with a bilobed flap in the same area.[8,16] As discussed previously, the addition of a third lobe adds an additional Z-plasty to the repair, which shortens the central limbs involved in the repair and the tension to transpose the flap. The primary lobe should be designed such that it is equal in size to the primary defect. Ideally, the secondary and tertiary lobes will be in progressively more flexible skin, if this holds true they can often be designed 85% to 90% and 75% to 80%, respectively, of the primary lobe diameter. This undersizing places these lobes under a small amount of tension, which helps to minimize pin-cushioning.[16,22] Finally, the pedicle base is generally wider in trilobed flaps, decreasing the risk of vascular compromise associated with rotation of a narrow pedicle.[8]

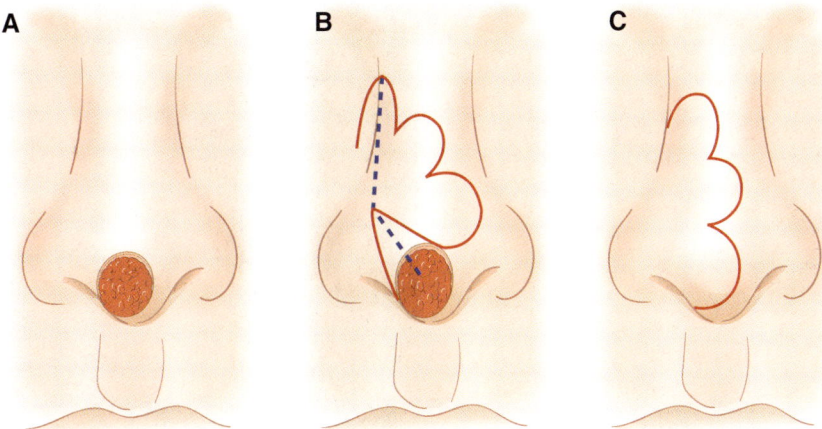

Fig. 7.15 The trilobed flap. The trilobed flap allows the surgeon to tap into tissue reserves at an even greater distance than the bilobed flap and works well on defects of the distal nasal tip. (A–C) The trilobed flap is designed in a similar manner as the bilobed flap with an additional lobe added to extend the arc of rotation to 120 to 150 degrees.

DORSUM OF THE NOSE AND THE NASAL SIDEWALL (Fig. 7.17)

The use of surrounding skin in transposition flaps helps maintain optimal color and texture match when repairing defects of the nasal dorsum or sidewall. The nose can be divided into several zones based on color, texture, sebaceous quality, and mobility. The skin of the nasal dorsum and sidewalls is thin, loose, and nonsebaceous. This area is designated zone I. Zone II consists of the thick, sebaceous, relatively immobile, and much less forgiving skin of the nasal supratip, tip, and ala. Zone III is a small area on the distal nose, including the soft triangles, columella, and infratip lobule, whether the skin again becomes thin, loose, and nonsebaceous.[16,32] The characteristics of zone I make it the best area to accommodate the added tension vectors of a transposition flap donor site. The less mobile skin of zone II often requires recruitment of tissue from the more distant, yet more mobile, skin of zone I.

Transposition flaps are more spatially confined than most other closures. On the nasal sidewall, they may be used to keep the closure within a single cosmetic unit/zone. In this area the free margins of the lower eyelid and nasal ala are particularly susceptible to distortion from adjacent forces. Keeping this in mind during the planning of repairs in these areas is essential. Tension vectors should be directed away from the free margins of these structures because distortion can lead to functional and aesthetic compromise. The mobility of the nasal tip should also be considered when repairing nasal defects. Occasionally, a favorable effect on the nasal tip can be achieved by correcting age-associated nasal tip ptosis during the repair of nasal defects. This is done by planning a repair where some of the tension produced by the repair is in a vertical orientation. To be aesthetically successful, the elevation of the nasal tip must be strictly vertical, which is often difficult to achieve if a rhombic flap is used off the nasal midline. Too much tip elevation and any lateral deviation are obviously cosmetically undesirable. When possible, it is best to place the tension-bearing defect over the bony nasal skeleton because

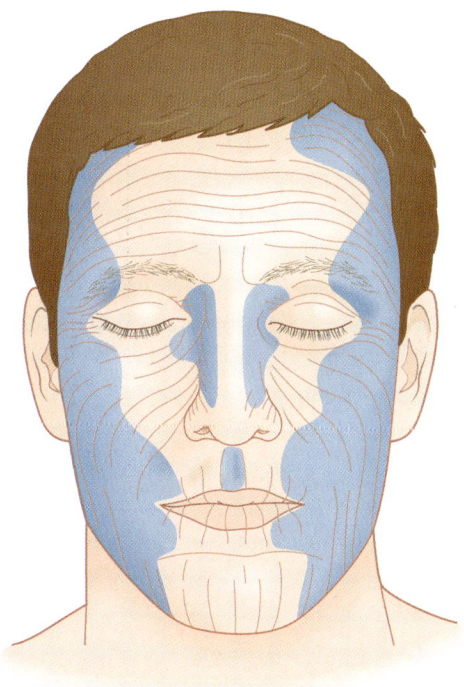

Fig. 7.16 Common locations, noted with shading, for the use of rhombic flaps.

General Applications of Transposition Flaps

The most common areas where transposition flaps are used include the nasal dorsum and sidewalls, the medial and lateral canthi, the lateral forehead, temple, cheek, the perioral region, the inferior chin, and the dorsal hand (Fig. 7.16). The following is a brief review of the rationale for choosing a transposition flap in these specific locations.

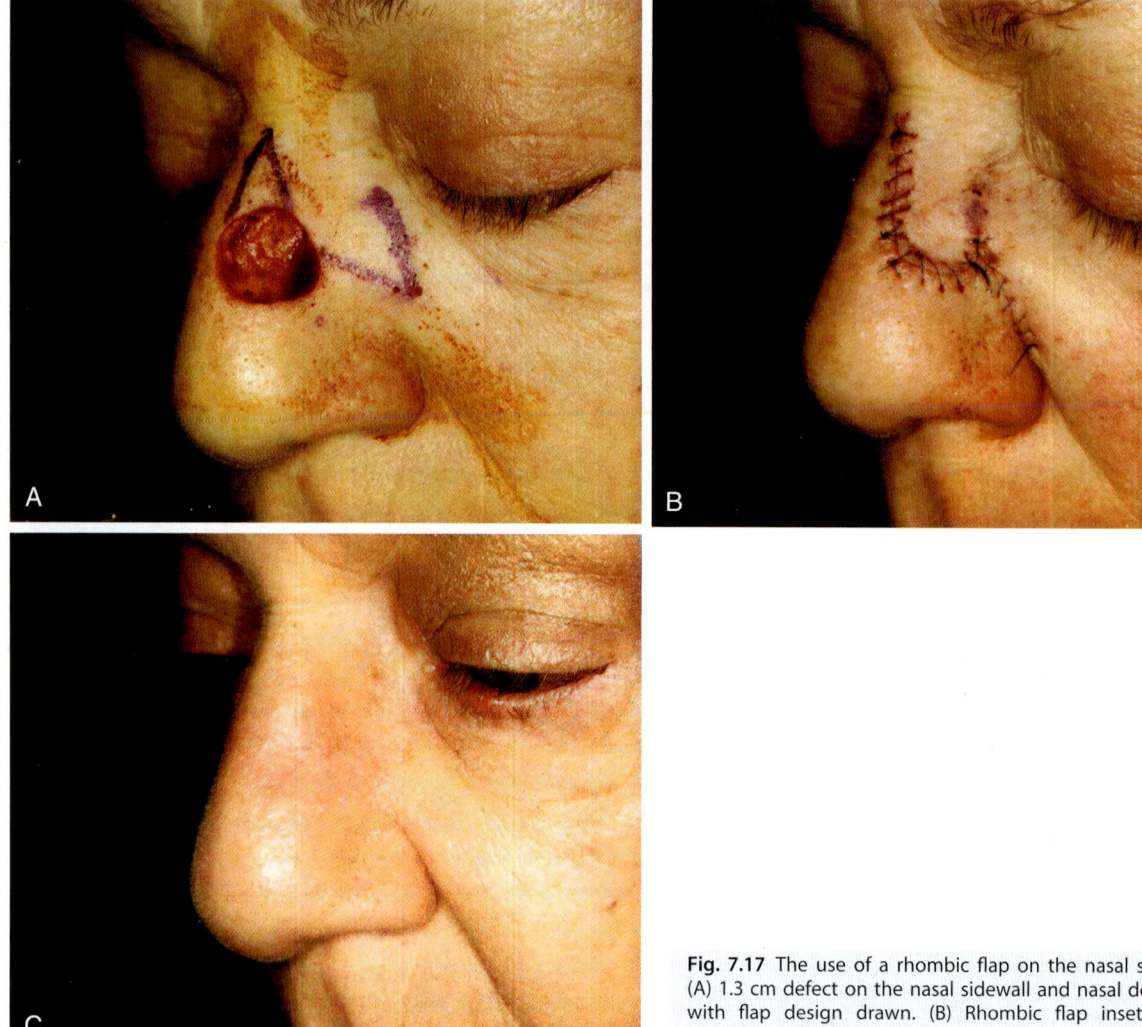

Fig. 7.17 The use of a rhombic flap on the nasal sidewall defect. (A) 1.3 cm defect on the nasal sidewall and nasal dorsum junction with flap design drawn. (B) Rhombic flap inset and sutured. (C) 3-month follow-up visit.

horizontal tension placed across the nasal dorsum can cause "cinching" of the dorsal nasal skin into the soft area overlying the upper lateral cartilages and cause a saddle nose deformity on lateral view.[16]

NASAL TIP

Bilobed and trilobed flaps are used extensively for the repair of defects of the nasal tip. The more proximal and lateral portions of the nasal tip are more amenable to bilobed flap repairs, whereas the distal nasal tip often requires a trilobed flap to prevent distortion of free margins.[22] For defects approximately 1 cm in size on the more proximal or lateral portions of the nasal tip, bilobed flaps are usually favored.[33,34] For defects larger than 1.5 cm on the nasal tip, the ability to displace the quaternary defect to the nasal dorsum and recruit tissue from zone I makes trilobed flaps an excellent option for many repairs.[22]

MEDIAL AND LATERAL CANTHI (Fig. 7.18)

The medial and lateral canthi are located near the highly mobile free margins of the eyelids. Care must be taken to redirect tension vectors to ensure that distortion of these structures does not occur after closure of the defect. Patients with lid margin laxity are particularly prone to distortion, which can lead to functional impairment of the eyelid. In addition, because some wound contraction inevitably occurs along the long axis of any wound, closures should be designed to minimize lines going across the concave contours of the inner canthus. The prominent lines of the crow's feet of the lateral canthi offer excellent hiding places for the acute angles generated by transposition flaps.

TEMPLE

Most defects in the temple can be closed primarily. However, when repairing large defects in this location, transposition flaps can be used to take advantage of the reservoir of excess skin over the cheeks, temple, and preauricular areas. In addition, for patients with a bleeding risk it is important to consider that significantly less undermining is needed for transposition flaps as compared with large sliding flaps.[16] A transposition flap may be designed to keep the closure of defects in the medial temple from extending into the periorbital cosmetic unit. The soft, supple skin of the temple and cheeks, although generous in its ability to take on additional tension, often is prone to pin-cushioning. Because of

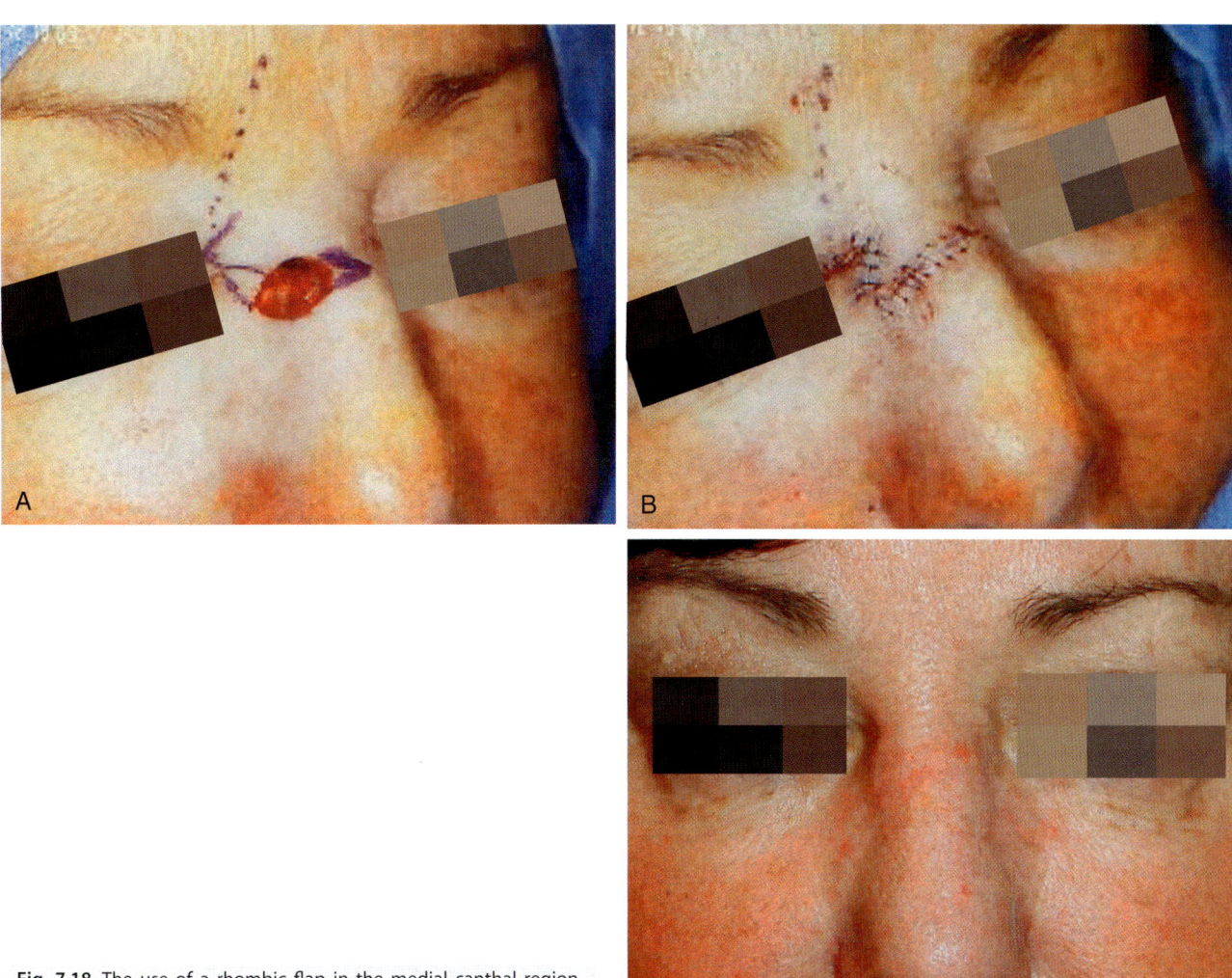

Fig. 7.18 The use of a rhombic flap in the medial canthal region. (A) 0.7 × 1.0 cm defect in the medial canthal region. (B) Rhombic flap inset and sutured in place. (C) 3-month follow-up visit.

this, it is important to undersize the flap slightly.[35] Caution should be used when undermining in this location because of the relatively superficial location of the temporal branch of facial nerve. Damage to the nerve can lead to ipsilateral paralysis of the frontalis muscle and a resultant brow ptosis.

CHEEKS (Fig. 7.19)

Although most small- and medium-sized defects on the cheeks may be closed primarily, transposition flaps can be used on larger defects or can even be used on smaller defects to leave geometric broken line scars instead of long linear scars. Transposition flaps are generally designed laterally, with the redundant tissue inferior to the primary defect. Positioning the scar laterally tends to make the scar less visible to the patient and observers. An inferiorly based flap provides better lymphatic drainage and may minimize the risk of flap engorgement and subsequent pin-cushioning. Bilobed flaps with or without Z-plasties may also be used in larger cheek defects.

PERIORAL AREA (Fig. 7.20)

Transposition flaps may occasionally be used in perioral defects. The adjacent skin folds, as well as wrinkles in various orientations, provide camouflage for the geometric scars of transposition flaps. The medial cheek often provides a good reservoir of lax skin. Care must be taken to properly orient the flap to ensure that the closure of the secondary defect does not result in any tension that may distort the lip.

CHIN (Fig. 7.21)

When repairing defects of the lateral and inferior chin, one may take advantage of the laxity of the medial cheek and submandibular area, as well as the many natural lines in this area, to hide the resulting scar. Care should be taken to minimize lines across the convex contour where the chin and neck meet, because scars in such situations tend to be quite visible and prone to hypertrophy.

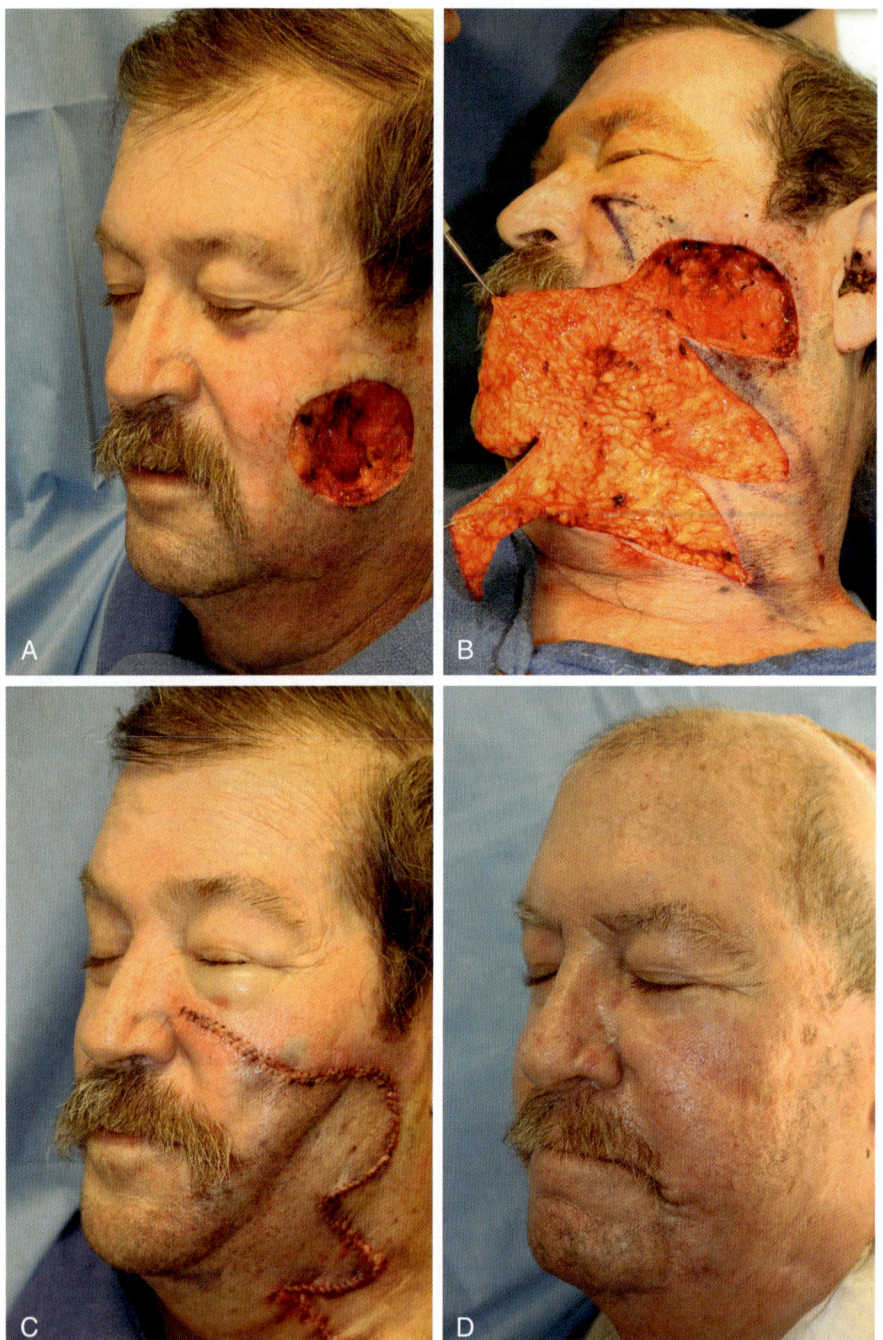

Fig. 7.19 Repair of cheek defect with trilobed flap. (A) 4.0 × 4.5 cm defect on the lateral cheek. (B) Trilobed flap raised. (C) Trilobed flap inset and sutured. (D) 3-month postoperative follow-up. (Photo courtesy of Dr. Joseph Sobenko.)

Complications

As with all repairs, a number of complications, such as postoperative hemorrhage, hematoma formation, infection, and wound dehiscence, may occur when using transposition flaps for closure of cutaneous defects. Most complications can be avoided with proper patient and repair selection, appropriate flap design, and careful surgical execution.

However, one surgical complication known as pin-cushioning is seen more frequently with transposition flaps than with other reconstructive alternatives. The term pin-cushioning, also known as the trapdoor deformity, refers to the protuberance of a flap or graft above the surface of the surrounding skin.[36] This can occur with all transposition flaps and occurs more commonly with the traditional banner flap and the bilobed flap. The development of the trapdoor deformity may be due to the additional peripheral contraction that occurs with the curved edge flaps versus flaps with geometric configurations. Another potential cause of pin-cushioning is excess subcutaneous fat under the flap. When raising the flap, care should be taken to

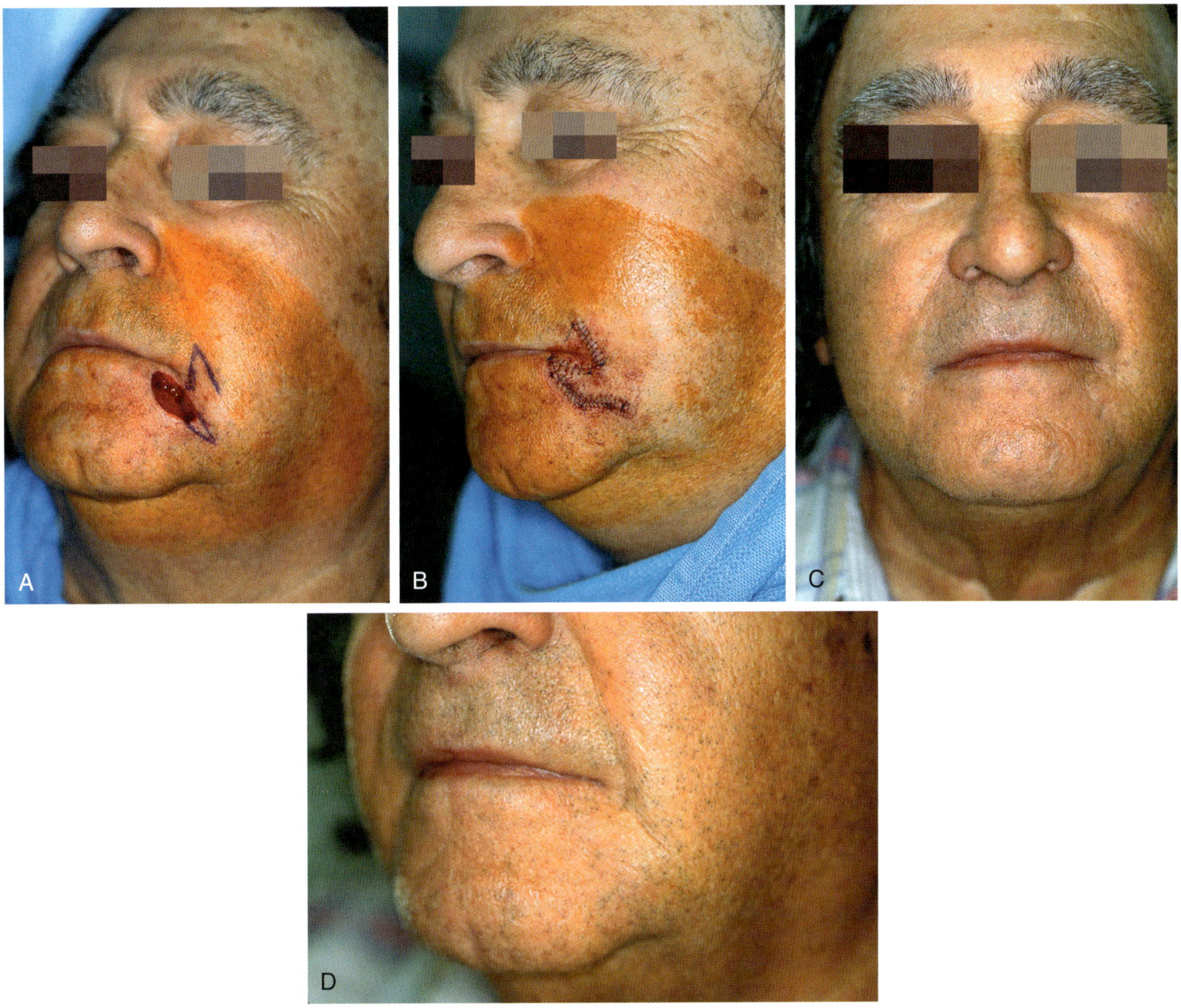

Fig. 7.20 Repair of a perioral defect using a transposition flap. (A) Intraoperative markings around the defect. (B) At the time of closure. (C, D) Appearance 3 months after closure.

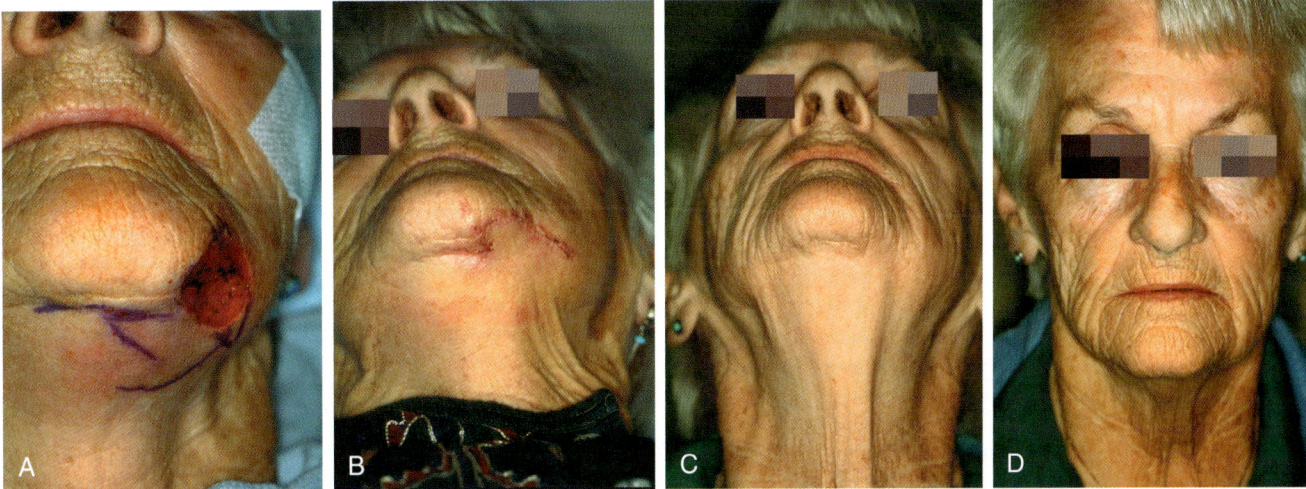

Fig. 7.21 Repair of a chin defect with a transposition flap. (A) Intraoperative markings around the defect. (B) At the time of closure. (C, D) Appearance 3 months after closure.

dissect at a consistent plane, adjusting the depth of dissection only to compensate for depth variations in the recipient bed. Pin-cushioning may also be due to lymphedema within a flap. At incision planes, the normal lymphatic drainage is altered, which can lead to thickening of a flap because of inability to drain properly. This is less likely when using inferiorly based flaps, which offer better dependent lymphatic drainage because the drainage channels at the pedicle of these flaps are largely intact and oriented to naturally drain the flap while the patient is in an upright position. Perhaps the most common cause of pin-cushioning is oversizing the flap. Careful inspection of the flap in the recipient space after the secondary or tertiary defect is approximated allows for proper sizing of the primary lobe. Judicious trimming of the primary lobe's leading edge should be performed at this point. Finally, a failure to establish contact between the undersurface of the flap and the recipient bed can lead to pin-cushioning. This occurs because no contact inhibition occurs at the base of the flap. This lack of contact inhibition causes excessive contraction at the wound bed.

Conclusion

Transposition flaps are powerful tools to produce excellent results in cutaneous reconstruction. As in the closure of any surgical defect, the goal should be to achieve the best possible functional and aesthetic result. This can only be accomplished by proper surgical planning. Every effort should be made to avoid distortion of the free margins of structures such as the nose and eyelids. Attempts to best camouflage incision lines within existing lines or creases, at the junction of cosmetic units, or at least parallel to lines of relaxed skin tension should be undertaken. A complete knowledge of the possible variations and modifications of these transposition flaps can help to fine-tune the execution of the flap to provide the patient with the best possible result. Good surgical technique and proper wound eversion through meticulous suture placement also help tremendously in consistently attaining aesthetically pleasing results. At the surgical bedside, an artistic eye should meet the science of cutaneous biomechanics (Box 7.1).

References

1. Sutton A, Brewer J. Tetralobed transposition flap: a novel repair for large surgical defects of the nasal tip. *Dermatol Surg.* 2014;40:197-200.
2. Limberg AA. Design of local flaps. In: Gibson T, ed. *Modern Trends of Plastic Surgery.* London: Butterworth-Heinemann; 1966:38-61.
3. Borges AF. The rhombic flap. *Plast Reconstr Surg.* 1981;67:458-466.
4. Larrabee WF Jr, Trachy R, Sutton D, Cox K. Rhomboid flap dynamics. *Arch Otolaryngol.* 1981;107:755-757.
5. Dufourmentel C. Le fermeture des pertes de substance cutanée limitées. "Le lambeau de rotation en L pourlosange" dit"LLL". *Ann Chir Plast.* 1962;7:61-66.
6. Webster R, Davidson T, Smith R. The thirty degree transposition flap. *Laryngoscope.* 1978;88:85-94.
7. Bray DA. Clinical applications of the rhomboid flap. *Arch Otolaryngol.* 1983;109:37-42.
8. Miller C. Design principles for transposition flaps: the rhombic (single-lobed), bilobed, and trilobed flaps. *Dermatol Surg.* 2014;40(suppl 9):S43-S52.
9. Lister G, Gibson T. Closure of rhomboid skin defects: the flaps of Limberg and Dufourmentel. *Br J Plast Surg.* 1972;25:300-314.
10. Dzubow L. Mohs surgery report: design of an appropriate rhombic flap for a circular defect created by Mohs microscopically controlled surgery. *J Dermatol Surg Oncol.* 1988;14:124-126.
11. McNay A, Ostad A, Moy R. Surgical pearl: modified rhombic flap. *J Am Acad Dermatol.* 1997;37(2 Pt 1):256-258.
12. Bullock J, Koss N, Flagg S. Rhomboid flap in ophthalmic plastic surgery. *Arch Ophthalmol.* 1973;90:203-205.
13. Rossi A, Jeffs JV. The rhomboid flap of Limberg—a simple aid to planning. *Ann Plast Surg.* 1980;5:494-496.
14. Walike JW, Larrabee WF Jr. The "note flap". *Arch Otolaryngol.* 1985;111:430-433.
15. Masson JK, Mendelson BC. The banner flap. *Am J Surg.* 1977;134:419-423.
16. Blake BP, Simonetta CJ, Maher IA. Transposition flaps: principles and locations. *Dermatol Surg.* 2015;41:255-264.
17. Borges AF. Choosing the correct Limberg flap. *Plast Reconstr Surg.* 1978;62:542-545.
18. Brobyn TJ, Cramer LM, Hulnick SJ. Facial resurfacing with the Limberg flap. *Clin Plast Surg.* 1976;3:481-490.
19. Fee WE Jr. Gunter JP, Carder HM. Rhomboid flap principles and common variations. *Laryngoscope.* 1976;86:1706-1711.
20. Dzubow LM. The dynamics of flap movement: effect of pivotal restraint on flap rotation and transposition. *J Dermatol Surg Oncol.* 1987;13:1348-1353.
21. Collins S, Dufresne RJ, Jellinek N. The bilobed transposition flap for single-staged repair of large surgical defects involving the nasal ala. *Dermatol Surg.* 2008;34:1379-1385.
22. Claiborne JR, Albertini JG. Trilobed flap for inferior-medial alar defect. *Dermatol Surg.* 2014;40:794-798.
23. Webster RC, Davidson TM, Smith RC. The thirty degree transposition flap. *Laryngoscope.* 1978;88:85-94.
24. Masson JK, Mendelson BC. The banner flap. *Am J Surg.* 1977;134:419-423.
25. Zitelli JA. Commentary on the Trilobed flap for inferior-medial alar defect. *Dermatol Surg.* 2014;40:799-800.
26. McGregor JC, Soutar DS. A critical assessment of the bilobed flap. *Br J Plast Surg.* 1981;34:197-205.
27. Morgan BL, Samiian MR. Advantages of the bilobed flap for closure of small defects of the face. *Plast Reconstr Surg.* 1973;52:35-37.
28. Esser JSF. Gestielte locale Nasenplastik mit zwewiplifgem Lappen, Deckung des sekundaren Defektes vom ersten Zipfel durch den zweiten. *Dtsch Z Chir.* 1918;143:385-390.
29. Cook J. Reconstructive utility of the bilobed flap: lessons from flap successes and failures. *Dermatol Surg.* 2005;31:1024-1033.
30. Cook JL. A review of the bilobed flap's design with particular emphasis on the minimization of alar displacement. *Dermatol Surg.* 2000;26:354-362.
31. Zitelli J. Comments on a modified bilobed flap. *Arch Facial Plast Surg.* 2006;8:410.

Box 7.1 Tips to Minimize the Risk of Developing Trapdoor Deformities With Transposition Flaps

- Use straight lines and geometric angles, avoiding curvilinear lines wherever possible to minimize circumferential contraction around the flap.
- Undermine widely beyond the base of the flap. Wide undermining creates a uniform "platelike scar"[a] and may minimize the elevation of the flap in any particular area.
- Appropriately size the flaps. Do not oversize the flaps.
- Maintain contact of the flap base with the recipient base to cause contact inhibition of flap contraction. If necessary (e.g., if going over a concavity), this may be facilitated by the use of an absorbable suture from the base of the flap to the recipient bed. The suture placed within the flap should be oriented parallel to the direction of the flap's blood flow to minimize the risk of inducing flap ischemia.
- Orient the flap to allow good lymphatic drainage and prevent lymphedema. Inferiorly based flaps allow favorable lymphatic drainage.

[a]Fee WE Jr, Gunter JP, Carder HM. Rhomboid flap principles and common variations. *Laryngoscope.* 1976;86:1706-1711.

32. Zitelli J. The bilobed flap for nasal reconstruction. *Arch Dermatol.* 1989;125:957-959.
33. Zitelli J. Design aspect of the bilobed flap. *Arch Facial Plast Surg.* 2008;10:186.
34. Steiger J. Bilobed flaps in nasal reconstruction. *Facial Plast Surg Clin North Am.* 2011;19:107-111.
35. Pletcher S, Kim D. Current concepts in cheek reconstruction. *Facial Plast Surg Clin North Am.* 2005;13:267-281.
36. Koranda FC, Webster RC. Trapdoor effect in nasolabial flaps. Causes and corrections. *Arch Otolaryngol.* 1985;111:421-424.

Further Reading

Brodland DG, Pharis D. Flaps. In: Bolognia J, Jorizzo J, Rapini R, eds. *Dermatology.* London: Mosby; 2003:2287-2303.

Converse JM, ed. *Reconstructive Plastic Surgery: General Principles.* 2nd ed. Philadelphia: WB Saunders; 1977:202-207.

Davidson TM, Webster RC, Gordon BR. *The Principles and Dynamics of Local Skin Flaps.* Chicago: American Academy of Otolaryngology Head and Neck Surgery; 1983.

Grabb WC, Myers MB, eds. *Skin Flaps.* Boston: Little Brown; 1975:111-131.

Lister GD, Gibson T. Closure of rhomboid skin defects: the flaps of Limberg and Dufourmentel. *Br J Plast Surg.* 1972;25:300-314.

Webster RC, Benjamin BJ, Smith RC. Closure of circular defects. *Laryngoscope.* 1978;88:534-538.

Webster RC, Benjamin BJ, Smith RC. Treatment of "trap door deformity". *Laryngoscope.* 1978;88:707-712.

Yotsuyanagi T, Yamashita K, Urushidate S, et al. Reconstruction of large nasal defects with a combination of local flaps based on the aesthetic subunit principle. *Plast Reconstr Surg.* 2001;107:1358-1362.

Videos for this chapter can be found online by accessing the accompanying Expert Consult website.

8 Staged Interpolation Flaps

TRI H. NGUYEN, MD, and JANET LI, MD

Interpolation flaps demand exquisite planning and execution. In return, their sophistication offers rich rewards, with a highly vascularized covering that may resurface complex defects, provide tissue bulk, nourish free cartilage grafts (CG), and restore lining or contour as needed. The terms *axial*, *indirect*, *interpolation*, and *staged flaps* are synonymous, and all are variations of transposition repairs. All interpolation flaps have these shared features: (1) vascular pedicle based on a named artery and or its tributaries, (2) donor location distant and noncontiguous from the defect, and (3) two or more stages for completion (stage I for flap creation and closure, stage II for pedicle division, and often additional stages for revisions).

The success of these flaps is dependent on adhering to three key principles. First, all margins must be definitively cancer free. Second, these flaps should be considered as heavy surface coverings (skin, subcutis, muscle), and a stable infrastructure must exist to support them. A large nasal defect, for example, cannot simply be covered without stable cartilage support and mucosal lining. Third, optimal repairs often require the reconstruction of an entire subunit.[1] Wounds that consume 50% or more of a subunit are best restored in total, with few exceptions. Patients with staged flaps require a complete preoperative consultation. Multiple visits and revisions, temporary physical deformities, and intensive wound care, as well as substantial activity and work restrictions, are the rule in staged repairs. In exchange for this demanding regimen, however, are surgical results that have no parallel. This chapter will discuss techniques for (1) paramedian forehead flap (PFF), (2) cheek-to-nose interpolation flap (CNIF), and (3) Abbé or lip-switch flap as applied to skin cancer reconstruction.

Paramedian Forehead Flap, Stage I

INDICATION

The PFF is a workhorse in facial reconstruction. Although it may close any wound on the central face, its best application is to the distal nose (tip, ala, and columella), where tissue thickness and sebaceous quality are closely matched by forehead skin.[2] The PFF is ideal for recreating the convexity and projection of the nasal tip. Subtotal nasal tip and/or alar defects may be candidates for the PFF. Proximal wounds on the nasal dorsum, sidewall, nasal root, and medial canthus have inherently thinner skin and may be incongruous for the much thicker PFF, unless a substantially deep defect is present.

ANATOMY

The primary and secondary vascular supply to the PFF is the supratrochlear (internal carotid system) and dorsal nasal artery (external carotid system), respectively. The supratrochlear artery (SA) is reliably located at the medial border of the eyebrow, on average 10.9 mm from the facial midline.[3] At the medial eyebrow, a glabellar crease (if present) delineates where the SA crosses the superior orbital rim to enter the forehead (Fig. 8.1). Below the orbital rim, the SA lies deep to the periorbital muscles (orbicularis oculi and frontalis) just above the periosteum. Above the rim, however, the SA pierces the corrugator supercilii muscle at 15–25 mm above the supraorbital rim and ascends superficially into the forehead, sandwiched between the frontalis muscle below and the subcutis above. Consequently, to preserve the SA near the orbital rim, dissection must be below the frontalis muscle and deep fascia. Transection of the SA during surgery is not always disastrous. The robust arterial perforators are often sufficient to nourish the flap. Indeed, histologic studies suggest that the PFF is sometimes a random pattern flap, with no discernible high caliber artery within the pedicle.

FLAP DESIGN

The ideal PFF is an aesthetic covering that restores normal contour and symmetry without creating a shapeless blob. Table 8.1 discusses the critical design issues in a PFF. The covering provided by a PFF requires a stable nasal infrastructure (cartilage support and mucosal lining). Structural cartilage grafts (SCGs) to prevent nasal valve collapse and alar rim contraction are usual considerations in PFF repairs. More neglected, however, are SCGs that restore contour to the nasal supratip. Contour grafts should be considered in patients that have thick nasal tip skin and supratip defects (Fig. 8.2). Without a contour graft in these patients, a PFF alone may be insufficient to restore normal tip projection.[4]

Measurements of the defect must be accurate—neither oversized nor undersized for the wound. The PFF template should be measured after the residual subunit has been outlined, but *prior* to the excision of any remaining skin (Fig. 8.3). This avoids an artificially enlarged dimension from a retracted wound edge. A template should also reflect the three-dimensional nature of the nose, especially if a defect extends to the infratip, columella, and ala (Fig. 8.4). If the vestibular mucosa is missing, the PFF may be extended and turned down to provide nasal lining. The thin soft nasal triangle is difficult to rebuild. Either second intention healing or a finely thinned PFF are options for this thin,

8 • Staged Interpolation Flaps

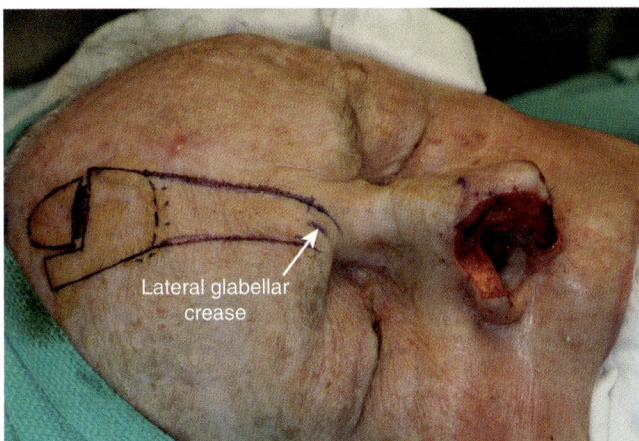

Fig. 8.1 Paramedian forehead flap—Supratrochlear artery location 1.5 cm lateral from midline at the medial eyebrow, marked by a lateral glabellar crease.

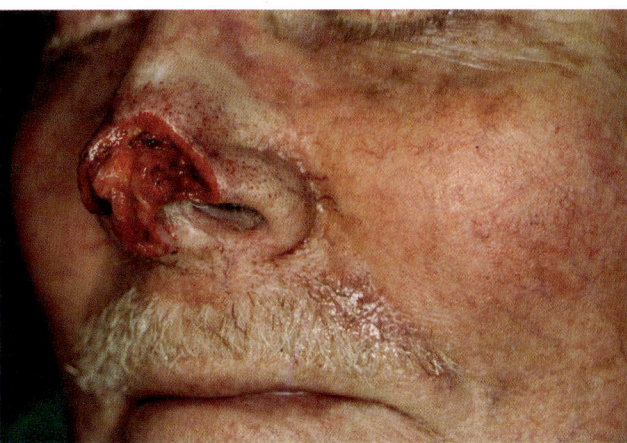

Fig. 8.2 Paramedian forehead flap—Supratip defect in a man with inherently thick nasal tip skin who would benefit from a contour cartilage graft.

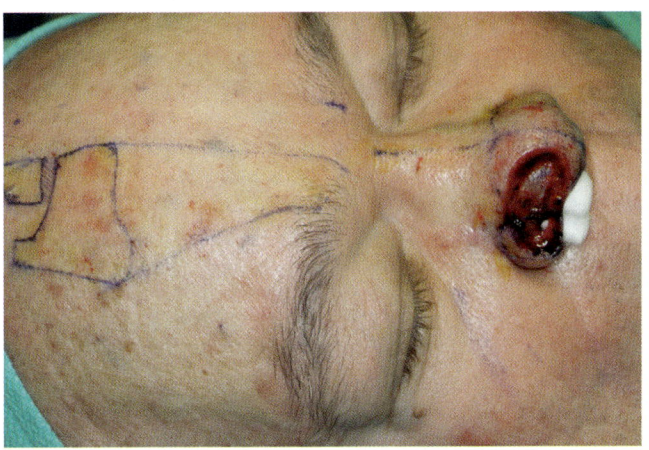

Fig. 8.3 Paramedian forehead flap—Flap template designed to include the eventual removal of nasal tip and alar subunit.

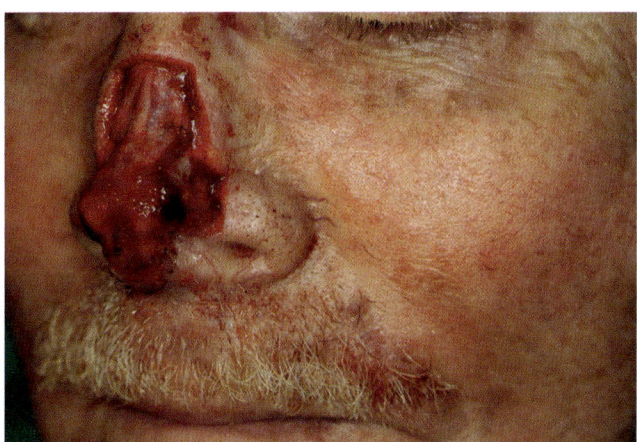

Fig. 8.4 Paramedian forehead flap—Complex Mohs defect of the nasal tip, soft triangle, and medial ala, necessitating a three-dimensional design.

Table 8.1 Issues in Paramedian Forehead Flap (PFF) Design for Distal Nose Defect (Nasal Tip and/or Ala)

Defect Considerations	Comments
Does this defect require lining support?	Replacing lining may require intranasal mucosal flaps prior to PFF execution.
Does this defect need cartilage support?	Cartilage grafts may be replacement or structural in nature. Replacement grafts restore missing cartilage or bone. Structural grafts add to stability and contour and prevent tissue contraction to an intact cartilage infrastructure.
Is the PFF sufficient to close this wound?	PFF may be combined with regional flaps, free cartilage grafts, and split- or full-thickness skin grafts for defects that extend onto multiple subunits.
Does the residual subunit need to be excised?	Cosmesis is often superior when entire subunits are resurfaced.
Flap Considerations	**Comments**
Has there been previous surgery at the proposed pedicle site?	Normal vascular anatomy may no longer be reliable and Doppler identification of a viable artery may be needed.
Does the flap template accurately account for the 3-dimensional contour of the nose and infratip?	A flexible template material (suture foil wrap, soft foam, Duoderm) is essential for accurately molding the template design. Two-dimensional defect measurements are inadequate.
Does the forehead's vertical height (from orbital rim to anterior frontal hairline) provide adequate length to reach the defect?	A short forehead height may require modifications to the template design and/or pedicle to optimize flap extension.

concave area. Whenever possible, the unaffected contralateral side should be used as a template to restore symmetry. A right-sided nasal tip and ala wound, for example, should be repaired based on the normal left tip and ala.

The vertical height of the forehead (from orbital rim to anterior frontal hairline) will determine the potential reach of this flap. If the vertical length is inadequate (short forehead height relative to distal defect), then the modifications listed in Table 8.2 will significantly extend a flap's distal reach.

Design considerations for the pedicle include its position and width. Identifying the SA pedicle may be done clinically, by using the anatomic landmarks mentioned earlier, or definitively by confirming with a manual Doppler (8–10 MHz frequency). However, 8% of supratrochlear arteries cannot by detected by Doppler.[3] Alternatively, PFF may be designed as a random flap based on the complex vascular plexus of the corrugator complex and frontalis.[5] The pedicle width therefore rarely needs to be greater than 1.5 cm.[6] Wider pedicles, in fact, are counterproductive and restrict flap mobility as well as vascular integrity (by increasing torque and compression on the artery during flap rotation). This author routinely develops a pedicle base of 1–1.5 cm. The glabellar frown line may be used as an anatomic landmark, with flap borders placed 8–9 mm lateral and 2–3 mm medial.[3] Another option is to base the template on a vertical line directly above the medial canthus, since the supratrochlear vascular pedicle has been shown to lie no more than 3 mm lateral or medial to the medial canthus.[7] The lateral pedicle incision stops at the eyebrow, whereas the medial incision should extend longer, often into the nasal root, to incorporate branches from the dorsal nasal artery (see Fig. 8.1). Traditionally the pedicle position is on the opposite side of where the defect is located. A left nasal tip defect, for example, would have been closed by a PFF based on the right SA. This concept applied when pedicles were much wider, to minimize twisting and tension. With more narrow pedicles (1.5 cm), there is less twisting during movement, and PFFs may be ipsilateral to the defect. Same side flaps are shorter in length than contralateral designs and conserve significant tissue.

ANESTHESIA

The PFF may be safely performed as an outpatient procedure under local anesthesia (LA). LA should be injected in stages. If a patient needs a CG and a PFF, then consider anesthetizing the ear and forehead first. Begin anesthetizing the nose when the forehead flap is incised. By administering LA in a stepwise fashion, the patient will be kept comfortable. Tumescent anesthesia (TA) is useful by rapidly anesthetizing large areas with minimal patient discomfort. With TA, however, waiting (at least 20 minutes) for the swelling to subside is advisable, as there is a pseudotension in tissue movement when it is edematous. LA may be supplemented by nerve blocks, oral benzodiazepines (lorazepam,

Table 8.2 Modifications to the Paramedian Forehead Flap for Extended Reach

Forehead Flap Design Modifications	Comment
Vertical extension of flap into the anterior frontal scalp	Potential transfer of terminal hairs onto the nasal defect. Potential disruption of frontal hairline and scarring alopecia if donor site closure is not complete.
Extension of flap lateral to midline	Potential compromise of vascular supply to lateral flap extension. Potential donor site morbidity with eyebrow elevation (scar contraction with second intention or distortion with complete closure).
Tangential flap design that crosses the midline	Flap becomes random pattern.
Pedicle Modifications	**Comment**
Keeping width of pedicle at its base between 1.0 and 1.5 cm	Wider pedicles (>1.5 cm) limit flap mobility. Wider pedicles increase vascular strangulation during flap rotation toward the distal defect.
Mobilizing base of pedicle below superior orbital rim	Incorrect elevation and undermining may lead to periorbital trauma and compromise vascular pedicle (supratrochlear artery). Limit incisions to the epidermis and dermis. Supraperiosteal undermining should be performed bluntly with a finger or cotton-tipped applicator. Alternatively, subperiosteal undermining of entire medial brow complex off of the superior orbital rim and arcus marginalis may be performed using a subperiosteal elevator. May extend flap reach by at least 2 cm. Pedicle division at stage II will require eyebrow repositioning for bilateral symmetry.
Relaxing incision at medial base of pedicle (toward glabella and nasal root)	Releases dermal attachments at the pedicle base that may enhance flap mobility. Incision must not extend past superficial dermis.
Superficial horizontal incisions in the undersurface of the pedicle	Allows for stretching of the pedicle. Incision must not extend into subcutaneous fat due to risk of transecting the supratrochlear artery.
Defect Modifications	**Comment**
Temporary alar suspension stitch	Suture is passed through the alar cartilages (if present) onto the glabella above. This suspends the nasal tip superiorly to meet the forehead flap, effectively extending flap reach. Suture is then removed at time of pedicle division. Prominent suture reaction at the glabella is predictable. Potential for weakening the alar cartilage integrity with excessive superior suspension.

midazolam), and oral analgesics. Rarely, conscious sedation may be needed and can be safely performed by dermasurgeons.[8,9] Appropriate credentialing for advanced cardiac life support and sedation are essential for the latter modalities.

EXECUTION

Prior to the first incision, all design elements should be measured and remeasured, and anesthesia must be complete. The execution sequence for this author is (1) cartilage support and nasal lining restoration (if needed), (2) flap harvesting and pedicle mobilization, (3) defect preparation, (4) flap preparation and inset, (5) donor site closure, and (6) postoperative care.

Suturing intranasally can be difficult both ergonomically and visually and is facilitated by Loupe magnification, a headlamp, Castroviejo needle drivers, Castroviejo delicate tissue forceps, or bayonet forceps.

Cartilage and Lining Restoration

CG and nasal lining are essential ingredients for a stable nasal architecture. CG are either structural (native cartilage present but additional CG needed for support; Fig. 8.5) or restorative (replacing missing cartilage). SCG serve to (1) support heavy flap tissue, (2) maintain airway patency of the internal nasal valve (priority in nasal reconstruction), (3) minimize scar contraction, and (4) restore contour projection (nasal tip). CG may be auricular (antihelix or concha; Fig. 8.6), nasal (septum), or costal in nature. Auricular cartilage harvest is easiest and may be performed from an anterior or posterior approach. Anterior incisions are more accessible, but scars are more visible than posterior incisions. Postauricular access often yields a larger cartilage piece than an anterior approach. The antihelix yields cartilage that is long but thin, ideal for alar support. The concha offers thick, curved, and large grafts that may be sculpted and divided into multiple grafts, ideal for the PFF.[10,11] The subject of nasal lining is beyond the scope of this chapter. General options, however, for smaller mucosal defects (<1 cm) include (1) turnover hinge flap, (2) turndown of a forehead flap extension, (3) full-thickness skin graft (FTSG), and (4) bipedicle vestibular skin advancement flap. Larger lining restoration may require (1) turnover forehead flap, (2) septal mucoperichondrial hinge flap, (3) composite septal chondromucosal pivotal flap, or (4) larger FTSG vascularized by an overlying PFF.[12]

Flap Harvesting and Pedicle Mobilization

The PFF may be mobilized at its superior edge to include just the skin and subcutis or down to underlying galea. The former approach facilitates flap debulking during inset but results in greater bleeding. A subcutaneous level is preferred if the flap is in the hair-bearing scalp, to expose terminal hair bulbs for depilation. The level of undermining, however, delves deeper into the subgaleal plane as one

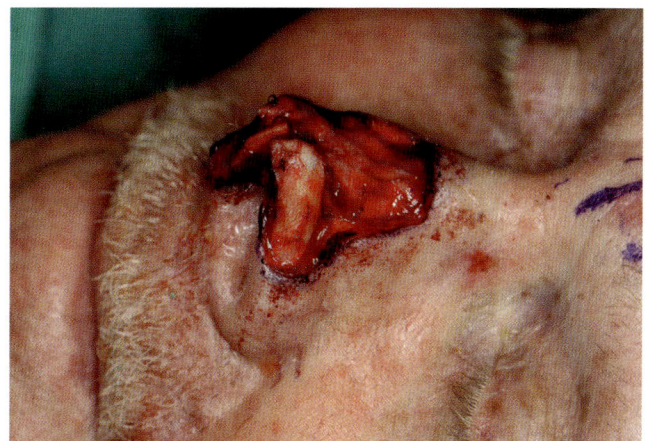

Fig. 8.5 Paramedian forehead flap (PFF)—Cartilage grafts: two alar battens and one columellar strut graft. Batten grafts placed close to the alar rim for stabilization and support of the overlying PFF.

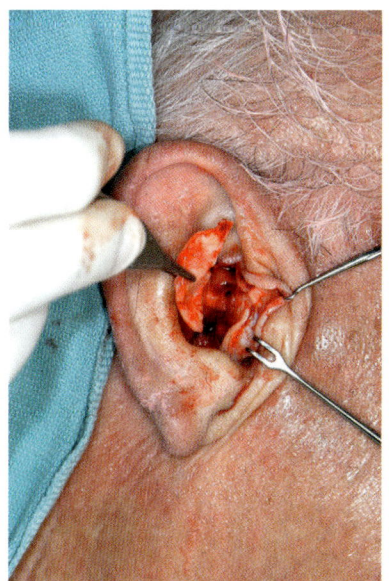 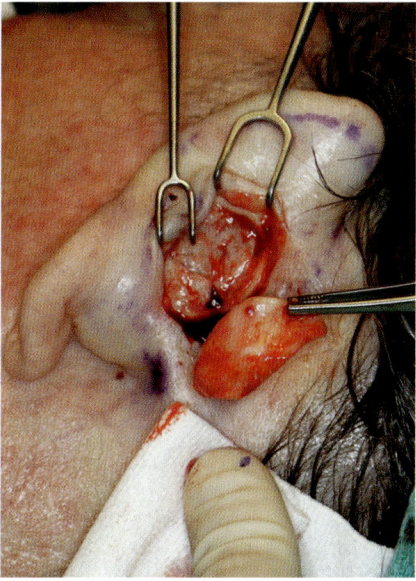

Fig. 8.6 Conchal cartilage harvested from either anterior or posterior approach.

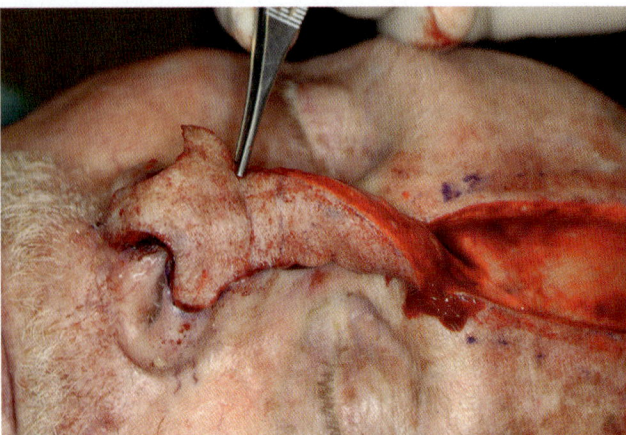

Fig. 8.7 Paramedian forehead flap lies without tension, draping to patient's columella.

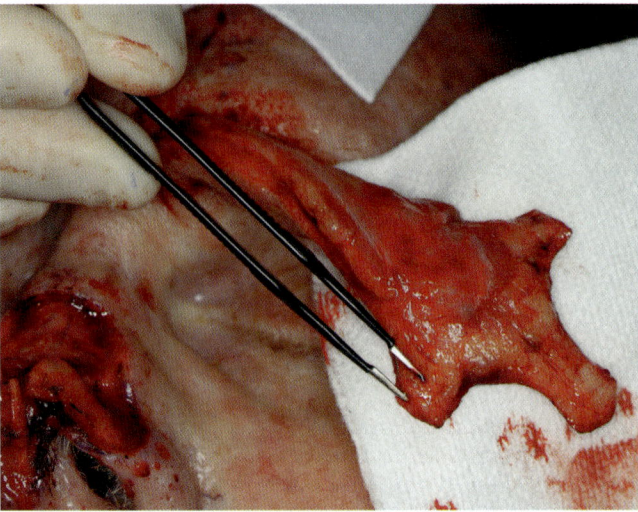

Fig. 8.8 Paramedian forehead flap—The distal forehead flap may be substantially debulked except for a thin subdermal fat layer.

approaches the eyebrow to preserve the SA. The transition from subcutis to subgalea should occur *at least* 3 cm above the orbital rim. Undermining past the orbital rim should be under direct visualization, as the SA is at risk of transection. Occasionally, subperiosteal release of the arcus marginalis and brow complex is required to enhance flap extension (see Table 8.2). The PFF should now overlie the defect without tension (Fig. 8.7).

Defect Preparation

With the flap reach and pedicle secured, the flap dimension is again compared with the defect plus any planned subunit enlargement. Only when adequate cover is ensured should the remaining subunit tissue be removed. Undermining is needed peripheral to the defect, and wound borders need to be trimmed. Beveled edges should be revised to be perpendicular except for the infratip, where a beveled edge is desirable to more smoothly approximate with the flap. The PFF's edge should correspondingly be reverse-beveled to fit the distal wound.

Flap Preparation and Inset

Prior to any suturing, the flap thickness must be revised to fit the defect. Aggressive debulking except for a thin subdermal layer is possible because of the excellent vascularity of the SA (Fig. 8.8). Constant reference to the defect is mandatory to prevent excessive thinning. Flap inset begins with interrupted epidermal sutures to secure its leading edge with the defect. If dermal-buried sutures are placed, this author prefers Poliglecaprone 25 (Monocryl, Ethicon) because of its minimal tissue reaction, a desirable feature on the sebaceous nasal tip.[13] Dermal sutures contribute to flap security and minimize incision line separation. The proximal flap as it abuts the nasal dorsum is not sutured until pedicle division.

Donor Site Closure

Donor areas are approximated as much as possible, and any remaining wound heals by second intention (Fig. 8.9). Patients may be reassured that this open portion will be significantly smaller because of inevitable wound contraction (Fig. 8.10). Tissue expansion and complex scalp flaps should be avoided, as they often lead to excessive morbidity

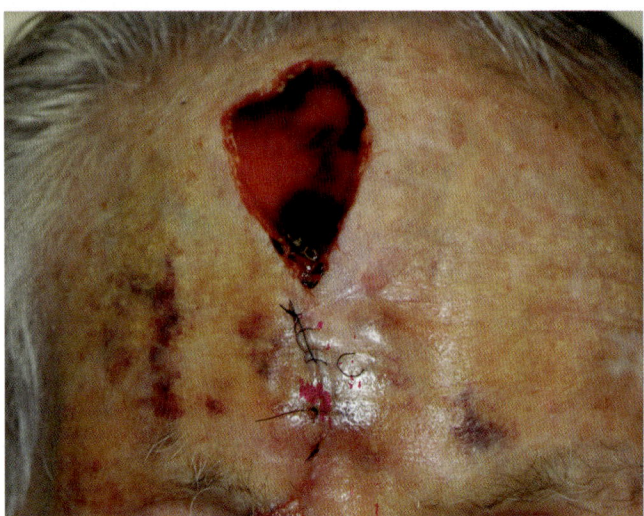

Fig. 8.9 Paramedian forehead flap—Second intention wounds at the midline or paramedian forehead heal exceptionally well. More lateral forehead wounds, however, are less predictable and usually result in poor donor site cosmesis.

on both donor and recipient tissue without cosmetic benefits. At most, unilateral or bilateral W-plasties along the frontal hairline may be considered for complete closure of the forehead wound, but excessive tension should be avoided.[6] Forehead tension (forced donor site closure) often leads to severe headache and nausea postoperatively.

POSTOPERATIVE CARE

Postoperative bleeding at the sides of the exposed pedicle is common and may be prevented with meticulous electrocoagulation. Bovine collagen matrix (BCM) may be sutured with 5-0 fast absorbing plain gut onto the exposed pedicle, followed by petrolatum gauze application. BCM is also applied to any remaining secondary defect at the forehead to aid second intention healing. BCM seals the exposed tissue, facilitates hemostasis, and is incorporated into the

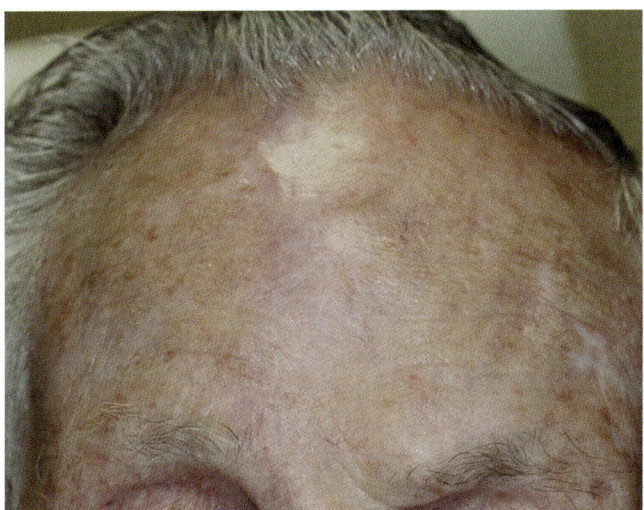

Fig. 8.10 Paramedian forehead flap (PFF)—1-year postoperative scar from primary closure and second intention healing of PFF donor site.

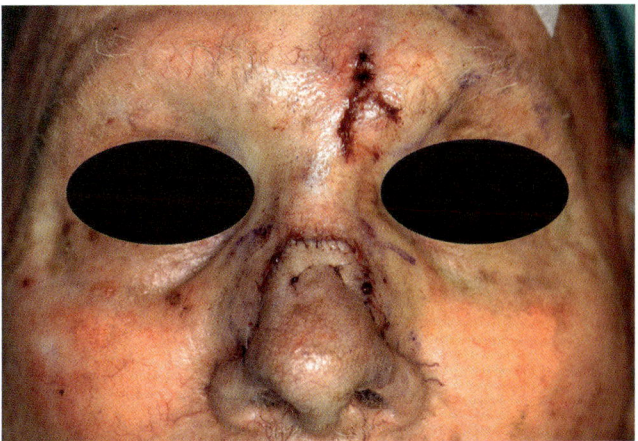

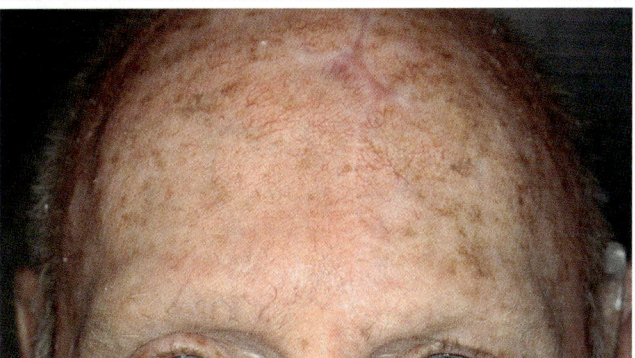

Fig. 8.11 Paramedian forehead flap—V–Y inset at stage II and long-term aesthetics.

pedicle as an epithelial covering.[14] Alternatively, the exposed pedicle may be wrapped with Surgicel or Surgicel Nu-Knit. This oxidized cellulose gauze promotes hemostasis and its removal causes less discomfort than Vaseline gauze.[15] Visual fields are blocked with pressure dressings, and the wearing of glasses is usually not possible without preoperatively customized devices. An optometrist may adjust the frame to temporarily fit over the dressing.

Postoperative observation for several hours is advisable, especially for patients at risk of bleeding. Hospitalization is not necessary, although patients must stay locally in the charge of a caretaker. Postoperative prescriptions include antibiotics (optional), analgesics, and antiemetics as needed. Wound care for the PFF may be intimidating and patients often express fear of detaching the pedicle. Detailed guidance with the first dressing change and the availability of a wound-dressing video will preempt much anxiety. A telephone call from the surgeon in the immediate perioperative period can also provide reassurance.

Paramedian Forehead Flap, Stage II

The second stage usually occurs approximately 3 weeks later and detaches the pedicle. Intermediate procedures may be needed (flap debulking and thinning) and should occur prior to the pedicle division. Stage II may be delayed for 4–6 weeks in patients at risk of flap compromise (heavy smokers), whereas earlier pedicle division (<3 weeks) may be safe but should not be performed routinely. In fact, the 6 weeks after stage I is a prime vascular period when revisions may be performed with impunity.

The approach to the pedicle stump after division varies. It may be closed primarily with a V–Y inset. A V–Y inset may be considered in patients who have a narrow glabellar width, or closely spaced eyebrows. The flap inset preserves the glabellar diameter and is camouflaged by existing rhytids (Fig. 8.11). Eyebrow repositioning is essential in all cases and may require a curvilinear ellipse for brow plasty.

Of greater consensus is the approach to proximal flap inset. The nasal dorsum is almost never excised (unless for tumor resection) to accommodate the proximal flap. Forehead tissue is invariably thicker than nasal dorsum and sidewall skin and excessive bulk is the rule unless the flap is appropriately thinned. Donor wounds healing by second intention will be significantly smaller by the time of pedicle division.

FINAL

After pedicle division, additional revisions may be needed, such as dermabrasion (6–8 weeks from stage I), depilation, and contouring (Fig. 8.12). After 8 weeks, however, further tuning should be deferred for several months to permit flap maturity and scar evolution. Early intervention for self-resolving issues only leads to unnecessary morbidity. A functional airway should always be evaluated prior to any intervention. The PFF is an extremely resilient and vascularized flap that has no equal in the aesthetic restoration of large complex nasal defects (Figs. 8.13 and 8.14).

Paramedian Forehead Flap Variations

THE FOLDED PARAMEDIAN FOREHEAD FLAP

The three-stage folded paramedian forehead flap (FPFF) is useful for full-thickness distal nasal defects involving the free margin.[16] It does not affect flap survival and may permit more aggressive flap thinning and the usage of skin grafts for nasal lining. It is also useful for patients at high risk of flap necrosis, such as heavy smokers, as thinning is delayed for an additional 3 weeks. In the first stage, a PFF with an extension is folded over to provide mucosal and soft tissue lining. At 3 weeks, the flap is elevated at the distal free margin, the nasal lining is debulked, and cartilage is inserted into the folded extension. At 6 weeks, the pedicle is divided and excess tissue thinned.

Stage I

A three-dimensional flap that folds into the nasal vestibule is designed by templating the mucosal portion and the epidermal portion separately (Fig. 8.15). Suture foil connected by Steri-Strips may be used to produce the templates and simulate the flap's folding movement. The width of the isthmus connecting the flap with its extension should be 2–3 mm for thinner forehead skin and 3–4 mm for thicker forehead skin. The distal flap margins should be elevated with a hyperbeveled thin 3–4 mm free edge, which matches well with the residual mucosal lining and distal infratip/columella or alar rim. Once the flap is elevated, the flap extension is folded, with its epithelium serving as the lining of the nasal vestibule. The mucosal and epithelial margins are approximated with 5-0 fast absorbing plain gut. The flap is sutured from inside to outside in the usual fashion, with knots facing intranasally (Fig. 8.16). Intranasal dressings are changed daily to help stabilize the flap and reduce edema.

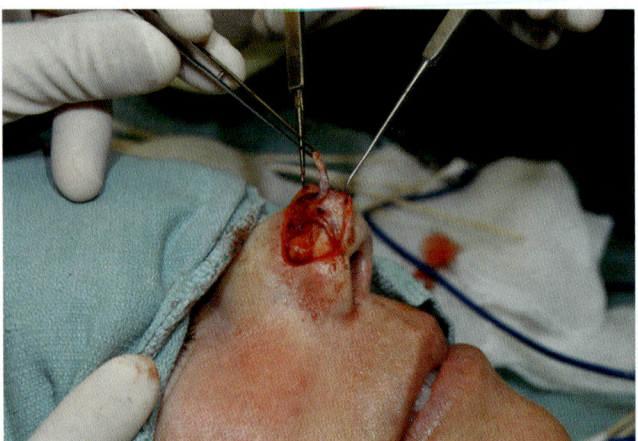

Fig. 8.12 Paramedian forehead flap—Flap contouring proceeds in incremental strips to prevent excessive thinning during revision procedure 5 months after stage I.

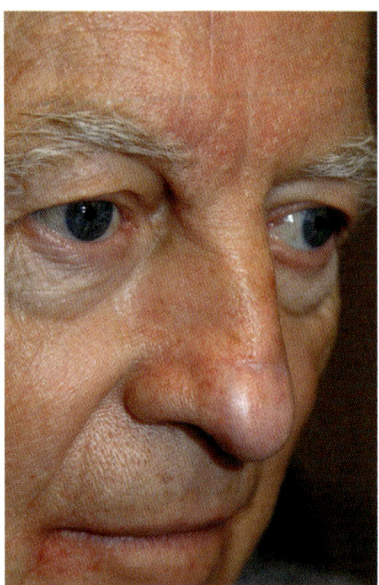

Fig. 8.14 Twelve-month result of a paramedian forehead flap *without* cartilage grafting.

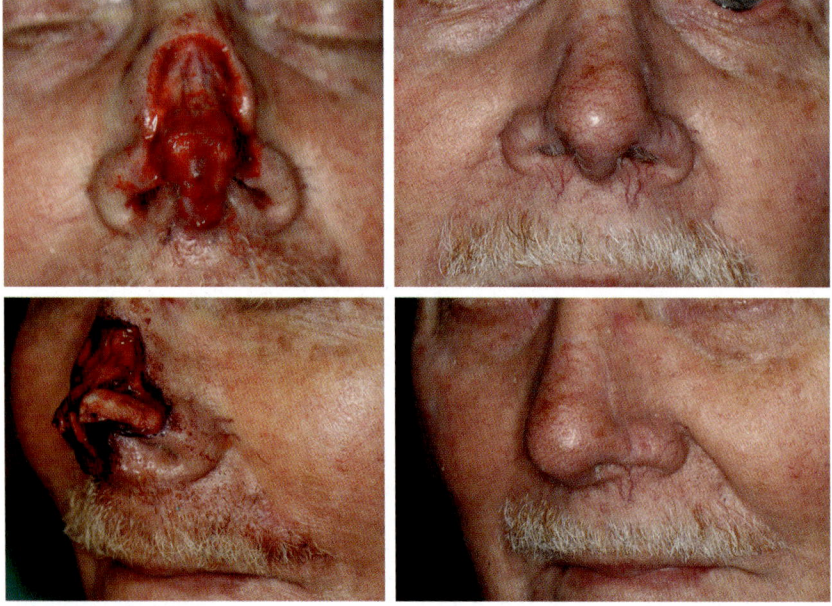

Fig. 8.13 Eighteen-month appearance of a paramedian forehead flap with cartilage grafting.

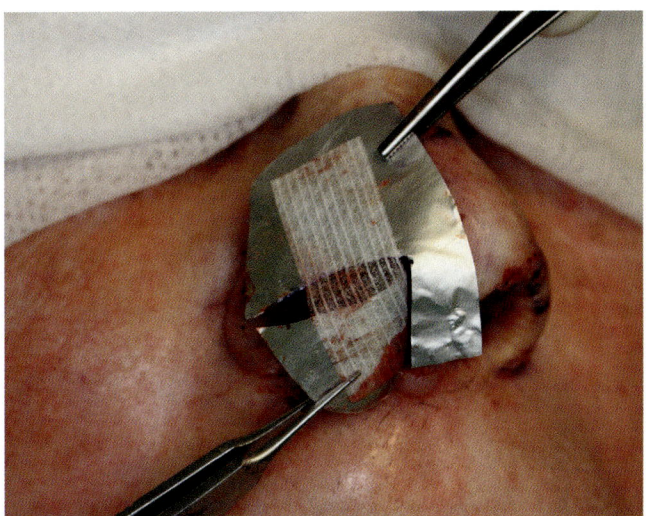

Fig. 8.15 Modular template for a folded paramedian forehead flap; includes surface covering and nasal lining. Steri-Strips simulate folded hinge.

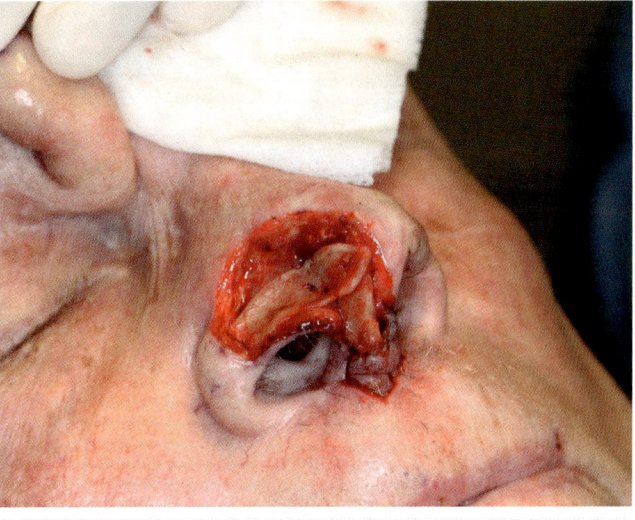

Fig. 8.17 Cartilage graft placement to support new nasal lining in Stage II of folded paramedian forehead flap.

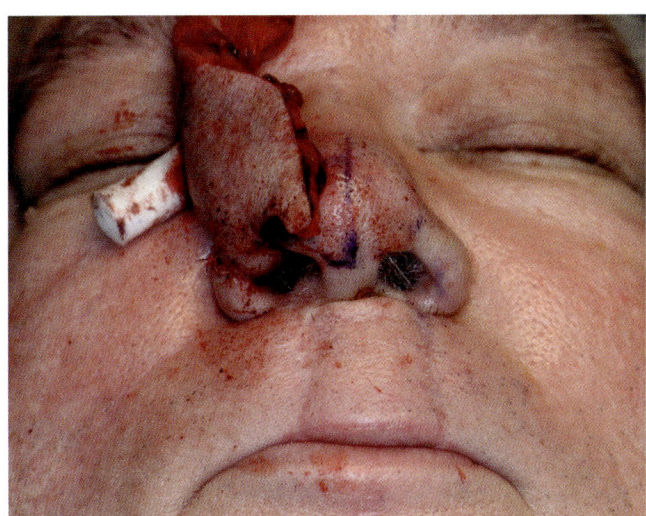

Fig. 8.16 Paramedian forehead flap with folded distal edge serving as nasal lining.

Stage II

At 3 weeks, the flap extension (now nasal lining) is adequately vascularized from the surrounding mucosa, which allows it to be detached from the main PFF and debulked. The repaired free margin is marked based on the normal contralateral side. The flap is sharply separated at the distal edge and the nasal lining is vigorously thinned, leaving only 1 mm of subdermal fat. Cartilage is harvested, sculpted to a thin tapered caudal edge, and inserted through pockets on either ends of the defect within 1–2 mm of the free margin (Fig. 8.17). The forehead flap is then reset over the new cartilage and nasal lining for an additional 3 weeks.

Stage III

Pedicle division and additional surface flap debulking and contouring occurs as in standard PFFs.

Heminasal Paramedian Forehead Flap

In the setting of a unilateral defect, a heminasal PFF with a midline scar may be performed. If the defect involves the entire width of the nasal sidewall, the template is based upon the contralateral heminasal unit and used to design an ipsilateral flap along the hairline. If the defect only involves the partial nasal sidewall, it may be enlarged to within 1 mm of the midline and then used to create the template.

Paramedian Forehead Flap With Vascular Delay

For patients at risk of vascular compromise, a PFF with vascular delay can be used to increase pedicle perfusion. The flap is incised while leaving proximal and distal portions intact and then sutured back into anatomical position. Several weeks later, the flap is reincised and elevated, and subsequently transposed according to standard recommendations. During this delay, the flap survives on its axial blood supply while the relative ischemia stimulates increased vascularization.[17]

Cheek-to-Nose Interpolation Flap

The CNIF is a two-stage flap with unique features. Its pedicle is based on tributaries from the angular artery, but the artery itself is not contained within. The vascular pattern, therefore, is more random than axial, and it is less reliable than other staged repairs. It is not a composite flap, in that only skin and subcutis are transferred and there is no muscle or fascia within the main flap body. Finally, the soft donor cheek will trapdoor easily (more so than other staged options) and a rounded convexity should be anticipated. This feature can be an asset in recreating the alar

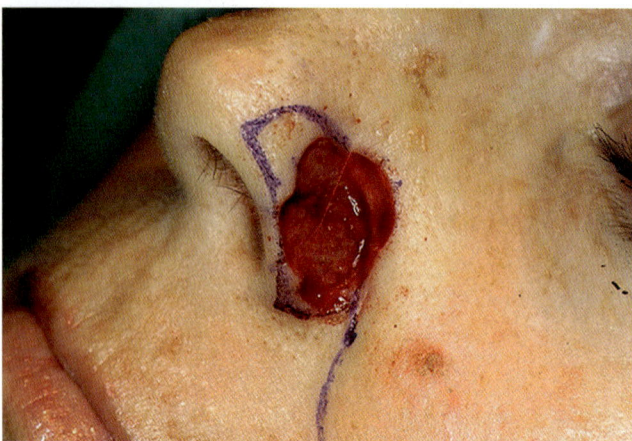

Fig. 8.18 Cheek-to-nose interpolation flap (CNIF)—Mohs defect consuming most of the ala, an ideal candidate for the CNIF.

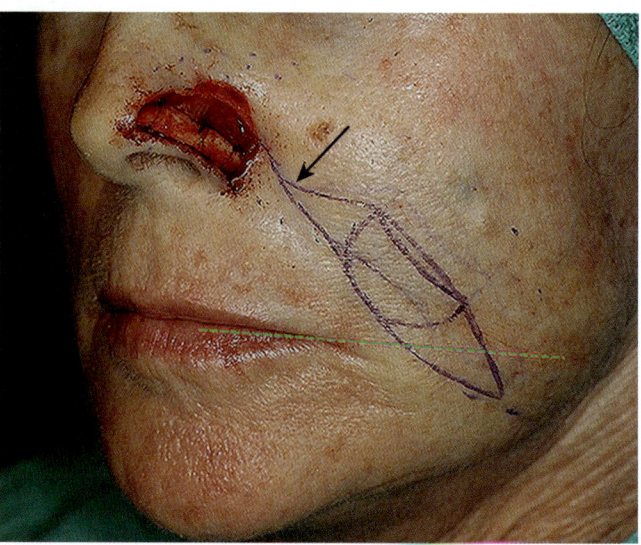

Fig. 8.19 Cheek-to-nose interpolation flap—Structural cartilage graft in place; note positioning of flap template slightly above oral commissure and narrow taper of upper flap triangle (arrow) below the alar-cheek sulcus.

lobule. The CNIF is an outpatient procedure and LA with or without an infraorbital nerve block is sufficient for patient comfort.

INDICATIONS

The CNIF is best at repairing small to medium-sized defects of the ala or infratip. The medial cheek donor skin is especially similar to the sebaceous texture of the ala. The CNIF is ideal for a deep defect (up to mucosa) that is confined to the ala and consumes 50% or more of this subunit (Fig. 8.18). Although other closures may be considered for such wounds (single-stage melolabial transposition flap), the CNIF is advantageous in preserving the alar groove and concealing donor scar within the melolabial fold.[18,19]

Single-stage buried island pedicle flaps and subcutaneous hinge flaps are also viable alternatives for strictly alar defects.[20,21] If a defect straddles both the ala and cheek, then the CNIF should resurface only the alar portion. The cheek wound may either heal by second intention (if small and shallow) or be repaired separately (cheek advancement).

ANATOMY

The flap is harvested from the skin and subcutis of the lower medial cheek and melolabial fold. In bearded men, transfer of terminal hairs is a potential disadvantage. The pedicle is proximal near the lateral alar groove and is nourished by arterial muscular perforators from the angular artery. Although the angular artery lies deep to the muscles of facial expression, its more superficial tributaries are oriented along the long axis of the flap, which contributes to its viability.[22]

FLAP DESIGN

Nasal infrastructure (cartilage and mucosal lining) requirements are stringent, as with the PFF. A CG for the CNIF is structural and not restorative (as cartilage is absent from most of the fibrofatty ala). Since the CNIF is not a heavy flap, antihelical cartilage is often sufficient. A CG braces the heavy CNIF and prevents alar retraction and adjacent nasal valve collapse (Fig. 8.19). Further, it restricts the inevitable flap contraction to create a soft convex alar lobule rather than a bulbous prominence. In width, the CG should be at least 5 mm and in length, beyond the alar defect by 3–4 mm at each end. The CG should be secured within 1–2 mm of the alar rim. Where the CG abuts the alar margin, the cartilage edges should be beveled to avoid a bulky rim. Pockets created on either side of the wound defect will secure the CG medially and laterally. When possible, the nasal lining should be lifted up to the overlying CG with a figure-of-eight suture.

The entire alar lobule should be resurfaced when possible. The remaining ala up to the alar groove, except for a 1-mm margin of alar base and rim, will eventually be excised in stage II for full subunit repair. Flap design should include this enlargement. Some even advocate a flap template that is 1 mm larger in all dimensions, partially to counteract wound contraction and partially to exploit the trapdoor effect and recreate a lobular convexity.[23] This mild oversizing may be achieved by incising on the outside edge of flap markings. The senior author has found that this enlargement is unnecessary in most cases.

Similar to the PFF, the contralateral normal side may serve as a model for template creation.

The template is now transferred to the medial cheek and lower melolabial fold and outlined, with the widest part of the flap positioned across or slightly above the oral commissure. Triangles are now drawn above and below the flap outline to create a curvilinear ellipse. The lower triangle will be excised full thickness to close the donor site. Proximally, the upper triangle must taper at least 0.5 cm below the lateral alar groove to avoid effacement of this landmark. Excessive tension lateral to the apical lip and alar sulcus can lead to webbed scars. Although this proximal triangle is drawn narrowly, the underlying pedicle is more wide and deep to maximize vascular supply. Flap reach should be confirmed with a stretched gauze that simulates actual

Table 8.3	Pedicle Variations for the Cheek-to-Nose Interpolation Flap	
Pedicle	Features	Comment
Myocutaneous	Pedicle contains skin, subcutaneous fat, and muscular fibers from the levator labii superioris alaeque nasi.	Easier to develop than myosubcutaneous design. Proximal skin is narrow in width superficially but underlying pedicle is wider. Overlying skin may restrict proximal flap movement unless relaxed with scoring incisions.
Myosubcutaneous	Pedicle is identical to above but is without the overlying proximal skin (epidermis and dermis).	Pedicle development is more challenging but movement is greater than with myocutaneous design.

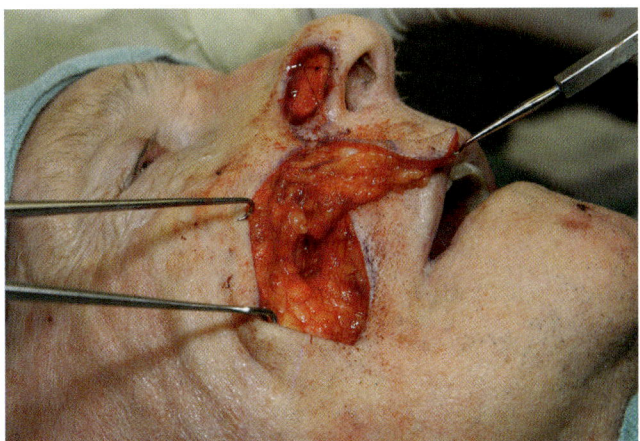

Fig. 8.20 Cheek-to-nose interpolation flap—Proximal pedicle requires deep dissection to incorporate muscle fibers at base that contain arterial perforators. The angular artery itself, however, is not within the pedicle.

movement. From the donor site, the flap transposes and rotates counterclockwise for a right-sided alar wound and clockwise for the left side. Template orientation must account for these directional distinctions.

EXECUTION

The CNIF pedicle may be developed to be either myocutaneous or myosubcutaneous. The myocutaneous design includes skin, subcutis, and muscle fibers of the levator labii superioris alequae nasi (LLSAN). The myosubcutaneous pedicle excludes the overlying dermis and epidermis, which is excised at the time of flap harvest. Features of both designs are discussed in Table 8.3.

Superficial incisions indelibly score the flap outlines and prevent the inaccuracies of blurred pen markings. The lower triangle is then fully excised and the distal flap sharply elevated with a 3- to 4-mm subdermal fat layer. As one nears the proximal pedicle, dissection delves deeper to incorporate muscle fibers of the LLASN (Fig. 8.20). Partial muscle inclusion is essential to preserving the arterial perforators for this flap. Hook retraction of the cheek laterally, the cutaneous lip medially, and the flap superiorly will expose these muscle fibers. Searching for the angular artery is to be avoided. Flap dissection is similar to that of an island pedicle flap in that excessive flap mobilization exacts the price of a smaller pedicle.

Resistance to flap movement may be alleviated by these maneuvers: (1) scoring incision (to dermis) at the proximal triangle (if a myocutaneous design was chosen), which frees proximal skin attachments tethering the flap; (2) closing the donor cheek in a superior oblique vector (northeast for the right cheek and northwest for the left), which progressively brings the flap medially and superiorly (Fig. 8.21); and (3) temporary suspension suture, lifting the flap to the upper cutaneous lip, which is removed in 1 week.

Once the flap reaches the defect with minimal tension, defect preparation begins with ensuring CG security and debeveling wound edges. The alar rim, however, should remain beveled, and likewise, the flap's margin at the alar

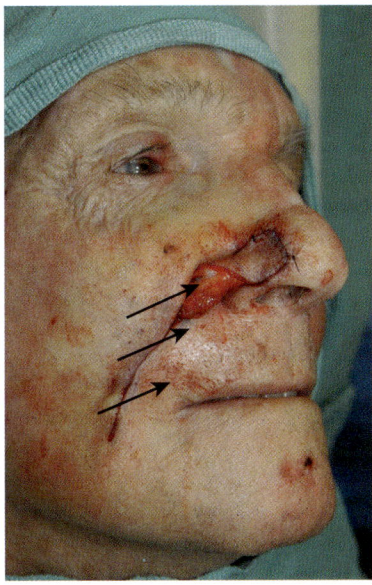

Fig. 8.21 Cheek-to-nose interpolation flap—Donor site closure in a superiorly oblique vector (arrows) progressively elevates the flap toward the defect and facilitates final closure.

rim must be reverse-beveled to achieve a flush closure. The lateral alar subunit is not resected by this author until pedicle division.

The flap must then be debulked of fat (except for a thin subdermal fat layer to preserve the superficial vascular plexus) to fit the defect. The first key sutures close the donor site, which progressively lifts the flap toward the defect. Epidermal sutures then align and inset the flap. If the flap covers the alar defect without tension, then buried dermal sutures are often not necessary. Throughout the execution phase, constant assessment of alar rim symmetry and airway patency must occur.

POSTOPERATIVE CARE

Wound care for the CNIF is less demanding than that for the PFF. Glasses may be worn and bandages are less

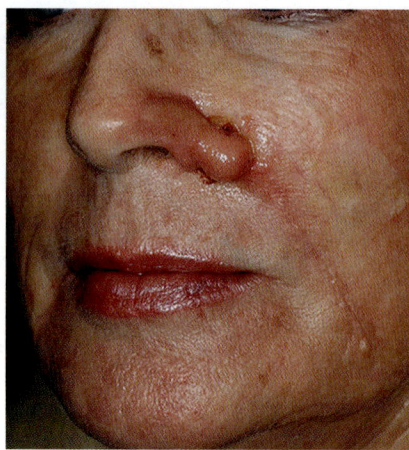
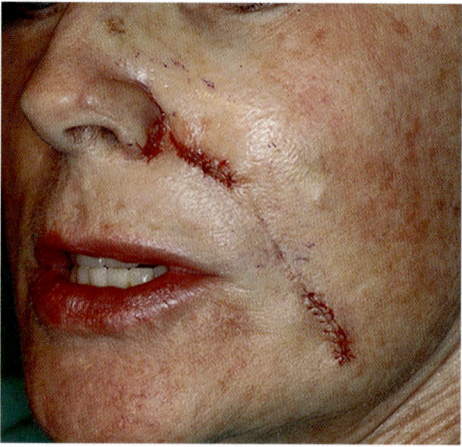

Fig. 8.22 Cheek-to-nose interpolation flap (CNIF)—Complete flap survival at 3 weeks, permitting pedicle division. CNIF-residual subunit excised except for 1–2 mm of the lateral alar base to anchor the flap.

cumbersome. A Xeroform gauze wraps around the exposed pedicle and another roll rests under it for support. Bleeding is uncommon at the pedicle edges, as the arterial supply is less vigorous. Intranasal dressings may be needed for bilayer support, especially if mucosal lining was repaired. Postoperative nausea is rare and pain, if any, is most often felt at the cartilage donor site. Postoperatively, respiration may be impaired despite nasal valve support because of transient surgical edema, which may require several weeks to subside.

Cheek-to-Nose Interpolation Flap, Stage II

Pedicle division in stage II should not be attempted prior to 3 weeks. Given the more tenuous pedicle, intermediate stages are not wise and longer deferment of stage II is preferred for smokers. If the flap survives completely at stage II, then the residual subunit may be excised, except for 1–2 mm of the alar base, which serves to anchor the flap and maintain the lateral alar groove (Fig. 8.22). Subunit enlargement must be attentive to the recently placed CG.

The pedicle base may be divided and the cheek closed primarily. Alternatively, it may be partially inset as a V-shaped section into the cheek to restore bilateral symmetry. Reinset is appropriate if either the donor cheek preoperatively was full or the flap was large. This author finds the V-shaped inset incongruous on the cheek unlike its more natural appearance at the glabella in the PFF.

With the pedicle severed and the residual subunit removed, the flap is trimmed and debulked to fit the defect. A beveled edge at the alar base and a reverse bevel at the lateral flap margin are helpful for a flush closure. Interrupted sutures complete flap inset and alar reconstruction. A tie-over bolster dressing at the alar groove may be helpful to compress and maintain this sulcus.

If necrosis is noted in stage II, then it is often seen at the distal flap margin and is usually due to a diminutive pedicle (Fig. 8.23). Gentle curettage will reveal the depth of necrosis (usually partial). Superficial necrosis is best approached with second intention healing and postponement of stage II. Deeper necrosis may be remedied with an excision of the failed margin and reclosure, if possible, with the healthy proximal flap (Fig. 8.24).

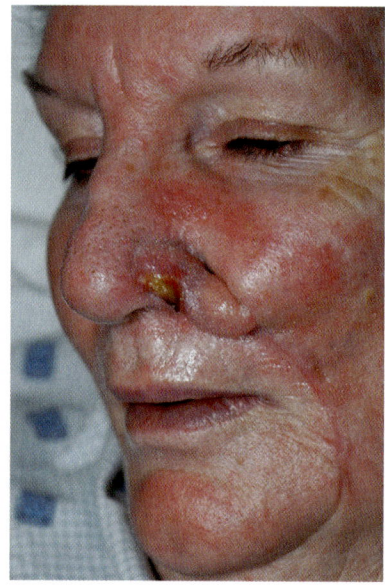

Fig. 8.23 Cheek-to-nose interpolation flap—Distal flap necrosis.

FINAL

Issues that may require revisions following stage II typically target the following: (1) flap trapdooring (intralesional steroids, surgical debulking), (2) alar groove definition (incising and debulking underlying scar at sulcus), (3) alar thickness (excising a wedge of fibrous scar via an intranasal approach), and (4) airway patency.

The CNIF's value as a staged repair lies in its tissue match with the lateral ala and distal nose. Donor scar is minimal and well camouflaged. The flap preserves important landmarks (alar groove) and meets high aesthetic standards (Fig. 8.25). It is flexible in its reach and may even extend to resurface the floor of the nasal vestibule. Compared with the PFF, the CNIF differs by (1) repairing smaller, less complex nasal defects; (2) being better suited for repair of

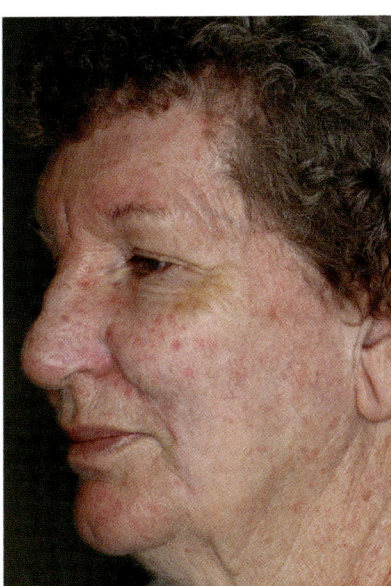

Fig. 8.24 Cheek-to-nose interpolation flap—6-month postoperative appearance with dermabrasion, a reasonable result despite partial flap necrosis.

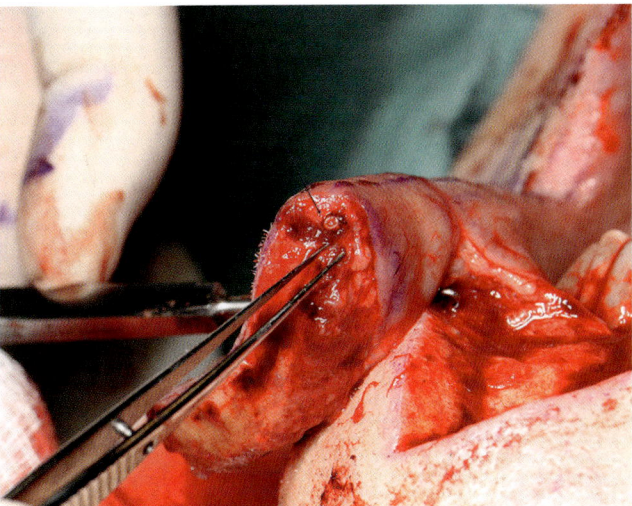

Fig. 8.26 Location of the inferior labial artery, sandwiched between the muscularis anteriorly and the mucosa posteriorly.

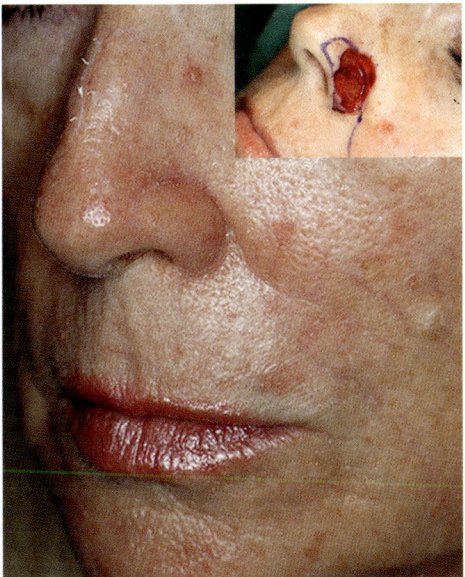

Fig. 8.25 Cheek-to-nose interpolation flap—1-year result, an excellent outcome relative to the original defect.

the lateral ala; (3) being less reliable in its vascularity; and (4) requiring less postoperative wound care and lifestyle restrictions.

Abbé (Lip-Switch) Flap

The Abbé flap is perhaps the most robust of all interpolation repairs. It is unique in several respects: (1) functional restoration is high as it includes muscle and mucosa from the donor flap, (2) pedicle survival is most dependable and flap viability is possible even with arterial transection, and (3) the same donor site may be harvested more than once if needed. The lip-switch terminology most commonly refers to the "switching" of a lower lip flap to reconstruct an upper lip defect. The reverse may also apply (upper lip flap to repair lower lip defect), although it is less ideal because of potential alterations on the philtrum. Further discussion will focus on the classic lip switch (lower lip to upper lip).

INDICATIONS

A number of flaps are applicable for medium to large full-thickness lip defects. These include the Abbé, Estlander, Karapandzic, Gilles fan flap, and McGregor repairs. Among these options, the Abbé is best at restoring neuromuscular function with the least disruption to the perioral anatomy.[24] Lip defects amenable for the Abbé are those that (1) are lateral to midline but do not involve the oral commissure (although wounds isolated to the philtrum are candidates), (2) consume one-third to one-half of the lip, and (3) involve significant loss of the orbicularis oris muscle. It is this last factor that demands functional muscle replacement, which is best provided by the Abbé procedure.

ANATOMY

Nourishing the Abbé is the inferior labial artery (ILA), which branches off the facial artery and has a variable course across the lower cutaneous and mucosal lip. At midline, the ILA is always posteriorly located within the mucosal lip (red lip) at the level of the vermilion border. Here it lies between the orbicularis muscle anteriorly and the mucosa posteriorly (Fig. 8.26). Lateral to midline, the ILA location is less predictable. Within the lip, the ILA may be found either within the orbicularis oris muscle (minority) or between the muscle and mucosa (majority).[25] The ILA is never located between the muscle and subcutis, a reassuring fact during flap creation.

FLAP DESIGN

The Abbé template is best positioned at midline where arterial location is most predictable and donor site symmetry

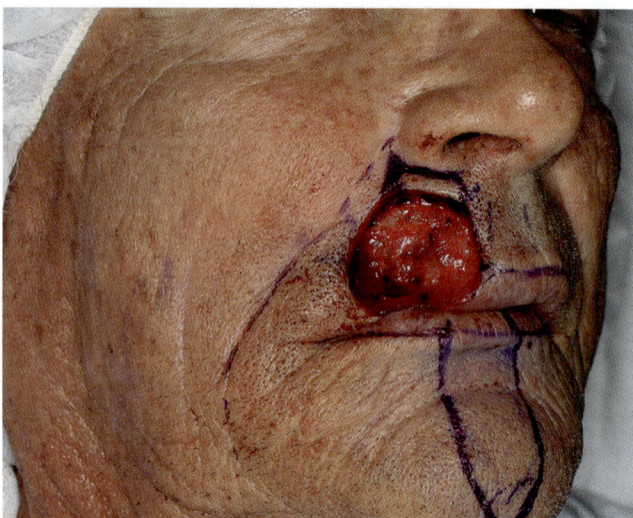

Fig. 8.27 Natural landmarks and subunit enlargement of defect are outlined prior to local anesthesia infiltration. Template is positioned midline and marked in solid line while dashed extension addresses the standing cutaneous cone and permits donor site closure.

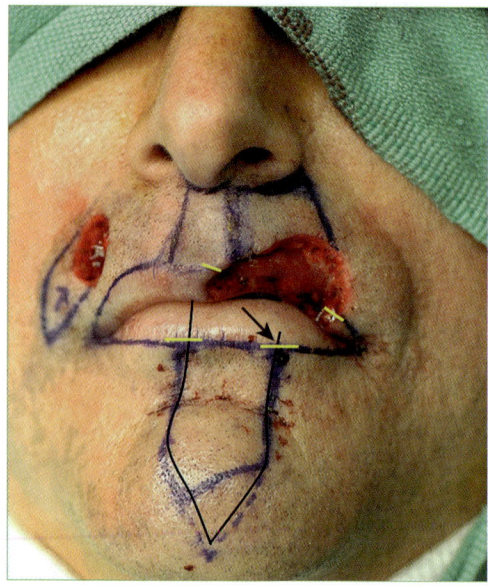

Fig. 8.28 Inferior labial artery on the side ipsilateral to the upper lip defect is preserved as the pedicle. Note anterior incision *(arrow)* extends beyond vermillion border and also note that upper lip defect enlargement to upper borders of subunit.

may be preserved. Paramedian locations may also be considered to match the vermilion border thickness between the donor and recipient lip. Extremely lateral flap designs, however, are contraindicated because of the potential distortion of the oral commissure. Donor site morbidity is low unless excessively resected, which may compromise stoma size.

Proper repair of the full-thickness defect in Fig. 8.27 requires its enlargement to the upper cutaneous lip borders. The template fashioned may be less than the defect as the inherent stretch of lip tissue compensates for a smaller flap size. The nasal sill and alar crease must be preserved with any flap design, and all landmarks (vermilion border, philtrum, etc.) must be outlined prior to LA and incision (Fig. 8.28).

EXECUTION

Table 8.4 details the execution sequence for the Abbé repair, which may be safely performed as an ambulatory procedure.

Inevitably, one side of the ILA must be transected to mobilize the Abbé flap. Determining which side to sacrifice is a critical decision. Generally, the ILA ipsilateral to the upper lip defect is preserved, while the other side is incised (see Fig. 8.28). This permits the widest oral stoma possible for eating and minimizes pedicle twisting during closure. Unlike the forehead flap, in which the SA is never seen, the ILA side that is incised serves as an excellent reference point during dissection to preserve the contralateral pedicle. The pedicle stump should be approximately 1 cm, smaller in front but wider posteriorly. A healthy wide cuff of posterior mucosa is essential, and perhaps even more critical for pedicle survival than arterial preservation. There are even reports of complete flap survival based solely on a mucosal attachment (inadvertent transection of artery).[26]

Suction should be used frequently both for patient comfort and for visibility in this highly vascular location. What may be counterintuitive is the need to excise all remaining lip layers (any remaining skin, muscle, mucosa) at the defect to create room for the Abbé. Without clearing the defect, the incoming Abbé will not fit well and become bloblike in its appearance. Similarly, the flap must be harvested in its full thickness to preserve all neuromuscular structures. Also counterintuitive is the need to enlarge the defect for subunit repair when possible. Superior aesthetic results, however, may be achieved with subunit replacement.

Closure begins with the donor site first, and suturing should approximate all lip layers in the following order: mucosa (absorbable gut), muscularis (polyglactin [Vicryl]), subcutis (Poliglecaprone [Monocryl]), and then cutaneous. Mucosal sutures should be soft (silk or polyglactin) to avoid irritation. Horizontal mattress sutures are advocated by some to prevent any gaps in the posterior mucosa, which may lead to fistulas and leaks from the minor salivary glands. The donor incision line externally should be well everted. Especially critical is the accurate approximation of the vermilion–cutaneous border, which is facilitated by (1) scoring incisions marking the horizontal free margin (see Table 8.4, Step 6) and (2) extending flap incision vertically on the pedicle side beyond the red lip border (see Table 8.4, Step 8; Fig. 8.29). This latter maneuver liberates an edge of the vermilion border and permits the accurate realignment of this free margin with the defect. Flap inset also proceeds in the order as described earlier (mucosa to cutaneous). A buried suture to align the vermilion border may help position the flap properly. The flap at the recipient site should lie flush with the surrounding skin.

POSTOPERATIVE CARE

Wound dressing with the Abbé is straightforward. The pedicle connecting the upper and lower lips is self-contained, and a circumferential dressing (like the PFF) is contraindicated. Patients are warned not to consume hot solids/liquids

Table 8.4 Abbé Flap Sequence for Classic Lip-Switch (Lower Lip Flap to Upper Lip Defect)

Steps	Comment
1. Outline all natural landmarks prior to local anesthesia.	Outline the philtrum, vermilion borders, nasal sill, alar groove, melolabial folds.
2. Enlarge defect outline if possible to permit subunit repair.	Extend defect to upper borders of cutaneous lip. Do not extend to oral commissures.
3. Fashion template and transfer to midline lower lip.	Template may be smaller than defect (50%–80% of defect width), as lip tissue will stretch.
4. Decide which side of the inferior labial artery will serve as the pedicle.	Preserve the pedicle side that will create the largest oral stoma postoperatively (usually the side ipsilateral to the defect).
5. Prepare the patient.	Administer oral prophylactic antibiotics (optional), mental nerve blocks, and local anesthesia. Wait at least 30 min for tissue distension from local anesthesia to subside prior to incising. Availability of suction is helpful.
6. Mark the vermilion–cutaneous borders on both lips with a scoring incision.	These superficial incisions will facilitate accurate realignment of the vermilion–cutaneous borders during closure. Do not rely solely on pen markings, which may be blurred intraoperatively.
7. Prepare the defect.	Excise all layers (skin, muscle, mucosa) of the remaining lip defect (and subunit if possible) to accommodate for the incoming Abbé flap.
8. Outline the flap with scoring incisions.	On the pedicle side, the scoring incision (to superficial dermis) should extend past the vermilion border, but not into the orbicularis muscle.
9. Perform a full-thickness incision on the side that will be mobilized.	Compress the ILA lateral to incision. Following transection, slow release of the ILA will confirm its location and serve as a reference when the contralateral side will be dissected as the pedicle.
10. Liberate the Abbé flap from all attachments.	Sharp resections of all attachments (mucosa, muscle, subcutis) are essential to completely mobilize the flap. Progress from the free end to the pedicle side.
11. Develop the Abbé pedicle.	Sharp dissection becomes blunt and spreading as one approaches the vermilion–cutaneous border on the pedicle side. Anterior surface incision should pass the vermilion border and is safe as long as muscle plane is not transgressed. Posterior surface mucosa must be preserved at the vermilion border level as the ILA lies just in front.
12. Close the donor site.	Partial closure of the donor site will facilitate flap movement. Initiate suturing at the mucosa with knots tied externally, facing the oral cavity.
13. Rotate the Abbé flap superiorly and inset into the defect.	The flap will require trimming and some debulking to fit the recipient site. Suture each lip layer separately and avoid burying knot within orbicularis oris muscle.
14. Final closure	Ensure that all vermilion–cutaneous borders are accurately approximated.

ILA, Inferior labial artery.

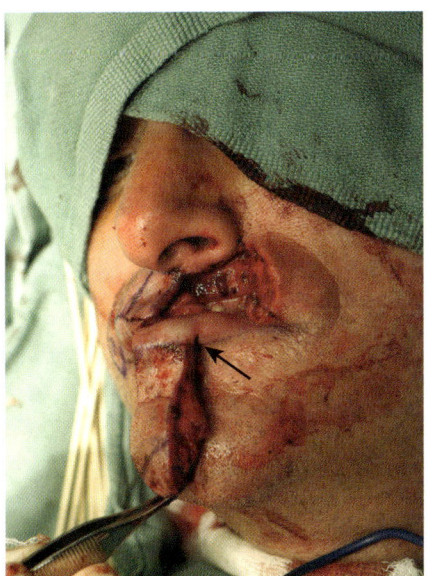

Fig. 8.29 Incision past the vermillion border on the attached pedicle side *(black arrow)* facilitates accurate margin alignment.

until anesthesia dissipates and semisolids or puréed foods may be needed. Patients may still converse. A standard postoperative regimen for this author includes antibiotics and analgesics in liquid formulations for ease of administration. Although nausea from surgery is uncommon, nausea and vomiting from the narcotic analgesics may occur, and a preemptive prescription is recommended. Antivirals are generally not necessary.

Abbé Flap, Stage II

Pedicle division occurs in 3 weeks or may be deferred longer for flaps with questionable viability. An intermediate stage prior to pedicle division is not risky but is rarely needed. Prominent flap edema, especially at the mucosal border, is normal and will subside with time (8–12 weeks) as lymphatic and venous drainage becomes reestablished (Fig. 8.30). Temptation to surgically intervene earlier should be resisted.

The vermilion–cutaneous borders should again be marked. LA to infiltrate the pedicle and adjacent skin on both ends will suffice. Patients are asked to slightly open

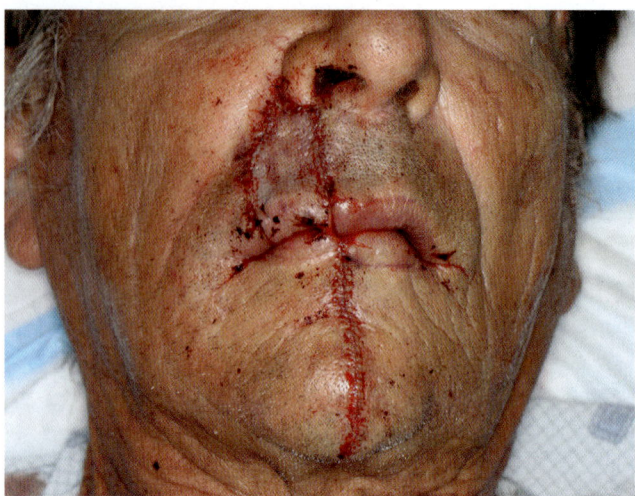

Fig. 8.30 Immediate postoperative appearance. Flap is flush with surrounding recipient lip.

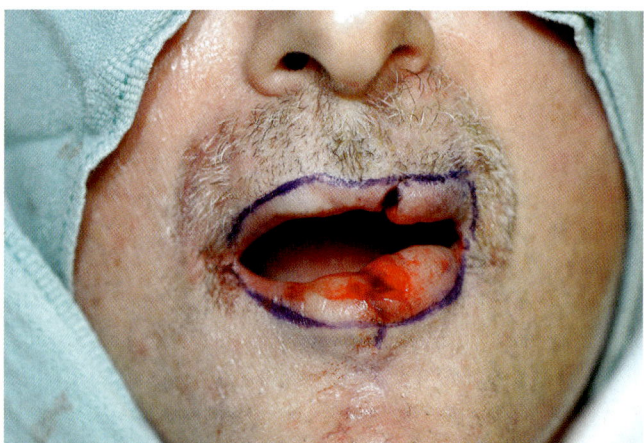

Fig. 8.32 Pedicle division creates a triangular defect on the upper lip, which is closed primarily and a pyramidal stump on the lower lip, which may be inset or excised.

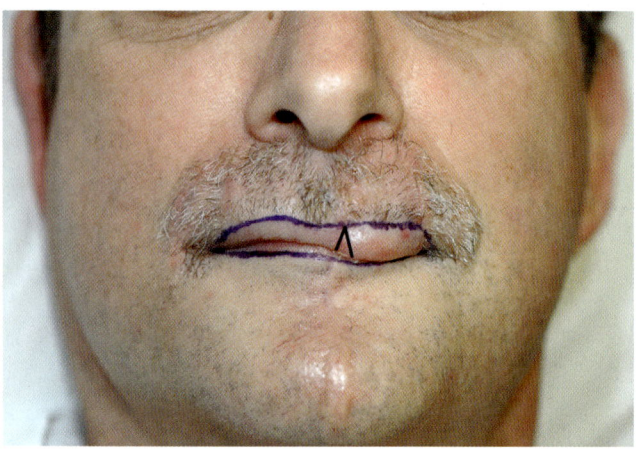

Fig. 8.31 Stage II-flap appearance at 3 weeks with prominent edema of lower flap margin. This transient edema resolves in time with lymphovascular reestablishment. An inverted V-shaped incision divides the pedicle with the base remaining on the lower lip.

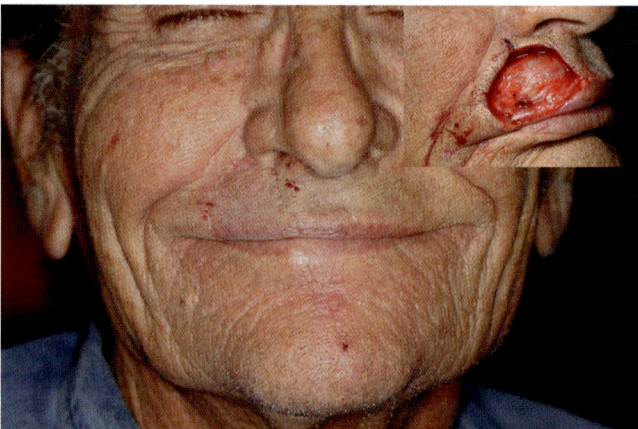

Fig. 8.33 Postoperative appearance at 4 months. Mucosal edema is almost resolved, and there is excellent symmetry of upper and lower lips, with accurate vermillion approximation.

their lips, a Q-tip is placed behind the pedicle, and two hooks should retract the upper and lower lip apart for stability and traction.

The first step creates an inverted V-shaped incision that divides the pedicle. Following separation, the upper mucosal lip will have a triangular defect, which may be sutured side to side (Fig. 8.31). The lower mucosal lip retains the triangular remnant of the pedicle, which may be either excised or resutured into the mucosal lip (Fig. 8.32). Reinset is appropriate if bulk is needed for donor site symmetry. As the mucosal lip heals exceptionally, the V-shaped inset blends well aesthetically, unlike that of its counterpart in the PFF and CNIF. If necessary, incisions may be carried into the recently sutured cutaneous lip on both ends for accurate tissue alignment.

FINAL

For male patients, any transferred hairs from the lower cutaneous lip and chin will continue to grow within the flap. The hair growth direction, however, will be reversed. Following stage II, revision surgery is rarely needed unless the vermilion border requires repositioning. Flap edema will resolve with time (Fig. 8.33). The time for neuromuscular recovery varies and can be age-dependent. Younger patients have almost full recovery within 6 months, whereas older patients may require 1 year or more. The Abbé repair is extremely flexible in its applications. Two or more Abbé flaps may be harvested from the same donor lip, provided that overall oral patency is not compromised. Abbé patterns extending into the submental region have been described with some designs tunneling under an intact upper vermilion border.[27,28]

These modifications may resurface large and complex central-facial defects. The lip-switch flap may also be combined with other repairs for subtotal lip restoration.[29,30]

Conclusion

Mastery of interpolation techniques requires a firm foundation in random pattern flaps. The subtleties of each procedure are many and cannot be learned superficially or casually. Some surgical principles are firm, such as (1) cancer-free margins, (2) function before cosmesis, (3) infrastructure support and restoration, and (4) subunit repair, when possible, although flexibility with subunit excision is key. Other positions are subjective and not to be taken as dogma. Properly performed, these staged techniques achieve both functional and aesthetic excellence for complex facial wounds. All specialties have valuable insights into these repairs, and dermatologic surgeons have contributed substantially to their refinement and enhancement.

COMPLICATIONS WITH SURGERY

Even with perfect planning and execution, surgical outcomes may still be suboptimal. The impact of failed (partial or total) staged repairs is devastating to both patient and surgeon. The authors' approach to these disappointments consists of four steps. Step 1 is an honest patient discussion, which begins with a sincere expression of regret. If identifiable factors for the complication are noted, then these may be avoided in subsequent surgeries. Patients, however, must never feel abandoned or blamed. Surgeons are human and imperfection is the plight of humanity. Step 2 assesses what revisions are needed. Fortunately, necrosis or dehiscence is often only partial with staged repairs, and thus some salvage is usually possible. The number of revisions needed and the timing of these surgeries are relevant issues. Patients must also be informed that revision plans may change, depending on the outcome of each intervention. Step 3 is a decision with the patient on who will be performing the revisions. Generally, the primary surgeon should also perform subsequent revisions, unless skill sets are not present. A referral externally (to a trusted and nonjudgmental colleague) is not a source of shame and is part of sound surgical judgment. Finally, a realistic appraisal of the eventual outcome is important but is not always possible.

The CNIF partially necrosed due to a shallow pedicle (minimal incorporation of muscle perforators at base). Fortunately, the necrotic area was small and superficial (gentle curettage of eschar). Pedicle division proceeded, and the shallow wound healed secondarily. Dermabrasion followed (6 weeks from stage I) and final results are shown in Fig. 8.24. An alternative approach would have been to delay pedicle division for an additional 2 weeks to allow for a better assessment of second intention healing. This necrosis exemplifies the need to defer subunit enlargement until stage II and only if flap survival is assured. Had the subunit been excised at stage I and had flap necrosis been more extensive at stage II, then an unfortunate outcome would have turned disastrous.

References

1. Burget GC, Menick FJ. The subunit principle in nasal reconstruction. *Plast Reconstr Surg.* 1985;76(2):239-247.
2. Sherris DA, Fuerstenberg J, Danahey D, Hilger PA. Reconstruction of the nasal columella. *Arch Facial Plast Surg.* 2002;4(1):42-46.
3. Vural E, Batay F, Key JM. Glabellar frown lines as a reliable landmark for the supratrochlear artery. *Otolaryngol Head Neck Surg.* 2000;123(5):543-546.
4. Burget GC, Menick FJ. The paramedian forehead flap. In: Burget GC, Menick FJ, eds. *Aesthetic Reconstruction of the Nose.* St. Louis, MO: Mosby; 1994:57-91.
5. Stigall LE, Bramlette TB, Zitelli JA, Brodland DG. The paramidline forehead flap: a clinical and microanatomic study. *Dermatol Surg.* 2016;42(6):764-771.
6. Quatela VC, Sherris DA, Rounds MF. Esthetic refinements in forehead flap nasal reconstruction. *Arch Otolaryngol Head Neck Surg.* 1995;121(10):1106-1113.
7. Ugur MB, Savranlar A, Uzun L, Kucuker H, Cinar F. A reliable surface landmark for localizing supratrochlear artery: medial canthus. *Otolaryngol Head Neck Surg.* 2008;138(2):162-165.
8. Otley CC, Nguyen TH. Safe and effective conscious sedation administered by dermatologic surgeons. *Arch Dermatol.* 2000;136(11):1333-1335.
9. Otley CC, Nguyen TH. Conscious sedation. *Dermatol Surg.* 2003;177-182.
10. Byrd DR, Otley CC, Nguyen TH. Alar batten cartilage grafting in nasal reconstruction: functional and cosmetic results. *J Am Acad Dermatol.* 2000;43(5 Pt 1):833-836.
11. Ratner D, Skouge JW. Surgical pearl: the use of free cartilage grafts in nasal alar reconstruction. *J Am Acad Dermatol.* 1997;36(4):622-624.
12. Baker SR. *Principles of Nasal Reconstruction.* 2nd ed. New York: Springer; 2011. http://www.columbia.edu/cgi-bin/cul/resolve?clio8850281.
13. Molea G, Schonauer F, Bifulco G, D'Angelo D. Comparative study on biocompatibility and absorption times of three absorbable monofilament suture materials (Polydioxanone, Poliglecaprone 25, Glycomer 631). *Br J Plast Surg.* 2000;53(2):137-141.
14. Wanitphakdeedecha R, Chen TM, Nguyen TH. The use of acellular, fetal bovine dermal matrix for acute, full-thickness wounds. *J Drugs Dermatol.* 2008;7(8):781-784.
15. Shinkwin CA, Beasley N, Simo R, Rushton L, Jones NS. Evaluation of Surgicel Nu-knit, Merocel and Vasolene gauze nasal packs: a randomized trial. *Rhinology.* 1996;34(1):41-43.
16. Menick FJ. A 10-year experience in nasal reconstruction with the three-stage forehead flap. *Plast Reconstr Surg.* 2002;109(6):1839-1855 [discussion 1856–1861].
17. Kent DE, Defazio JM. Improving survival of the paramedian forehead flap in patients with excessive tobacco use: the vascular delay. *Dermatol Surg.* 2011;37(9):1362-1364.
18. Fader DJ, Baker SR, Johnson TM. The staged cheek-to-nose interpolation flap for reconstruction of the nasal alar rim/lobule. *J Am Acad Dermatol.* 1997;37(4):614-619.
19. Baker SR, Johnson TM, Nelson BR. The importance of maintaining the alar-facial sulcus in nasal reconstruction. *Arch Otolaryngol Head Neck Surg.* 1995;121(6):617-622.
20. Hairston BR, Nguyen TH. Innovations in the island pedicle flap for cutaneous facial reconstruction. *Dermatol Surg.* 2003;29(4):378-385.
21. Johnson TM, Baker S, Brown MD, Nelson BR. Utility of the subcutaneous hinge flap in nasal reconstruction. *J Am Acad Dermatol.* 1994;30(3):459-466.
22. Hynes B, Boyd JB. The nasolabial flap. Axial or random? *Arch Otolaryngol Head Neck Surg.* 1988;114(12):1389-1391.
23. Burget GC, Menick FJ. The superiorly based nasolabial flap: technical details. In: Burget GC, Menick FJ, eds. *Aesthetic Nasal Reconstruction.* St. Louis, MO: Mosby; 1994:93-115.
24. Burget GC, Menick FJ. Aesthetic restoration of one-half the upper lip. *Plast Reconstr Surg.* 1986;78(5):583-593.
25. Schulte DL, Sherris DA, Kasperbauer JL. The anatomical basis of the Abbe flap. *Laryngoscope.* 2001;111(3):382-386.
26. Millard DR Jr. McLaughlin CA. Abbe flap on mucosal pedicle. *Ann Plast Surg.* 1979;3(6):544-548.
27. Kriet JD, Cupp CL, Sherris DA, Murakami CS. The extended Abbé flap. *Laryngoscope.* 1995;105(9 Pt 1):988-992.
28. Naficy S, Baker SR. The extended Abbe flap in the reconstruction of complex midfacial defects. *Arch Facial Plast Surg.* 2000;2(2):141-144.
29. Kroll SS. Staged sequential flap reconstruction for large lower lip defects. *Plast Reconstr Surg.* 1991;88(4):620-625 [discussion 626–627].
30. Filimon S, Richardson K, Hier MP, Roskies M, Mlynarek AM. The use of a modified abbé island flap to reconstruct primary lip defects of over 80. *J Otolaryngol Head Neck Surg.* 2016;45(1):35.

Videos for this chapter can be found online by accessing the accompanying Expert Consult website.

9 Skin Grafts

GERARDO MARRAZZO, MD, and JOHN ALBERTINI, MD

Introduction

Skin grafts are autologous portions of skin completely divided from their blood supply and transplanted into a recipient wound. Skin grafts vary in their thickness, composition, and intended purpose, and can be categorized broadly as either full-thickness skin grafts (FTSGs) or split-thickness skin grafts (STSGs). Used for thousands of years in a variety of clinical settings, the popularity of skin grafts has waned with the advancement of local flap design.[1] When used in the appropriate setting, however, skin grafting remains a superb choice rivaling the results attained by local flaps.[2] This chapter will instruct the reader on successful graft site selection and surgical technique, and prepare the surgeon for the management of proper postoperative care, revision, and complications.

Full-Thickness Skin Graft

SKIN GRAFT PHYSIOLOGY

FTSGs, if used selectively, can provide a very good match of color, thickness, and texture.[3-8] FTSGs are composed of epidermis and the full thickness of dermis, and therefore are relatively resistant to contracture and are replete with adnexal structures. The inclusion of adnexae provides the matured graft a much more natural and camouflaged appearance relative to its split-thickness brethren, although final appearance is more variable than with a flap. The full-thickness nature of this graft is not without its detractions, however, as it has significant nutritional requirements, and requires a rich vascular supply both to promote neovascularization and to develop a new collagenous matrix by which it adheres to the recipient site. Grafts are also constrained by their limited thickness and can only cover relatively shallow defects without appearing depressed.

Through careful study, three stages of wound healing have been identified in skin grafting.[9] Imbibition is the first stage, and is a period of relative ischemia that occurs during the first 2 days.[10] As the name suggests, the graft survives by imbibing nutrients from the plasma exudate of the wound bed via passive diffusion. Beginning on the second to third day and lasting as long as 10 days, inosculation, the second stage, marks the beginnings of true revascularization.[11-14] During this phase the dermal vessels of the graft anastomose with the vessels of the recipient bed. It is for this reason that unsuccessful inosculation and graft failure may follow full-thickness skin grafting of exposed bone or cartilage. The final step in graft survival, typically beginning concurrently with inosculation, is neovascularization.[10] A new microvascular plexus grows into the graft from the recipient bed, supplementing the anastomosed native vessels.

Several host and iatrogenic factors contribute to the success of a graft.[15-17] The vascular and nutritional demands of a graft may not be met in a patient with diabetes mellitus, nutritional deficiencies, heavy alcohol consumption, or tobacco dependence. Graft failure due to hematoma or prohibitive clotting may occur in those with inherited or acquired bleeding disorders, uncontrolled hypertension, or iatrogenic anticoagulation. Wound beds harboring high microbial loads and immunosuppression may also interfere with graft survival. Therefore these factors must be analyzed when considering an FTSG for the repair of a defect.

Graft Selection

The donor site selection is critical to the long-term aesthetic result of skin grafting, given the concept of donor dominance that describes how FTSGs retain those native characteristics like texture and hair growth attributable to preserved adnexal structures. The surgeon must understand both the epidermal and dermal qualities of a cadre of potential donor sites as one aims to provide optimal match. This analysis must extend further to the sebaceous qualities, relative dyschromia, telangiectases, and epidermal texture, as it compares with the recipient wound, of any potential donor site.[3-5,7,8] The following section will serve a guide to the surgeon on possible donor sites based on anatomic location of the recipient wound.

When reconstructing a wound on the nose with an FTSG, tremendous attention to the qualities of the skin and the individual cosmetic units of the nose is paramount. In general, the skin of the upper two-thirds of the nose (Zone 1) is thin and mobile relative to the thick, sebaceous lower third (Zone 2). This transition is highly variable among patients and must be closely studied prior to the design of a repair. Additionally, the nose is divided into cosmetic subunits based on convexities, concavities, natural borders, and the quality of skin. In certain instances, wounds may be extended so as to graft an entire subunit.[18] The cephalad two-thirds of the nose lends itself quite well to skin grafting. The dermis in this region is of medium thickness, and the skin of the preauricular cheek lateral to the sideburn or the postauricular sulcus (if the skin of the recipient site is notably thin) are good matches (Fig. 9.1). In males, an area of approximately 1.5 to 2 cm in the horizontal dimension can be harvested from the preauricular cheek without

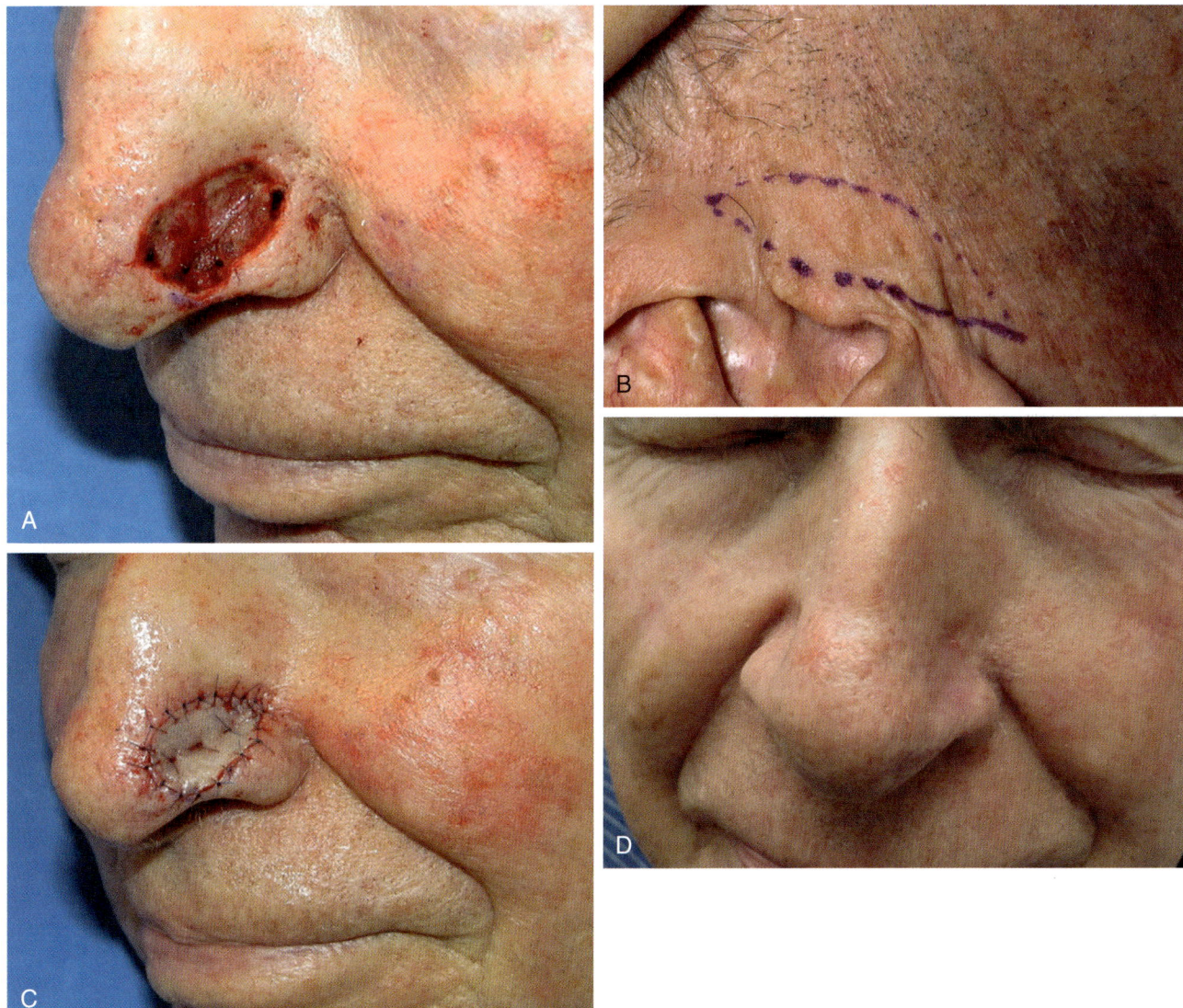

Fig. 9.1 Harvesting a full-thickness skin graft (FTSG). (A) Defect following Mohs micrographic surgery for basal cell carcinoma. (B) The preauricular donor site. (C) The FTSG sutured into place with interrupted 6-0 polypropylene sutures; note the tacking sutures within the alar crease. (D) Three-month follow-up view of an FTSG.

incorporating the terminal hairs of the sideburn. In women, the graft can be larger, but will likely include delicate vellus hairs that may detract from the cosmesis of the final appearance. In larger repairs, a defect template can be halved vertically, and two grafts can be harvested from the glabrous skin of a single preauricular donor site (Fig. 9.2). The two grafts heal as one, especially if sutured together along the midline or along a cosmetic subunit. When sizable defects are involved, supraclavicular skin can be used, but caution must be taken to thin the dermis to an appropriate thickness to avoid a patchlike blob of tissue.

The distal third of the nose is significantly more sebaceous, and is better matched by a conchal bowl, forehead, or nasolabial skin.[19] In women, the submental crease provides another excellent option. Grafts chosen for soft triangle and alar rim defects are often buttressed with cartilage to avoid notching. A Burow graft from a cephalad vertical triangle of skin can be harvested and transplanted into a more caudal defect.[20–22] When designing a Burow graft, the triangle of skin should be of sufficient height so as to avoid significant tension in closing donor site when the graft is repositioned in its more caudal position. Failure to do so may lead to contralateral alar flare when using the Burow graft to repair nonmidline defects. A Burow graft can also be used to repair complex wounds spanning the medial cheek and nasal sidewall.[23] First, a template of the defect confined to the nasal sidewall is created. The entirety of the medial cheek defect to its junction with the nasal sidewall is closed with a rotation or fusiform advancement flap, ensuring that the distal standing triangle is of sufficient size to serve as an FTSG for the nasal sidewall. The FTSG is then transplanted to the nasal sidewall defect and sutured into place. Defects of the columella are also well suited to repair with an FTSG.

Wounds of the ear are also commonly repaired by FTSG. Many superficial wounds of the auricle, not involving the helical rim or sulcus, lobule, tragus, or antitragus, heal beautifully with second intention healing and require no

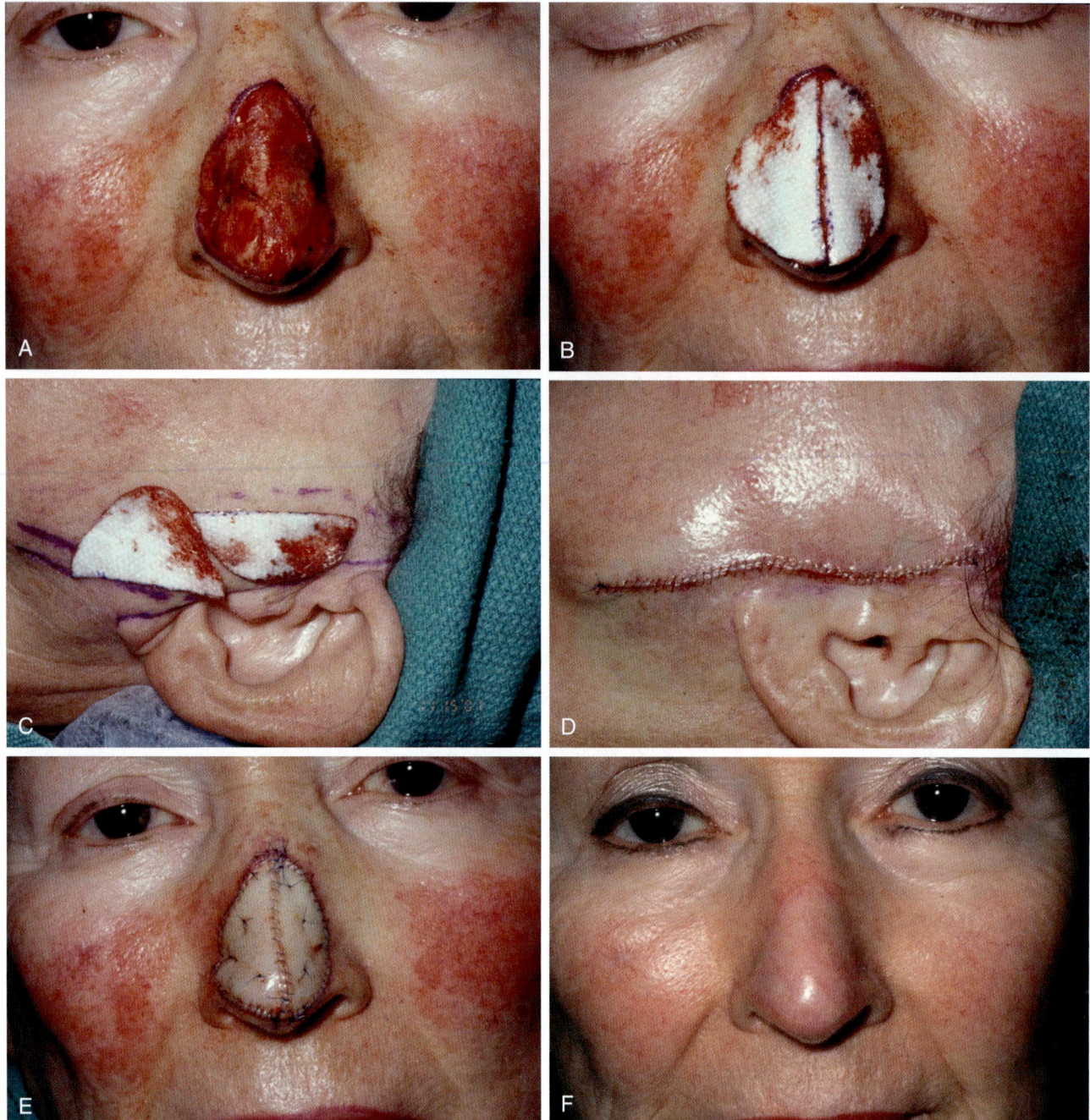

Fig. 9.2 (A) Sizable but shallow defect following Mohs micrographic surgery (MMS) for basal cell carcinoma. (B) A template of the wound divided exactly at the midline of the nasal dorsum and tip. (C) The two templates positioned on the preauricular cheek, oriented to facilitate linear closure. (D) Donor site closed linearly. (E) Two grafts positioned and sutured in place with running 6-0 polypropylene sutures and multiple basting sutures. (F) Follow-up view of the nasal full-thickness skin graft.

reconstructive intervention. Wounds of the helical rim, however, often heal with perceptible notching. Similarly, defects involving the sulcus between the helix and antihelix can web and distort anatomic landmarks. Broad wounds of the auricle with exposed perichondrium can be resurfaced with a thin FTSG. In broad wounds with exposed perichondrium, strips of cartilage can be excised from the triangular fossa, antihelix, and concha prior to placing an FTSG over the entirety of the defect.[24] This allows for imbibition and eventual anastomosis to arise from the skin and subcutaneous tissues of the medial ear. The auricle is best grafted with tissue from the postauricular sulcus, and the graft must be adequately thinned so as not to obscure the intricate topography of the ear. Thin freehand grafts harvested with double-edged razor blades from the mastoid process can be used to cover broad, thin wounds. The donor site is then allowed to heal secondarily.[25]

Eyelid defects involving exclusively the anterior lamella can be reproducibly reconstructed with FTSG. Defects of the eyelid are best repaired using FTSG of the upper eyelid or

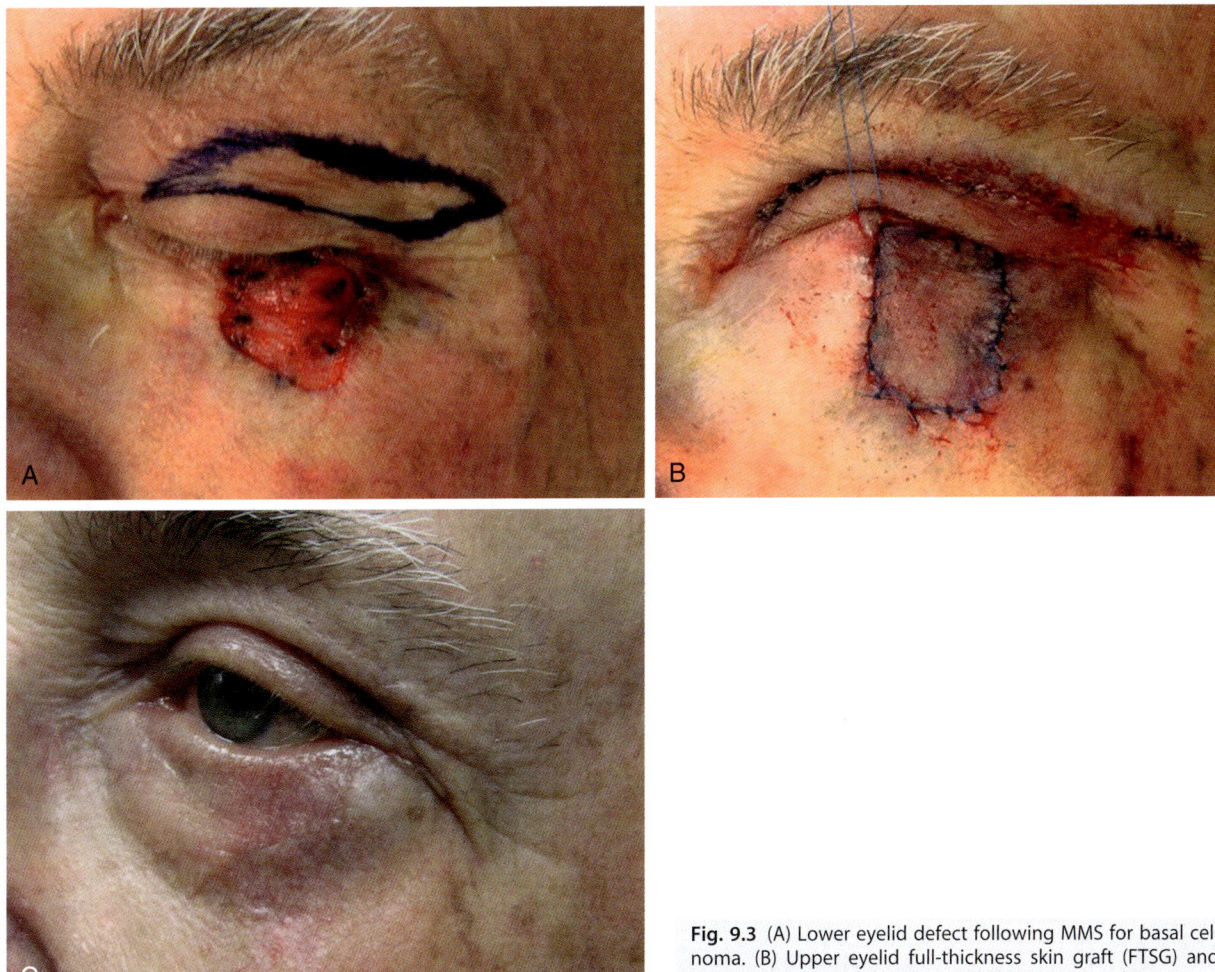

Fig. 9.3 (A) Lower eyelid defect following MMS for basal cell carcinoma. (B) Upper eyelid full-thickness skin graft (FTSG) and Frost suture in place. (C) Three-month follow-up view of FTSG.

postauricular sulcus. Judicious use of Frost sutures when reconstructing periorbital defects is recommended to avoid ectropion (Fig. 9.3).[26] An option for large defects abutting the lower eyelid is to use guiding sutures to reduce defect size and optimize tension vectors in combination with FTSG, but leaving the guiding sutures intact during the healing phase. Careful postoperative observation is critical in the grafting of eyelids, and small aliquots of high-potency intralesional triamcinolone into early hypertrophic scarring will often stave off or reverse ectropion. This observation, coupled with the selective use of the Frost suture to suspend the lower lid by its tarsal plate, can significantly reduce the risk of eyelid malpositions.[26] FTSG of the medial canthus is an excellent reconstructive choice because the graft can be appropriately thinned and made to fit into the contours of the defect with tacking sutures or a well-placed bolster. Local flaps, by contrast, tend to recruit excessive bulk. Grafts for the medial canthus are often obtained from the preauricular cheek or postauricular sulcus.

Grafts can be used throughout the face, although their use is less common than in ear, eyelid, and nose reconstruction. Their less frequent use is likely attributable to the availability of local tissue to closed primarily or with a local flap and the increased variability of the final cosmesis of grafts. Still, they are arguably less taxing on the patient and can be revised or even surgically extirpated at follow-up, and may represent the best choice for many patients. When encountered with massive defects of the forehead, temple, and cheek, the reconstructive surgeon is occasionally left no option but to repair all or part of a defect with an FTSG. In the cheek, FTSG, harvested either from the supraclavicular fossa or regionally (in the form of a standing triangle) can be paired with a rotation, rhombic, or V-to-Y advancement to repair sizable defects.[27] The forehead, given its relatively inelastic nature, is less forgiving than the cheek. The forehead is most frequently repaired with an FTSG from the supraclavicular fossa or from a Burow graft of the temple or frontal scalp (in an alopecic male). A novel method of FTSG for the upper forehead and scalp, presented by Dr. David Brodland, is the marriage of a simple purse string closure with an FTSG. The defect is initially partially closed with purse string, and a template of the new, smaller defect is made. The FTSG, often harvested from the supraclavicular fossa, is sewn into place. The purse string is then released, drawing the graft over the defect like a drum head. This repair both reduces the size of the grafted area and provides a taut appearance to the FTSG that replicates the appearance of normal forehead or scalp. Grafting on the lip can prove invaluable in select scenarios. Very superficial defects involving delicate structures such as the philtral ridges can

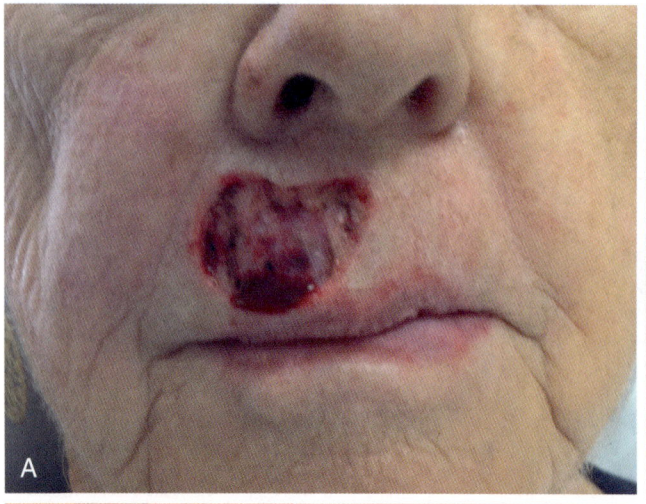
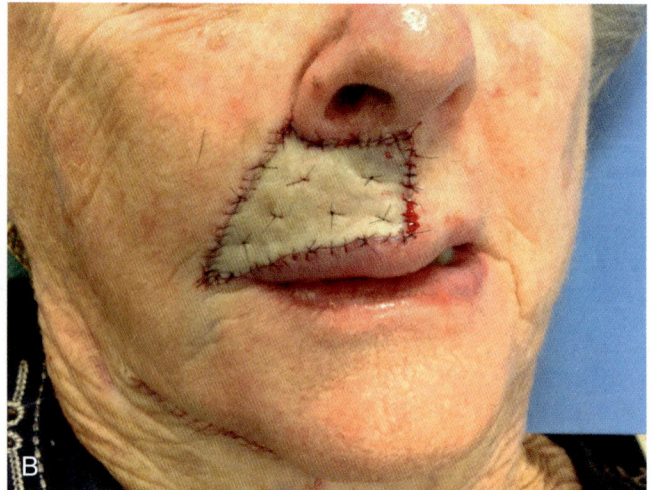
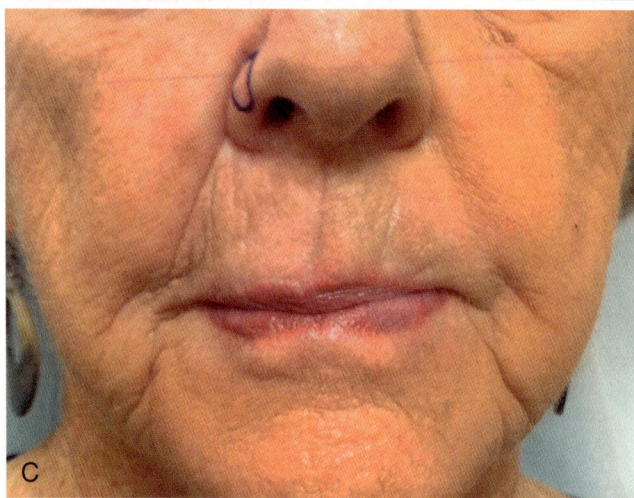

Fig. 9.4 (A) Shallow cutaneous lip defect following MMS for basal cell carcinoma. (B) The entire cosmetic subunit following excisional preparation and grafting by a submental full-thickness skin graft (FTSG). (C) Three-month follow-up view of FTSG.

be grafted with thin FTSGs, often from the postauricular sulcus. If an entire cosmetic subunit has been extirpated, it can be redraped with a more sizable graft. As the lip is a very dynamic anatomic structure, the use of basting sutures and bolster dressings can aid in graft survival (Fig. 9.4).

Full-Thickness Skin Graft Technique

There are multiple techniques for templating, harvesting, and insetting an FTSG. The following reflects the authors' preferred techniques, with mention of other valuable alternatives.

The first step of performing an FTSG is creating a template of the defect. The foil suture packaging, cut with scissors, allows the surgeon to sculpt his template and produce a three-dimensional representation of the defect. Alternatively, the wound edge can be inked with a waterproof pen, and a Telfa pad can be pressed to the defect and ink to create a template.[28] Advocates of this method suggest oversizing the graft 5% to 10% to avoid an undersized FTSG; we prefer to precisely match the size while accounting for convexities and concavities that can cause sizing errors.[4] Grafts should be placed under the same surface tension as the native skin elasticity to prevent pincushioning or distortion of free margins. Once completed, the template is then transferred to the donor site, and the skin underlying the template is excised to the subcutaneous fat. The graft is excised in as atraumatic a fashion as possible, with the authors' preference being a single skin hook grasping the leading edge of subcutaneous fat and dermis. The harvested graft can be transferred to normal saline as the donor site is closed. With rare exceptions, most donor sites can be closed in a fusiform fashion. The graft can survive 1 to 2 hours in normal saline at room temperature without increased necrosis or failure.[8] Similarly, the use of lidocaine with epinephrine at the donor site does not lead to poor outcomes.[29]

Once the donor site has been closed, attention is redirected to inset of the graft into the recipient wound. The graft is stripped of subcutaneous fat, exposing the glistening white underbelly of the dermis. This is most commonly achieved by draping the graft over the digital pulp of the surgeon's nondominant second digit, and tangentially snipping fat with sharp scissors. In deeper defects of the nose, some have achieved success leaving 1 to 5 mm of subcutaneous fat to add bulk and volume to match the defect.[29] The authors recommend tie-over bolster dressing rather than bolster sutures for this type of less viable FTSG to improve adherence and take. This variation should be approached with caution in active or even former tobacco smokers. Conversely, the dermis can be thinned if necessary to match the depth of a thin defect, but this may damage adnexae and deter from the final cosmesis of the graft.

Once thinned, the graft is placed in the recipient wound. The wound must not be actively bleeding, as any seroma can cause graft necrosis and failure. The bevel of the recipient site is left as is, and the dermal edge of the graft can be slightly reverse-beveled by trimming with the scissors. Initially, one to four interrupted 5-0 or 6-0 sutures are placed in four quadrants, typically at 12, 3, 6, and 9 o'clock. Interrupted or running vertical epidermal sutures are then placed along the entire periphery of the graft. A vertically oriented bite through the epidermis and dermis of the graft, coupled with a slightly oversized bite through the wall of the recipient wound edge, ensures that the graft's wound edge is closely apposed to its recipient wound bed.

Direct contact with the wound bed and strict immobilization are important to the survival of the graft. While there are several reports demonstrating bolster dressings may not be necessary, many surgeons use them. Numerous methods including basting sutures, bolsters, and thermoplastic casts have been used singly or in combination to achieve this goal.[30] The authors' technique is described herein. The graft is covered in a generous layer of petrolatum ointment. A tightly folded nonstick dressing or Vaseline impregnated gauze shaped to extend millimeters beyond the graft edge is held in place with dressing forceps by the surgical assistant. For bolsters in the periocular area, one should avoid the yellow Vaseline impregnated gauze that contains bismuth, because this is a known irritant to the conjunctival tissues. The dressing is then secured by as many bolster sutures as necessary (typically one or two) to securely position the bolster and prevent movement (Fig. 9.5). A conventional pressure bandage is placed over the bolster. The patient removes the pressure dressing in 48 hours, and the bolster is left in place for 1 week.[31] The patient must be instructed to avoid any strenuous activities that may risk trauma to the graft site, as the graft is at risk to be sheared from the wound bed for the first month.

COMPLICATIONS AND MANAGEMENT

The principal complications in the immediate postoperative period are partial and complete graft necrosis. Causes for necrosis include hematoma, seroma, and trauma leading to disruption of graft-bed apposition, infection, smoking, and excessive electrocoagulation of the wound base. At 1 week, the graft is ideally pink in color, but may be varying shades of purple and blue secondary to edema and ecchymosis. Gray and black tones imply at least partial necrosis. Partial necrosis, or death of at least the epidermis and typically some dermis, often heal well via re-epithelialization from the wound edge and adnexae. Regardless of presumed depth of necrosis, the eschar should not be debrided, as it serves as a natural dressing for healing. Most contour irregularities can be repaired with a combination of skin resurfacing and/or intralesional corticosteroids. Ablative lasers, dermabrasion, or dermasanding is optimally performed in the 6 to 8 weeks following surgery during wound remodeling, but can be delayed many months with excellent results depending on patient preferences.[32] Intralesional

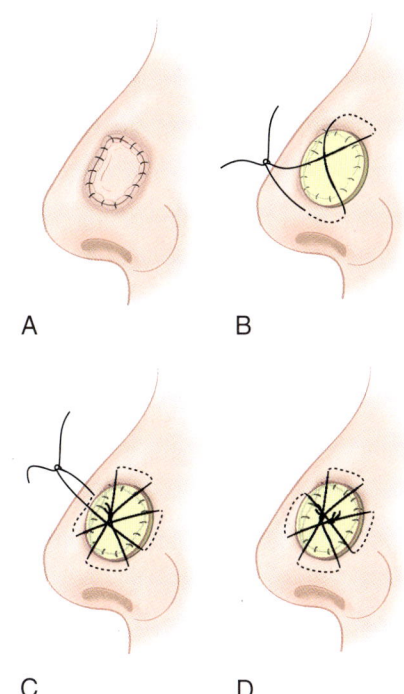

Fig. 9.5 Schematic view of a tie-over bolster: (A) Graft sutured into place. (B) A single figure-of-eight silk suture placed above the graft. The graft is covered in white petrolatum prior to introduction of compressive nonstick bolster material (xeroform gauze or TELFA). (C) Often multiple figure-of-eight sutures are required to fully secure the bolster. (D) Final appearance of bolster, which is left in place for 1 week.

corticosteroids are particularly helpful in mitigating hypertrophic scarring and pincushioning as a result of recipient wound contraction, and should be undertaken within the first 2 months, which corresponds with the period of maximum wound contraction. This is particularly critical with the grafting of free margins such as the eyelid and lip, which tend to experience these two phenomena. A variety of techniques, including delayed dermal or cartilage grafting, filler, and microliposuction injection have been used to elevate depressed nasal graft scars.[33]

Modifications of the Full-Thickness Skin Graft

Composite grafts are modifications of the FTSG and are grafts consisting of tissue from two germ layers. In dermatologic surgery, the term composite graft almost invariably means chondrocutaneous graft, an FTSG connected to its underlying cartilaginous base by perichondrium. Traditionally described in the repair of small full-thickness defects of the nasal ala, composite grafts have a variety of applications, including the lining of nasolabial and forehead flaps, and the repair of nasal, auricular and eyelid defects.[34–37] Its use in dermatologic surgery is primarily in nasal reconstruction, and the following discussion will center on this application.

Composite chondrocutaneous grafts of the ear lend themselves very well to the repair of the alar rim. The helical root in particular is of similar color, contour, sebaceous quality, and rigidity to reconstruct a small full-thickness alar defect. Additionally, its cartilaginous core is generally resistant to contraction and free margin distortion. Excision of the helical root also allows for additional cutaneous grafting from the preauricular cheek, should the need exist. The helical root can be repaired elegantly and without notable scarring for the patient[38,39] and is often the choice for the alar rim, especially in a thinner and delicate naris. Composite grafts from the conchal bowl are often chosen for defects of the columella and alar body.[38,40] This can often be shaped as an inverted pyramid, with the broad base representing epidermis and its progressively thinning apex representing cartilage. This configuration contributes to the survivability of the graft (Fig. 9.6).

As with FTSG, composite grafts are dependent on the recipient wound bed for initial nutritional support and eventual revascularization. Since they are used in many instances to reconstruct full-thickness defects, they often are exclusively dependent on the lateral wound edges. For this reason, composite grafts are typically limited to 1 to 2 cm in size, so no part of the graft is significantly farther than 0.5 cm from wound edge.[6,38] Despite adherence to these limitations in graft size, their inherent thickness and limited nutritional supply lead to greater rates of partial and full failure. Survival of composite grafts are lower in smokers and diabetics, as well as in previously irradiated sites and scar tissue, and should be approached with caution in these scenarios.[38]

In selecting a donor site for the composite graft, careful examination of the contralateral ala allows for selection of skin with the appropriate thickness, sebaceous quality, and contour. A template of the defect is then made, and transferred to the donor site for excision. The graft is often oversized by approximately 5% to allow for contraction.[41] The outline of the graft is incised with the scalpel, and the remaining dermis and cartilage is freed with iris scissors. Alternatively, the graft can be oversized 2 to 3 mm on each side. The epidermis and dermis is trimmed away so that the cutaneous component matches the defect, and pockets are made in the recipient wound to fit the struts of cartilage at either end.[42] This design both anchors the graft and places more of the avascular cartilage in direct apposition with its well-vascularized wound bed (Fig. 9.7). Another option to improve vascularization is to expand the cutaneous defect on the nose, thereby creating a greater surface area of FTSG component to support the underlying cartilage component

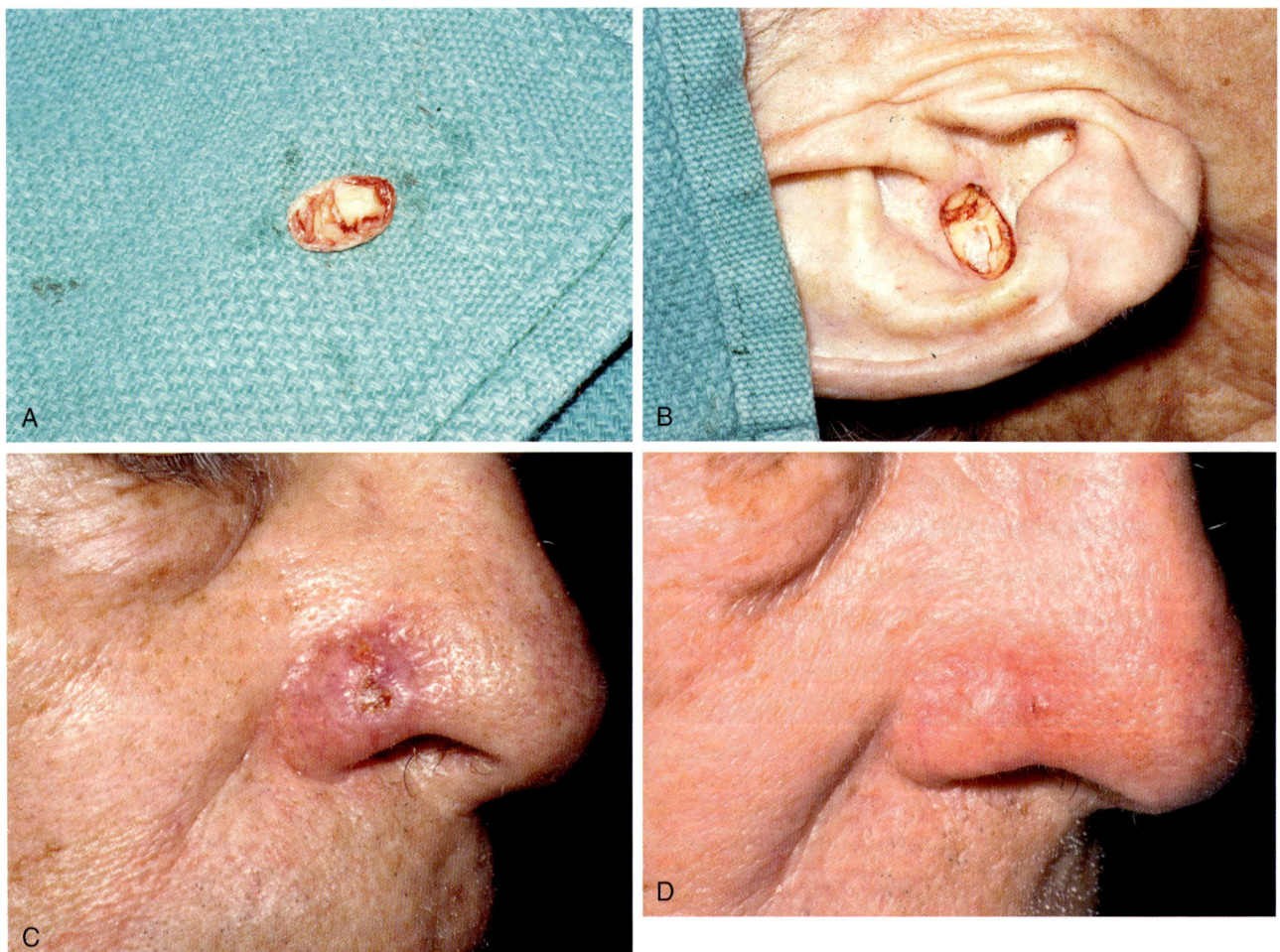

Fig. 9.6 (A) Chondrocutaneous composite graft harvested from the conchal bowl (note the inverted pyramid shape). (B) The donor site is filled with white petrolatum, packed with a nonstick dressing, and allowed to heal secondarily. (C) Short-term follow-up reveals inflammation and epidermal sloughing indicative of the graft's increased metabolic demand. (D) Three-month follow-up view of chondrocutaneous composite graft.

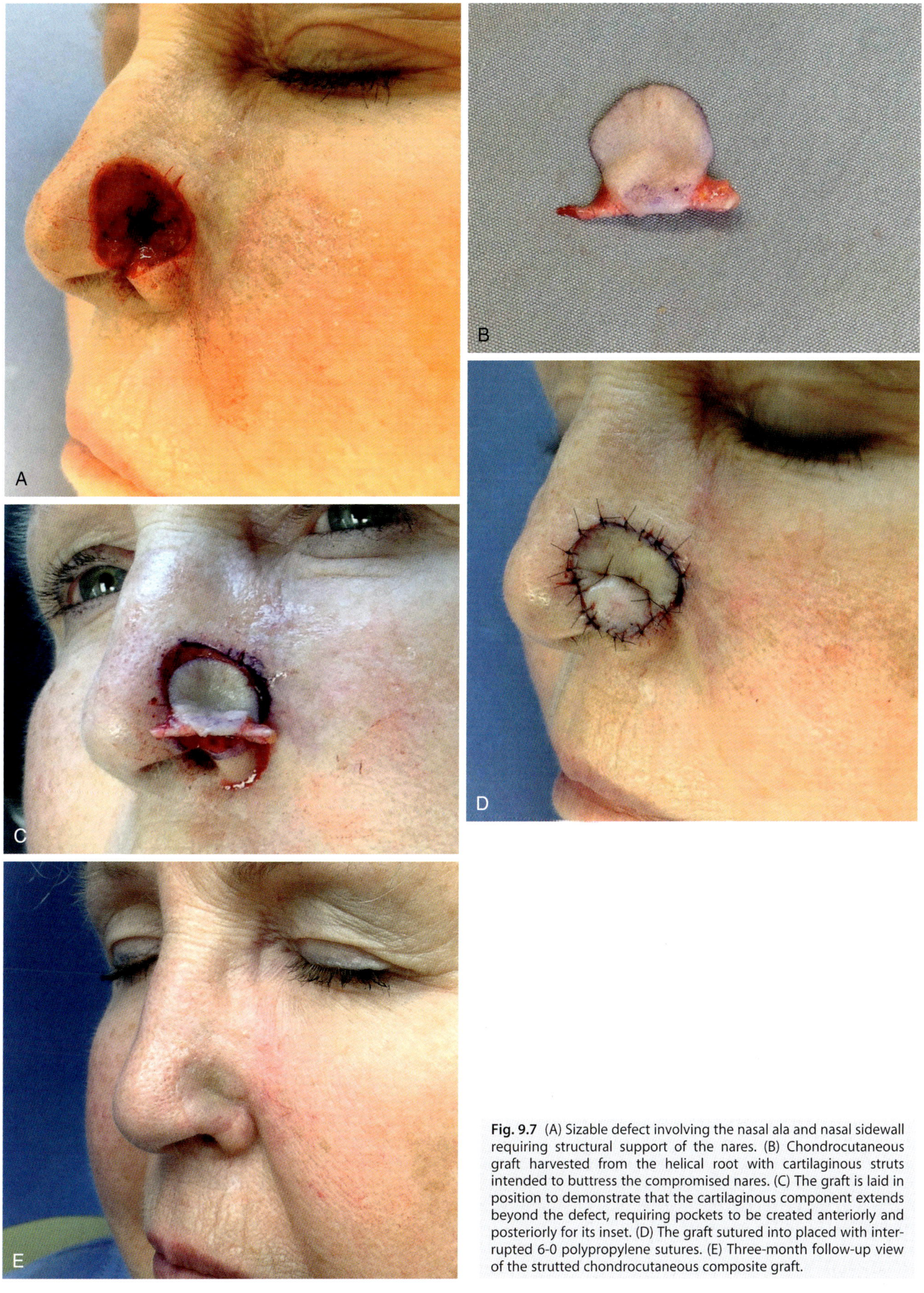

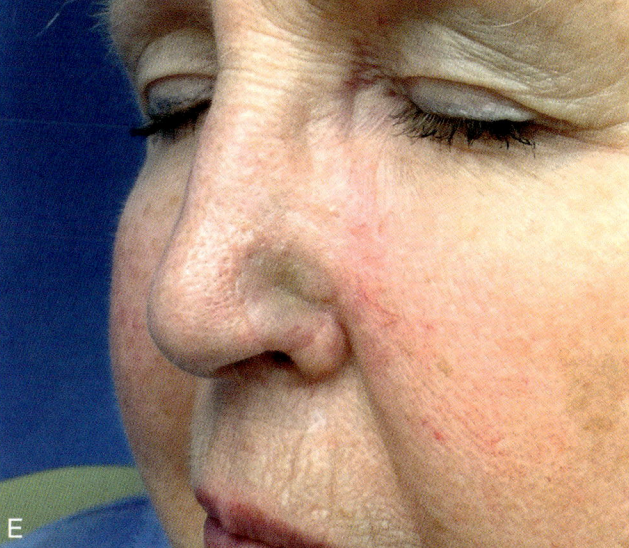

Fig. 9.7 (A) Sizable defect involving the nasal ala and nasal sidewall requiring structural support of the nares. (B) Chondrocutaneous graft harvested from the helical root with cartilaginous struts intended to buttress the compromised nares. (C) The graft is laid in position to demonstrate that the cartilaginous component extends beyond the defect, requiring pockets to be created anteriorly and posteriorly for its inset. (D) The graft sutured into placed with interrupted 6-0 polypropylene sutures. (E) Three-month follow-up view of the strutted chondrocutaneous composite graft.

metabolic demand. Ideally a ≥3:1 ratio of skin to cartilage can improve composite graft survival. The graft is secured to the nasal vestibule with interrupted chromic or fast-absorbing gut sutures. The delayed knot tying technique can also improve visualization and suture placement into the nasal lining.[43] The cutaneous surface of the graft is then closed with interrupted sutures. The cartilage does not require buried suturing. The graft can then be secured in place with a thermoplastic cast or intranasal packing coupled with a traditional cutaneous dressing.[44]

It is critical to stress the delicate nature of the graft to the patient, and to have the patient return for regular follow-up in the immediate postoperative period. Patients should be instructed to stop smoking prior to their arrival for surgery, and should maintain smoking cessation for at least 2 weeks postoperatively. Because of the high bacterial load within the nares, the dressings are coated with antibiotic ointment at initial bandaging, and the patient is typically placed on a week-long course of oral antibiotics. The cast or intranasal packing typically is left in place for 1 week, although some authors advocate leaving the intranasal packing in place for 2 weeks.[45]

Simultaneous Free Cartilage and Full-Thickness Skin Grafting

In complex defects approximating free margins, such as the alar rim and helical rim, there exist the limited options of local flaps, interpolated flaps, and combination cartilage and FTSG for reconstruction. The benefits of this combination over composite grafts are multiple.[46] First, the combination of independent grafts is metabolically less demanding and less prone to necrosis than composite grafts. Since they are independent grafts, the FTSG component can be harvested from any donor site and can therefore be used to repair sizable cutaneous defects. This combination of grafts should be considered every time the surgeon considers a graft but is concerned about free margin distortion.

Cartilage grafts maintain contour and prevent contraction and batten grafts harvested from the antihelix are the preferred cartilaginous substrate.[46] Depending on the desire for a flat or curved batten graft, an appropriate location is identified on the ipsilateral ear so the patient has one side of the face free of wounds and bandages. An incision is made along the antihelix, 2 to 3 mm longer than the length of the desired cartilaginous strut. The dermis is lifted from the perichondrium with gentle blunt dissection. The skin is then retracted as the desired cartilage graft is incised with the scalpel and then bluntly dissected from the dermis of the posterior auricular skin. The cartilage graft should be slightly longer than the defect. This allows for inset of the graft within two dermal pockets created at the lateral edges of the defect. Once hemostasis is achieved and the donor site is closed with running absorbable stitches, the graft is then secured in position. This can be achieved via a buried absorbable suture that loops around the cartilage graft and secures it to the dermis of the free margin. Alternatively, a nonabsorbable suture can pass through the skin of the nasal vestibule, then loop around or pierce through the cartilage graft, and then exit to the nasal vestibule adjacent to the first bite. This knot is external and removed at 1 week.

The cutaneous defect is templated in the same manner as when an FTSG is utilized alone. The graft is then harvested, thinned, and secured with perimeter sutures. Once the graft has been inset in its typical fashion, through-and-through sutures parallel to the long axis of the cartilage strut are placed along the cartilage graft on the side opposite the free margin. The purpose of these sutures is to prevent cartilage graft migration and ensure the FTSG is closely apposed to the wound bed in area of inherent tenting. In small defects, it is recommended the cartilage graft be narrowed so that it represents less than 50% of the wound bed surface.[46] This decreases the proportion of the FTSG dependent on vascular bridging and improves FTSG survival.

Split-Thickness Skin Grafts

Split-thickness skin grafts provide the surgeon a means to cover massive and even avascular defects and are a rarely used but important arrow in the quiver of the reconstructive surgeon. They are less metabolically demanding than their full-thickness brethren, and can be used to repair defects overlying the wound bed of tumors at high risk for recurrence, as they allow early visualization of local recurrence. STSGs consist of epidermis and only a portion of the dermis, meaning they lack adnexae. The absence of adnexal structures leads to a taut, shiny, and often depigmented final cosmetic appearance. Thickness of an STSG varies with the arbitrary classifications of thin (0.013 to 0.033 cm), medium (0.033 to 0.046 cm), or thick (0.046 to 0.076 cm), depending on the amount of dermis included.[8] Regardless of thickness, it is estimated that STSGs contract up to 70%, limiting their utility in areas close to a free margin.[47] Additionally, they are fragile relative to other reconstructive options and create a sizable donor wound that must be bandaged for several weeks and leave cosmetically displeasing scars. For these reasons, they are often viewed as a repair of last resort. Despite these limitations, STSGs are useful in the postoperative repair of select scalp, auricular, and lower extremity defects.

GRAFT SELECTION

When choosing a donor site for STSG, matching of donor and recipient skin plays little to no role in selection. The selection hinges on identifying a donor site with easy accessibility for the patient during wound care that will cause minimal interference with sleep and other activities. Other factors that influence donor site selection include the desired graft's size and method of harvesting. The most common donor sites are the lateral and medial thighs. In patients with a high cosmetic demand, the buttocks are an ideal donor site because they can be hidden under most clothes and bathing suits.[48] The authors, however, generally advocate the lateral occipital and/or mastoid scalp areas as ideal donor sites. The density of hair follicles ensures complete reepithelialization of these donor sites within 2 weeks, significantly reducing morbidity. The scalp donor site is used extensively in burn wound treatment, and thin STSGs can be reharvested repeatedly due to rapid healing. The hair shaft fragments do not persist long term.

Split-Thickness Skin Graft Technique

There are multiple manual and mechanically assisted methods of harvesting STSGs.[49] This section will cover the authors' preferences for graft harvesting.

Once the donor site has been selected, the area is shaved of hair to aid in the handling of the graft. The area to be harvested is then outlined with a surgical pen and anesthetized, most commonly with local 1% lidocaine with epinephrine. If harvesting from the lateral thigh, a nerve block of the lateral femoral cutaneous nerve can be employed that provides regional anesthesia.[50]

Pinch grafting is a form of split-thickness skin grafting that serves as an accelerant for the host's own re-epithelialization. Often it is used in the follow-up period after an individual has allowed a lower extremity or scalp defect to granulate. The base of the wound is debrided of fibrinous exudate and crust. Superficial blebs of lidocaine are made at the donor site, which is usually the lateral thigh, and thin 4 to 5 mm grafts are harvested by tangentially excising the superficial skin of each bleb.[51] The pinch grafts are then placed in the bed of the wound, spaced 1 to 2 cm from each other. The entire wound is covered with petrolatum gauze dressing, and then a tape bolster is used to immobilize the wound. At 2-week follow-up, there are often slightly elevated pinch grafts with peripheral rims of new epidermis. The wound is kept moist with petrolatum jelly and nonstick dressings until the wound has completely re-epithelialized. One of the detractions of this technique is that there is often a textural and pigmentary discrepancy between the pinch grafts and the surrounding new epithelium within the healed wound, but this typically improves significantly with time.

Harvesting of small medium-to-thick STSGs for use on the face can be achieved using a freehand STSG harvesting method. A template of the defect is transferred to the mastoid process and scored using a #15 scalpel blade. The surgical assistant then holds the area with firm lateral tension as the surgeon harvests the graft. The scalpel blade is held parallel to the skin surface and is advanced with a careful combination of pushing and downward cutting. This technique can be utilized with very thin defects of the face, in which repair may damage delicate anatomic structures (such as the philtral ridge or helical sulcus), but secondary intention healing may cause slight distortion. It can also be used in repair of auricular defects sparing the helix.

Harvesting of medium-sized STSGs can be achieved with a Weck blade. The Weck blade is a relatively inexpensive handheld surgical instrument that allows the surgeon to harvest an STSG of uniform thickness. It requires a relatively flat surface. A rough estimate of the required STSG size is outlined on the donor site surface. The donor site is lubricated with mineral oil. The assistant provides tension on the medial and lateral edges of the donor site. The surgeon then applies downward pressure with the Weck blade on the donor area until the surface skin flattened against the blade is the same as the desired graft width. The surgeon then advances the blade with a back and forth sawing motion, taking care to maintain the correct downward pressure to maintain the desired graft width. When the graft has achieved the correct length, the surgeon continues the back and forth sawing motion but releases the downward pressure. The appearance of the graft is often experience dependent, and may be saw-toothed at the lateral edges. Harvesting of large STSGs is best achieved with pneumatically powered dermatomes. Among the various options, the Zimmer dermatome is often the preferred device due to its ease of use and ability to harvest uniform, consistent grafts at various predetermined widths, and thicknesses.[8] Prior to harvesting, the donor site is lubricated. The assistant holds lateral pressure on the donor site, most commonly the thigh or buttock, providing the surgeon with a relatively flat surface area for harvesting. The surgeon then presses the dermatome against the patient donor skin and guides the unit forward at a 30- to 45-degree angle. The graft will emerge from the posterior surface of the dermatome and is gently tented from the device with forceps by an assistant. Once the desired graft has been obtained, the dermatome is lifted from the skin, freeing the graft.

Once the STSG has been harvested, it is immediately placed in normal saline as attention is turned to the recipient wound. Often, STSGs are used in delayed repairs so that the recipient wound can at least partially granulate. Prior to insetting the graft, care must be taken to remove all fibrinous exudate and crust. Some surgeons advocate scoring of the underlying granulation tissue as a method to reduce STSG contraction and wrinkling.[52] In cases in which the calvarium is exposed, it is often desirable to allow the wound to granulate so that the patient experiences less volumetric loss. If this is not possible or desirable, then small windows of the outer table should be chiseled or burred away to expose the vascularized cancellous bone of the diploic space.[52] Patients should be placed in the Trendelenburg position, and surgeons should be well experienced when manipulating the calvarium so as to avoid the incidence of air embolus and stroke.[53] When grafting over moderate or large defects with exposed auricular cartilage, scattered 2 to 4 mm fenestrae or larger windows in nonstructural areas through the auricular cartilage supply the graft with improved vascular support.

Once the recipient site is readied, the graft is then placed into the wound. When securing a topographically complex wound, it is often preferred to tack an edge of the graft in place with an interrupted absorbable suture, trim the graft a few millimeters, and then tack again with the suture. In less demanding regions such as the scalp, the graft can be tacked in place, and then trimmed and secured with absorbable suture, staples, or cyanoacrylate.[54] Once the periphery is secured, pie-crust incisions with a #11 or #15 blade help prevent underlying hematomas or seromas that may cause graft failure. Similarly, basting sutures can help prevent accumulation of fluid beneath the graft, and can also be at least partially protective against shearing forces. Basting sutures most commonly take the form of interrupted basting sutures placed at evenly spaced intervals across the graft surface (Fig. 9.8).

Various dressings have been used successfully in the bandaging of the STSG and donor site. The STSG, however, can essentially be dressed in the same fashion as an FTSG. The goals are the same—provide constant downward pressure to secure the STSG to its wound bed and prevent fluid accumulation, and prevent shearing forces that lead to graft

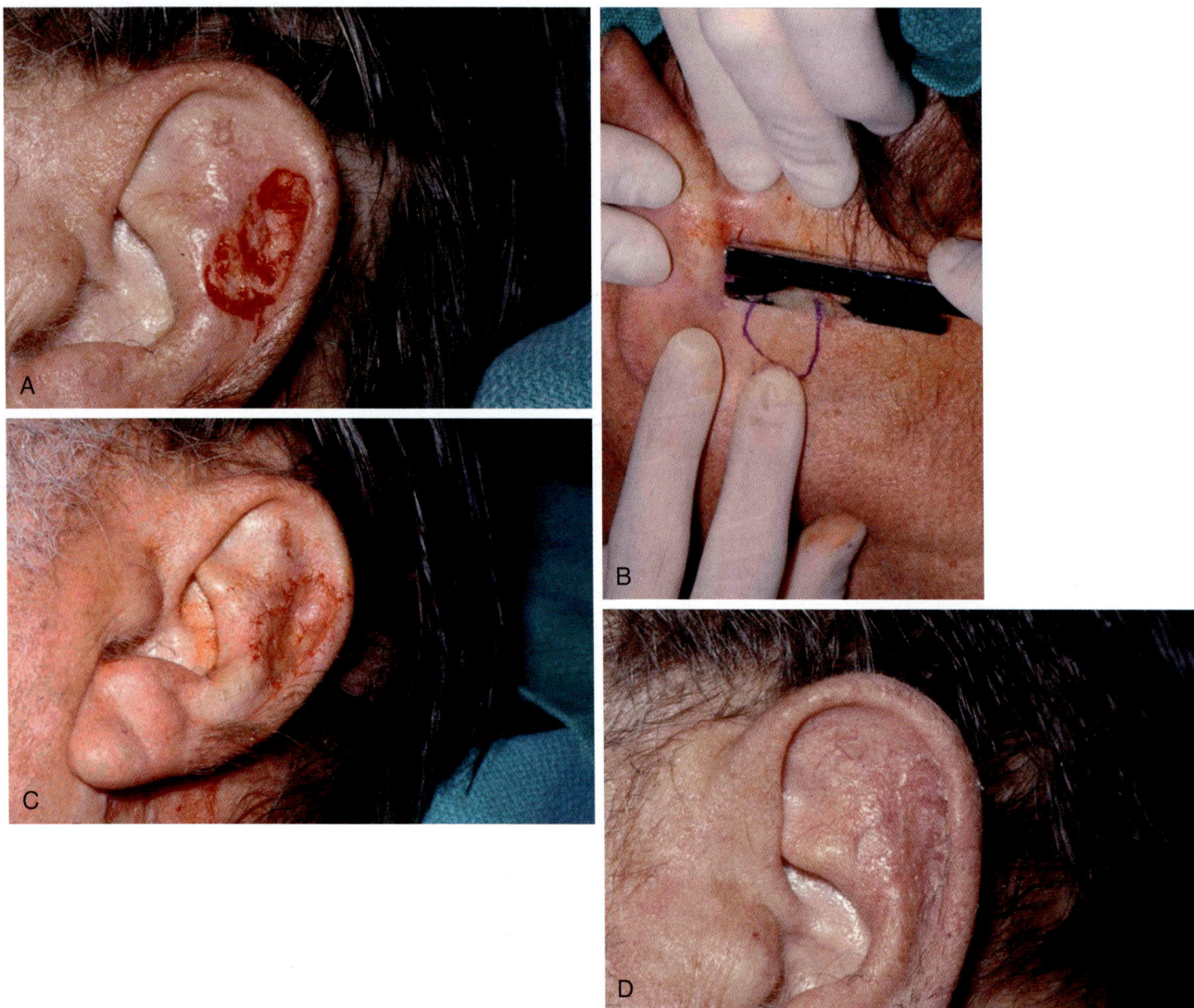

Fig. 9.8 (A) Shallow defect involving the scaphoid fossa and antihelix. (B) Harvesting a split-thickness skin graft (STSG) from the mastoid process with a Weck blade. (C) STSG sutured in place with interrupted 5-0 fast absorbing gut suture. (D) Three-month follow-up view of STSG.

failure. The donor site can be dressed in a variety of ways, with the emphasis on maintaining a moist wound environment that is conducive to re-epithelialization. The dressing that has garnered the most interest of late in dermatologic surgery is a transparent, vapor-permeable dressing called Opsite (Allerderm Laboratories, Inc., Petaluma, California). Opsite allows drainage at the donor site to collect and keep the wound moist, shortening healing times to 2 to 3 weeks.[55,56] These dressings are inexpensive and associated with a decreased incidence of infection and lower levels of pain. They are also waterproof, so the patient is able to immediately bathe after the procedure.

COMPLICATIONS AND MANAGEMENT

Complications are slightly less common with STSGs than with FTSGs, but are still principally partial or complete necrosis. Shearing of the graft from its recipient bed, even if minimal, interferes with revascularization. If this trauma occurs after the first 24 hours of graft placement, the STSG has a high likelihood of failure.[52] The process of revascularization of an STSG takes approximately 3 to 5 days, and the initial bulky bandage is kept in place for 1 week. Following the first bandage change, the patient should be further warned of the graft's fragility, especially within the first postoperative month. The final cosmetic appearance is highly variable and unpredictable, and the patient must be appropriately informed of this prior to the procedure. Contraction is similarly unpredictable but is typically maximal in the first 2 months. If contraction arises, especially adjacent to a free margin, intralesional corticosteroids can be started 4 to 6 weeks postoperatively and repeated every 4 to 6 weeks as needed.[52] The graft can be massaged with an emollient such as Aquaphor as soon as 6 to 8 weeks, which can have the dual benefit of reducing contraction and preventing accumulation of scale.[48] Practicing aggressive sun protection and using daily broad-spectrum sunscreens on both FTSG and STSG and donor sites is of the utmost importance to prevent hyperpigmentation

The donor site is frequently the primary source of patient complaint, typically from pain or excessive drainage. Pain can be handled with the same analgesics as typical dermatologic postoperative pain and often improves considerably in the first 24 hours. Excessive drainage beneath a semipermeable bandage is evacuated with a needle or syringe or pierced with a scalpel blade and then resealed with the same bandage material (without removing bandage and placing the immature and delicate STSG at risk). The donor site may be treated with pulsed dye laser to reduce erythema and improve texture.

Conclusion

Skin grafting is a frequently used and invaluable tool in the armamentarium of the dermatologic surgeon. Success hinges upon simultaneously analyzing several patient, defect, and donor site factors. Knowledge of the advantages, disadvantages, and limitations of each graft type can prevent reconstructive misadventure, and lead to satisfying cosmetic and functional outcomes for patients.

References

1. Hauben DJ, Baruchin A, Mahler A. On the history of the free skin graft. *Ann Plast Surg*. 1982;9:242-245.
2. Sapthavee A, Munaretto N, Toriumi DM. Skin grafts vs local flaps for reconstruction of nasal defects: a retrospective cohort study. *JAMA Facial Plast Surg*. 2015;17(4):270-273.
3. Johnson TM, Ratner D, Nelson B. Soft tissue reconstruction with skin grafting. *J Am Acad Dermatol*. 1992;27:151-165.
4. Christensen DR, Arpey CJ, Whitaker DC. Skin grafting. In: Robinson JK, Hanke CW, Sen gelmann RD, Siegel DM, eds. *Surgery of the Skin: Procedural Dermatology*. 1st ed. Philadelphia, PA: Elsevier Mosby; 2005:309-325.
5. Ratner D. Skin grafting. From here to there. *Dermatol Clin*. 1998;16:75-90.
6. Jewett BS. Skin and composite grafts. In: Baker SR, ed. *Local Flaps in Facial Reconstruction*. Philadelphia, PA: Elsevier/Saunders; 2014:339 367.
7. Wheeland RG. Skin grafts. In: Roenigk RK, Roenigk HH, eds. *Dermatologic Surgery: Principles and Practice*. New York, NY: Marcel Dekker; 1996:879-896.
8. Ratner D. Skin grafting. *Semin Cutan Med Surg*. 2003;22:295-305.
9. Smahel J. The healing of skin grafts. *Clin Plast Surg*. 1977;4:409-424.
10. Converse JM, Uhlschmid GK, Ballantyne DL Jr. "Plasmatic circulation" in skin grafts. The phase of serum imbibition. *Plast Reconstr Surg*. 1969;43:495-499.
11. Converse JM, Smahel J, Ballantyne DL Jr, Harper AD. Inosculation of vessels of skin graft and host bed: a fortuitous encounter. *Br J Plast Surg*. 1975;28:274-282.
12. Birch J, Branemark PI, Nilsson K. The vascularization of a free full thickness skin graft. 3. An infrared thermographic study. *Scand J Plast Reconstr Surg*. 1969;3:18-22.
13. Zarem HA, Zweifach BW, McGehee JM. Development of microcirculation in full thickness autogenous skin grafts in mice. *Am J Physiol*. 1967;212:1081-1085.
14. Clemmesen T, Ronhovde DA. Restoration of the blood supply to human skin autografts. *Scand J Plast Reconstr Surg*. 1960;2:44-46.
15. Goldminz D, Bennett RG. Cigarette smoking and flap and full-thickness graft necrosis. *Arch Dermatol*. 1991;127:1012-1015.
16. Harris DR. Healing of the surgical wound. II. Factors influencing repair and regeneration. *J Am Acad Dermatol*. 1979;1:208-215.
17. Pollack SV. Wound healing: a review. IV. Systemic medications affecting wound healing. *J Dermatol Surg Oncol*. 1982;8:667-672.
18. Burget GC, Menick FJ. The subunit principle in nasal reconstruction. *Plast Reconstr Surg*. 1985;76:239-247.
19. Rohrer TE, Dzubow LM. Conchal bowl skin grafting in nasal tip reconstruction: clinical and histologic evaluation. *J Am Acad Dermatol*. 1995;33:476-481.
20. Zitelli JA. Burow's grafts. *J Am Acad Dermatol*. 1987;17:271-279.
21. Chester EC Jr. Surgical gem. The use of dog-ears as grafts. *J Dermatol Surg Oncol*. 1981;7:956-959.
22. Chester EC Jr. Closure of a surgical defect in a nose using island grafts from the nose. *J Dermatol Surg Oncol*. 1982;8:790-791.
23. Kim KH, Gross VL, Jaffe AT, Herbst AM. The use of the melolabial Burow's graft in the reconstruction of combination nasal sidewall–cheek defects. *Dermatol Surg*. 2004;30:205-207.
24. Mellette JR Jr, Swinehart JM. Cartilage removal prior to skin grafting in the triangular fossa, antihelix, and concha of the ear. *J Dermatol Surg Oncol*. 1990;16:1102-1105.
25. Hexsel CL, Loosemore M, Goldberg LH, Awadalla F, Morales-Burgos A. Postauricular skin: an excellent donor site for split-thickness skin grafts for the head, neck, and upper chest. *Dermatol Surg*. 2015;41(1):48-52.
26. Connolly KL, Albertini JG, Miller CJ, Ozog DM. The suspension (Frost) suture: experience and applications. *Dermatol Surg*. 2015;41(3):406-410.
27. Moyer JS, Baker S. The use of skin grafts with local flaps. In: Baker SR, ed. *Local Flaps in Facial Reconstruction*. Philadelphia, PA: Elsevier/Saunders; 2014:368-384.
28. Putterman AM. Blotter technique to determine the size of skin grafts. *Plast Reconstr Surg*. 2003;112:335-336.
29. Hubbard TJ. Leave the fat, skip the bolster: thinking outside the box in lower third nasal reconstruction. *Plast Reconstr Surg*. 2004;114:1427-1435.
30. Fish FS, Hilger PA. Aquaplast thermoplastic (Opti-Mold): a unique moldable tie-down dressing for full-thickness skin grafts. *J Dermatol Surg Oncol*. 1994;20:239-244.
31. Salasche SJ, Winton GB. Clinical evaluation of a nonadhering wound dressing. *J Dermatol Surg Oncol*. 1986;12:1220-1222.
32. Robinson JK. Improvement of the appearance of full-thickness skin grafts with dermabrasion. *Arch Dermatol*. 1987;123:1340-1345.
33. Hambley RM, Carruthers JA. Microlipoinjection for the elevation of depressed full-thickness skin grafts on the nose. *J Dermatol Surg Oncol*. 1992;18:963-968.
34. Gillies HD. A new free graft applied to the reconstruction of the nostril. *Br J Surg*. 1943;30:305.
35. Maves MD, Yessenow RS. The use of composite auricular grafts in a nasal reconstruction. *J Dermatol Surg Oncol*. 1988;14:994-999.
36. Yildirim S, Gideroglu K, Akoz T. Application of helical composite sandwich graft for eyelid reconstruction. *Ophthal Plast Reconstr Surg*. 2002;18:295-300.
37. Manson PN. Algorithm for nasal reconstruction. *Am J Surg*. 1979;138:528-532.
38. Raghavan U, Jones NS. Use of the auricular composite graft in nasal reconstruction. *J Laryngol Otol*. 2001;115:885-893.
39. Cook JL. Optimal repair of the composite graft donor wound at the root of the helix. *Dermatol Surg*. 2010;36(10):1588-1591.
40. Keck T, Lindemann J, Kuhnemann S, Sigg O. Healing of composite chondrocutaneous auricular grafts covered by skin flaps in nasal reconstructive surgery. *Laryngoscope*. 2003;113:248-253.
41. Bennett JE. Reconstruction of lateral nasal defects. *Clin Plast Surg*. 1981;8:587-598.
42. Ratner D, Katz A, Grande DJ. An interlocking auricular composite graft. *Dermatol Surg*. 1995;21:789-792.
43. Albertini JG, Ramsey ML. Surgical pearl: delayed intranasal knot tying for composite grafts of the ala. *J Am Acad Dermatol*. 1998;39(5 Pt 1):787-788.
44. Conley J. Intranasal composite grafts for dorsal support. *Arch Otolaryngol*. 1985;111:241-243.
45. Adams DC, Ramsey ML. Grafts in dermatologic surgery: review and update on full- and split-thickness skin grafts, free cartilage grafts, and composite grafts. *Dermatol Surg*. 2005;31(8 Pt 2):1055-1067.
46. Ewanowski CD, Cook J. Using cartilage and skin grafts concurrently: an alternate route to repair. *Dermatol Surg*. 2009;35(11):1809-1817.
47. Skouge JW. Techniques for split-thickness skin grafting. *J Dermatol Surg*. 1987;13:841-849.
48. Pitkanen JM, Al-Qattan MM, Russel NA. Immediate coverage of exposed, denuded cranial bone with split-thickness skin grafts. *Ann Plast Surg*. 2000;45:118-121.
49. Glogau RG, Stegman SJ, Tromovitch TA. Refinements in split thickness skin grafting technique. *J Dermatol Surg Oncol*. 1987;13:853-858.

50. Cook J, Cook J. The lateral femoral cutaneous nerve block. *Dermatol Surg*. 2000;26:81-83.
51. Wheeland RG. The technique and current status of pinch grafting. *J Dermatol Surg Oncol*. 1987;13:873-880.
52. Ceilley RI, Bumsted RM, Panje WR. Delayed skin grafting. *J Dermatol Surg Oncol*. 1983;9:288-293.
53. Goldman G, Altmayer S, Sambandan P, Cook JL. Development of cerebral air emboli during Mohs micrographic surgery. *Dermatol Surg*. 2009;35(9):1414-1421.
54. Field LM. More surgical gems. *J Dermatol Surg Oncol*. 1980;6:690-691.
55. James JH, Watson AC. The use of Opsite, a vapour permeable dressing, on skin graft donor sites. *Br J Plast Surg*. 1975;28:107-110.
56. Rakel BA, Bermel MA, Abbott LI, et al. Split-thickness skin graft donor site care: a quantitative synthesis of the research. *Appl Nurs Res*. 1998;11:174-182.

Videos for this chapter can be found online by accessing the accompanying Expert Consult website.

10 Scalp Reconstruction

JUSTIN J. LEITENBERGER, MD, and KEN K. LEE, MD, PC

Although the scalp represents one of the most visually and anatomically homogeneous regions of the head and neck, its unique anatomic characteristics and subtleties, however, can often make reconstructive surgery in this area quite challenging. The distribution of underlying muscle and the compartmentalization of the scalp by the galea aponeurotica, the presence of terminal hairs, and the skin biomechanics are features that must be taken into consideration. These characteristics of the scalp provide both benefits and drawbacks during reconstructive planning. Primary closures, flaps, and grafts can all be utilized to reconstruct the scalp, although their application techniques can be very different when compared to their uses on other parts of the face. The broad, inelastic nature of the galea, encompassing the scalp as a tendonlike sheath under constant tension, lends the scalp its relative immobility. As such, in comparison to facial skin, extensive undermining and longer incisions are often necessary during scalp reconstruction in order to achieve only small degrees of tissue movement. A thorough understanding of these aspects of the scalp is mandatory for attaining the best surgical outcome.[1]

Scalp Surgical Anatomy

The scalp extends from the superior nuchal line posteriorly to the superior border of the frontalis muscle and is delineated by the pinnae bilaterally. The scalp is composed of five layers: skin, subcutaneous connective tissue, galea, subaponeurotic loose areolar tissue, and pericranium. The skin is tethered to the underlying subcutaneous connective tissue and galea by muscle and fibrous bands. Local flaps commonly incorporate the outer three layers of the scalp, and flap undermining is easily performed through the subgaleal space, a relatively avascular plane.[1]

The galea consists of a thick membranous tendon (galea aponeurotica) that completely encases both the frontalis muscle anteriorly and the occipitalis muscle posteriorly. These muscles are joined in the midline by posterior and anterior extensions of the galea. The galea tightly wraps over the skull because of the antagonistic actions of the frontalis and occipitalis muscles. The temporoparietal muscles originate from the superficial temporal fascia and insert into the lateral border of the galea aponeurotica. Whereas the frontalis/galea/occipitalis are at the depth of the muscles of facial expression, the temporoparietalis is at the deeper level of the muscles of mastication. The subgaleal space lies over the pericranium on the crown of the scalp but extends over the temporoparietalis muscle laterally. This is important, as undermining should be performed in the relatively avascular subgaleal plane above the temporoparietalis muscle and under the frontalis and occipitalis muscles. The scalp areas associated with muscle and fascia exhibit greater mobility than the central regions that consist only of dense underlying galea. As such, more distensible flaps arise from the peripheral scalp, where the skin overlies the frontalis, occipitalis, and temporalis muscles (Fig. 10.1).[2]

Blood vessels and sensory nerves traverse the scalp in a centripetal fashion through the subcutaneous connective tissue layer above the galea. The scalp's abundant arterial supply is derived from the internal carotid system anteriorly (supraorbital and supratrochlear arteries) and from the external carotid system laterally and posteriorly (occipital, postauricular, and superficial temporal arteries). The extensive vascular anastomoses allow a single superficial temporal artery to provide sufficient blood supply to virtually the entire scalp; however, the midline scalp possesses a relative watershed zone where perfusion may be less predictable. The scalp lymphatic filtration system interlaces with medium-sized blood vessels in the subdermal and subcutaneous layers. Since the scalp lacks lymph nodes, there are no barriers to lymph flow. Lymph flows in a centrifugal pattern toward the parotid, occipital, preauricular, and postauricular areas.[3]

The ophthalmic branch of the fifth cranial (trigeminal) nerve provides sensation to the anterior scalp. The occipital nerve, a second cervical nerve derivative, supplies the posterior scalp. The auriculotemporal and maxillary nerves are responsible for sensation to the temple area, while the great auricular nerve supplies the postauricular area.[1] Infiltrating local anesthetic around the scalp's periphery (through which all the sensory nerves traverse) can produce total scalp anesthesia.

Evaluation of the Scalp Defect

When presented with a scalp defect or a lesion to be excised, the surgeon must evaluate the various reconstructive options that will result in the optimal surgical outcome.

The following questions need to be considered:

What is the depth of the wound? Is the wound through the skin, galea, or pericranium?

Some superficial wounds can appropriately heal by second intention and may even have hair regrowth if the depth of the wound does not extend below the level of the terminal hair bulbs. Most full-thickness wounds will require undermining in the subgaleal plane for tissue movement. Without an intact periosteum, a skin graft will not likely

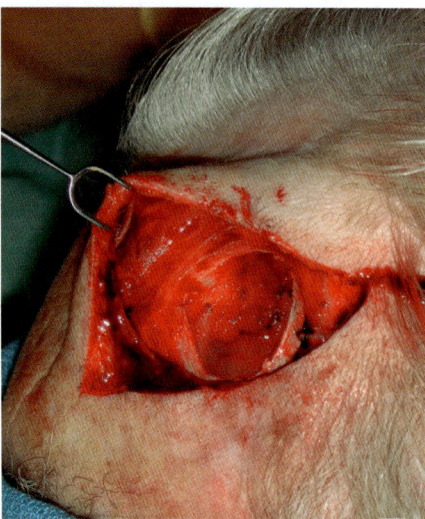

Fig. 10.1 In this wound in the temporoparietal area, note that beneath the galea and subgaleal space lie the temporalis fascia and the temporoparietalis muscle, which inserts into the cranium. Pericranium is seen superiorly.

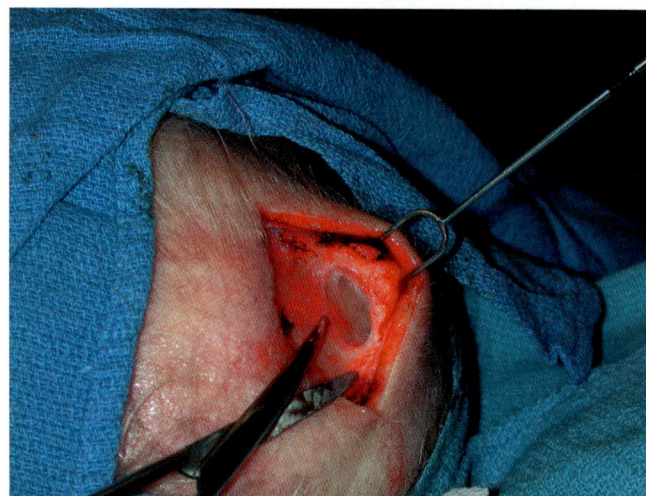

Fig. 10.2 Subgaleal space. The loose aponeurotic connective tissue layer is bluntly dissected with wide scissor undermining. Note the avascularity of this tissue plane.

survive unless the underlying bone is burred to induce pinpoint bleeding.[4]

Is the defect surrounded by hair-bearing or glabrous skin?

On a bald scalp, second intention healing or skin grafting may be reasonable options, as the resulting scars will be less conspicuous on hairless skin. If the defect is surrounded by dense terminal hair growth, either primary closure or flap alternatives should be considered in order to avoid focal alopecia.

How much tissue laxity is present?

Scalp laxity can significantly vary by age and location, and from person to person. Scalps in infants, for example, are quite loose and mobile. As one ages, scalp mobility can change dramatically. The crown of the scalp usually is the least mobile area, whereas the peripheral scalp is more distensible. When evaluating for scalp laxity, one can be deceived by the amount of movement obtained by simply squeezing the sides of the defect together. This movement is partly due to the laxity of the dermis, and the actual movement of the surrounding scalp will be dictated by the galea, which is far stiffer and more immobile.

Can adequate anesthesia be obtained with local infiltration and/or nerve blocks for the type of reconstruction planned?

The degree of undermining required for a scalp closure is far greater than that in many other facial regions. These undermining requirements need to be evaluated before a reconstruction under local anesthesia is initiated. Even with adequate local anesthesia, scalp reconstruction can be quite difficult when patients hear and feel the pressure sensation of the undermining conducted through the underlying bone. General anesthesia may be more suitable for some anxious patients.

Basic Reconstruction Concepts

Accessing the subgaleal space is paramount in scalp reconstruction, as this plane is relatively avascular, making it ideal for atraumatic undermining (Fig. 10.2). Blunt dissection of the subgaleal space is all that is needed, and this can be achieved by scissor dissection or by simply using one's gloved finger. This relative ease of undermining can be very deceptive, however, as the degree of additional movement afforded by wide undermining can be surprisingly small. For the best reconstructive outcome, the galea must be fully reapproximated. It is common for less experienced surgeons, particularly when confronted with very tense wounds, to not fully reapproximate the galea. In these cases, the final reapproximation of the wound's edges involves stretching the overlying skin. The undesirable tension placed on the epidermal edges results in spread and inverted scars (Fig. 10.3). It is therefore important that the galea is reapproximated by reaching underneath the leading edge of the defect and grabbing a large bite of galea with the suture needle (Fig. 10.4). The strength of a properly realigned galea allows for minimal tension on the overlying skin, which leads to a more aesthetically appropriate scar.[1] If proper wound eversion is not achieved, the final scar will likely be less than ideal.

When confronted with an immobile scalp, the surgeon can enhance the movement of the scalp by performing a galeotomy. The classic galeotomy technique is accomplished by making linear scalpel incisions through the galea from within the essentially avascular subgaleal space. These incisions should be oriented parallel to the wound edge and, if possible, parallel to the course of the underlying vascular supply. The fenestrations expose overlying subcutaneous fat and allow the galea to effectively stretch. Galeotomies can be performed on large flaps without difficulty, as the skin is easily lifted to expose the flap's undersurface. However, without special equipment such as scalp retractors, galeotomies are more difficult to perform during primary closures. In this setting, angling the scalpel blade to place fenestrations through the galea away from the wound edge is challenging because of limited exposure of the scalp's undersurface. An electrosurgical apparatus set in the cutting mode can be utilized to reach farther back.

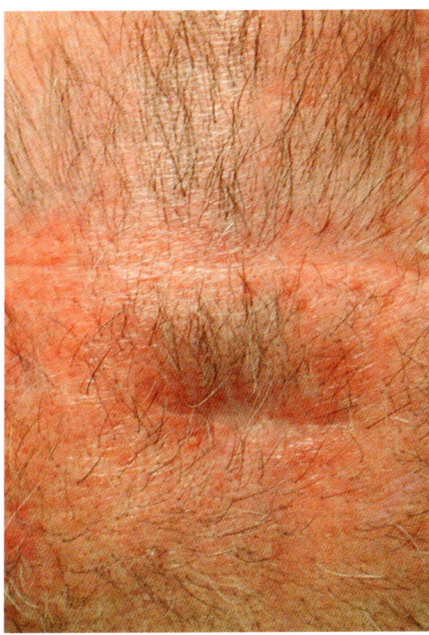

Fig. 10.3 There are two linear scars on this scalp. The inferior scar is inverted and spread, a likely result of insufficient undermining and failure to reapproximate the galea at the time of wound closure. The superior scar is well approximated and more aesthetically appropriate.

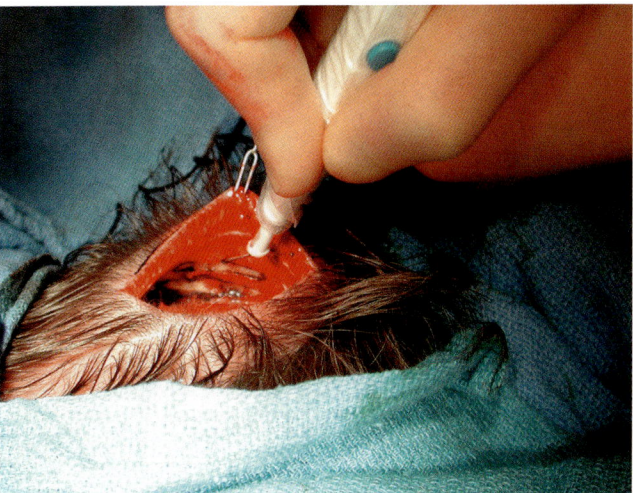

Fig. 10.5 The electrocautery set on cutting mode is pointed upward to provide galeotomy incisions. Incisions are made approximately 1 cm apart along the length of the wound. These fenestrations in the galea allow for greater scalp movement. Care must be taken not to cut too deeply, as the subcutaneous vessels may be damaged. Galeotomy incisions should be at least 1 cm away from the wound's leading edge, so that the galea does not rip when sutured.

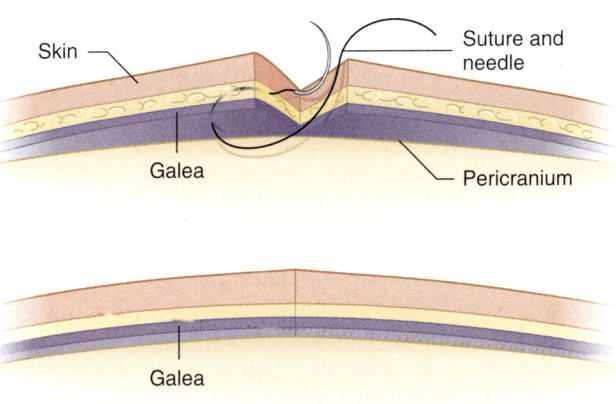

Fig. 10.4 The galea typically retracts back into the wound. For proper suture technique, a larger bite needs to be taken in order to reapproximate the galea and reduce the overlying skin tension. Note that only the galea (without the skin) has been sutured.

The needle can be bent slightly upward to assist with this maneuver (Fig. 10.5).

When performing galeotomies, one must take care not to incise too vigorously, as the deeper vessels in the subcutaneous fat are in close proximity to the galea. The incisions should be made at least 1 cm from the wound edges, or the galea may tear when sutures are used to subsequently reapproximate the surgical defect.

Second Intention Healing

Dermatologic surgeons are accustomed to letting many wounds granulate. Second intention healing is indicated in patients who may not tolerate or desire extensive reconstructive surgery. Allowing the wound to heal by second intention can sometimes be the most appropriate wound management strategy for wounds on alopecic scalps. Often the resultant scars are particularly cosmetically acceptable in these areas of the scalp where hair is absent.[5]

Surprisingly, even deeper scalp wounds allowed to heal by second intention can often fill in to nearly the level of the surrounding skin, and the resulting scars usually look better than alternative split-thickness skin graft or scars from side-to-side or flap repairs. One of the main disadvantages of second intention healing is the prolonged duration of wound healing. These defects often take more than 1 month to completely granulate. If the underlying calvarium is exposed at the base of the wound, the duration of second intention healing can be much longer, but this option remains relatively safe and successful.[6,7] One must be sure that the patient or a caretaker is able to provide proper wound care.

In older patients with atrophic scalp skin, the healing process can uncommonly arrest after the initial period of granulation. In these instances, the use of delayed split-thickness skin grafts can be helpful in achieving final epithelialization.

Primary Closure

Primary linear closure is often the best option for the reconstruction of smaller scalp wounds. The maximum defect diameter that can be closed by primary closure varies from patient to patient, but it is generally less than 3 cm (Fig. 10.6). The surgeon can estimate whether a wound will close primarily by pushing on the sides of the defect. However, as mentioned earlier, this often overestimates the amount of actual tissue availability.

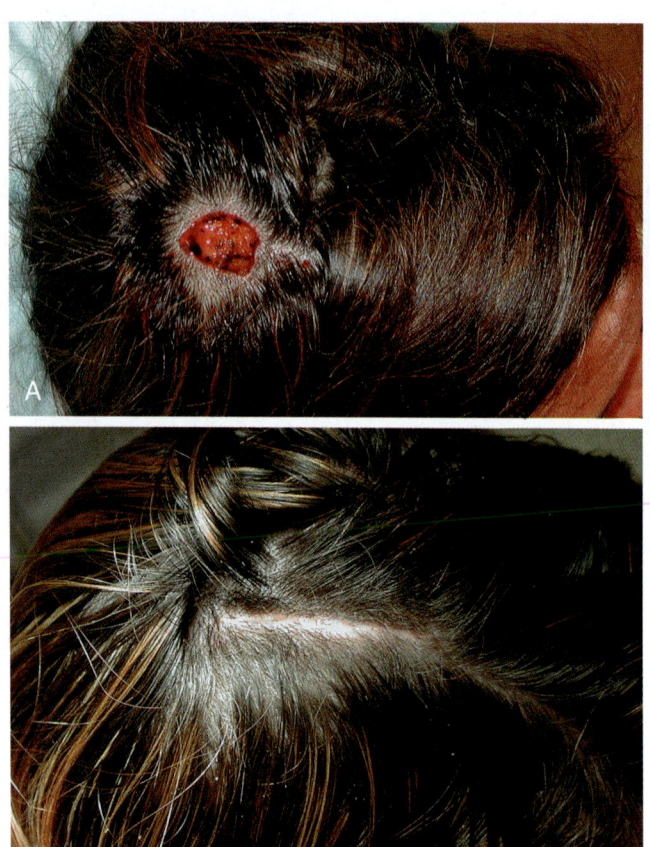
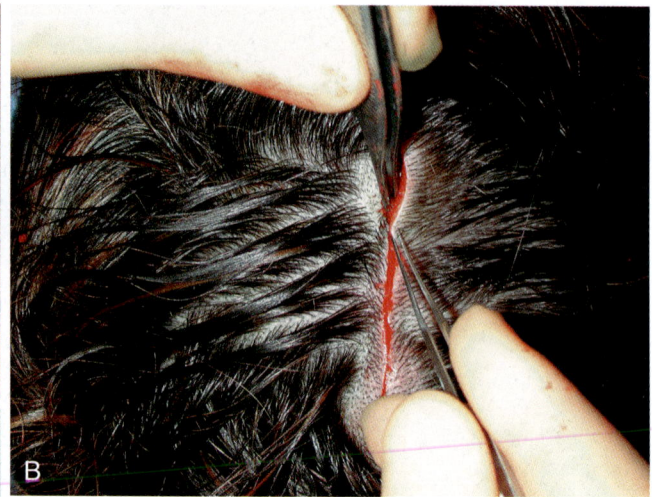

Fig. 10.6 (A) Full-thickness cutaneous defect. Intact galea needs to be removed prior to reconstruction. (B) The wound has been closed primarily with galeal sutures only. Note the eversion and the lack of tension on the skin edges. (C) Two months postoperatively. Note some degree of alopecia over the surgical scar despite appropriate wound closure.

If the defect involves only the skin, the base of the wound should be deepened by removing the galea prior to closing the wound primarily. This deepening of the wound allows proper wide undermining in the subgaleal space. Wound closure tensions should be minimized, and galeotomies should be placed if appropriate. Spread scars resulting from unacceptably high wound closure tensions can be particularly noticeable in hair-bearing scalps, because there is an absence of hair within the scars. Proper surgical technique can reduce this complication. Hair shafts on the scalp do not commonly grow directly perpendicular to the skin. When appropriate, incisions in the scalp should be angled along the direction of hair growth in order to transect the fewest follicles. This will lead to more viable hair follicles at the scar's edge. When bringing the wound edges together, the surgeon needs to initially reapproximate the galea in order to reduce tension on the overlying skin. It is helpful to use a suture such as 2-0 Vicryl (Ethicon Corp) on a PS-4 needle, as the smaller needle size facilitates grasping only the galea. One should not pass the suture needle through both the galea and dermis in one bite, as this may lead to a more inverted wound. In fusiform elliptical closures, it may be helpful to place all the galeal sutures prior to tying them. Once in place, they can be tied starting from the ends of the wound so that the tension is reduced in the middle. The superficial skin can then be closed with staples, as they are occasionally easier to remove than sutures in hair-bearing regions. In the occipital scalp, however, sutures are occasionally preferred, since staples tend to be less comfortable than sutures when they are compressed during sleep.

Split-Thickness Skin Grafts

Split-thickness skin grafts (STSG) are convenient modes of reconstruction for larger defects on the scalp. Beyond the convenience, however, such grafts have a number of disadvantages. The cosmetic appearance of STSGs is often less than ideal because the grafts are typically depressed, shiny, and hairless (Fig. 10.7). When healed, STSGs are often bound down to the underlying bone, and they therefore do not mimic the mobility of the normal scalp. The grafts are also sometimes quite fragile and susceptible to shearing forces. Often a second intention scar has a better cosmetic appearance and is stronger than the STSG alternative.

The STSG does fill an important role in scalp reconstruction by allowing rapid coverage of larger surgical defects. The healing time of an STSG is typically less than the time required for a wound to granulate. In defects resulting from aggressive tumors, STSGs also allow for better tumor surveillance of the wound bed than flaps. For the graft to survive, the recipient bed needs to be well vascularized. If the periosteum is absent, the vascularity of the underlying intact calvarium is insufficient to allow graft survival. In such cases, the outer table of the cranium needs to be sufficiently removed to produce bleeding for graft nourishment.

This can be performed with the use of a chisel and hammer[8] or with a high-speed drill. After burring the calvarium's outer table, the STSG can then be placed in an immediate or delayed fashion or after placement of a dermal regeneration template.[9] Delaying the graft placement enables the wound bed to partially granulate, potentially allowing for increased graft survival.

The defect size can also be slightly decreased by a purse-string closure prior to the application of the STSG. Although the amount of tissue movement produced by the purse-string closure is often relatively minimal, the diameter of the wound may be reduced by 10% to 30%. There are numerous variations to the purse-string technique. One method that works well on the scalp is the use of 2-0 Vicryl absorbable suture, where bites of the galea are taken in a circumferential fashion, tying the suture off within the wound so that it does not need to be removed at a later time. The STSG is then placed in the center of the remaining defect (Fig. 10.8).[4]

Skin Substitute Reconstruction

Artificial dermal grafts, often composed of bovine collagen, provide a dermal matrix for which serves as a dermal regeneration template promoting cellular ingrowth.[10] Atop a bilayer wound matrix is often a silicone layer serving as an epidermal substitute to provide mechanical protection and moisture modulation of the wound. The application of a bilayer dermal regeneration template is often used to promote granulation for 14 to 21 days, after which time the silicone is removed and a delayed STSG may be applied. Using a dermal xenograft alone can improve the appearance of the scar with less contraction and better pliability, when compared with STSG performed immediately after skin cancer removal.[11] Moisture modulation is paramount to promote early granulation and faster healing for extensive scalp wounds not amenable to other reconstructive options.

Full-Thickness Skin Grafts

Full-thickness skin graft is a less applicable reconstructive option on the scalp than in other areas of the head and neck. One of the main reasons is that suitable donor sites having hair-bearing skin are difficult to find. Additionally, larger full-thickness skin grafts thick enough to contain terminal hair have high metabolic demands, and such grafts therefore have much greater risks of ischemic necrosis. The Burow skin graft, however, is an often-overlooked reconstructive technique for the scalp. The Burow graft is taken

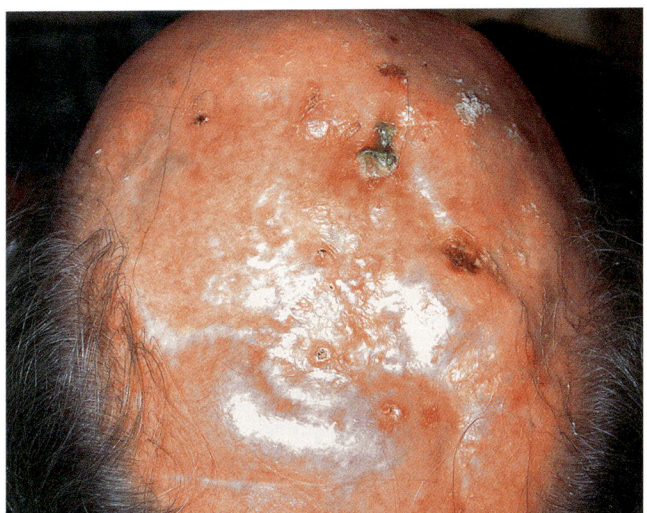

Fig. 10.7 The split-thickness skin graft on the crown has a bound down, shiny, atrophic appearance. There is extensive sun damage and possible persistent tumor at the graft's periphery.

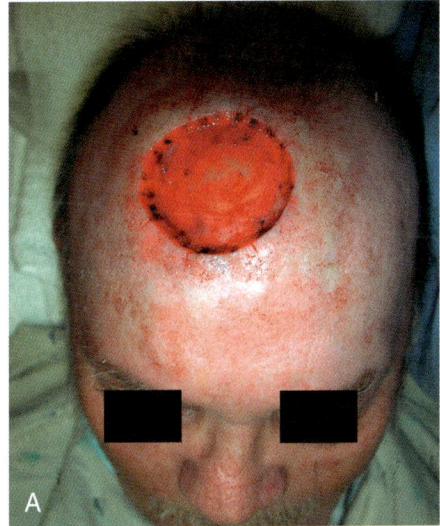 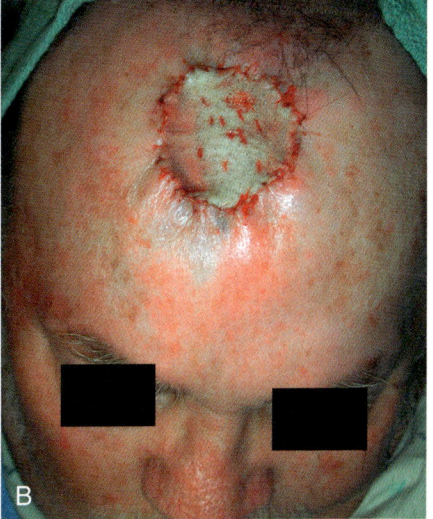

Fig. 10.8 (A) Defect of the forehead/frontal scalp that extends to the underlying galea. (B) After purse-string closure and split-thickness skin grafting (STSG). The defect size has been partially reduced by the purse-string closure, resulting in a smaller STSG.

from the redundant triangle that is removed when a circular defect is converted into a fusiform ellipse. The ellipse is then "zippered" closed from both ends until the escalating tension does not allow for further closure of the center portion of the wound. The remaining central defect is usually significantly decreased in size. The small full-thickness graft is placed in the remainder of the defect after trimming off the fat with careful attention to avoid undue trauma to hair follicles located in the deep dermis. Because the Burow graft is typically quite small, the hair in the graft often survives, thereby restoring a cosmetically acceptable appearance. The advantage of this technique is that medium-sized defects that cannot be closed primarily can be closed without the use of a larger flap. There is, however, a risk of graft failure, leading to an alopecic scar. If this does occur, the resulting scar can be excised at a later time when the surrounding tissue has relaxed and stretched through tissue creep.[12]

Random Pattern Cutaneous Flaps

The varied nomenclature for local cutaneous flaps can be confusing. One major classification scheme for cutaneous flaps utilizes descriptive terms of the flaps' major motions. In this manner, flaps are traditionally divided into advancement, rotation, and transposition. An alternative, simplified nosological approach is to divide flaps into sliding (advancement and rotation) and lifting (transposition) to describe their primary motions.

Regardless of classification schemes, flaps share common features that must be understood. The primary defect is the wound, often resulting from tumor removal, which is to be closed. The secondary defect is the defect created by the movement of the flap to close the primary defect. Secondary defects are more difficult to close in the relatively inelastic scalp. The primary motion is the predominant direction in which the flap is moved to close the primary defect. The secondary motion is the resultant motion on the surrounding skin caused by the primary motion. These concepts of primary and secondary motion (the effect of the flap on the surrounding skin) are very important in understanding the applications and limitations of local cutaneous flaps.[13]

ADVANCEMENT FLAPS

Pure advancement flaps are not commonly used in head and neck reconstruction, because there is great limitation in the amount of tissue movement in a linear vector. In other words, wounds that cannot be closed in a simple linear manner will not often be amendable to closure using a unidirectional advancement flap, as the tension directions and magnitudes are essentially identical. One place where a traditional advancement flap is applicable is the frontal scalp region, where the flap's incision lines can be hidden within the anterior hairline. The use of bilateral advancement flaps with the incisions placed along the hairline can nicely camouflage the inevitable scars. In order to minimize the standing cutaneous deformities that accompany tissue advancement, the incisions of the advancement flaps need to be long. The redundant Burow triangles can be removed to improve flap contour, but the required incisions will be perpendicular to the ideal horizontal incisions. Another technique that can reduce the "dog-ear" protrusions is the inward curving of the flap incisions to create wounds of unequal lengths. By doing so, the surgeon removes some of the dog-ear redundancy from the body of the flap instead of "pushing" the dog-ear laterally, where it must be excised vertically in order to achieve proper flap contour. One must make incisions into the body of the flap with care, as overzealous removal of tissue from these areas can compromise the flap's vascular supply.[14]

A variation of the pure advancement flap, the O-to-T advancement flap is also useful on the upper forehead/frontal scalp region (Fig. 10.9). The flap is particularly useful when the defect abuts the frontal hairline. The flap's relaxing incisions are made bilaterally along the hairline, and the flap is elevated at the level of the subgaleal space, which in this case is underneath the frontalis muscle. For proper tension-free movement of the flap, the undermining needs to be extensive, and galeotomies are sometimes needed when tissue movement requirements are great. When the limbs of the O–T flap are advanced, a dog-ear redundancy will be present at the inferior aspect of the defect. This triangle is removed in a vertical direction to form the final incision lines in the shape of a "T." Vertical scars on the forehead often spread less than horizontal scars and therefore remain aesthetically appropriate.

ROTATION FLAPS

Variations of the traditional rotation flap are commonly used for medium- to large-sized scalp defects. The curvature of the dome-shaped scalp lends itself to the long arced incisions of the rotation flap. As with most other scalp reconstructive options, the incisions of rotation flaps are required to be long in order to compensate for the relative immobility of the scalp, and the incision should extend into an area of scalp mobility (e.g., over the temporoparietal fascia). The single rotation flap is designed by extending a curvilinear incision from the defect edge (Figs. 10.10 and 10.11). The incision is carried through the galea so that the flap is elevated at the level of the subgaleal space. The flap is rotated around a pivot point that is typically 180 degrees from the incision point on the defect. A common error in the design of a rotation flap, especially on the scalp, is to make the flap's arc too curved or narrow. This results in excess tension at the pivot point, which consequently limits flap movement and perfusion. For this reason, the flap's curved incision needs to start almost straight, elongate the leading edge, and then arc gently. When the flap is rotated into the primary defect, the flap's motion typically creates a Burow triangle redundancy near the pivot point. This Burow triangle usually needs to be removed to prevent unsightly tissue bulging, but the dog-ear excision can be done anywhere along the arc of the flap's motion. Although the Burow triangle is typically removed near the flap's pivot point, for larger rotation flaps, the triangle's excision can be placed anywhere there is lax skin or areas to conceal the required incision.

In medium to larger defects, a single rotation flap often recruits insufficient tissue to close the wound under sufficiently low tension, and the use of a double rotation flap, also called an O-to-Z closure, can be required (Fig. 10.12).

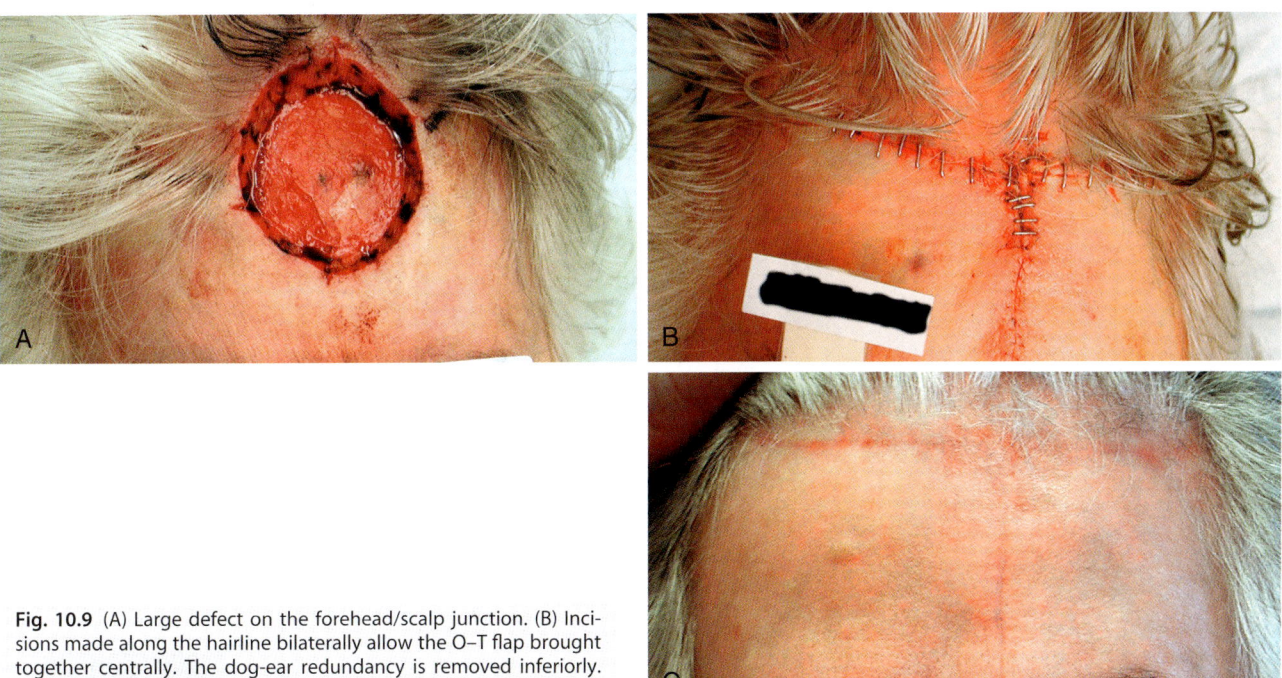

Fig. 10.9 (A) Large defect on the forehead/scalp junction. (B) Incisions made along the hairline bilaterally allow the O–T flap brought together centrally. The dog-ear redundancy is removed inferiorly. (C) Six weeks postoperatively.

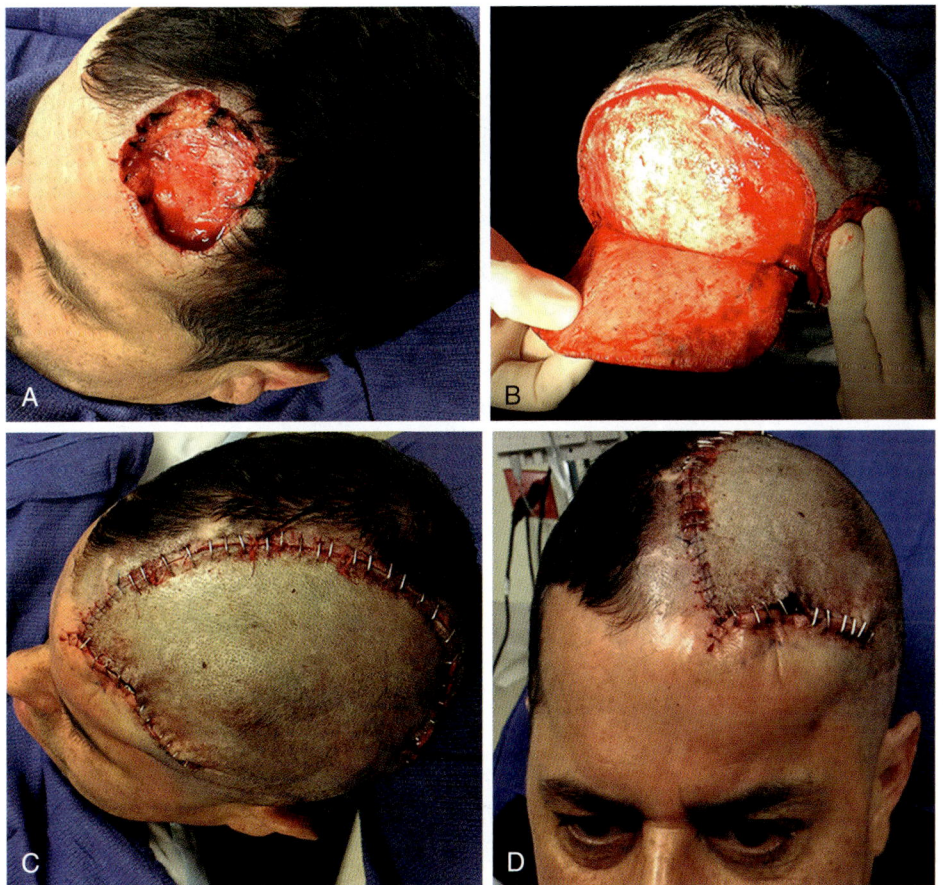

Fig. 10.10 (A) Defect on frontal scalp and forehead at hairline. (B) Elevation of unilateral rotation flap in subgaleal space. (C, D) Final closure.

152 **10 • Scalp Reconstruction**

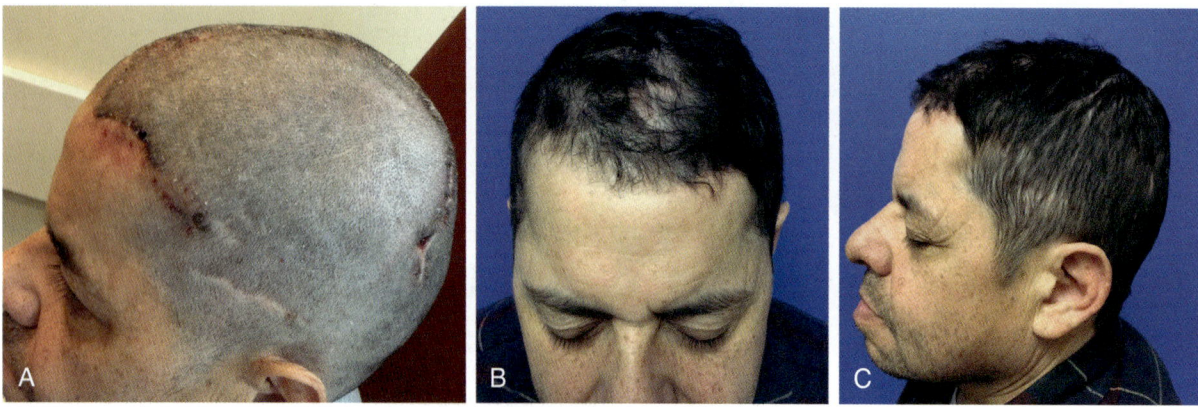

Fig. 10.11 (A) One week postoperatively. (B, C) Three-month follow-up appearance.

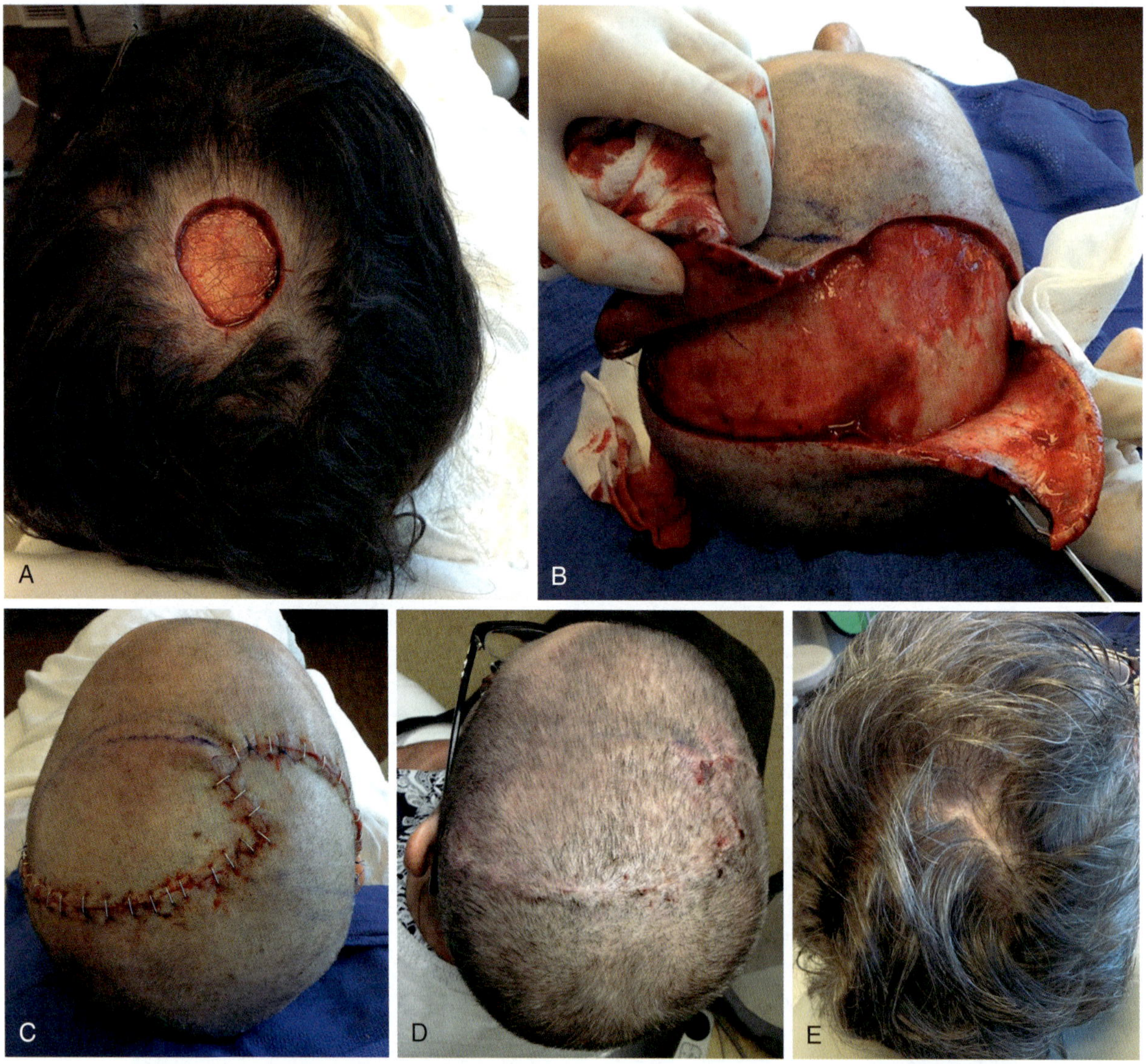

Fig. 10.12 (A) Defect on the crown of the scalp. (B) Two long, gently arcing incisions are made in clockwise directions to form an O–Z bilateral rotation flap. (C) The flaps are advanced and rotated into place. (D) Ten-day postoperative follow-up at staple removal. (E) One-year follow-up appearance.

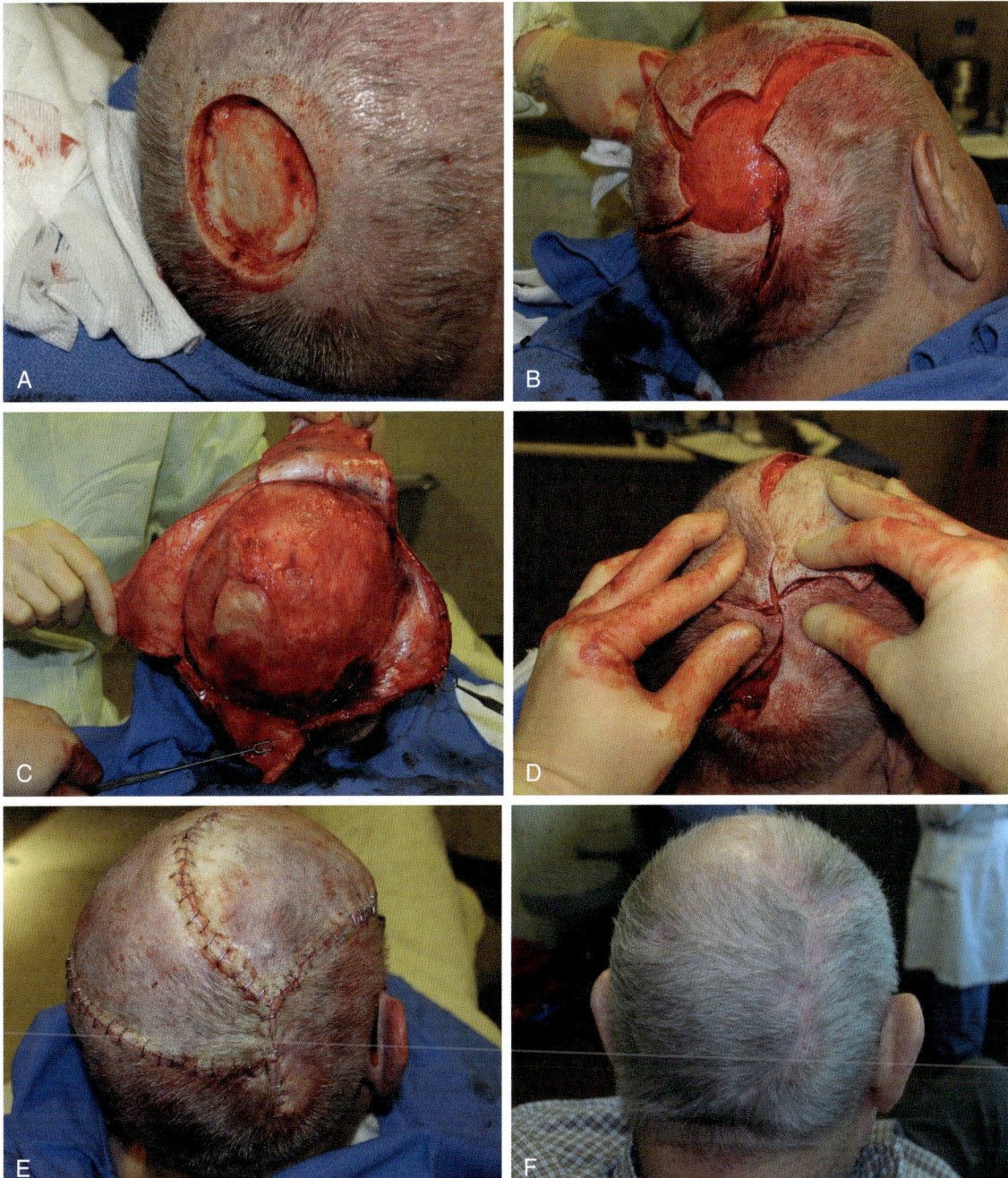

Fig. 10.13 (A) Large defect on the occipital scalp. (B) Many arcing incisions are made around the defect to create multiple rotation flaps. (C) Wide undermining necessary for mobility. (D) All flaps are rotated until they meet at one point in the center. (E) Final closure. (F) Six-week follow-up appearance.

Defects on the crown of the scalp are especially amenable to this closure technique. Although the two incisions are on the opposite sides of the defect, the arcs should curve in the same direction. In other words, they should both be designed to move either clockwise or counterclockwise. The two flaps are elevated then rotated from opposing directions, forming a "Z" shape (see Fig. 10.12). A back-cut at the distal end of the incision may be useful to help facilitate mobilization.

When the defect is large or the tissue is very inelastic, multiple rotation flaps may need to be used. The flaps' incisions are placed equidistantly on the circumference of the circular defect with the arcs curving in the same direction. Multiple incisions can be placed, but three to six flaps are typically designed. The final appearance of the multiple rotation flaps is that of a pinwheel (Fig. 10.13).[15]

TRANSPOSITION FLAPS

Transposition flaps are also called lifting flaps because the donor skin is lifted over intervening skin to fill the primary defect. These flaps are helpful in moving skin from a more mobile area such as the lateral scalp into a more immobile

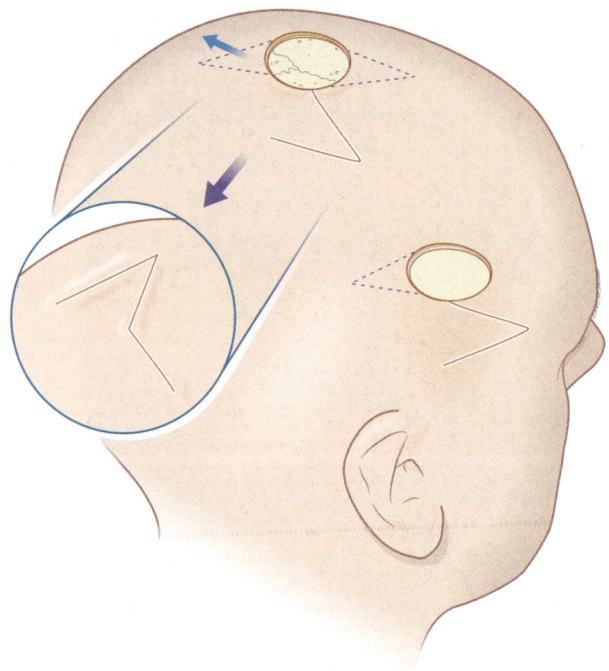

Fig. 10.14 A rhombic transposition flap is designed to transfer the loose lateral scalp onto a surgical defect on the crown. The secondary defect is closed first, which allows for the flap to drape into the primary defect. In this case, the flap is narrower than the width of the defect, and part of the defect will therefore be closed by undermining and advancing from the vertex side of the defect (secondary motion).

area such as the crown (Fig. 10.14). The rhombic transposition flap and its variations are commonly used flaps in facial reconstructive surgery. The classic rhombic flap has the primary defect in the shape of a rhombus. The flap's limb is projected at 120 degrees from one of the corners of the defect, and the flap angle width is 60 degrees. The disadvantage of this traditional flap design is that the transposition angle of 120 degrees produces excess tension and a larger dog-ear removal. The DuFourmentel and Webster variations of the rhombic flap are more practical techniques because the angles at the flap apices are smaller (60 degrees and 30 degrees, respectively), making the closure of the secondary defects much easier.[16] When evaluating the suitability of a wound for a transposition flap repair, the skin around the defect is squeezed to see where there is maximal tissue laxity. In scalp reconstruction, tissue availability is typically located laterally. The origination of transposition flaps within loose skin will allow for easier closure of the secondary defect. After the flap is incised and lifted, the secondary defect is closed initially, which is distinct from the technique typically used with sliding flaps. Initial closure of the secondary defect effectively "pushes" the flap into the primary defect and allows the flap to easily drape into the primary defect under minimal tension. A dog-ear will need to be removed opposite the secondary defect. Care must be taken not to make this incision across the flap's base.

Although the flap may be sutured under minimal tension, wide undermining of the defect is recommended in order to minimize the potential development of the trapdoor deformity. Transposition flaps typically trapdoor more than sliding flaps. Wide undermining of the flap's recipient site allows the scar base to circumferentially contract, and placement of buried sutures around the flap may minimize the risk of flap protrusion during healing.[17]

Conclusion

Reconstruction of the scalp can be one of the most challenging endeavors in head and neck surgery. The tautness of the scalp and the desire to maintain terminal hair patterns make the closure of even the smallest scalp defects sometimes difficult. With a thorough understanding of anatomy and surgical principles, the experienced surgeon can make scalp reconstruction more predictable and successful.

References

1. Panje WR, Minor LB. Reconstruction of the scalp. In: Baker SR, Swanson NA, eds. *Local Flaps in Facial Reconstruction*. St Louis, MO: Mosby; 1995:481-484.
2. Salache SJ, Bernstein G, Senkarik M. Scalp. In: Salache SJ, Bernstein G, Senkarik M, eds. *Surgical Anatomy of the Skin*. Norwalk, CT: Appleton & Lange; 1988:151-162.
3. Field LM. Scalp flaps. *J Dermatol Surg Oncol*. 1991;17:190-199.
4. Glogau RG, Haas AF. Skin grafts. In: Baker SR, Swanson NA, eds. *Local Flaps in Facial Reconstruction*. St Louis, MO: Mosby; 1995:247-271.
5. Converse JM. The technique of closure of scalp defects. *Clin Neurosurg*. 1977;57:1011-1021.
6. Snow SN, Stiff MA, Bullen R, Mohs FE, Chao WH. Second-intention healing of exposed facial-scalp bone after Mohs surgery for skin cancer: review of ninety-one cases. *J Am Acad Dermatol*. 1994;31:450-454.
7. Becker GD, Adams LA, Levin BC. Secondary intention healing of exposed scalp and forehead bone after Mohs surgery. *Otolaryngol Head Neck Surg*. 1999;121(6):751-754.
8. Vanderveen EE, Stoner JG, Swanson NA. Chiseling of exposed bone to stimulate granulation tissue after Mohs surgery. *J Dermatol Surg Oncol*. 1983;9(11):925-928.
9. Koenen W, Goerdt S, Faulhaber J. Removal of the outer table of the skull for reconstruction of full-thickness scalp defects with a dermal regeneration template. *Dermatol Surg*. 2008;34(3):357-363.
10. Gonyon DL Jr, Zenn MR. Simple approcate to the radiated scalp wound using Integra skin substitute. *Ann Plast Surg*. 2003;50:315-320.
11. Wilensky JS, Rosenthal AH, Bradford CR, Rees RS. The use of a bovine collagen construct for reconstruction of full-thickness scalp defects in the elderly patient with cutaneous malignancy. *Ann Plast Surg*. 2005;115:1010-1017.
12. Argenta LC. Controlled tissue expansion in facial reconstruction. In: Baker SR, Swanson NA, eds. *Local Flaps in Facial Reconstruction*. St Louis, MO: Mosby; 1995:517-544.
13. Swanson NA. Basic techniques. In: Swanson NA, ed. *Atlas of Cutaneous Surgery*. Boston: Little, Brown; 1987:69-112.
14. Dzubow LM. Advancement flaps. In: Dzubow LM, ed. *Facial Flaps Biomechanics and Regional Application*. Norwalk, CT: Appleton & Lange; 1990:22-30.
15. Vecchione TR, Griffith L. Closure of scalp defects by using multiple flaps in a pinwheel design. *Plast Reconstr Surg*. 1978;62:74-80.
16. Bray DA. Rhombic flaps. In: Baker SR, Swanson NA, eds. *Local Flaps in Facial Reconstruction*. St Louis, MO: Mosby; 1995:151-164.
17. Webster RC, Benjamin RJ, Smith RC. Treatment of "trapdoor deformity." *Laryngoscope*. 1978;88:707-711.

11 Forehead and Temple Repair

MARY L. STEVENSON, MD, and JOHN A. CARUCCI, MD, PHD

Successful treatment of the skin cancer patient revolves around three goals: (1) tumor-free surgical margins; (2) preservation of function; and (3) restoration and optimization of cosmesis. Before conceptualizing any repair, the surgeon must keep in mind that the primary goal of the oncologic surgeon is achievement of a tumor-free plane. Residual tumor will lead to recurrence, which can be devastating functionally and cosmetically, and potentially life threatening with aggressive tumors. One must understand tumor biology and relevant anatomy in order to be successful in this endeavor. From an aesthetic perspective, reconstructions planned according to the cosmetic unit principle provide optimal cosmesis.

The forehead, which includes the temple region, is defined superiorly and laterally by the natural anterior hairline and inferiorly by the zygomatic arch, eyebrows, and nasal root. It may be subdivided into five subunits: the central forehead, which is contiguous with the scalp; the bilateral temples; and the hair-bearing eyebrows (Fig. 11.1).[1] Relaxed-skin tension lines (RSTLs) run horizontally in the central forehead, perpendicular to the underlying frontalis musculature, and curve laterally as the temple is approached (Fig. 11.2). Convex centrally, the lateral subunit of the temple is relatively concave. Composed of moderately sebaceous skin, the central forehead is relatively immobile, with adherence to the underlying frontalis muscles. The temple subunit is more mobile, as it is loosely adherent to the underlying temporal fascia. The paired frontalis muscles insert into the inferior musculature and the brow without muscle directly midline. Inferiorly, the procerus muscle acts centrally, with bilateral corrugator supercilii muscles, and more laterally the superior aspects of orbicular oculi (Fig. 11.3). The superficial musculoaponeurotic system (SMAS), which underlies the dermis and subcutaneous tissue superiorly, is composed of the galea aponeurotica of the scalp, which invests the frontalis muscle and orbicularis oculi. Laterally, the galea is contiguous with temporoparietal fascia. In the temporal region, the superficial temporal fascia lies just beneath the subcutaneous tissue and is contiguous with the galea superiorly, the frontalis muscle, and the SMAS. Deep to this layer is the innominate fascia. Concern in this region must be taken for preservation of the temporal branch of the facial nerve, which generally runs just beneath the superficial temporal fascia within the SMAS creating a relative "danger zone," though some consider this branch to course deeper in the innominate fascia.[2,3] This region is generally defined inferiorly by a line drawn from the earlobe to the lateral brow and superiorly by a line drawn from the tragus to the lateral aspect of the highest RSTL on the forehead, with the nerve being most superficial and at risk as it crosses the midzygomatic arch (Fig. 11.4).[2]

Vascular supply to the majority of the forehead is supplied by the dorsal nasal artery, supratrochlear artery, and supraorbital artery, all branches of the internal carotid artery. The supratrochlear artery, which is most medial, is the axial artery for the paramedian forehead flap. Laterally, the temple region is supplied by the superficial temporal artery, which arises from the external carotid artery (Fig. 11.5). This artery runs within and then above the SMAS layers of the lateral forehead. Generally, two undermining planes may be defined on the forehead—above the frontalis muscle and below the muscle and deep fascia. This latter plane provides a relatively bloodless plane but can result in transection of the major vessels and requires repair of the frontalis muscle.[4] Sensory innervation mirrors the vasculature medially and arises from the supratrochlear and supraorbital branches of the ophthalmic division of the trigeminal nerve (Fig. 11.6). These nerves divide into four to six terminal branches collectively and may have variable anatomy, but notably these nerves quickly penetrate the muscle and enter the superficial subcutaneous plane after leaving their foramens.[5] As a result, horizontal closure in this area may result in a fan-shaped area of numbness superior to the closure that is usually temporary. Laterally the temple receives sensory innervation from the zygomaticotemporal nerve, a branch of the maxillary division of the trigeminal nerve. Motor innervation is provided predominantly by the temporal branch of the facial nerve. Contraction of the frontalis muscle causes brow elevation, and denervation results in brow ptosis. The paired corrugator supercilii muscles are also innervated by the temporal branch of the facial nerve and act to pull the brow medially and downward while the central procerus muscle is innervated by the zygomatic branch of the facial nerve and acts to depress the brow. Laterally the paired orbicular oculi muscles are innervated by the temporal branch of the facial nerve and act to close the eyes.

As in the case of surgical defects in any location, various repairs may be considered on the forehead. Generally a poor match for skin grafts, secondary intention, primary linear closure, M-plasty, advancement flaps including rotation flaps, and transposition flaps may all be considered in this subunit. Which type of repair is optimal depends on the size and location of the defect, as well as the patient's individual anatomy. Maintenance of brow position is of utmost importance with respect to cosmesis, and consideration of tension placed on the eyelid must be observed more laterally in the temple region.

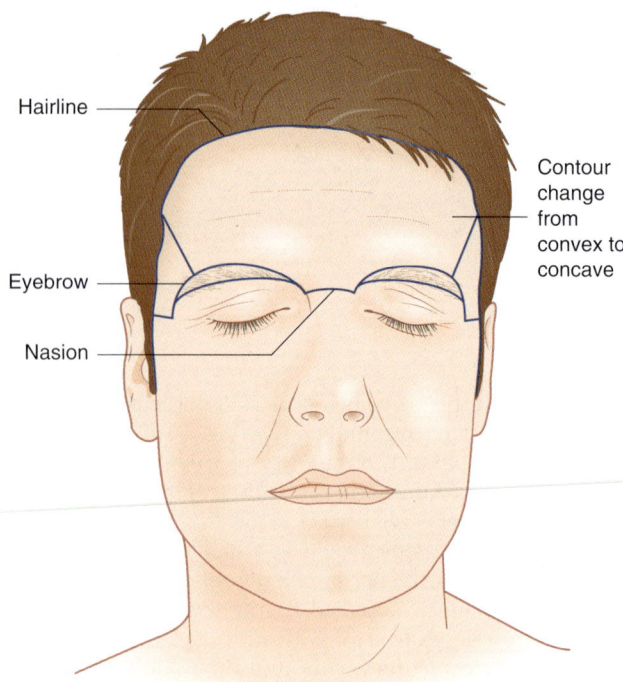

Fig. 11.1 Cosmetic units. The cosmetic units of the forehead and temple area can be divided into five subunits: the central forehead, the paired lateral foreheads or temples, and the paired eyebrows.

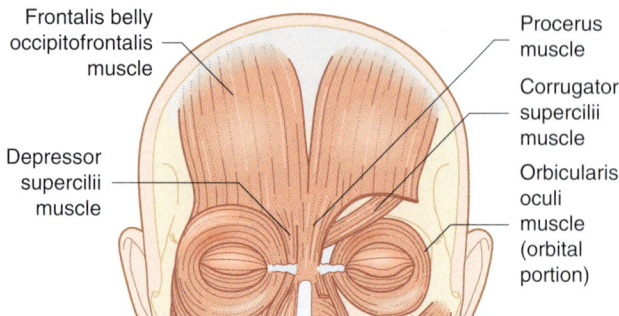

Fig. 11.3 Musculature anatomy. The frontalis muscle is shown as it interdigitates with the procerus, orbicularis oculi, corrugator supercilii, and depressor supercilii. The frontalis muscle also interdigitates with the skin of the eyebrow inferiorly. Portions of the frontalis, orbicularis oculi, and depressor supercilii have been dissected to reveal the corrugator muscle.

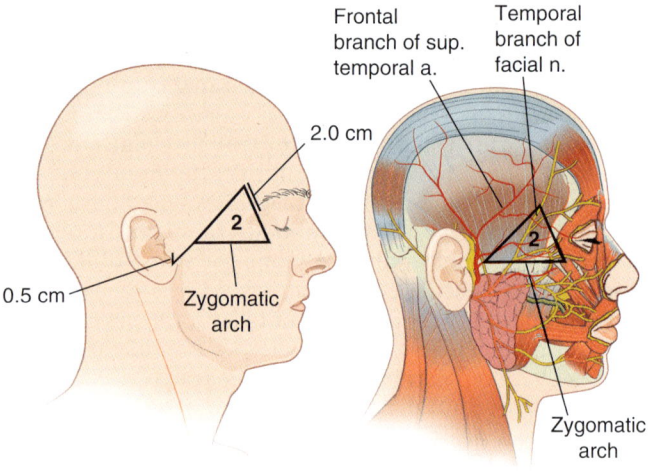

Fig. 11.4 Temporal nerve danger zone. The temporal branches lie between two lines drawn from the earlobe to the lateral brow and to the lateral end of the highest forehead crease. From the time the nerve exits the parotid and enters the frontalis, it lies in the superficial musculoaponeurotic system (SMAS), just below the subcutaneous fat.

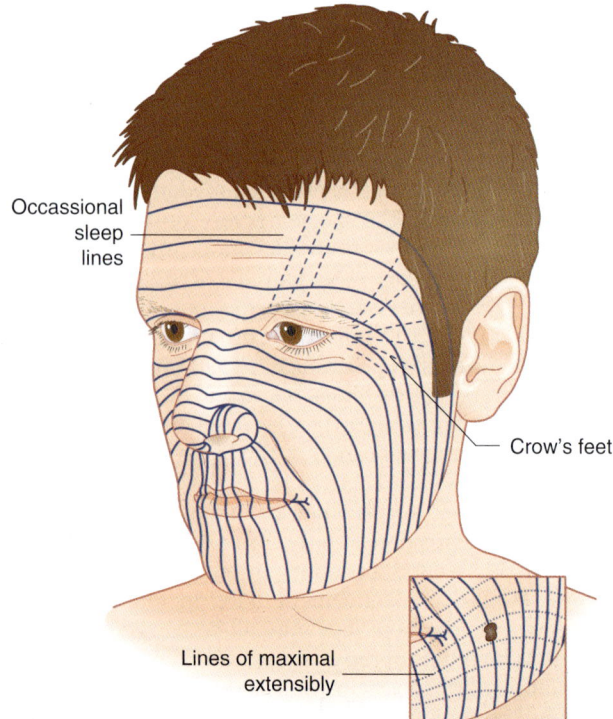

Fig. 11.2 Relaxed-skin tension lines (RSTL). The RSTL run horizontally in the central forehead and curve inferiorly as the temple is reached perpendicular to the underlying musculature.

Reconstructive Principles

SECONDARY INTENTION

Surgical defects on the concave aspect of the lateral temple generally heal significantly better than the convex central forehead when allowed to granulate.[6,7] Wound healing by secondary intention results in flat or slightly depressed, hypopigmented scars. The risk of hypertrophic scarring and brow or eyelid distortion is rare if the defect is not too large.[8] Additionally, healing by secondary intention may prolong wound care, and patients should be seen at regular intervals to ensure proper wound care is being performed.[9] Biologic dressings are an option for forehead closure to stimulate granulation tissue, especially if the defect has areas of exposed bone (Fig. 11.7). Currently the authors favor porcine xenograft sutured with 5-0 or 6-0 fast absorbing gut in these cases.

PRIMARY LINEAR CLOSURE

Horizontal and vertical primary linear closures are the mainstays for reconstruction of the forehead. Vertical closures are especially well suited to prevent elevation of the brow, and can be hidden in RSTLs created by the procerus and corrugator supercilii for centrally based forehead defects. In addition, vertical closure may prevent the numbness that can be temporarily produced with horizontal closures. Horizontal closures, on the other hand, are significantly masked in the RSTLs created by the frontalis muscle (Fig. 11.8). In general, forehead defects measuring up to 1.0 cm in diameter may be closed in a horizontal fashion with minimal risk of permanent change in brow position, depending upon several anatomical factors such as skin laxity, brow ptosis, eyelid redundancy, and the location of the defect. The higher the location of the defect on the forehead, the less likely brow distortion is to occur. The brow may elevate when the wound edges are approximated during reconstruction of even these smaller defects;

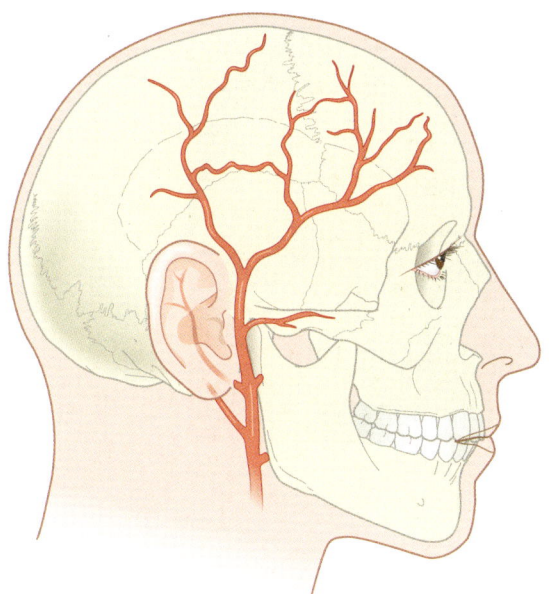

Fig. 11.5 Temporal artery. The temporal artery runs within and above the superficial musculoaponeurotic system (SMAS) layer of the lateral forehead. The branches of this artery can be localized by palpation. When possible these vessels should be dissected and ligated before severing, thereby decreasing the risk of postoperative hematoma.

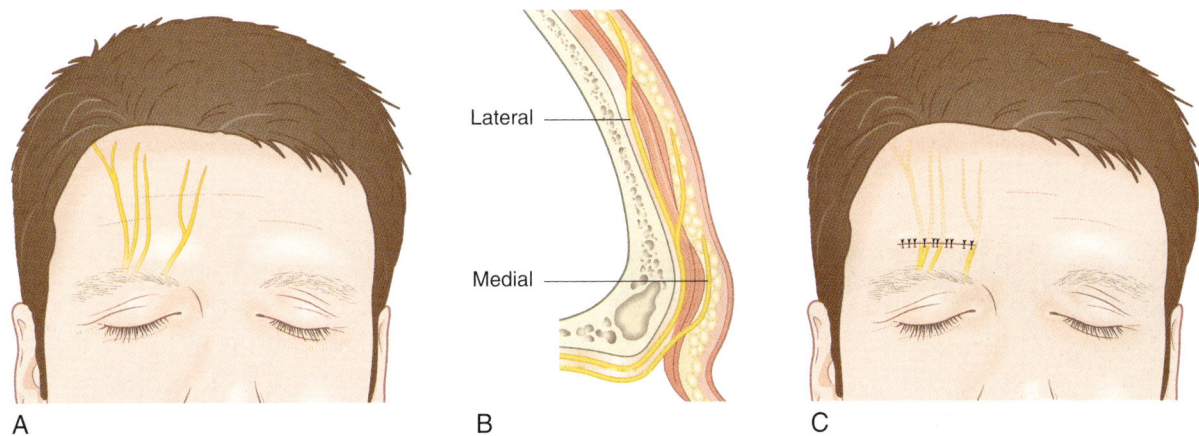

Fig. 11.6 (A) Medially positioned supratrochlear and laterally positioned supraorbital nerve; (B) sagittal view of supraorbital and supratrochlear nerves; (C) schematic demonstrating how sacrifice of supraorbital and supratrochlear nerves can result in a fan-shaped sensory deficit.

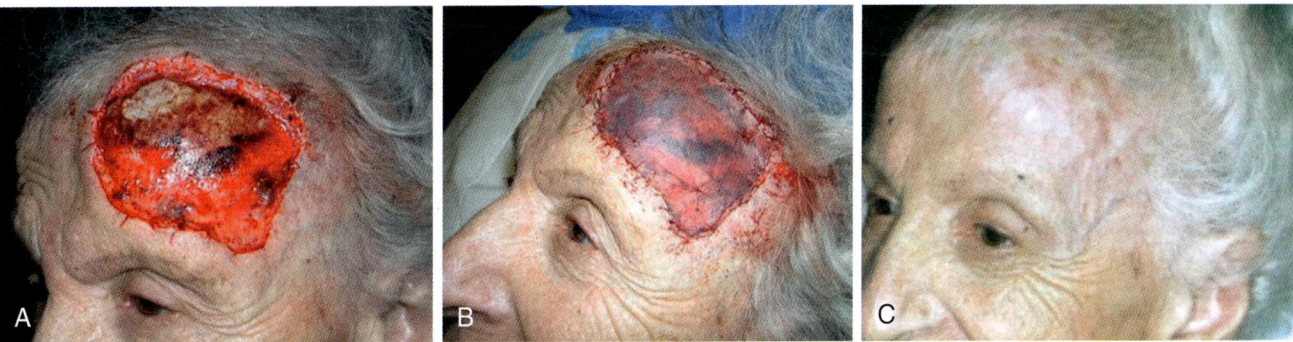

Fig. 11.7 Defect to bone repaired with human cadaveric allograft to facilitate granulation with improved contour. Today the authors favor the use of porcine xenograft. (A) Defect. (B) Repair. (C) Six-month follow-up.

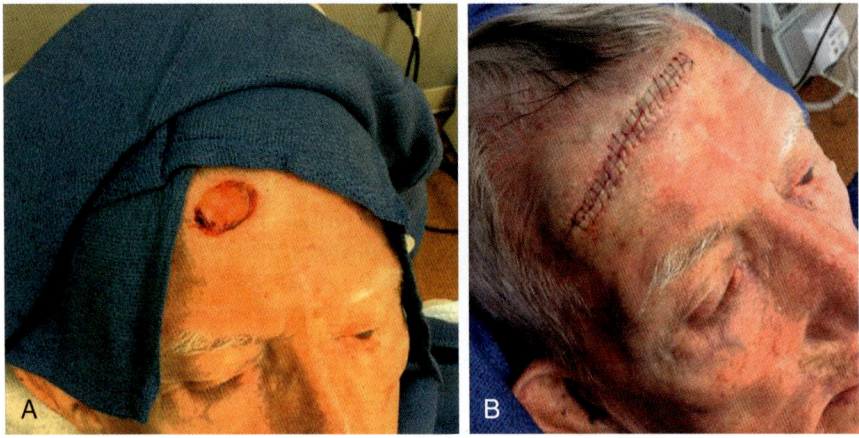

Fig. 11.8 Horizontal closure. One of the most commonly utilized closure for the forehead is the horizontally oriented linear closure. This is optimally used for defects that are situated higher on the forehead. (A) Defect. (B) Repair.

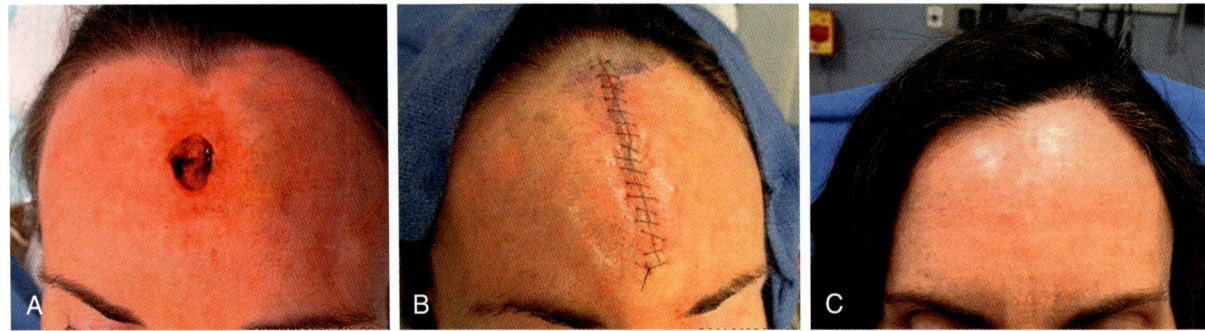

Fig. 11.9 Vertically oriented linear closure on the forehead can be an option for defects that cannot be closed horizontally within frontalis generated relaxed-skin tension lines (RSTLs) without causing free margin distortion. (A) Defect. (B) Closure. (C) Four-month follow-up.

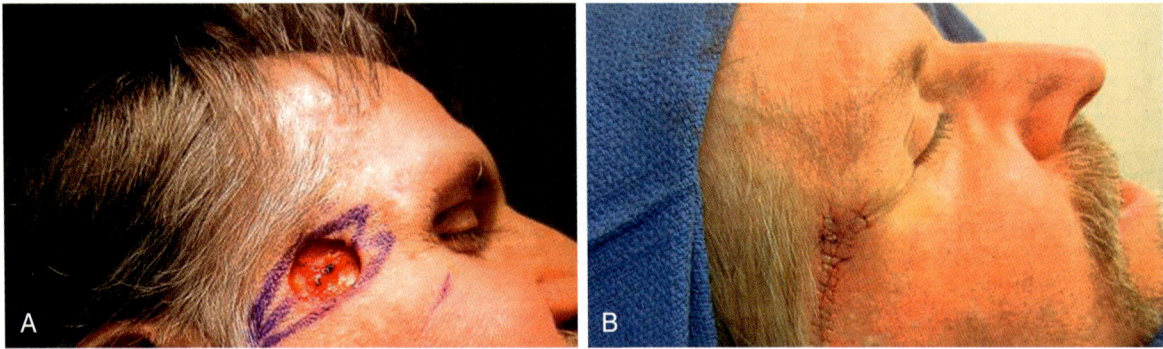

Fig. 11.10 M-plasty to facilitate placement of incision lines within crows' feet. (A) Defect. (B) Repair.

however, this elevation is usually temporary. Typically, the brow will return to its normal or near-normal position 1 to 2 months following surgery. When considering whether vertical or horizontal repair is optimal, consideration should be given to use of RSTLs, the closure of which will place minimal tension on the wound, and brow placement (Fig. 11.9). In the lateral region of the temple, radial orientation of the orbicularis oculi muscle should prompt consideration for closure in a radial direction (Fig. 11.10).[10] Finally, modification of the standard elliptical closure using an M-plasty is particularly useful in the temple to avoid the lateral canthus (Fig. 11.11; Box 11.1).[11]

ADVANCEMENT, ROTATION, AND TRANSPOSITION FLAPS

Various advancement, rotation, transposition, and combination flaps may be used to close moderate to larger defects on the forehead and temple.[9] Bilateral advancement flaps including H-flaps and A-to-T advancement flaps can be

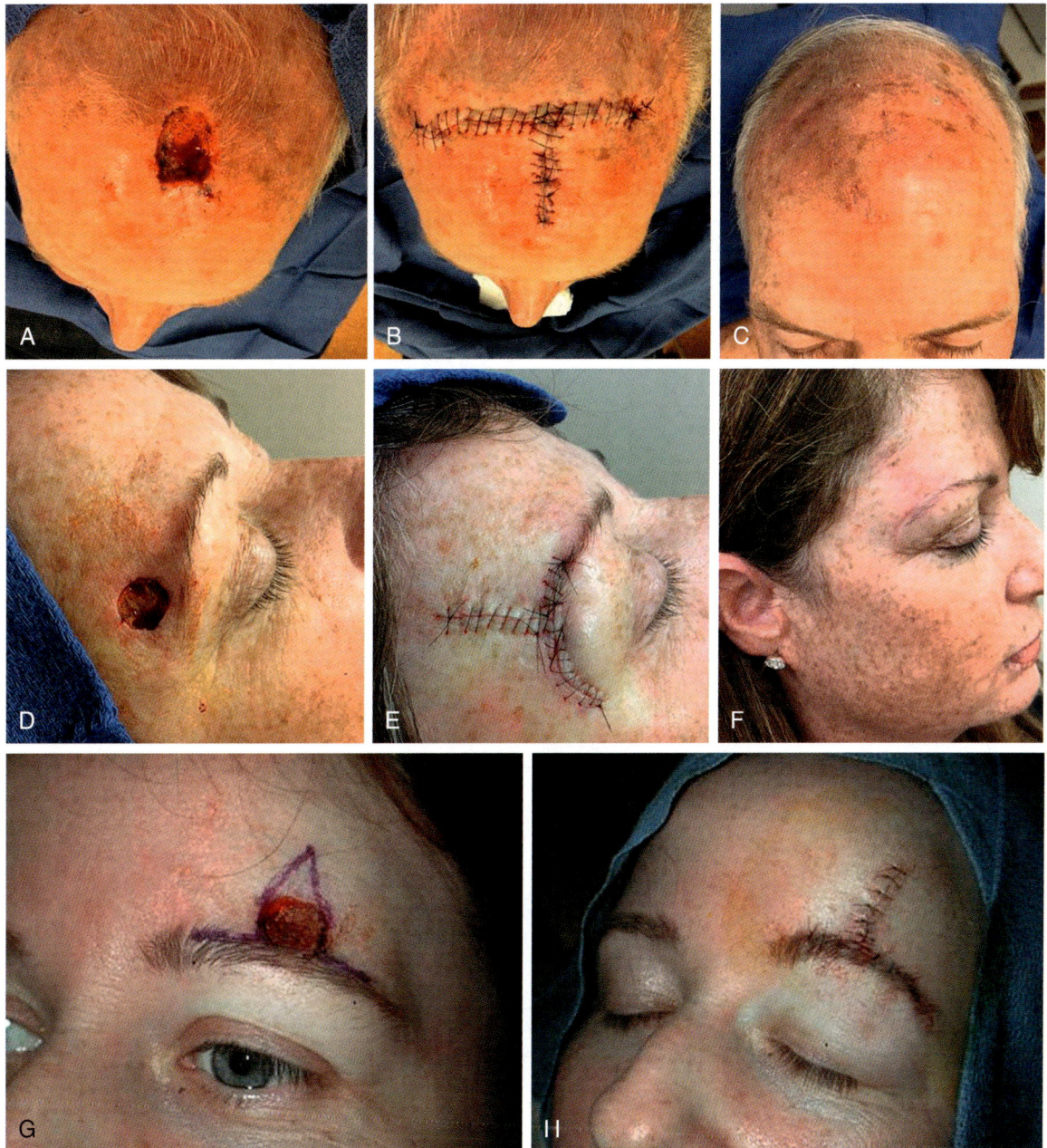

Fig. 11.11 A-to-T advancement flaps. (A) Defect on the border of forehead and scalp. (B) Repair. (C) Three-month follow-up. (D) Defect on the lower lateral forehead. (E) Repair. (F) Three-month follow-up. (G) Defect on the mid eyebrow border. (H) Repair.

good repair choices for moderate to large wounds on the central forehead. These repairs tap into laxity on both sides of the wound and can increase movement of tissue in a relatively immobile region of the forehead.[12]

The authors tend to favor A-to-T flaps higher on the forehead or lower on the forehead near the brow (see Fig. 11.11). They may incorporate an element of rotation that is key in restoration of contour (Fig. 11.12). A-to-T flaps may also be used to prevent brow distortion in medium-sized defects of the lower mid forehead (Fig. 11.13). Placement of the horizontal limb in RSTLs or along the anterior hairline improves cosmesis.[13] Burow triangles may also be incised back into the hairline. This shortens the length of the scar on the forehead, though extension into the hairline may also be used (Fig. 11.14; Box 11.2). The A-to-T repair may be reoriented in a radial fashion for closure of the temple.

In H-plasty bilateral advancement flaps, the superior and inferior limbs are designed to be roughly three to four times the width of the defect in total and to lie within RSTLs, with the vertical component centered on the midline of the defect (see Fig. 11.14).[14] Burow triangles are traditionally excised from the lateral aspects of the superior and inferior limbs. H-plasty may also be useful in order to preserve the eyebrow (Fig. 11.15). Unilateral advancement flaps, rather than H-plasty flaps, may also be used (Fig. 11.16). Laterally

Box 11.1 Vertical Versus Horizontal Closure

Vertical Closure

Advantages

Prevention of brow distortion
Avoids V-shaped area of numbness
Well hidden in RSTL of glabella and mid-forehead, if present

Disadvantages

Possibility of white vertical scar
Care must be taken to realign horizontal RSTL

Horizontal Closure

Advantages

Well hidden in RSTL that run across forehead

Disadvantages

Large defects or unfavorable anatomic features can elevate brow
V-shaped area of numbness above excision and extending onto scalp

Box 11.2 Primary Closure Versus A-to-T Closure

Primary Closure

Advantages

Decreased length of scar line
Scar line extends to scalp
Less undermining

Disadvantages

Inadequate for closure of large defects

A-to-T Closure

Advantages

Scar line extends up to scalp

Disadvantages

Increased length of scar line
If hairline recedes, possibility of complete scar line revealed

RSTL, Relaxed-skin tension line.

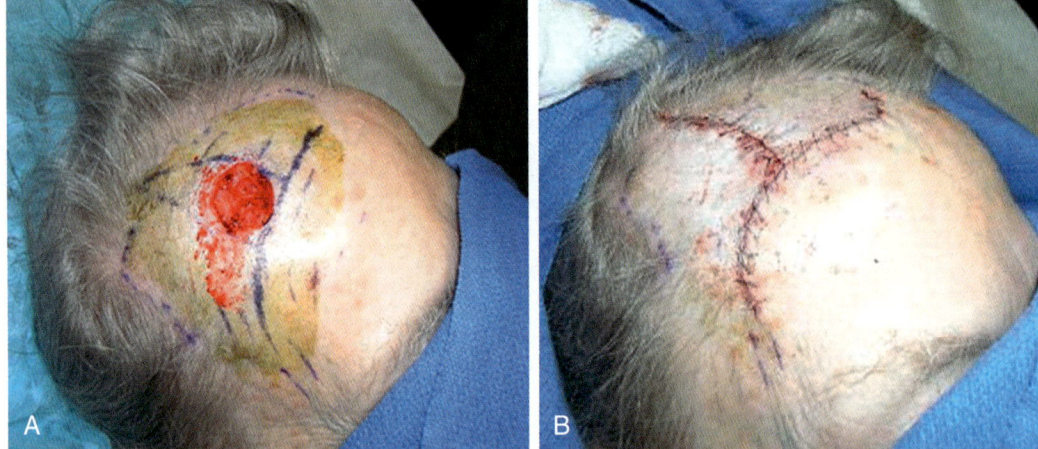

Fig. 11.12 Bilateral advancement flap incorporating element of rotation to restore contour. (A) Defect (B) Repair.

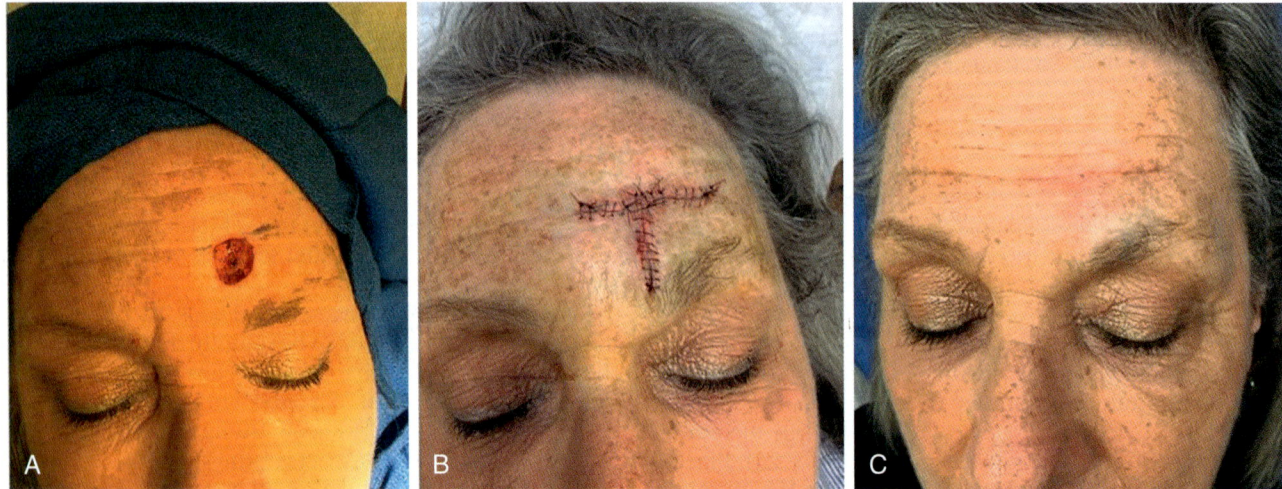

Fig. 11.13 Bilateral advancement flap taking advantage of horizontal and vertical relaxed-skin tension lines (RSTLs) for medium-sized defect of mid low forehead. (A) Defect. (B) Repair. (C) Six-week follow-up.

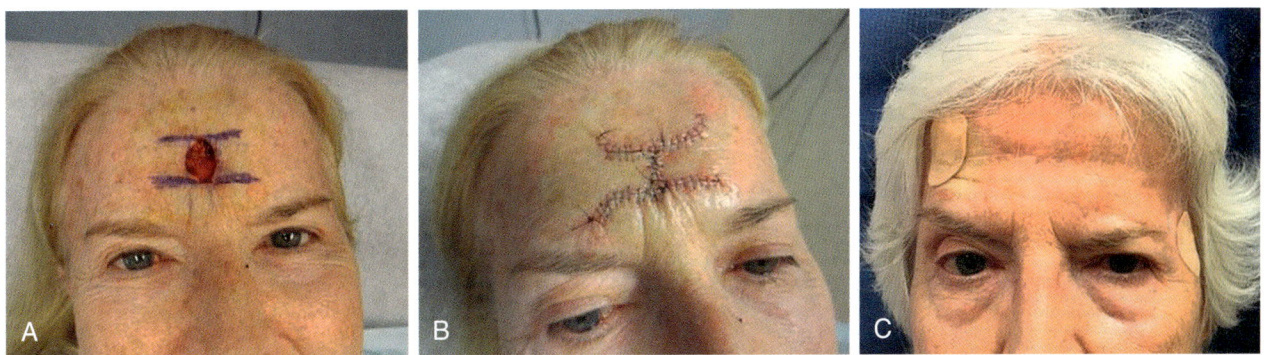

Fig. 11.14 H-plasty bilateral advancement. (A) Defect. (B) Repair. (C) One-year follow-up.

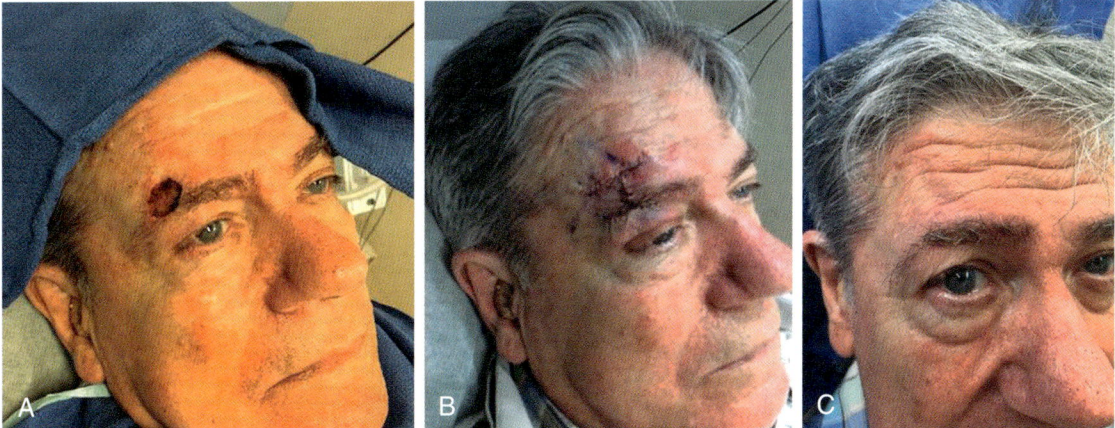

Fig. 11.15 Bilateral H-plasty advancement is useful near the eyebrow. (A) Defect. (B) Repair. (C) Four-month follow-up.

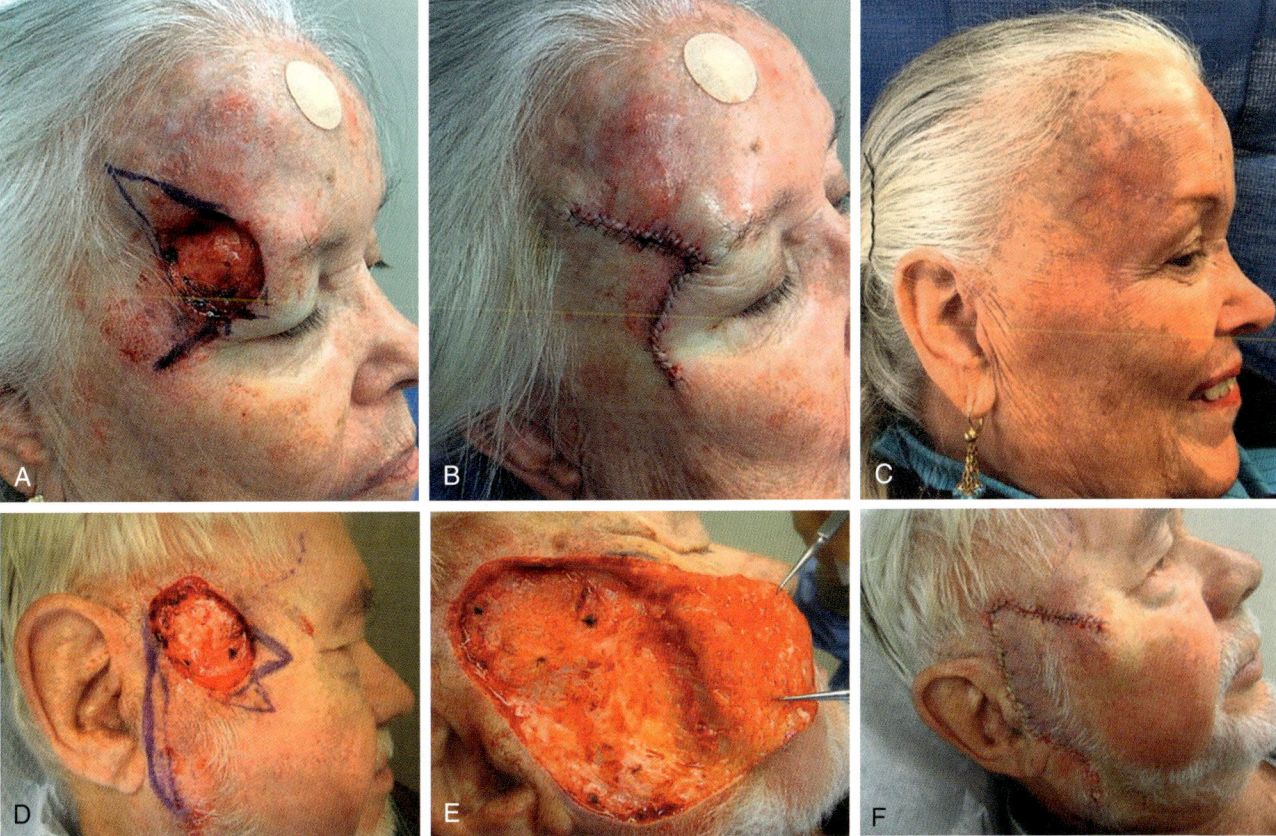

Fig. 11.16 Unilateral advancement is a less frequently used option. Erythema present after postoperative radiation for large-caliber nerve invasion by squamous cell carcinoma (SCC). (A) Defect. (B) Repair. (C) Three-month follow-up. (D) Temple defect with temporal artery visible. (E) Undermining planes. (F) Repair.

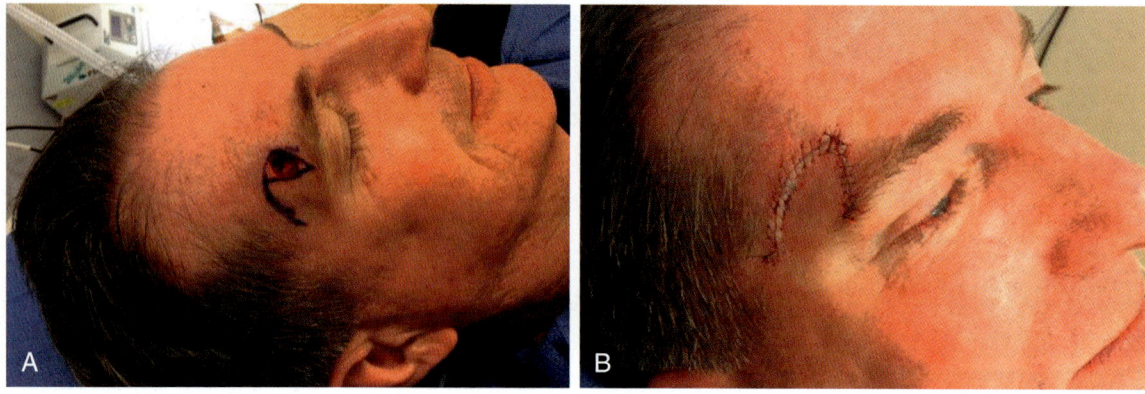

Fig. 11.17 Laterally based rotation flaps may be useful in avoiding brow elevation. (A) Defect. (B) Repair.

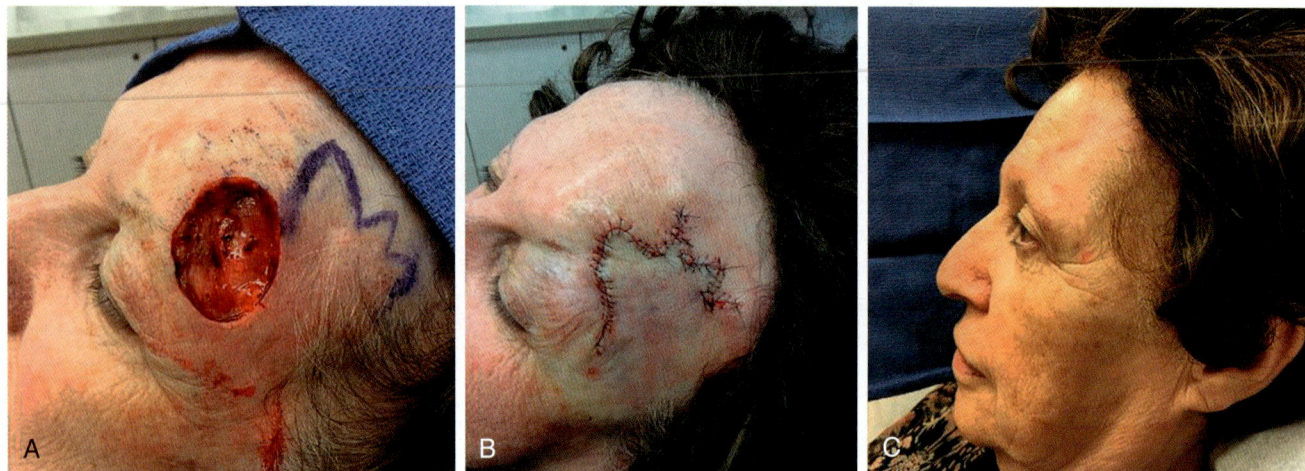

Fig. 11.18 Trilobed flap for closure of deep temple defect. (A) Defect. (B) Repair. (C) Six-month follow-up.

based rotation flaps may be useful in avoiding brow elevation (Fig. 11.17). This flap is generally performed above the frontalis muscle for smaller defects and below the deep fascia in a relatively bloodless plane for larger defects, in what has been termed the contralateral subgaleal sliding or CLASS flap.[15]

In the temple region, while rarely used, the bilobed and trilobed flaps may also be utilized. The blood supply of this flap is anteriorly based, allowing for lateral and radial rotation of tissue to cover defects of this area (Fig. 11.18).[16] Birhombic transposition flaps have also been described as useful in the lateral forehead or temple region.[17] Bilateral advancement flaps, including classic Burow wedge advancement, may also be used in the lateral forehead and temple.[18] The main axis is often on an arc, and may be buried within the hair-bearing eyebrow, or in a radial fashion mirroring the radial array of orbicularis oculi. For large defects of the temple and lateral forehead, transposition flaps may be used (Fig. 11.19). The addition of Z-plasty facilitates movement of the leading edge of the flap while placing lengthy incisions within RSTLs.

Flap-graft combinations can be used in select cases. The Burow triangles created in flap (Fig. 11.20) movement are an excellent color and texture match and can be used to minimize the size of the flap and cover areas that will otherwise not close on the generally inelastic forehead.

Complications

Complications that are not unique to the forehead and temple include infection, bleeding, flap failure, and scarring. Various studies have cited either infection or bleeding as the most common complication of office-based Mohs micrographic surgery.[19,20] Given the vasculature supply of the forehead, repairs under the deep fascia and frontalis muscle may predispose to hematoma formation if care of larger vessels is not considered in this plane. Additionally, the superficial temporal artery should be considered in lateral forehead repairs, as it is in the subcutaneous tissue. This vessel may be palpated and traced with a surgical marking pen prior to repair to avoid transection. When transected, bleeding is controlled by the following process: (1) the assistant applies pressure around both ends of the cut artery to allow better visualization of the cut vessel; (2) the surgeon clamps the transected artery; and (3) the vessel is ligated using a 4-0 absorbable polyglactin suture placed in a figure-of-8 fashion. Damage to the temporal branch of

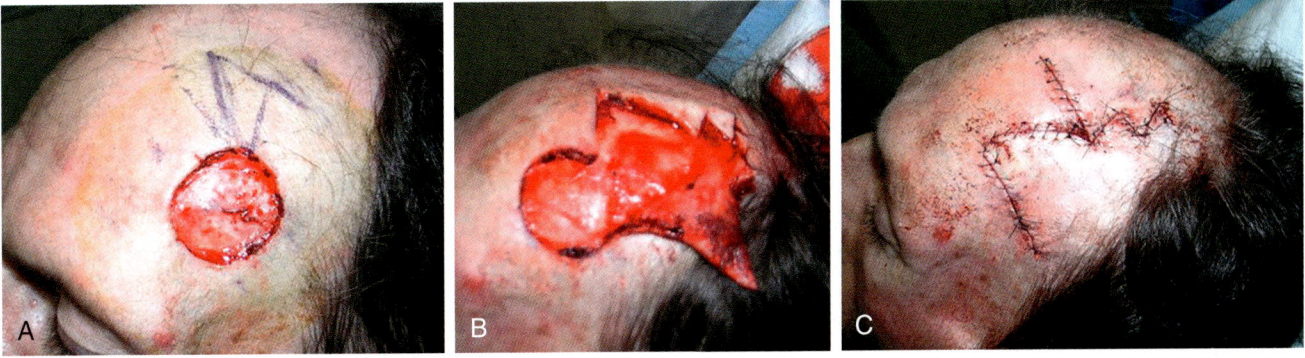

Fig. 11.19 Transposition flap closure for forehead defect. Addition of Z-plasty facilitates movement of the leading edge of the flap while placing lengthy incisions within relaxed-skin tension lines (RSTLs). (A) Defect. (B) Intraoperative view demonstrating flap depth. (C) Repair.

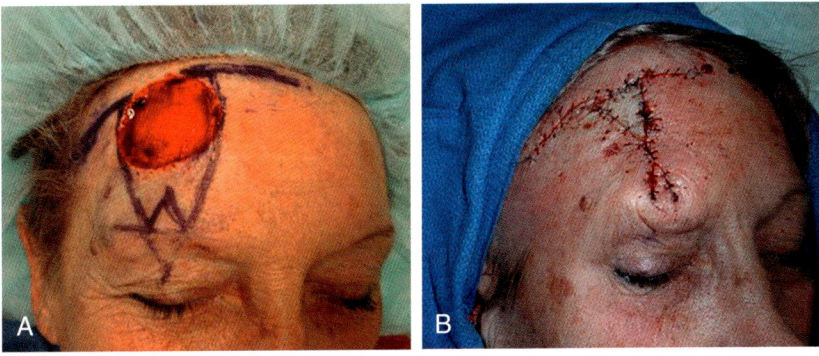

Fig. 11.20 (A) Defect. (B) Advancement flap with inferiorly placed W-plasty.

Box 11.3   Complications and How to Avoid Them

Temporal Nerve Damage

Be aware of danger zones and undermine in the superficial subcutaneous plane.
Use closures needing the least amount of undermining.

Hematoma

Palpate the superficial temporal artery and trace its path with a surgical marker.
Avoid the vessels when possible. Dissect and then ligate vessels before severing them.

Nerve Injury

Expect sensory loss superior to incisions and inform patient of this preoperatively.
Be patient if motor deficits are present. Wait approximately 12 months before embarking on corrective procedures.

---

the facial nerve may result in brow ptosis, and care in this "danger zone" should be maintained (Box 11.3). If brow ptosis occurs, a unilateral brow lift may improve symmetry but does not return expression to this region. Branches of the supratrochlear and supraorbital nerves, which course superficially in the subcutaneous tissue, can result in numbness if transected. New sensation is established over 3 to 24 months, with most patients experiencing some dysesthesia as the nerves regenerate.[21] Patients should be warned of this predictable complication prior to any surgery in this area.

Conclusion

The forehead, including the subunit of the temple, poses unique challenges to repair. The best option of wound closure is one that is under minimum tension, maintains symmetry and does not distort free margins, and hides incision lines in RSTLs or along the cosmetic unit junctions (hairline and eyebrow). Maintenance of the anterior hairline and brow position is essential in this region.

References

1. Larrabee W Jr, Sherris D. Forehead. In: *Principles of Facial Reconstruction*. Philadelphia, PA: Lippincott-Raven; 1995:18-33.
2. Flowers F, Breza T Jr. Surgical anatomy of the head and neck. In: Bolognia J, Jorizzo J, Schaffer J, eds. *Dermatology*. 3rd ed. New York: Elsevier; 2012.
3. Agarwal CA, Mendenhall SD, Foreman KB, Owsley JQ. The course of the frontal branch of the facial nerve in relation to fascial planes: an anatomic study. *Plast Reconstr Surg*. 2010;125(2):532-537.
4. Goldman G, Dzubow L, Yelverton C. Forehead. In: Goldman G, Dzubow L, eds. *Facial Flap Surgery*. China: McGraw-Hill Companies, Inc.; 2013: 263-281.
5. Fatah MF. Innervation and functional reconstruction of the forehead. *Br J Plast Surg*. 1991;44(5):351-358.

6. Goldwyn RM, Rueckert F. The value of healing by secondary intention for sizeable defects of the face. *Arch Surg.* 1977;112(3):285-292.
7. Mott KJ, Clark DP, Stelljes LS. Regional variation in wound contraction of Mohs surgery defects allowed to heal by second intention. *Dermatol Surg.* 2003;29(7):712-722.
8. Zitelli JA. Wound healing by secondary intention. *J Am Acad Dermatol.* 1983;9(3):407-415.
9. Grigg R. Forehead and temple reconstruction. *Otolaryngol Clin North Am.* 2001;34(3):583-600.
10. Goldman G, Dzubow L, Yelverton C. Temple. In: Goldman G, Dzubow L, eds. *Facial Flap Surgery*. China: McGraw-Hill Companies, Inc.; 2013: 282-291.
11. Webster RC, Davidson TM, Smith RC, et al. M-plasty techniques. *J Dermatol Surg.* 1976;2(5):393-396.
12. Harahap M. The modified bilateral advancement flap. *Dermatol Surg.* 2001;27(5):463-466.
13. Field LM. The forehead V-to-T plasty (Dieffenbach's winged V-plasty). *J Dermatol Surg Oncol.* 1986;12(6):560-562.
14. Rose V, Overstall S, Moloney DM, Powell BW. The H-flap: a useful flap for forehead reconstruction. *Br J Plast Surg.* 2001;54(8):705-707.
15. Hussain W. The contralateral subgaleal sliding flap for the single-stage reconstruction of large defects of the temple and lateral forehead. *Br J Dermatol.* 2014;170(4):952-955.
16. Sutton AE, Quatela VC. Bilobed flap reconstruction of the temporal forehead. *Arch Otolaryngol Head Neck Surg.* 1992;118(9):978-982 [discussion 983].
17. Johnson TM, Wang TS, Fader DJ. The birhombic transposition flap for soft tissue reconstruction. *J Am Acad Dermatol.* 1999;41(2 Pt 1): 232-236.
18. Seline P, Siegle R. Forehead reconstruction. In: Brown M, ed. *Advanced Surgical Reconstruction Techniques*. Philadelphia: Saunders; 2005:1-11.
19. Cook JL, Perone JB. A prospective evaluation of the incidence of complications associated with Mohs micrographic surgery. *Arch Dermatol.* 2003;139(2):143-152.
20. Alam M, Ibrahim O, Nodzenski M, et al. Adverse events associated with Mohs micrographic surgery: multicenter prospective cohort study of 20,821 cases at 23 centers. *JAMA Dermatol.* 2013;149(12): 1378-1385.
21. Lutz ME, Otley CC, Roenigk RK, Brodland DG, Li H. Reinnervation of flaps and grafts of the face. *Arch Dermatol.* 1998;134(10):1271-1274.

12 Periocular Reconstruction

ANDREA WILLEY, MD

Introduction

Mastering the fundamental techniques of periocular surgery is essential for the Mohs and reconstructive surgeon. The eye holds immeasurable value, visual and aesthetic, that demand understanding and expertise to ensure successful surgical outcomes. The mobile nature of the eyelids and their bipolar suspension creates tensional forces that must be appreciated and actively managed during surgical repairs. Numerous surgical techniques have been described throughout the decades. In this chapter, fundamental principles and select reconstructive techniques that reliably produce optimal results and minimize complications are presented.

Preoperative Assessment

For most patients, a preoperative examination assessing visual acuity, intraocular pressure, and tear film/dryness is generally recommended within a year before surgery. Consultation with an oculoplastic surgeon is prudent for patients with preexisting eye disease and defects close to involving the lid margin. Imaging with computed tomography or magnetic resonance imaging may be indicated for tumors in the medial canthus and complex tumors that may extend into the orbit. Management or cessation of blood-thinning medications is indicated for tumor extirpations or repairs that extend into the orbital septum to minimize risks of retrobulbar hemorrhage. Meticulous intraoperative control of bleeding and postoperative observation and counseling are essential. Assessment and control of blood pressure in hypertensive patients is also important to minimize risks of bleeding. In addition, anxiolytic medications with adequate monitoring can be useful during periocular surgery.

Specialized Instrumentation

Although many periocular repairs can be performed with standard facial repair trays, specialized instrumentation can be useful, particularly for defects involving the lid margins.

Specialized instrumentation for periocular surgical trays:

Corneal shields protect the globe and shield the light
Bishop-Harmon forceps for handling delicate tissue
Spring scissors for accurate cutting of fine tissues
Tenotomy scissors for cutting tarsus
Castroviejo needle drivers for grasping and placing fine sutures
Fine tissue hooks
Beaver blade and blade holders
Bipolar unit for hemostasis in a wet field
5-0 and 6-0 polyglactin sutures spatulated needles
6-0 polypropylene sutures
Proparacaine ophthalmic drops
Erythromycin ophthalmic ointment
Nonstick eye pads

Anatomy

The unique anatomy of the eyelids and supporting structures present unique challenges to the periocular surgeon. The eyelids are conceptually divided into anterior and posterior lamella for purposes of reconstruction.[1] The posterior lamella, composed of mucosa and tarsus, also houses numerous glands vital for producing the tear film, which is essential for clear vision. The anterior lamella is composed of the orbicularis oculi muscle and skin, with minimal retinaculum in between. The orbicularis oculi is contiguous with the lateral canthal tendon, a fibrous tissue that tethers the tarsal plates to the bony orbit. The lateral canthal tendon attaches to the inside of the orbital rim at Whitnall tubercle, a bony prominence where additional suspensory ligaments, essential for opening and closing the lids, also converge. Whitnall tubercle can be palpated manually and is an important point of fixation for suspension and fixation of the of the lateral canthal tendon fundamental to many periocular repairs (Fig. 12.1). The medial canthal tendon bifurcates into anterior and posterior limbs, which diverge around the lacrimal sac to facilitate the lacrimal pump before attaching to the anterior and posterior aspects of the bony lacrimal crest. Familiarity with the complex anatomy of the medial canthal region is essential to preserve lacrimal drainage.

The vascular supply of the periorbital region is ample and facilitates a low infection rate and rapid healing of repairs in this area. The internal and external carotid arteries and veins provide vascular supply to the eyelids and surrounding tissue via numerous branches, including the dorsal nasal artery medially and the temporal and transverse facial arteries laterally that anastomose to form the marginal arcades of the eyelids. The sensory nerves of the eye emanate from ophthalmic and maxillary branches of the trigeminal nerve. Motor innervation required for both

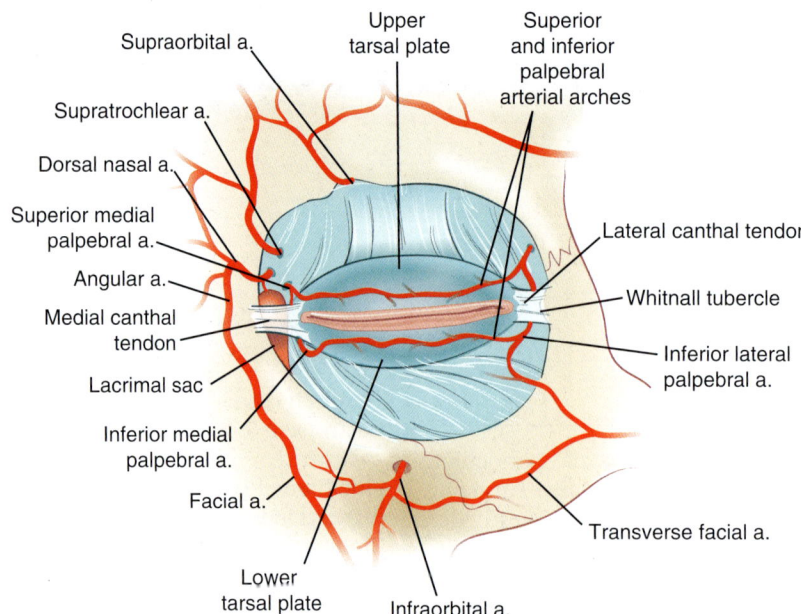

Fig. 12.1 Anatomy of the eye.

movement and constitutive tone of the periocular muscles is supplied by branches of the facial, oculomotor, and sympathetic nerves.

Tension

Preoperative, intraoperative, and postoperative assessments of the tensional forces around the eye are essential to prevent complications that may impact vision and cosmetic outcomes. Indeed, even the smallest tensional forces on the lid margin, created primarily or secondary to adjacent wound contraction, can lead to ectropion and webbing. The limits of tension can be assessed preoperatively by performing a "snap test," in which the lid is pulled away from the globe and watching the rate of return, which correlates with the degree of laxity. Assessing maximal tension intraoperatively is also prudent, so that adjustments can be made and suspension sutures used to ensure tensional limitations are not exceeded. Forceps can be used to approximate wound edges prior to closure and tension assessed again after key sutures are placed. Maximal tension can be assessed by asking the patient to look up while opening the mouth widely (see Fig. 12.3). If the lid pulls away from the globe, then adjustments can be made before the surgery is completed. Additional support can be achieved intraoperatively by placing deep sutures in the cutaneous retinaculum and fascia to reinforce horizontal support and minimize downward pull on the eyelid. However, most importantly, the power of suspension sutures placed in the fascia, periosteum, and canthal support tissues to minimize tension around the eye cannot be overstated.[2] Examples of periocular suspension sutures will be highlighted throughout this chapter.

Periocular Repairs

There are many ways to approach the repair of defects located around the eye. Keeping incisions perpendicular to the lid margin and designing flaps that push tissue towards the lid margin and limit downward pull is the cornerstone of avoiding ectropion in periocular surgery (Figs. 12.2 and 12.3). It is also important to oversize flaps and grafts adequately to accommodate for convexities, eye movement, and facial expression. The choice of closure often depends on a number of factors, including the size, depth, location of the defect and tissue reservoirs, skin laxity, and stability of the canthal tissues. Despite these variables, fundamental principles and techniques of reconstruction in the periocular area can be followed to optimize outcomes and avoid complications of webbing and ectropion (see Fig. 12.3).

Linear Repairs

Repairing wounds in a linear fashion around the eye often requires a balance of obscuring incisions in relaxed skin tension lines (RSTLs) and directing tension parallel to the lid margin. Below the lid, vertical incisions can be designed increasingly oblique to the lid margin from medial to the lateral where incisions become more horizontal (see Fig. 12.2), excepting the medial canthus, where horizontal incisions are strictly avoided to prevent webbing. M-plasty repairs can also help to manage redundant cones near the lid margin when needed. Below the eye, removing less of the redundant tissue at the apex of the ellipse can also help to protect against ectropion. Small defects located on the upper lid crease can often be repaired with a crescent-shaped incision along the natural crease similar to a

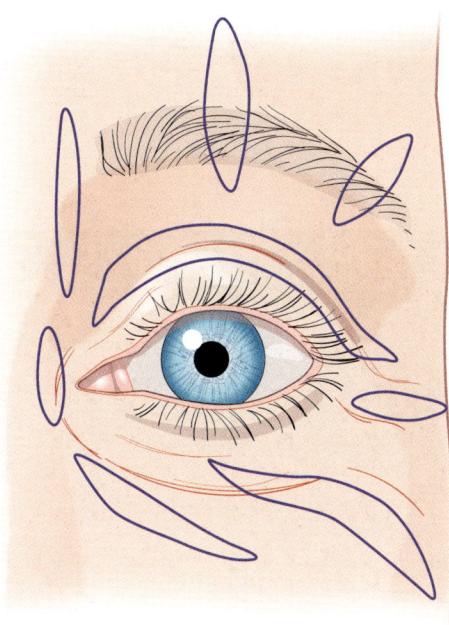

Fig. 12.2 Linear repairs: incision lines are perpendicular to the lid margin superior and laterally, except the lid crease and medial canthus where incisions are horizontal. Below the lid margin incisions are placed obliquely in relaxed skin tension lines (RSTLs) to balance tension and obscure scars.

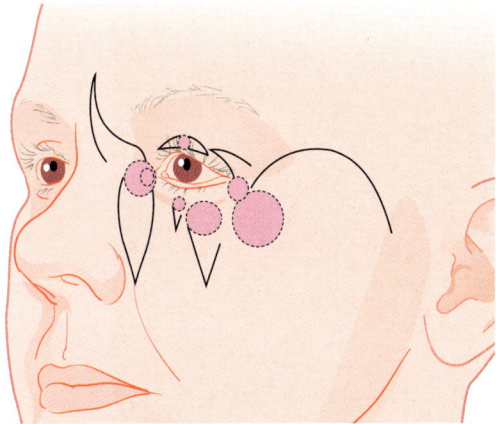

Fig. 12.3 Flap repairs: structured repairs that reliably avoid complications include (1) rhomboid transposition flaps below the lid margin, (2) Trippier flaps for small lateral defects, (3) rotation flaps for medium lateral defects, (4) blepharoplasty advancement flaps on the upper lid, (5) hatchet and island pedicle flaps in medial canthus, (6) lid advancement flaps inside the orbital rim, and (7) cheek rotation and advancement flaps for larger defects below the lid and in the medial canthus.

traditional blepharoplasty (keeping incisions medial to the caruncle to avoid webbing and extending beyond the lateral canthus when hooding is present).

Skin Grafts

Full-thickness skin grafts can be useful when primary closures are not possible but must be well designed and supported in the perioperative period. In general, skin grafts must be oversized by 30% to allow for wound contracture and avoid ectropion. More precise sizing can be achieved by putting the eyelid on stretch and using a sterile nonstick gauze pad as a blotter to create a graft template. The ideal donor site is the ipsilateral or contralateral upper lid and can be harvested with a typical blepharoplasty incision. Larger grafts can be harvested from the preauricular, supraclavicular, and inner arm area. Grafts can be thinned, fenestrated, and tacked to the base to optimize inosculation. Canthopexy sutures can be useful to prevent ectropion. Frost sutures can be helpful to support the low lid immediately postoperatively.[9] Dental wax or petroleum gauze bolsters can be useful to provide gentle pressure. Split thickness skin grafts are generally not recommended due to skin contraction.

Flap Repairs

DEFECTS BELOW THE LID MARGIN

Rhomboid transposition flaps that "push" tissue towards the lid margin are a staple for repairing small and medium defects located below the eyelid (Fig. 12.4). Rhomboid flaps must be adequately sized to accommodate for upgaze, maximal tension, and wound contraction to reliably avoid complications of ectropion. Tension-free incisions heal well and are often obscured, despite crossing cosmetic unit boundaries and rhytids, owing to ample vascular supply and rapid healing. Transposition flaps based on skin within the orbit are useful for central defects that are very close to the lid margin, where they soundly direct tension superiorly (Fig. 12.5). More lateral defects can be repaired with transposition flaps based on the redundant skin of the upper lid crease (Fig. 12.6).[3] Canthal suspension sutures can be used to provide additional support when indicated. Laterally based rotation flaps can be useful for defects exceeding the limits of the upper lid reservoir (Fig. 12.7).

Rotation/advancement flaps that use the ample cheek skin are reliable for larger defects below the lid margin (Fig. 12.8).[4] Ideally, cheek rotation flaps are designed with incisions along the subcilliary skin, extending at or above and lateral to the lateral canthus so that vertical tension originates lateral to the lid margin. Incision lines can be partially obscured in RSTLs. Inferiorly based cheek advancement flaps with ample mobility from malar fat pads are also useful for repairing medial defects below the lid (Fig. 12.9).

DEFECTS ON THE UPPER LID

Defects on the upper lid can often be efficiently repaired with flaps and grafts based on the adjacent or contralateral lid, which provide like tissue and robust vascularity for rapid wound healing. "Blepharoplasty advancement flaps" are ideal for superficial defects on the upper lid where the incision lines are made along the natural lid crease. Just as in a simple blepharoplasty, incisions are kept medial to the caruncle and may extend beyond the lateral canthus when hooding is present (Fig. 12.10). Blepharoplasty grafts can be designed similarly from the contralateral lid. Full-thickness

Text continued on p. 175

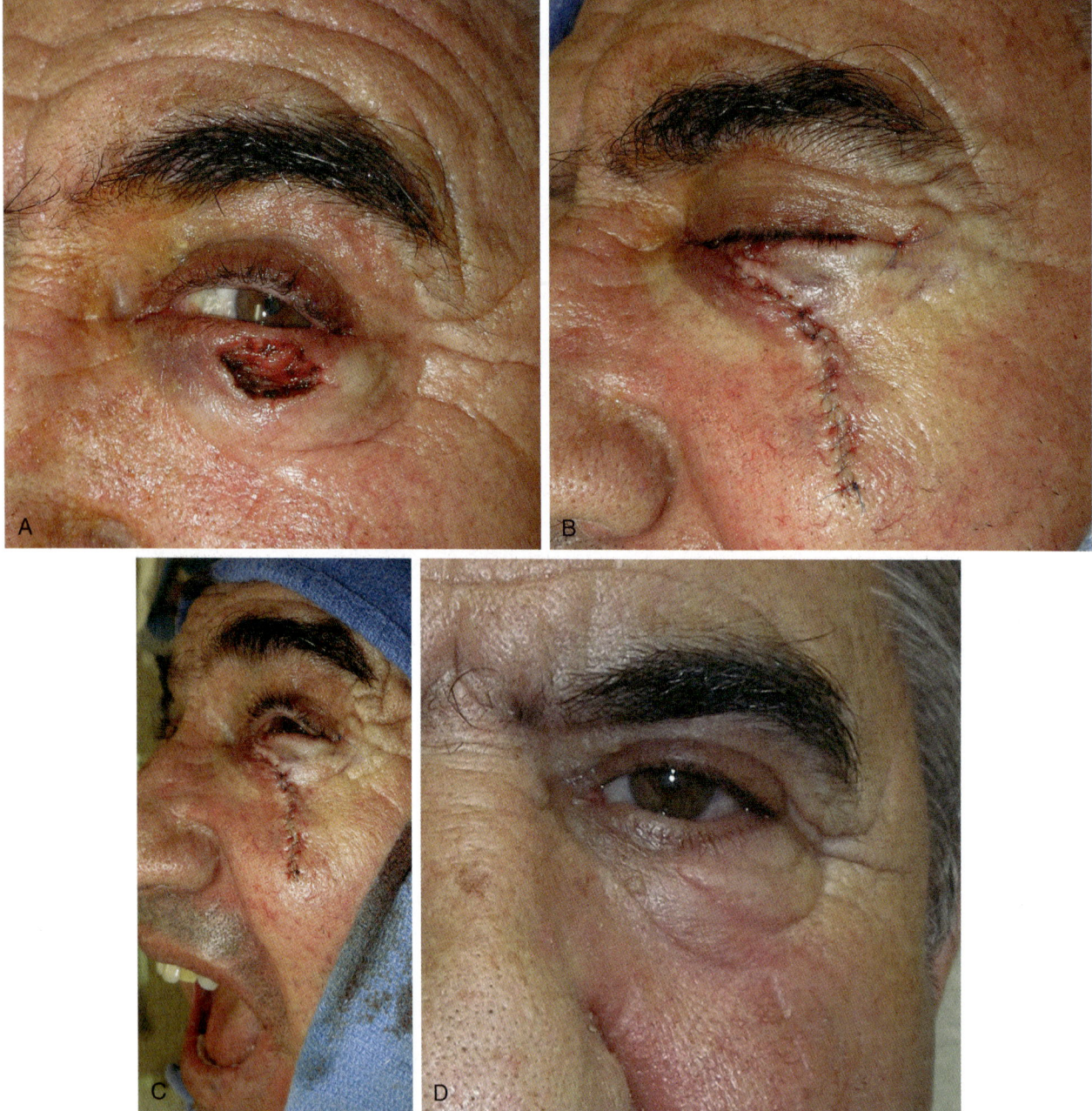

Fig. 12.4 Rhombic transposition flap. (A) Medium-size defect below the lid margin. (B) Flap oversized to minimize vertical tension and prevent ectropion. (C) Lid snug against the globe with maximum tension postoperatively. (D) Tension-free flap 3 months postoperatively.

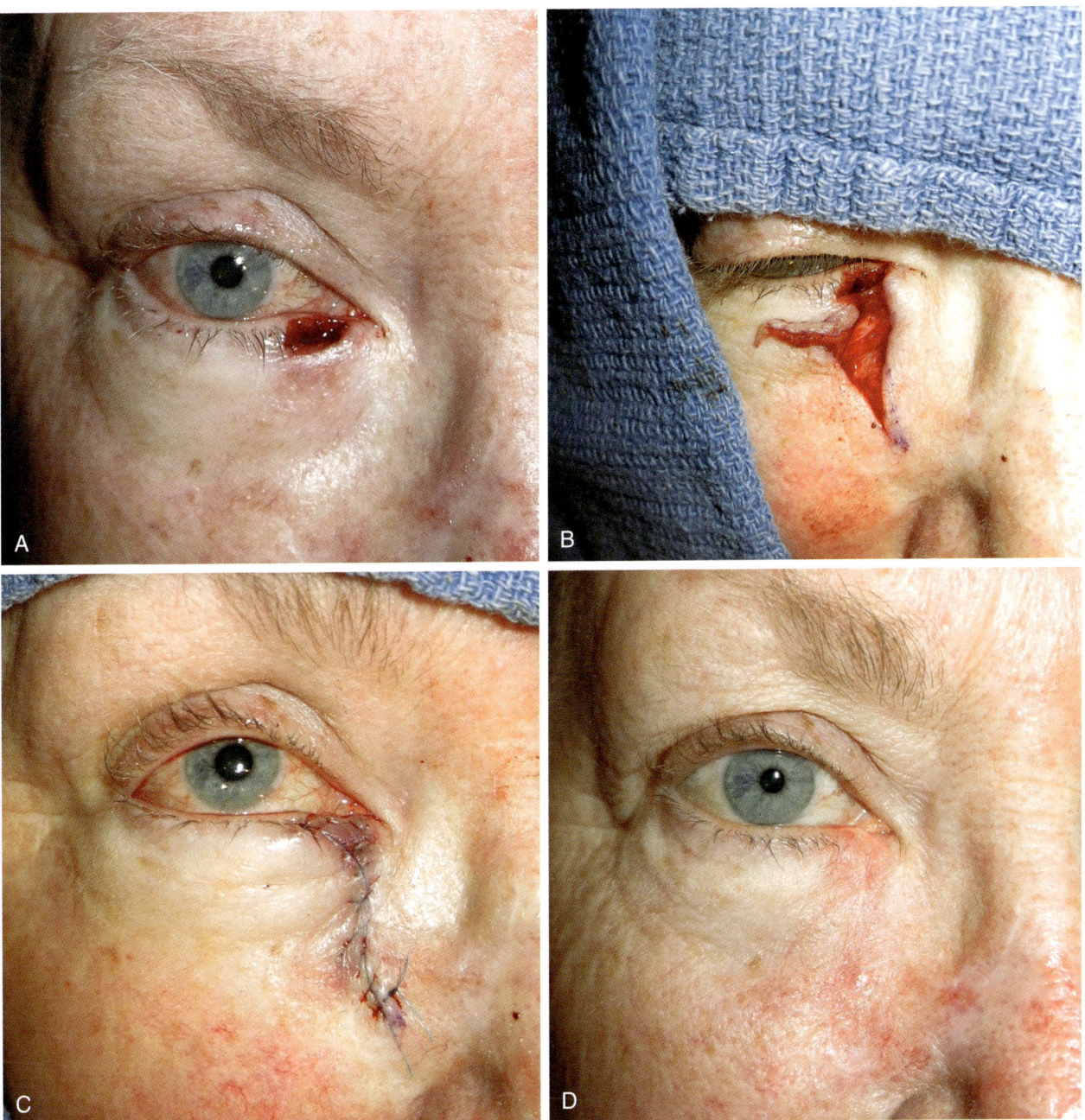

Fig. 12.5 Rhombic transposition flap. (A) Small defect close to the lid margin. (B) Flap undermined. (C) Lid snug against the globe with flap in place intraoperatively. (D) Tension-free flap 3 months postoperatively.

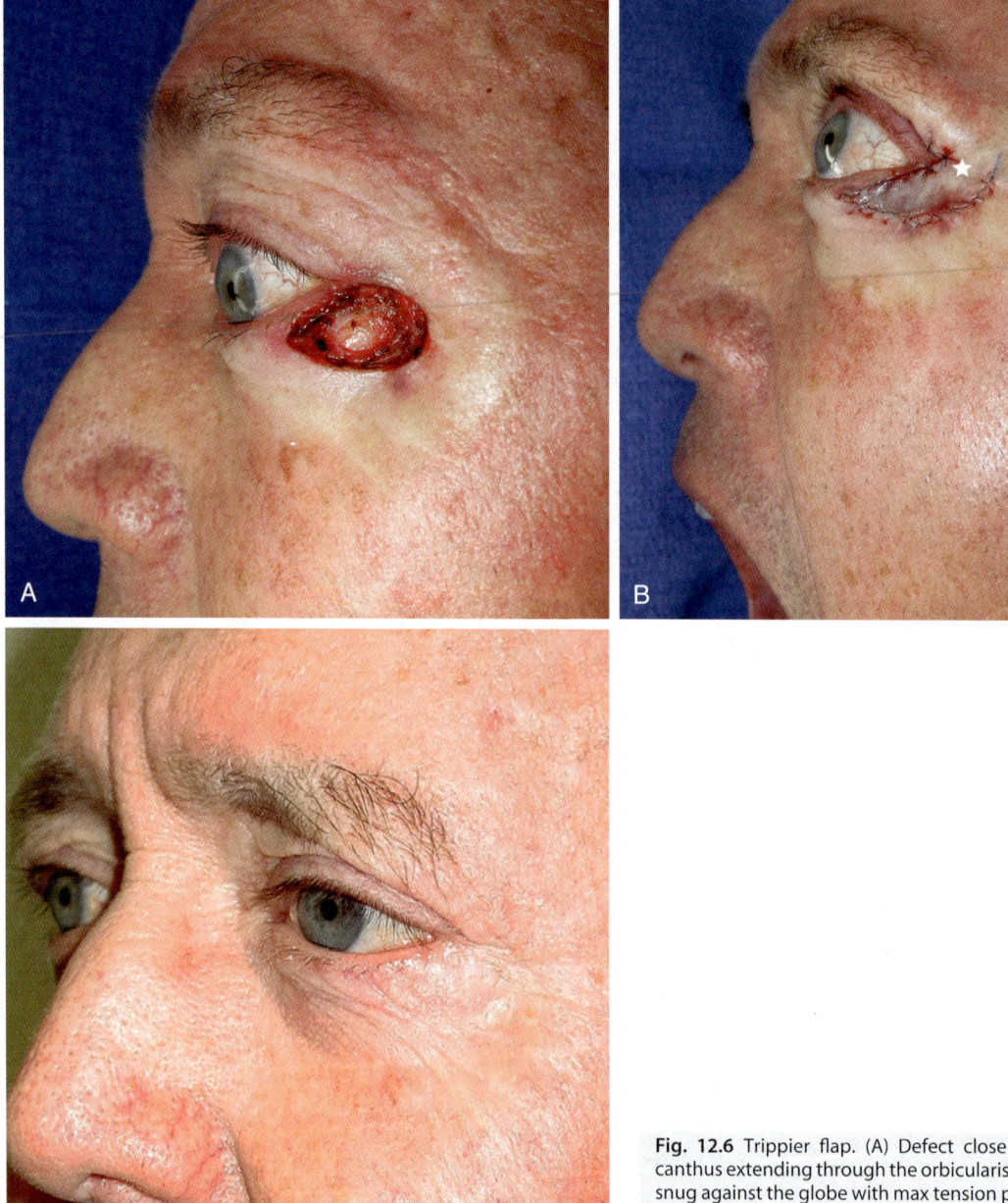

Fig. 12.6 Trippier flap. (A) Defect close to the lateral canthus extending through the orbicularis. (B) Lid margin snug against the globe with max tension postoperatively (*star* indicates periosteal suspension suture). (C) Tension-free flap 6 months postoperatively.

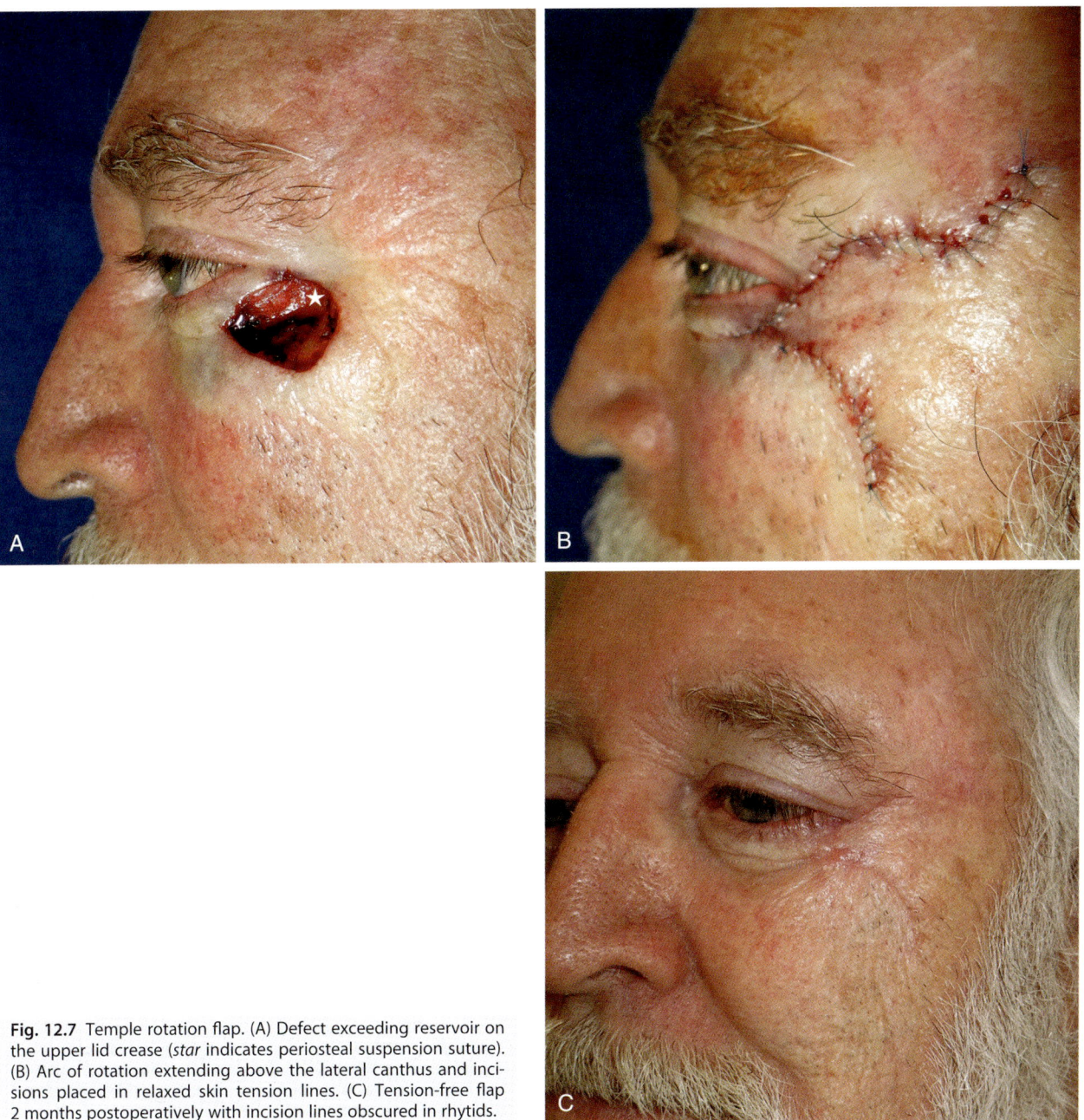

Fig. 12.7 Temple rotation flap. (A) Defect exceeding reservoir on the upper lid crease (*star* indicates periosteal suspension suture). (B) Arc of rotation extending above the lateral canthus and incisions placed in relaxed skin tension lines. (C) Tension-free flap 2 months postoperatively with incision lines obscured in rhytids.

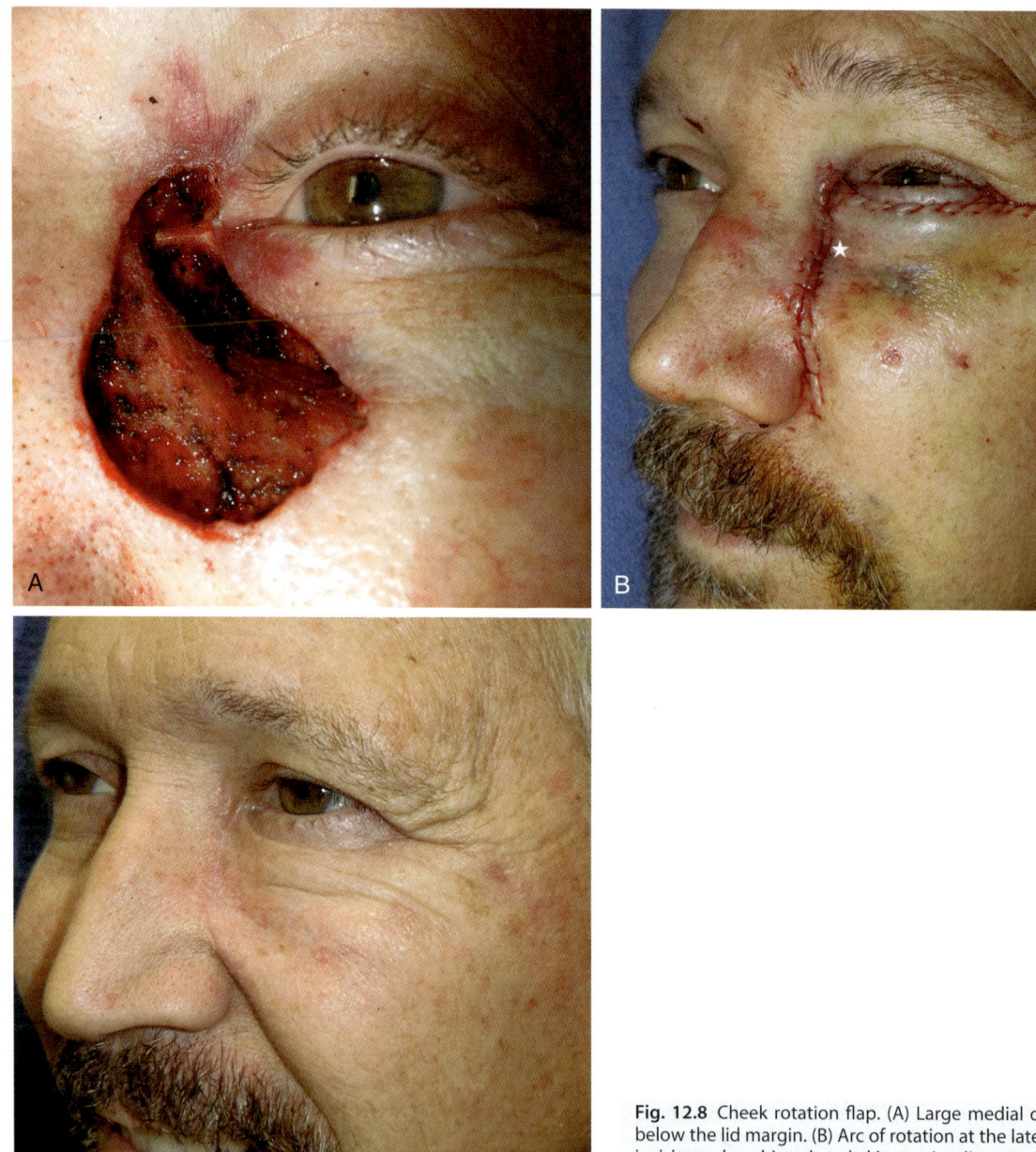

Fig. 12.8 Cheek rotation flap. (A) Large medial defect extending below the lid margin. (B) Arc of rotation at the lateral canthus with incisions placed in relaxed skin tension lines and ample tissue in the medial canthus (*stars* indicate periosteal suspension sutures). (C) Tension-free flap 5 months postoperatively.

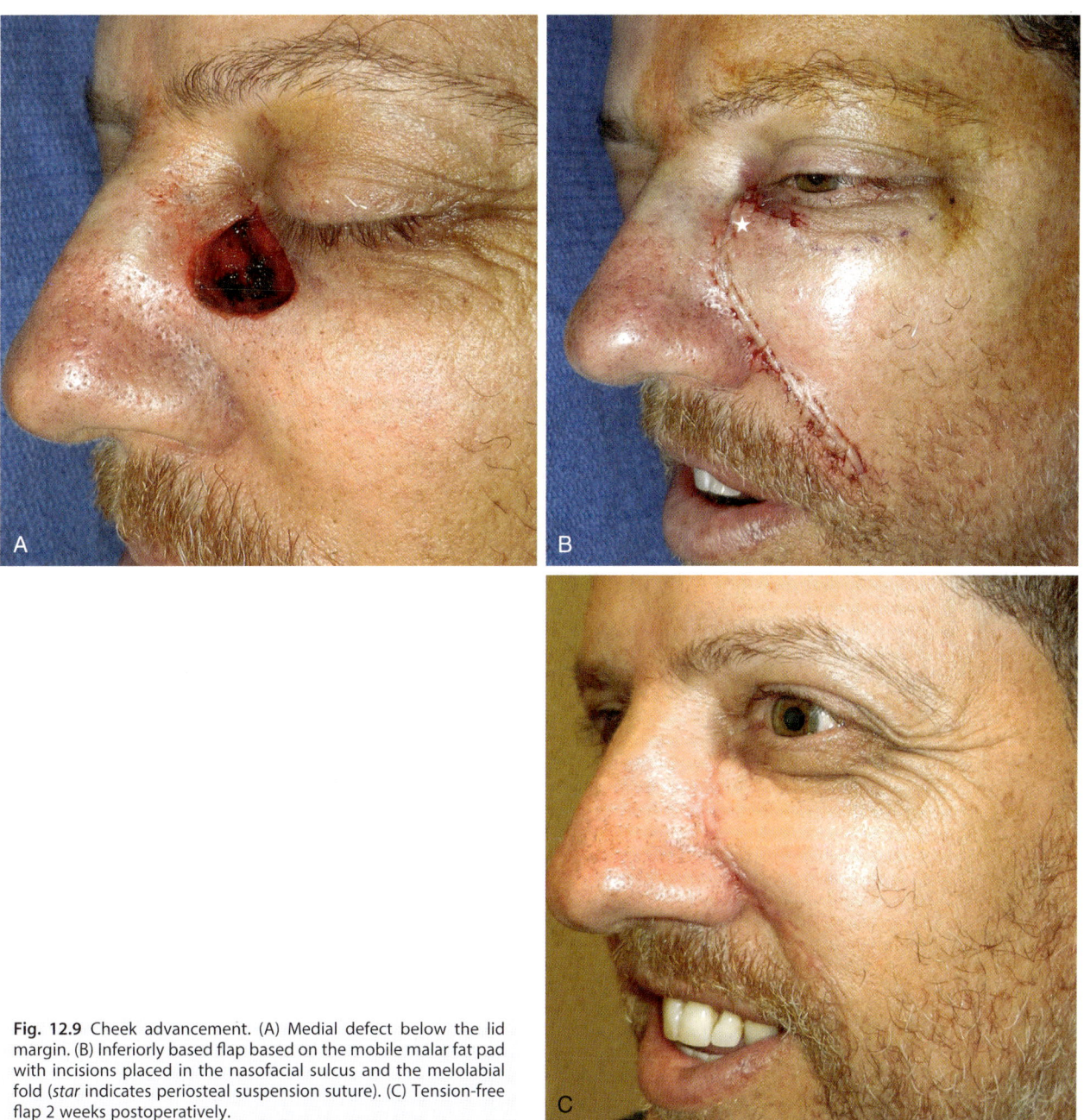

Fig. 12.9 Cheek advancement. (A) Medial defect below the lid margin. (B) Inferiorly based flap based on the mobile malar fat pad with incisions placed in the nasofacial sulcus and the melolabial fold (*star* indicates periosteal suspension suture). (C) Tension-free flap 2 weeks postoperatively.

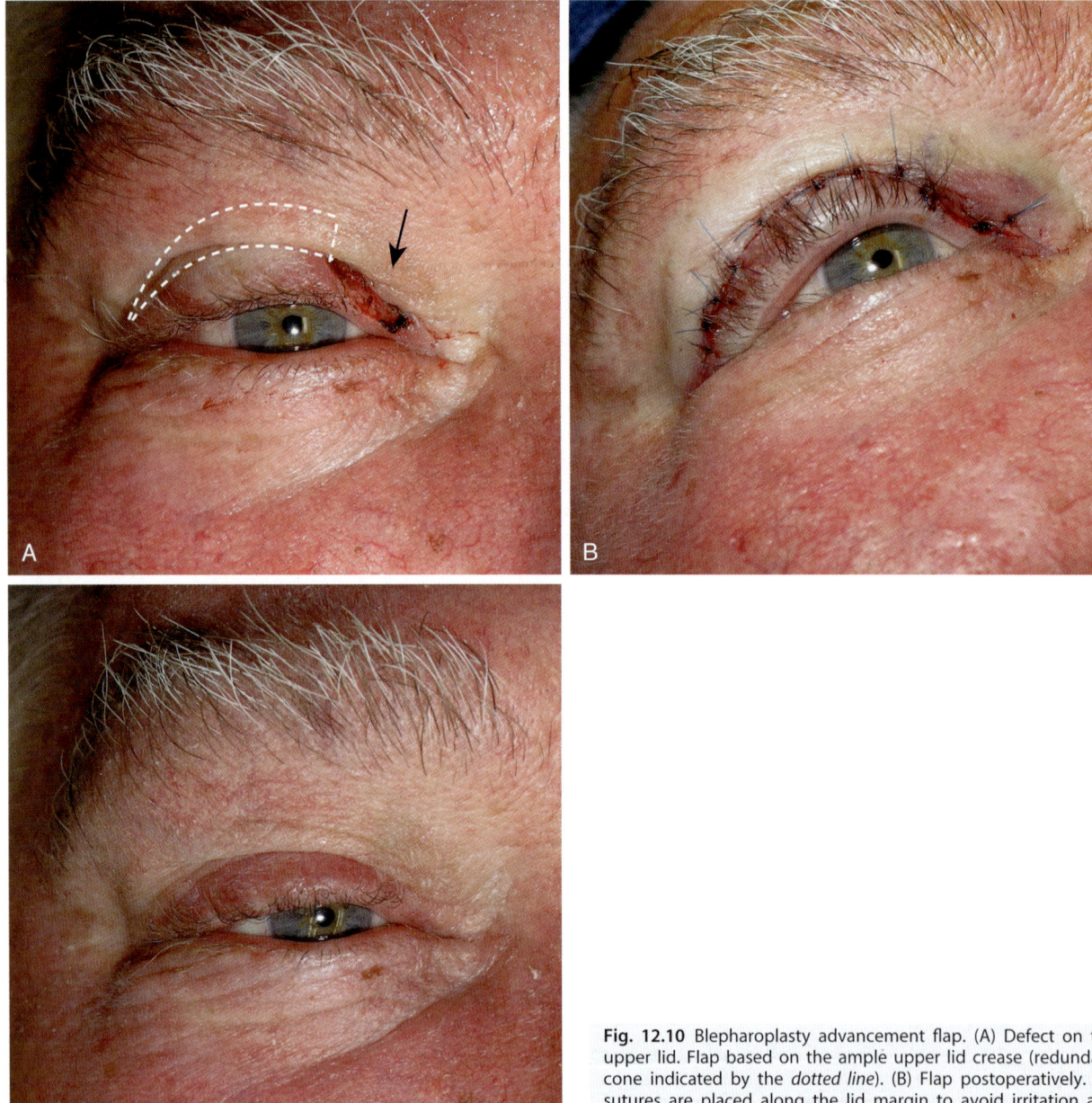

Fig. 12.10 Blepharoplasty advancement flap. (A) Defect on the upper lid. Flap based on the ample upper lid crease (redundant cone indicated by the *dotted line*). (B) Flap postoperatively. No sutures are placed along the lid margin to avoid irritation and corneal abrasion. (C) Tension-free flap with punctum snug against the globe 2 weeks postoperatively.

defects of the upper lid often require the expertise of an oculoplastic surgeon to preserve the functional components of the upper lid.

MEDIAL CANTHAL DEFECTS

The complex anatomy of the medial canthus poses distinct challenges for the periocular surgeon. Webbing across the canthus occurs readily if not actively prevented, owing to the concave contour, need for the vertical movement of the brows, and the thin mobile skin inside the orbital rim adjacent to the relatively thicker bound skin of the cheek and nose. Prevention of webbing relies on designing flaps with adequate tissue to accommodate vertical movement, suspending flaps to the periosteum or medial canthal tendon, and combining flaps when necessary.[5] Medial canthal subunits are approximately defined by the osteocutaneous attachments of the orbital rim and the horizontal apex of the canthus (see Fig. 12.14A).[5]

Small superficial defects centered around the apex of the canthus are often left to heal by secondary intention. Full-thickness skin grafts are also commonly used to repair canthal defects. Flap repairs in the medial canthus are often preferred to optimize outcomes and avoid the drawbacks and limitations of grafts and laissez-faire healing.

Hatchet rotation flaps based on the glabellar skin are ideal for defects that are located at or superior to the canthal apex (Fig. 12.11). Incisions can be obscured in natural

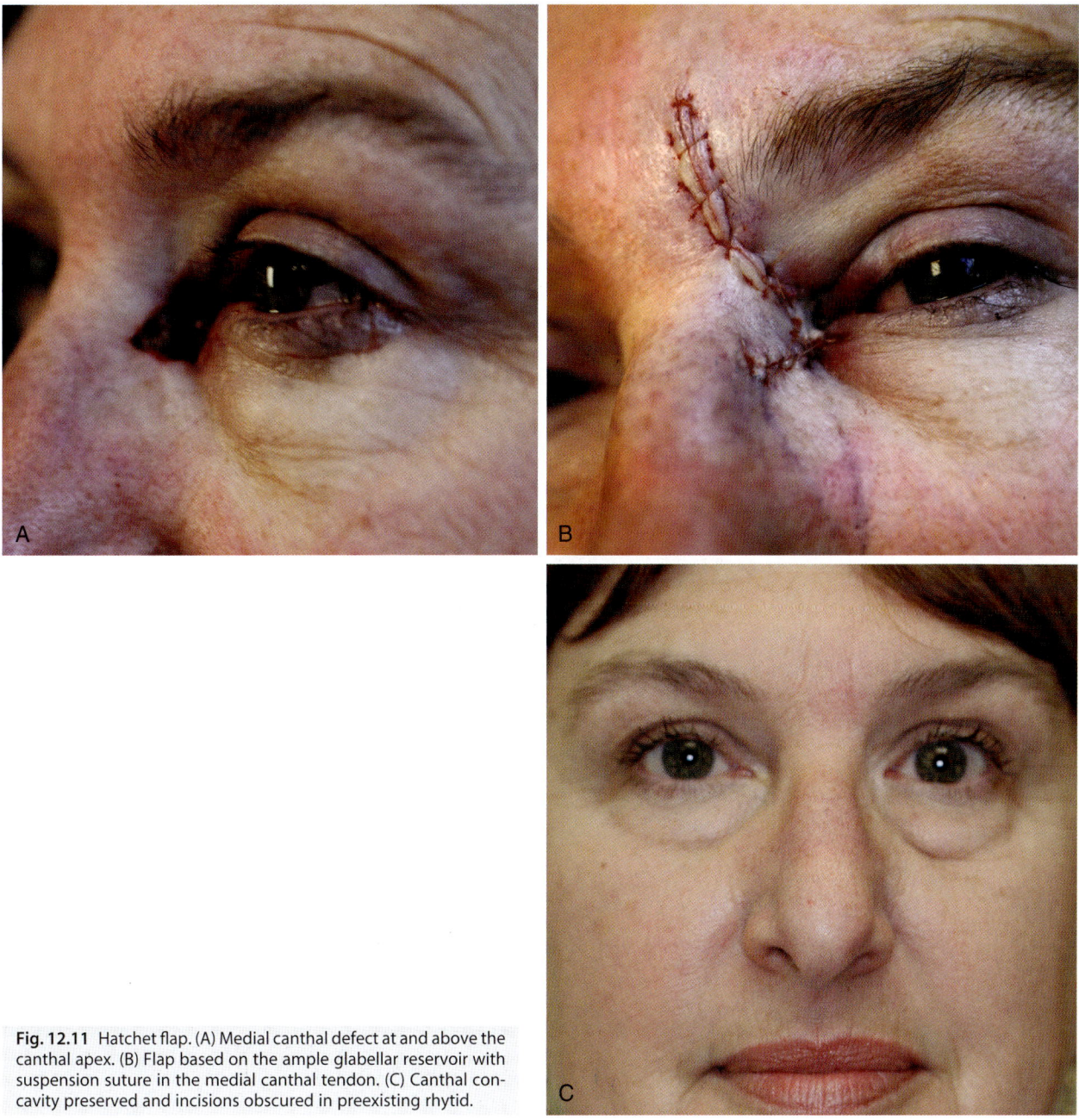

Fig. 12.11 Hatchet flap. (A) Medial canthal defect at and above the canthal apex. (B) Flap based on the ample glabellar reservoir with suspension suture in the medial canthal tendon. (C) Canthal concavity preserved and incisions obscured in preexisting rhytid.

rhytids, and the tissue reservoir is ample so that flaps rotate freely into the canthus. Flaps can be easily suspended to the medial canthal tendon to recreate the canthal concavity.

Defects located at or below the canthal apex can be efficiently repaired with an island pedicle advancement flap based on the medial cheek skin where malar fat allows for flap movement, and incision lines can be partially obscured in the shadow of the nasofacial sulcus (Fig. 12.12). Island flaps are suspended to the medial canthal tendon to preserve the contour of the canthus. Larger defects can be repaired with a combination of these two flaps to avoid webbing (Fig. 12.13). Bilateral rhomboid transposition flaps designed so that redundant cones are directed towards the canthus are also a staple for larger canthal defects.

Lid advancement flaps based on the lax lid skin are ideal for smaller defects close to the lid margins (Fig. 12.14). Incisions are made close to the lash line and advanced horizontally to minimize risk of webbing.

FULL-THICKNESS LID DEFECTS

Primary Lid Repair

Full-thickness lid defects up to one-third of the lid width can often be repaired primarily (Fig. 12.15). Repair of

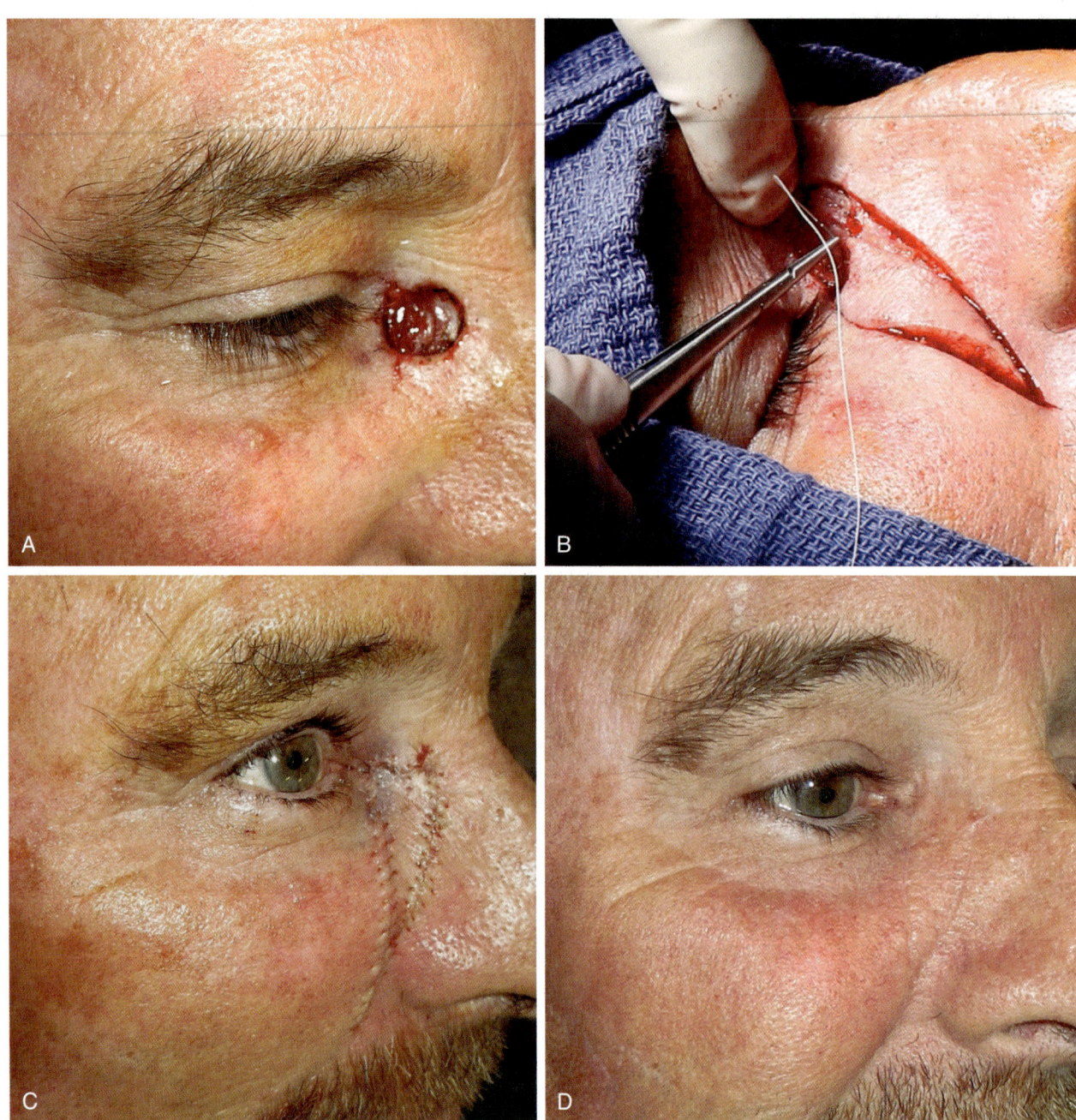

Fig. 12.12 Island pedicle flap with canthal suspension. (A) Medial canthal defect at and below the canthal apex. (B) Suspension suture is placed with a shallow suture through the medial canthal tendon. (C) Flap suspended with concavity preserved postoperatively. (D) Tension-free flap 2 months postoperatively.

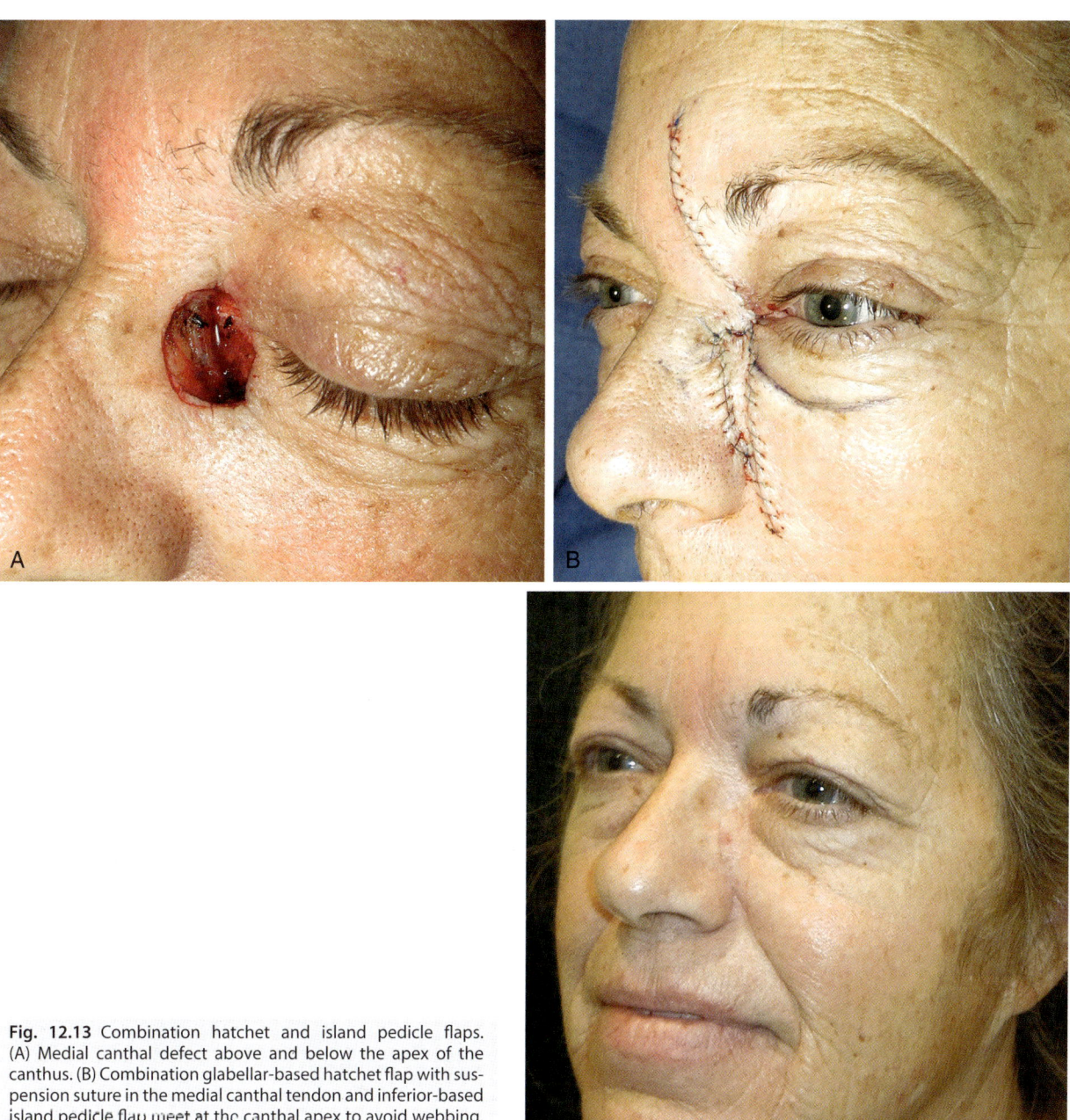

Fig. 12.13 Combination hatchet and island pedicle flaps. (A) Medial canthal defect above and below the apex of the canthus. (B) Combination glabellar-based hatchet flap with suspension suture in the medial canthal tendon and inferior-based island pedicle flap meet at the canthal apex to avoid webbing. (C) Tension-free flap 2 months postoperatively.

full-thickness marginal lid defects requires the robust apposition of the posterior and anterior lamella and meticulous alignment of the lid margin. Less than adequate execution of either of these can lead to notching, malalignment, or torsion of the lid margin. Tension on the lid margin is first minimized by creating a defect in the shape of a pentagon, with slightly inward sloping edges on each side. Redundant skin of the anterior lamella can also be excised obliquely along the natural RSTLs, if preferred. Primary lid closures are classically described with tarsal sutures placed horizontally across the wound to appose the tarsus followed by two or three marginal sutures to ensure alignment. More recently, numerous techniques have been described to optimize primary closures to avoid notching and complications associated with marginal sutures. The diagonal tarsal suture technique is one such adaptation, reliable and easily executed, that provides robust apposition of the tarsus and accurately aligns the lid margin so that marginal sutures are not necessary.[6] After the margins of the defect are perfected, the first tarsal suture is placed by entering the tarsus 2 mm below the lash line and exiting at the superior apex of the lid margin where it meets the conjunctiva (see Fig. 12.7). The mirror image of this suture is placed on the opposing lid margin and tarsus. A traditional horizontal tarsal suture is placed below this, and the orbicularis is repaired with a traditional deep suture. The skin is closed

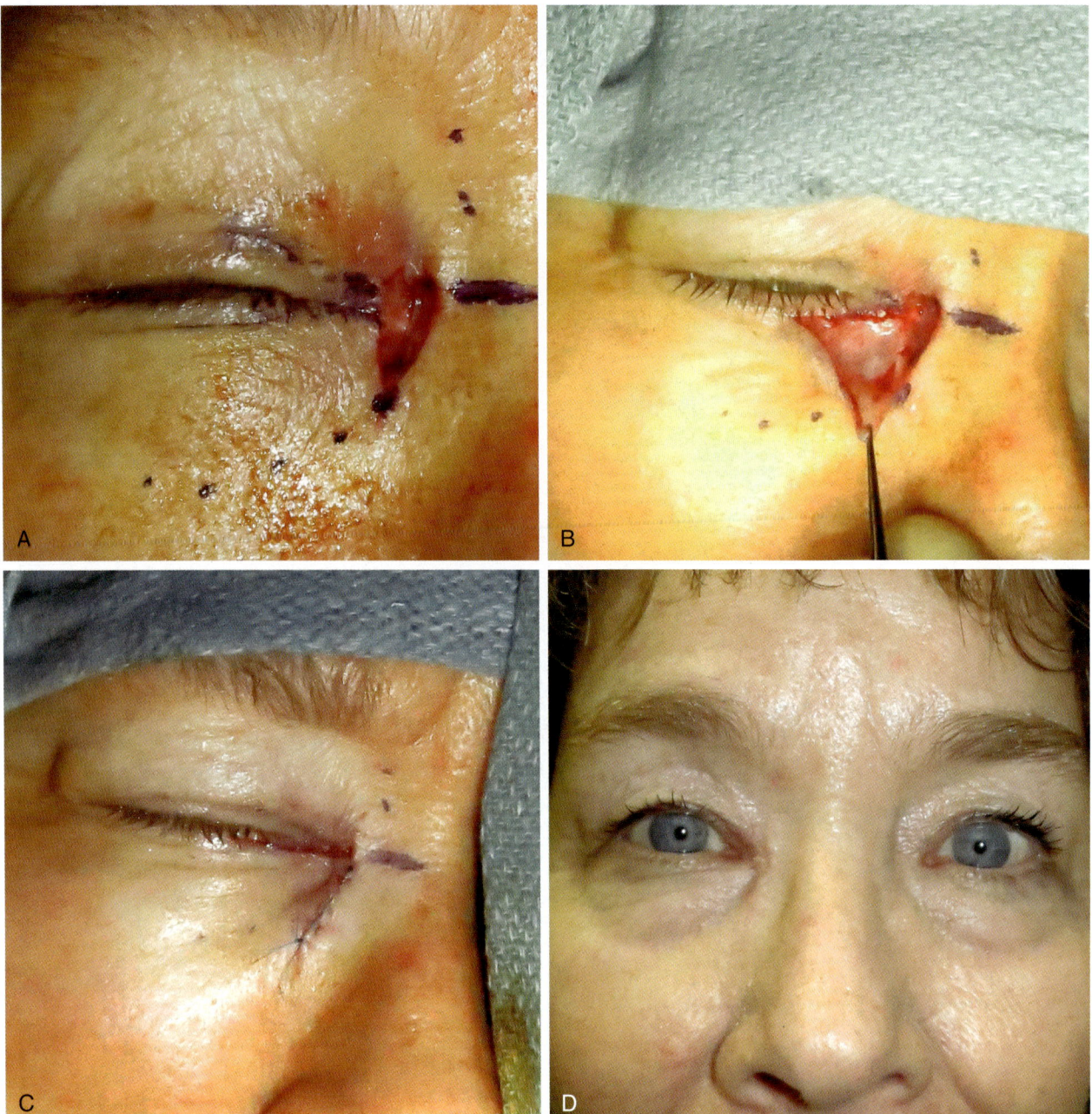

Fig. 12.14 Lid advancement flap. (A) Medial canthal defect located inside the orbital rim (medial canthal cosmetic unit boundaries drawn in purple). (B) Inferior flap with subcilliary incision. (C) Flap in place with medial canthal suspension suture. (D) Flap with no horizontal tension 2 weeks postoperatively.

with a simple running suture placed below the lash line that may be clipped short or sewn into the running suture to minimize irritation.

Lateral Canthotomy

Defects one-third to one-half the width of the lid margin can often be repaired primarily when combined with a lateral canthotomy. A lateral canthotomy incision can be made by making a small superficial incision at the lateral commissure followed by a slight nibbing of the inferior lateral canthal tendon to provide just enough mobility to close the defect without tension. Some tension will remain to ensure the lid is snug against the globe and will usually loosen naturally to the ideal degree with time.

Tenzel Semicircle Flap

Slightly larger, full-thickness lid defects one-half the width of the lid margin can be repaired with a semicircle rotation flap (Fig. 12.16).[7] Tenzel semicircular flaps are ideally performed when a small bit of lid is preserved at the lateral canthus that will allow for a seamless apposition to the medial defect margin. The flap is designed by incising the skin and orbicularis in the shape of a semicircle, beginning at the lateral canthus and extending upward (for lower lid

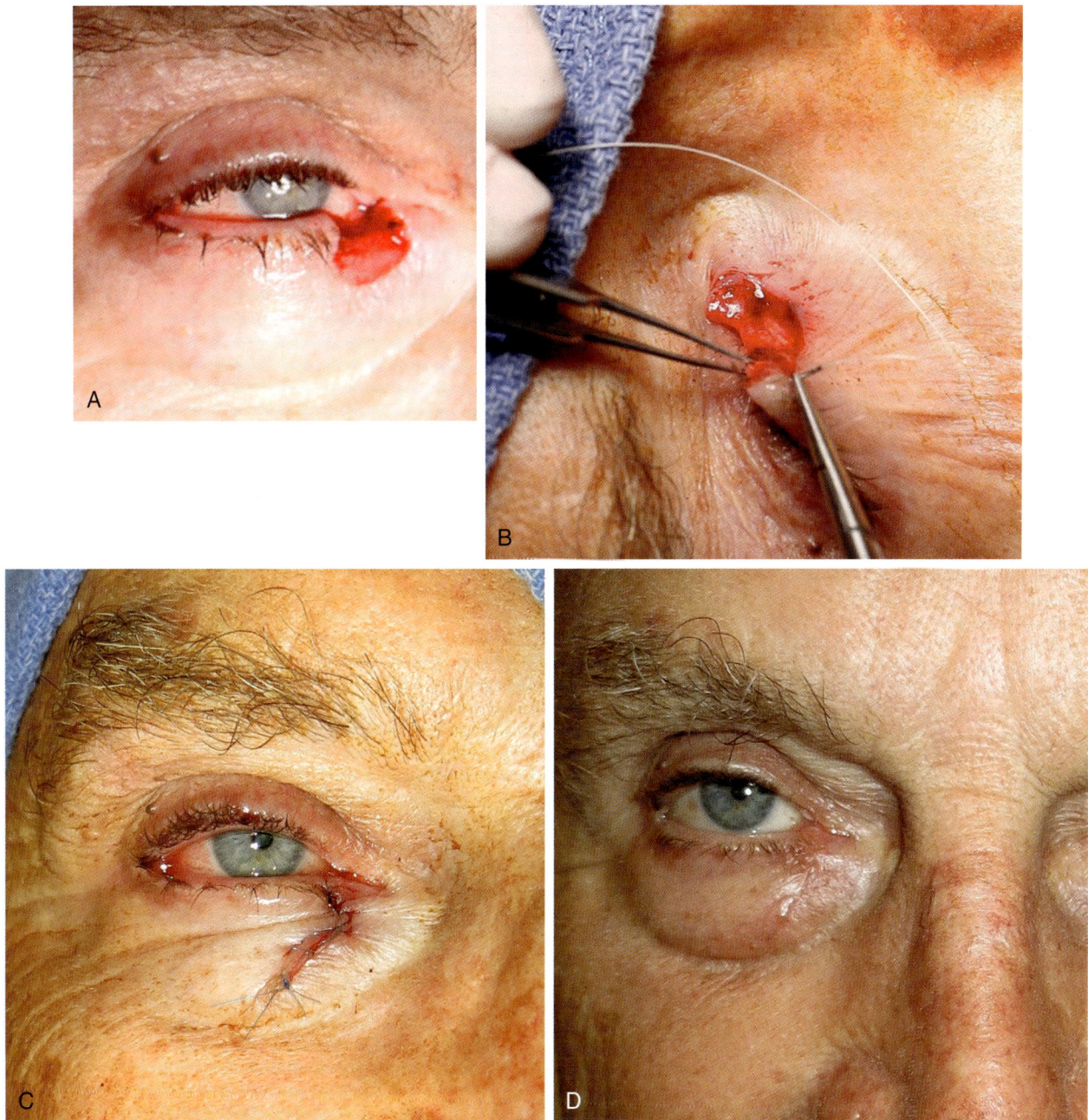

Fig. 12.15 Primary lid repair: diagonal tarsal suture sine marginal sutures. (A) Full-thickness defect involving more than one-third of the lid margin. (B) Diagonal tarsal suture entering the tarsus 2 mm below the lash line and exiting at the posterior apex of the lid margin to robustly approximate the tarsal edges. (C) Primary lid closure postoperatively, robustly approximated and accurately aligned without need for marginal sutures. (D) Primary lid repair well healed without notching 3 months postoperatively.

defects) for a full 180 degrees. The semicircular shape allows for full rotation of the tissue to minimize horizontal tension created by broader arcs. Designing the flap above the commissure ensures vertical tension is above and lateral to the canthus. The inferior limb of the lateral canthal tendon is then severed (while preserving the superior limb) to allow horizontal movement of the lid margin. The lid margin is opposed as described previously for repair of primary lid defects and the skin flap sutured in the usual manner.

Although some shallow full-thickness defects of the lower lid can heal with a laissez-faire approach, a two-stage tarsoconjunctival flap is often required to reconstruct the anterior and posterior lamella (Fig. 12.17).[8]

Tarsoconjunctival Flap

The upper and lower lid mucosa and skin, including a small area on the brow to anchor the lid during the flap design, are infiltrated with local anesthesia. The upper lid is everted and secured to the brow area during flap creation. The mucosa and tarsus are incised 5 mm from the lid margin horizontally and vertically to the end of the tarsal plate. Meticulous hemostasis is maintained with the judicial use

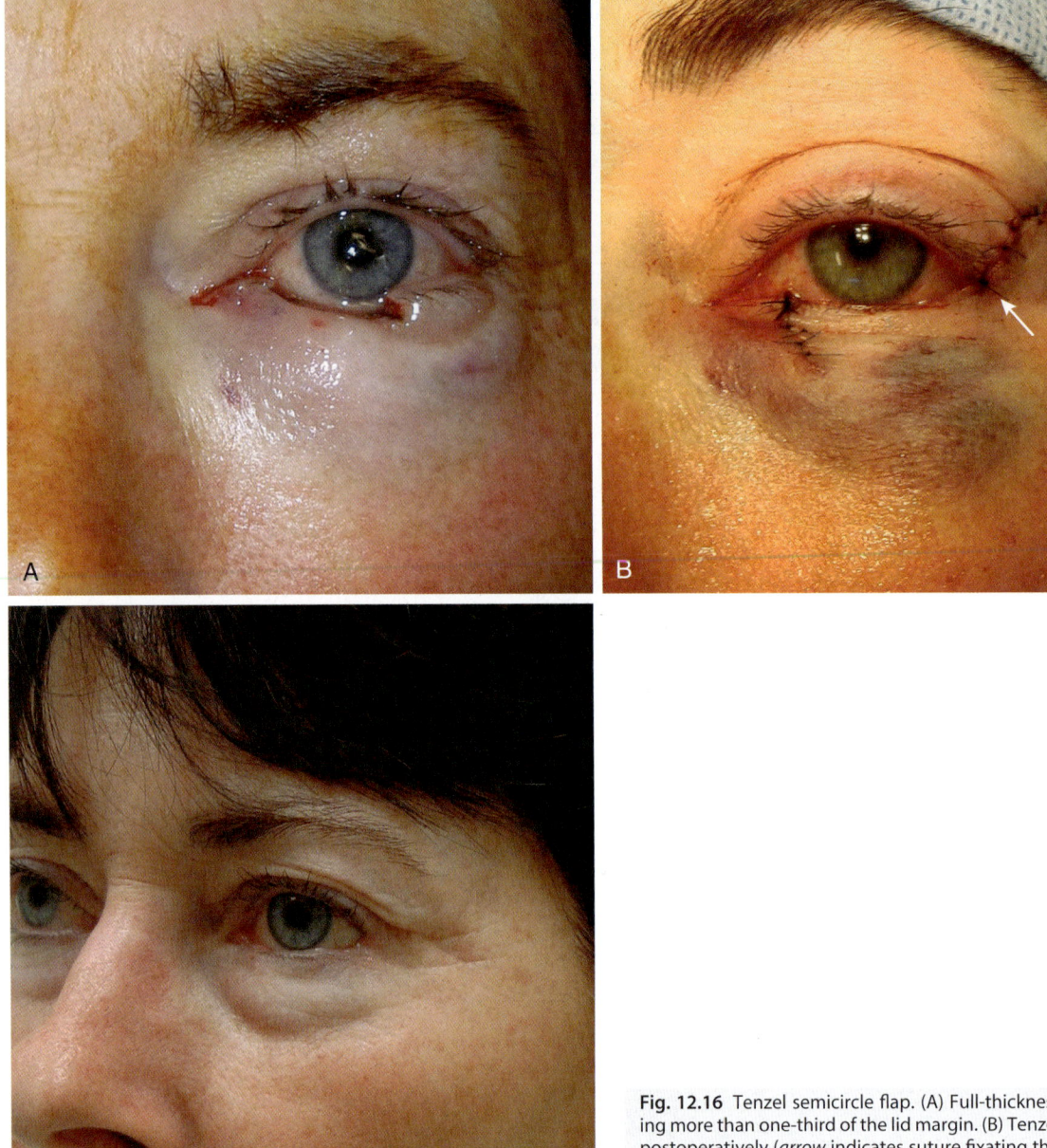

Fig. 12.16 Tenzel semicircle flap. (A) Full-thickness defect involving more than one-third of the lid margin. (B) Tenzel semicircle flap postoperatively (*arrow* indicates suture fixating the flap margin to the lateral canthal tendon). (C) Six months postoperatively (note absence of lashes at the new lid margin).

of cautery. The flap is then further mobilized by loosening its attachment to the levator aponeurosis with blunt dissection. The free edge of the tarsus is then sutured to the mucosal edge of the residual lid within the fornix with 6-0 polyglactin interrupted sutures. These sutures are tightly secured inferior to the corneal surface within the fornix. The lateral edges of the tarsus are placed with care to avoid extension through the conjunctiva and secured so that the knots are facing anteriorly so as not to abrade the cornea. After the tarsoconjunctival flap is secured, the anterior lamella is reconstructed. A full-thickness skin graft may be used; however, an inferiorly based advancement flap is efficient and often preferred, especially in procedures performed under local anesthesia where expediency is desired.

The low lid advancement is undermined below the orbicularis directly inferior to the defect and dog-ears removed at the subciliary line on both sides of the flap incision to allow mobility. The lateral edges of the skin and muscle flap are then sutured into place. The marginal edge of the flap is tacked to the tarsoconjunctival flap if necessary. The flap is left in place approximately 3 weeks before takedown.

The flap is taken down in approximately 3 weeks under local infiltration and corneal anesthesia. The flap is severed with a guide in place to protect the cornea a few millimeters above the lid margin to allow for contraction when the flap is released. Excessive tarsus can be sculpted with cautery if necessary. After the flap is released, it may be necessary to loosen the base of the flap origin to prevent bunching of the posterior upper lid.

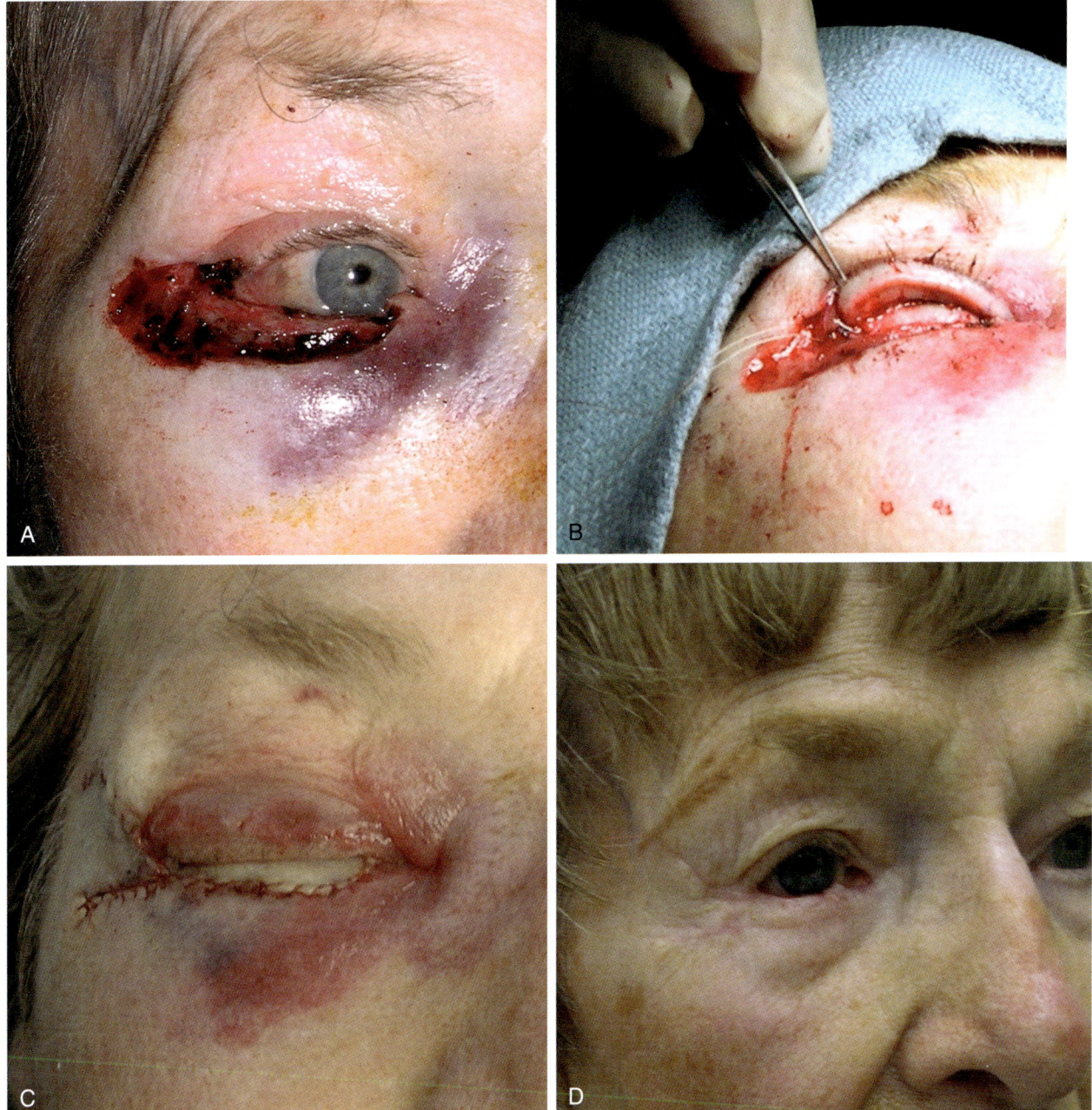

Fig. 12.17 Hughes tarsoconjunctival flap. (A) Full-thickness defect involving 90% of the low lid and 10% of the upper lid. (B) Lateral canthal fixation after the inferior tarsoconjunctival flap was secured to the fornix. (C) Tarsoconjunctival flap with a full-thickness skin graft replacing the anterior lamella of the low lid and a rotation flap to recreate the lateral canthus. (D) Three months after flap takedown with lid margin fully granulated over tarsal flap.

Postoperative Considerations

Observation is essential in the postoperative period to identify potential complications early and ensure success. Because pressure cannot be applied to the eye directly, meticulous hemostasis during surgery is required. It is also prudent to ensure hypertensive patients continue management of blood pressure. For patients who are at high risk of bleeding, leaving a small opening in the wound for drainage can be helpful. Postoperative dressings that are tension bearing can help to offset tension associated with swelling and administration of local anesthetics. Defects close to or involving the lid margin are often dressed with an eye pad placed over a closed lid and covered with an eye shield to protect the eye from trauma. It is often prudent to apply ice and observe the area while elevated for 20 minutes before patients leave the office to ensure hemostasis and comfort. Complex wounds with full-thickness lid loss that will be transferred to the care of an oculoplastic surgeon may require a temporary tarsorrhaphy to ensure the cornea is protected until they are repaired.

Wounds should be kept clean, and erythromycin ophthalmic ointment is usually applied to primary lid repairs to reduce infection risk and keep the eye moist during the immediate postoperative period. Follow-up evaluation in 24 to 48 hours is generally recommended for complex eye repairs. Early epiphora can occur in the early postoperative period, indicating that eye moisture must be managed to prevent excessive dryness.

Ectropion and webbing are best prevented with fundamental surgical techniques and tension management, including appropriate flap design, suspension sutures, and frost sutures when indicated.[9] Both ectropion and webbing tend to occur 2 to 4 weeks postoperatively during maximal with wound contraction. Correction usually requires flap or graft revision and canthopexy procedures.[10,11] Webbing is often easily corrected with a Z-plasty procedure in which the web is incised directly and two 60-degree flaps are transposed to create vertical length along the canthus.[12]

References

1. Bergin DF. Anatomy of the eyelids, lacrimal system, and orbit. In: McCord CD, Tanebaum M, eds. *Oculoplastic Surgery*. New York: Raven Press; 1987:41-72.
2. Harris GJ, Perez N. Anchored flaps in post-mohs reconstruction of the lower eyelid, cheek, and lateral canthus. *Ophthal Plast Reconstr Surg*. 2003;1:5-13.
3. Tripier L. Lambeau musculo-cutané en forme de pont. Appliqué à la restoration des paupières. *Gazette des Hôpitaux de Paris*. 1889;62:1124-1125.
4. Mustardé JC. Problems in eyelid reconstruction. *Ann Ophthalmol*. 1972;4:883-901.
5. Harris GJ, Logani SC. Multiple aesthetic unit flaps for medial canthal reconstruction. *Ophthal Plast Reconstr Surg*. 1998;5:352-359.
6. Willey A, Caesar RH. Diagonal tarsal suture technique sine marginal sutures for closure of full-thickness eyelid defects. *Ophthal Plast Reconstr Surg*. 2013;29:137-138.
7. Tenzel RR, Stewart WB. Eyelid reconstruction by the semicircle flap technique. *Ophthalmology*. 1978;85:1164-1169.
8. Hughes WH. Reconstruction of the lids. *Am J Ophthalmol*. 1945;28:1203-1211.
9. Connolly KL, Albertini JG, Miller CJ, Ozog DM. The suspension (frost) suture: experience and applications. *Dermatol Surg*. 2015;41:406-410.
10. Wesley RE, Collins JW. McCord procedure for ectropion repair. *Arch Otolaryngol*. 1983;109:319-322.
11. Lemke BN, Cook BE, Lucarelli MJ. Canthus-sparing ectropion repair. *Ophthal Plast Reconstr Surg*. 2001;3:161-168.
12. Field LM. Repair of cicatricial epicanthal fold by a double Z-plasty. *J Dermatol Surg Oncol*. 1982;8:215-217.

13 Cheek Reconstruction

RICHARD G. BENNETT, MD

As with other facial areas, the goal of cheek reconstruction is to create the "illusion of normality and the perception that all is as it was."[1] Normality on the cheeks is defined as symmetrical contour, color, and texture. The face is centered by the nose, eyelids, and mouth, and framed by the forehead, chin, and cheeks. Thus reconstruction on the peripheral cheeks will not be as apparent as on the central nose.

Cheek defects are generally repaired by side-to-side closures or flap closures, if possible. Flap closures are used frequently because of the abundant loose cheek tissue, and generally lead to optimal cosmetic results. Grafts and healing by second intention (granulation, contraction, and epidermization) often produce inferior cosmetic results and, except in unusual circumstances that will be discussed later in this chapter, are not commonly used on the cheek.

Like other body areas, cheek reconstruction takes into consideration a number of factors that include the following: location of relaxed skin tension lines (RSTLs); surface anatomy; skin texture; subcutaneous anatomy; patient's age and medical problems; size, depth, and location of the cheek defect; and previous surgery, radiation, and scars. This chapter will discuss the author's approach to repair of cheek defects.

Regional Reconstruction Principles

RELAXED SKIN TENSION LINES

As discussed in Chapters 1 and 2, the RSTLs generally run inferiorly and posteriorly over the cheek surface. If possible, the long axis of wounds should be directed parallel to these lines, particularly because these wounds will eventuate into scars that run parallel to the wrinkle lines. Also, scars are best placed within the lines and grooves of the cheek borders in the cosmetic unit junctions, such as the preauricular fold, melolabial fold, and nasofacial angle. It should be noted, however, that flap incisions on the cheek rarely spread, even when placed perpendicular to the RSTLs. The reason for this is that in the cheek, although the inherent pull in the direction of the RSTL is more than the pull in the direction perpendicular to the RSTL, it is not very much more.

SURFACE ANATOMY

The cheek boundaries are the preauricular crease, the superior border of the zygomatic arch and malar eminence, the inferior orbital rim, the nasofacial angle, the melolabial crease, and the inferior border of the mandible. The cheek may be roughly divided into seven somewhat overlapping and poorly demarcated subunit areas for the purpose of discussion. These seven areas include the medial, anterior (maxillary), infraorbital, zygomatic, buccal, lateral/preauricular, and mandibular. In each of these areas some flap types are more preferable than others. Many repairs in the cheek cross over and include more than one of these subunits. In some peripheral borders on the cheek, for instance the cheek and eyelid boundary, the border is best not transgressed by a single flap, but rather two flaps, one from the upper eyelid and one from the cheek, so as to reestablish the boundary between the cheek and eyelid zones.[1]

Repairs on the face may be regional (e.g., the whole cheek), as emphasized by Gonzalez-Ulloa,[2] or local (e.g., small flaps on only a portion of the cheek). The subunit principle applied by Burget and Menick[3] to the nose is not as critical on the cheek because the subunits are less distinct. The only defining grooves are at the periphery of the cheek along the cosmetic unit junctions.

The cheek is not a flat surface, but is concave medially, as it extends into the nasofacial sulcus; it is convex over the malar eminence. Only in the lateral cheek and preauricular area is the cheek flat. This uneven topography is important for the surgeon to be mindful of, as cheek reconstruction is three dimensional.

Abundant loose skin exists on the cheeks for flap repairs. This abundant tissue is usually found inferior and lateral to defects to be reconstructed. With age, cheek skin begins to sag, and thus more loose tissue becomes available for repairs. However, in the elderly who have had a facelift procedure or in the young, this normally loose tissue is generally not plentiful. Additionally, if prior surgery has been done on the cheek, the underlying anatomy may have been altered and tissue may not move normally.

SKIN TEXTURE

Skin surface characteristics may vary enormously on the cheek from individual to individual and also within the cheek on the same individual. In patients with very oily skin and patulous pores, it may be more difficult to get a good cosmetic result than in patients with smooth nonoily skin. Elderly patients with great skin laxity and a plethora of wrinkles will be easier to reconstruct than the young, who have great elastic skin recoil and no wrinkles. Furthermore, wrinkles afford camouflage for linear, arciform, and flap incision lines. Because of the unique texture of cheek skin,

skin grafts in this location generally provide a poor color and texture match. Skin grafts on the cheek appear as patches and should be avoided if possible. The texture of cheek skin may also vary from one cheek region to another. The beard area in a man needs to be kept in mind. The wrong skin in the wrong place may lead to a less than optimal cosmetic result.

SUBCUTANEOUS ANATOMY

Beneath cheek skin lies an investing fibrous layer, the submuscular aponeurotic system (SMAS). This layer lies between and is attached to the dermis above and the muscles below. Inferiorly SMAS is continuous with the platysma muscle.[4] Deep to the SMAS lies the parotid gland and its duct, facial nerve branches, and superficial muscles of facial expression. All these muscles are supplied by branches of the facial nerve (VII). The buccal branches of the facial nerve over the cheek ramify to such a great extent that any motor loss after reconstruction is usually temporary. The sensory supply to the cheek is mostly from the trigeminal nerve (V). The medial cheek is supplied by the second division (V_2) through the infraorbital nerve. The lateral cheek to the mandible is innervated by third division (V_3) of the trigeminal nerve. A small lower area of the posterior cheek near the lower ear is supplied by the anterior cutaneous nerve of the neck and by the great auricular nerve, which originates from the cervical plexus (C_2, C_3).[5]

The arteries and veins in the cheek generally need not be taken into account to any great extent when performing superficial cheek flaps. There is such an abundant vascular supply on the head and neck that cheek flaps can be randomly placed in relationship to underlying arteries and nerves. The arterial supply to the cheek is from the external carotid artery, which gives rise to the transverse facial artery and the facial artery. Venous drainage is via the anterior facial vein.[5]

There are, however, two motor nerve branches that are superficial in part of their course on the cheek and that one needs to be wary of. The first is the temporal branch of the facial nerve, which may be superficial as it crosses the zygomatic arch. The second is the marginal mandibular nerve, which crosses over the mandibular artery as it courses along the lower edge of the mandible.[5]

SPECIAL ANATOMIC STRUCTURES

There are two special anatomic structures in the cheek worth noting: the buccal fat pad and the parotid duct. The buccal fat pad is a large well-defined area in the central cheek with a large amount of fat. Its importance is that it is a good landmark for Stenson duct, which is the main drainage channel for the parotid gland. The duct courses over the buccal fat pad and descends anterior to it. If Stenson duct is transected and a flap repair done over the leaking area, there will be salivary drainage at the flap edge. Sometimes a Stensen duct partial transection will be difficult to see and is unavoidable. However, should clear fluid drainage occur from the Stensen duct transection, the drainage will generally slow down and go away after a few months.[6] If one sees salivary gland leakage, recanalization of the duct may be attempted with a Silastic tube prior to flap repair; however, in the author's experience, this procedure is often unsuccessful.

WHICH RECONSTRUCTIVE PROCEDURE?

Faced with a cheek defect, how does one select the optimal repair? Generally, healing by second intention on most of the cheek will lead to a noticeable scar, except in the preauricular area. In this latter area, even a very large wound may be allowed to heal by granulation, often resulting in a healed scar with an excellent cosmetic appearance. As mentioned earlier, a skin graft is generally not used on the cheek. A skin graft matches poorly with the surrounding and contralateral cheek skin in color, texture, and degree of hair growth.[7] Furthermore, a skin graft often will not completely fill in a subcutaneous defect, and provides less protection to underlying vessels and nerves than a skin flap. There are, however, two exceptions as to when a skin graft may be useful. The first is to repair a defect that resulted from excision of an aggressive tumor (e.g., angiosarcoma or sebaceous gland carcinoma). In this case, a split-thickness graft can be used immediately to repair the wound defect and prevent contraction. When healed the graft provides a window through which a tumor recurrence could be seen (Fig. 13.1). The second circumstance for placing a split-thickness graft would be to repair a very large defect, which could not be repaired in any other way. Prior to the development of large cheek flaps and cheek–neck rotation flaps, multistaged cheek rotation flaps[8] or large skin grafts were commonly used to repair cheek defects.[9] For a large deep cheek wound with extensive bone exposure, a free flap may be considered. However, a free flap in this area always evenutates into a poor cosmetic result, its thickness will bury tumor, and it requires a prolonged (8–10 hour) operation under general anesthesia. For a very extensive cheek defect that is superficial, a tissue expander could also be considered.[10]

The single largest decision when contemplating a cheek reconstruction is whether to repair a wound with a side-to-side linear closure (complex repair) or a skin flap. The same defect that may be repaired side-to-side in an elderly person with excess skin and wrinkles may require a skin flap for closure in a young person to avoid scar spreading from excess tension.

This author has found empirically that the best way to determine whether a complex repair or a skin flap could be done easily is to lift with skin hooks the ends of the wound up along the RSTLs (see Fig. 13.19B). If the central wound edges come together easily across the wound with the skin hooks tenting up the wound at the superior and inferior ends, then a side-to-side linear repair may be done. Sometimes, however, a side-to-side repair may be possible, but distortion of the melolabial fold may occur. In this instance, a flap may be preferable. When possible, however, one should close a wound with a side-to-side linear repair, since it will result in fewer incision lines than those from a skin flap.

RECONSTRUCTION PHILOSOPHY

In reviewing the literature on cheek reconstruction, this author was struck by three trends. The first is that surgeons

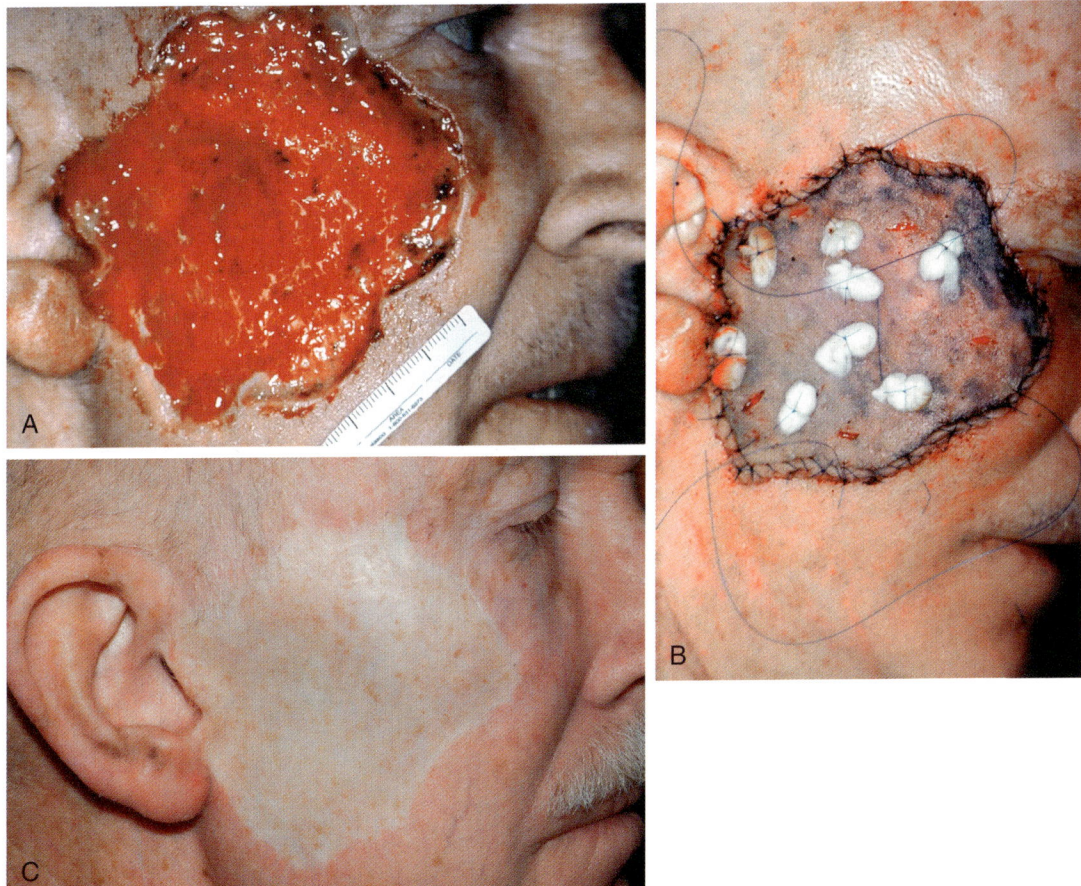

Fig. 13.1 (A) Large wound on right cheek after excision of multiple recurrent level II lentigo maligna. (B) Medium, split-thickness skin graft sutured into wound. Note bolster sutures to tack graft onto recipient wound so as to keep graft from slipping during healing. (C) Healed result 6 months postoperatively.

like to do one specific flap type for one specific defect; the second is that surgeons prefer to close the entire wound at one time. These issues have been raised by other authors.[1,11] Part of the reason for this approach has been that surgical training programs dogmatically emphasize repairing the whole wound at one time; leaving part of the wound open to heal by granulation is thus unacceptable. The third trend is that even medium-sized wounds on the cheek are repaired by rather large flaps extending into the neck and shoulder, when these same wounds could have been closed with an equally good or better result by smaller, less complicated local flaps. The trend of using cervical neck or cervical pectoral flaps results in excessive surgery. This is not to say there is not a time and place for such flaps, but many of the case examples presented in the literature show medium-sized wounds that could be repaired in other ways.[12]

FLAPS TO AVOID

On the cheek, two flaps that this author avoids are the subcutaneous island pedicle flap and the bilateral advancement flap. The former usually results in a puffy flap that does not lie flat[13]; the latter produces too many straight lines that are easily seen. However, some authors continue to recommend these flaps despite showing photographs that demonstrate excessive poorly placed incision lines and a puffy flap.[14]

Flaps by Cheek Region

MEDIAL CHEEK

The medial cheek usually has abundant skin laxity. If the wound is small to medium in size and its long axis is oriented obliquely, a side-to-side repair may be done easily (Fig. 13.2).[15] If possible, repairs in this area are closed along or parallel to the nasofacial angle or melolabial fold. Although some authors[9] advise deep "periosteal" tacking sutures for side-to-side linear closures in the nasofacial angle, this author does not do this and feels it is usually unnecessary. For long obliquely oriented wounds on the medial cheek that cannot be closed without excessive tension on the wound edges, the rhombic transposition flap with a double Z-plasty is useful (Fig. 13.3). This flap takes advantage of the inferiolateral loose tissue available on the cheek. The double Z-plasty helps increase the extension of the rhombic flap.[16] The angulated incisions of the rhombic flap and Z-plasties generally blend in well to the surrounding skin over time.

For a medial cheek wound with its long axis oriented horizontally, a side-to-side linear closure obliquely oriented along the RSTLs would lengthen the closure line considerably. Therefore it might be best to consider a flap closure. There are three main flap choices for such a wound in this

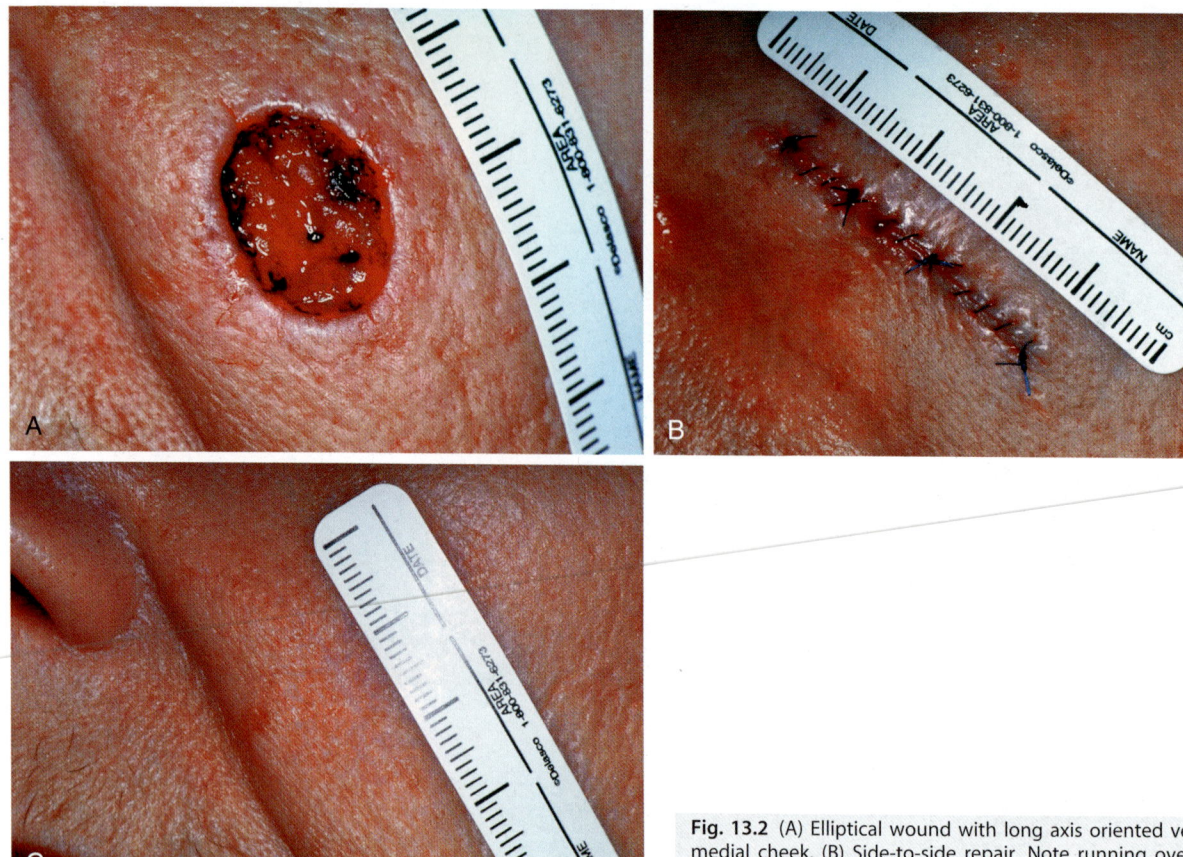

Fig. 13.2 (A) Elliptical wound with long axis oriented vertically on medial cheek. (B) Side-to-side repair. Note running over-and-over stitch. (C) Healed result 1 year postoperatively.

area: the subcutaneous island pedicle flap, the rhombic transposition flap (Fig. 13.4), and the advancement flap with a back-cut (Fig. 13.5). This author does not like the subcutaneous island pedicle flap for large wounds in this location, as this flap is often puffy, even many months later. When this happens, the puffiness is difficult to correct.[13] Nevertheless, the subcutaneous island pedicle flap may be considered for small wounds just above or within the melolabial fold.[14]

The rhombic transposition flap works well for medium-sized wounds in the medial cheek (see Fig. 13.4). As emphasized by Borges,[17,18] it is important to design the rhombic flap so the base of the flap (i.e., the base of the flap triangle) is perpendicular to the RSTLs on the cheek. Also, as Becker[19] points out, the main rhombic flap tension is at the donor area, and these flaps on the cheek are generally laterally and inferiorly based. Cabrera and Zide[20] further recommend that one base the rhombic flap inferiorly, as this orientation tends to minimize the trapdoor effect due to fluid accumulation, which may or may not be true.

Horizontally oriented defects in the medial cheek are often best repaired with a rotation/advancement flap from the inferior direction (see Fig. 13.5).[21] An incision line is made inferiorly along the melolabial crease line, often with a back-cut. The tissue is rotated and advanced superiorly and the back-cut triangle is excised. The incision down the melolabial crease with excision of a Burow triangle rather than a back-cut was described by Imre.[22] I prefer the back-cut triangle because the resultant scar will be well camouflaged by the melolabial crease. Another alternative to the Burow triangle excision is to excise an ellipse at the inferior end of the flap with the lateral side longer than the medial side.[23] On closure the lateral wound edges are displaced superiorly and medially. One problem with the advancement/rotation flap with a back-cut is that medial canthal tenting may occur, particularly when this flap is used to repair horizontally oriented defects high in the medial cheek. To help prevent this problem, Jelks and Jelks[24] advise de-epithelializing the flap tip and fixing it to the medial canthal tendon. The tenting, if bothersome, may be released by a V-to-Y or Z-plasty. For a very large advancement/rotation flap in the medial cheek, one should also place a deep buried "periosteal" suture to hold the downward weight of the flap and decrease wound tension (Fig. 13.6). Another alternative to the inferior cheek advancement flap is the O-to-Z flap.[25] In this case both an inferior and a superior incision are made from opposite sides of the wound. Thus after undermining, advancement and rotation occurs but in opposite directions. To enhance flap movement a back-cut can be made in one or both ends of the O-to-Z flap. As the wound size increases, so does the complexity and difficulty of the flap. For large defects (especially those oriented obliquely) in the medial or anterior cheek area, a whole cheek advancement/rotation flap may be created from the lateral cheek. Using the entire cheek lateral to a large defect as a single flap is considered by some physicians

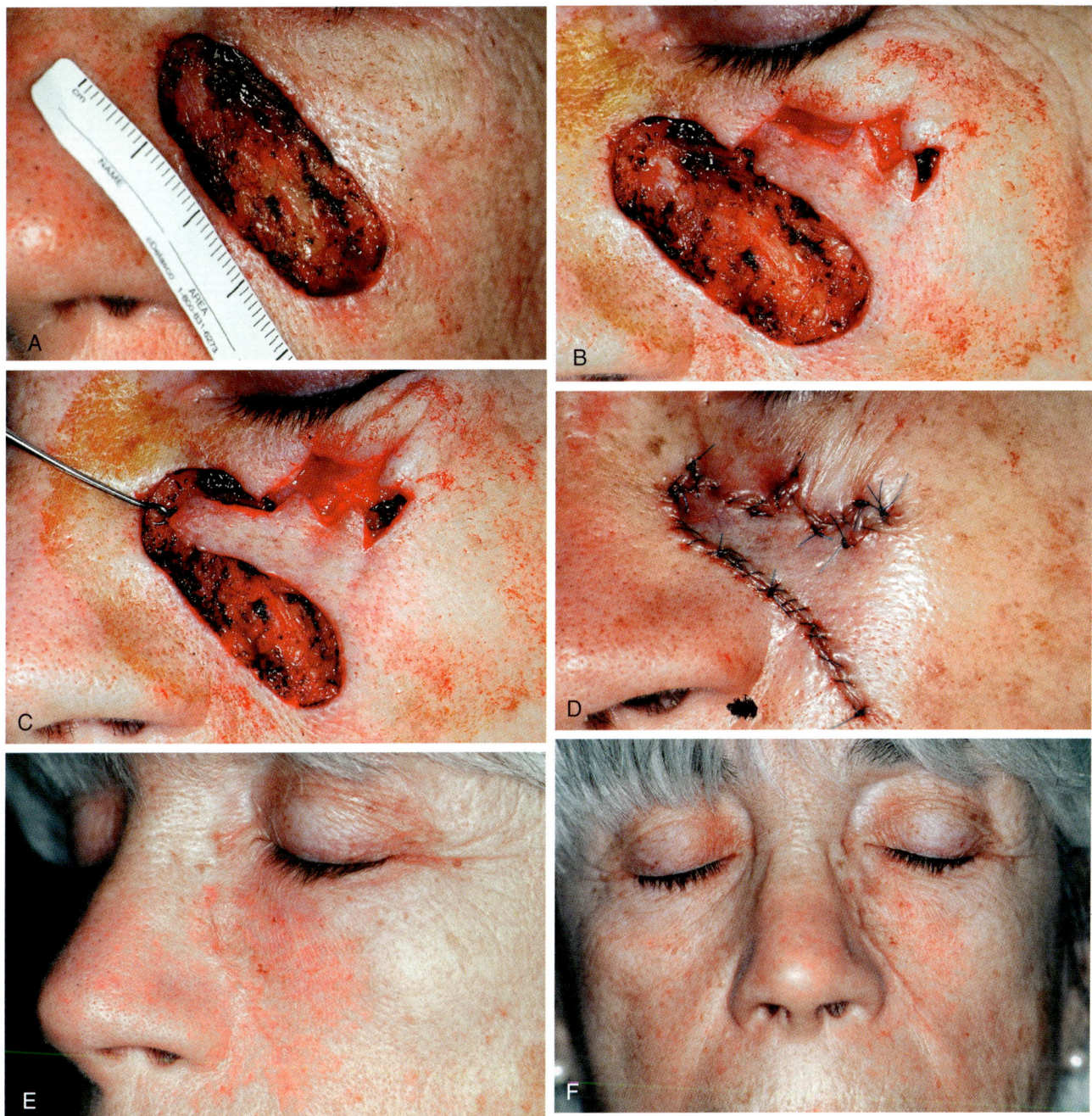

Fig. 13.3 (A) Large elliptical wound on medial cheek with long axis oriented vertically. (B) Rhombic flap with double Z-plasty cut and undermined. (C) Flap transposed into wound. (D) Flap sutured into defect. (E, F) Healed result 6 months postoperatively.

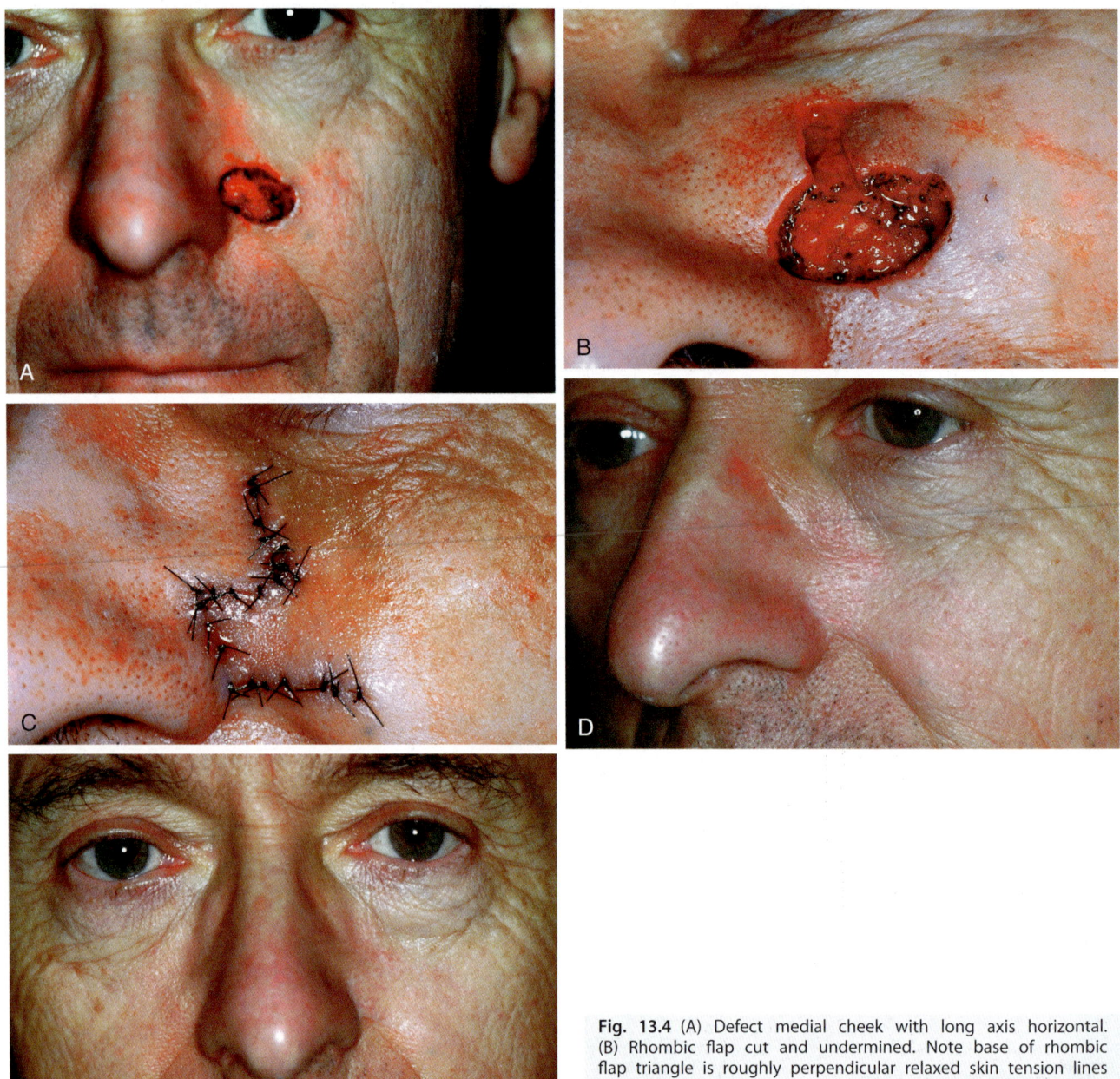

Fig. 13.4 (A) Defect medial cheek with long axis horizontal. (B) Rhombic flap cut and undermined. Note base of rhombic flap triangle is roughly perpendicular relaxed skin tension lines (RSTLs). (C) Flap transposed and sutured. (D, E) Healed result 1 year postoperatively.

to be ideal because its scar will be less noticeable compared to scars from smaller flaps, which may cross the lines and natural creases of the face.[12,26] Furthermore, this flap is a very vascular and therefore a safe flap, which rarely has tip necrosis.

The lateral cheek advancement flap has a medial inferior base and a forward and medial destination. The initial incision for a cheek rotation/advancement flap is made horizontally and laterally from the cheek defect extending on top of the orbital rim; as it progresses laterally at the point of the lateral canthus, it is gently curved superiorly above the zygomatic arch to at least the level just above that of the lateral canthus to decrease the chance of ectropion (Fig. 13.7). This latter incision places the vector of any scar contraction in an upward posterior direction so that it will counteract any inferior pull on the lower eyelid. If this flap stops above the zygomatic arch in the temple, it is similar to the Tenzel flap used to close defects on the lower eyelid.[27]

For very large defects of the medial or anterior cheek, the incision should be carried over the zygomatic arch and down the preauricular crease to a point 2 to 3 cm below the earlobe. Here a Burow triangle may be excised and hidden behind the earlobe (Fig. 13.8).[28] The flap is then rotated medially as it is advanced superiorly. It is critical to place tacking sutures along the lateral and inferior lateral orbital rim and the malar eminence to support the heavy flap and prevent ectropion. It is also important to thin the subcutaneous tissue along the superior flap border to match the skin thickness of the lower eyelid.

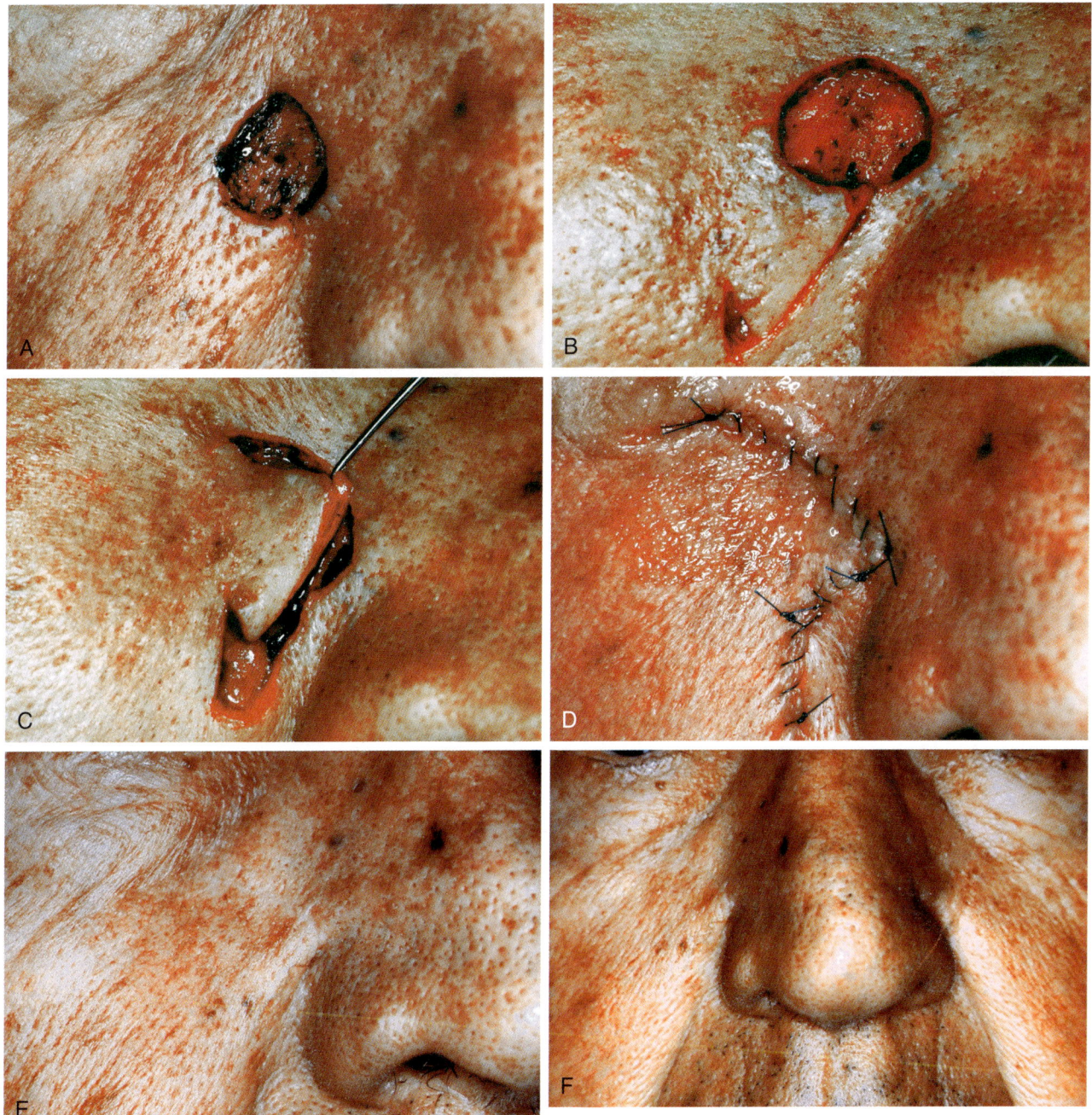

Fig. 13.5 (A) Round defect medial cheek. (B) Advancement flap from inferiorly cut with back-cut. (C) Advancement flap advanced superiorly. The back-cut triangle will be cut off. (D) Flap sutured into place. (E, F) Healed result 2 years postoperatively.

An alternative to the lateral cheek advancement/rotation flap is a 180-degree transposition flap (Fig. 13.9). I have found this flap to be particularly useful for large medial cheek wounds extending into the medial canthus. As shown in Fig. 13.9, a transposition flap is created in the medial cheek and then transposed 180 degrees. Because of the extreme flap shortening with rotation, this flap should be approximately 40% longer than the height of the recipient wound. The 180-degree transposition flap results in a high standing cone that is generally removed 4 to 8 weeks later at a second operation.

For large defects in the medial or anterior cheek, some authors[12,29] prefer the cheek–neck (cervical facial) rotation flap. The flap incision on the cheek is similar to that of the cheek rotation flap just described. The incision follows the orbital rim laterally and at the lateral canthus is arched superiorly. The incision is continued posteriorly along the temporal hairline and preauricular crease. At the inferior lobule of the ear, the incision is then continued either inferiorly and anteriorly into a neck crease along the sternocleidomastoid muscle or posteriorly around the lobule and along the lateral inferior hairline.[30,31] The extended

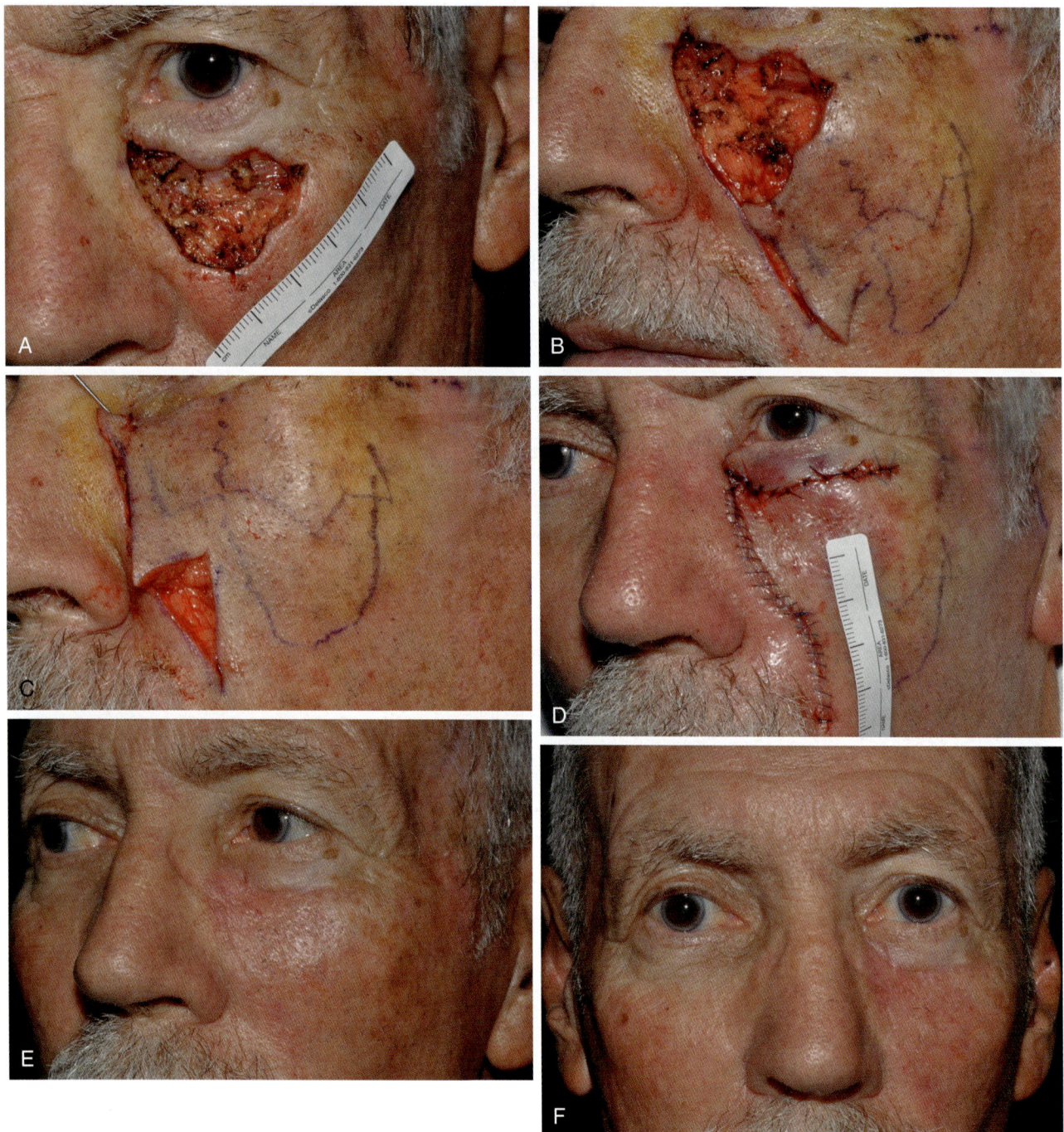

Fig. 13.6 (A) Wound on medial cheek with long axis horizontally. (B) Advancement flap with back-cut incised and undermined. (C) Advancement flap advanced and rotated superiorly. (D) Flap sutured into place. Tacking sutures placed in concavity of nasofacial angle and near flap tip to prevent inner canthal tenting. (E, F) Healed result 1 year postoperatively.

incisions allow recruitment of tissue from the neck and retroauricular areas. Undermining is done in the midsubcutaneous level (the face-lift plane) with sufficient fat maintained to ensure adequate blood supply and adequate tissue thickness. As the flap is rotated, tacking sutures are placed into the deep tissues of the medial and lateral orbital rim to prevent inferior lid displacement. Tacking sutures are also advisable along the line between the lateral eyebrow and the superior attachment of the ear.[32] Even though this flap may extend over the entire cheek, drains or suction catheters are rarely needed.[33]

For even larger defects on the medial and anterior cheek, the incision may be carried further down the neck to recruit even more tissue. Instead of bringing the incision anteriorly into a neck crease, as in the cervical facial rotation flap, the incision continues along the posterior border of the trapezius muscle and then medially at the end of the clavicle either along the clavicle or more inferiorly into the pectoral

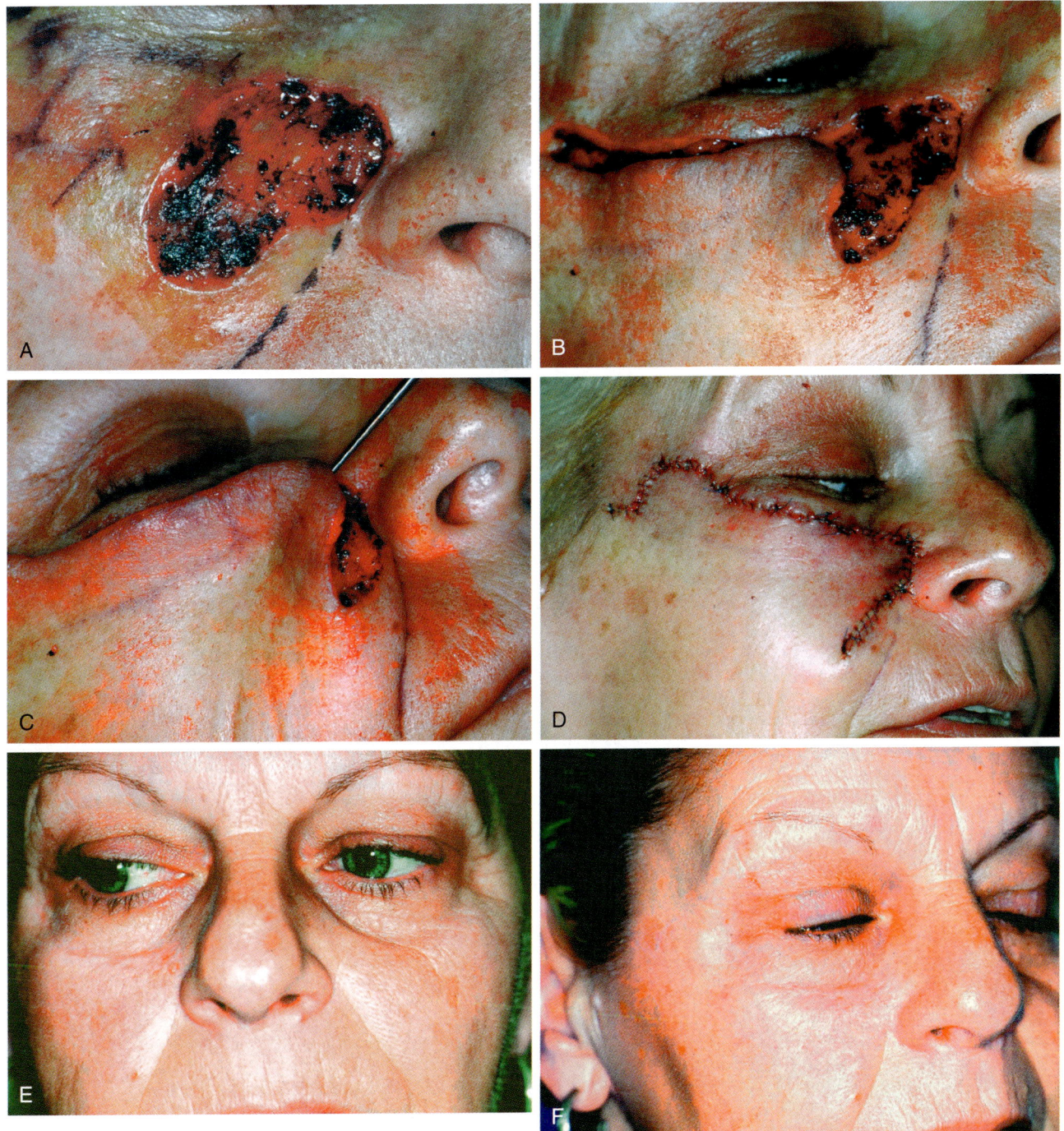

Fig. 13.7 (A) Large irregular wound with widest diameter oriented almost vertically. (B) Flap incision extending laterally over cheek. Note that laterally, it arches superiorly at the lateral canthus. (C) Flap advanced medially. (D) Flap sutured into defect. (E, F) Healed result 1 year postoperatively.

chest (cervicopectoral flap).[34] If one makes the incision on the posterior border of the trapezius muscle, there will be little likelihood of scar contracture or hypertrophy. Although the cervicopectoral flap has been considered a safe flap, some authors would disagree, particularly if the flap is under considerable tension.

As an alternative to basing the cheek advancement/rotation flap medially, some authors[20,35–37] have suggested a laterally based cheek advancement/rotation flap, in which an incision is made down the melolabial fold and onto the neck. This flap would mostly advance tissue superiorly with little rotation (thus the name the "hike flap"). Most of the blood supply to this latter flap would come from branches of the facial artery as it crosses over the inferior border of the mandible, where it can be palpated. In addition, if one includes the platysma muscle in the flap, the blood supply will be further enhanced.[38] However, because of the forces of gravity on this flap, great care needs to be taken to

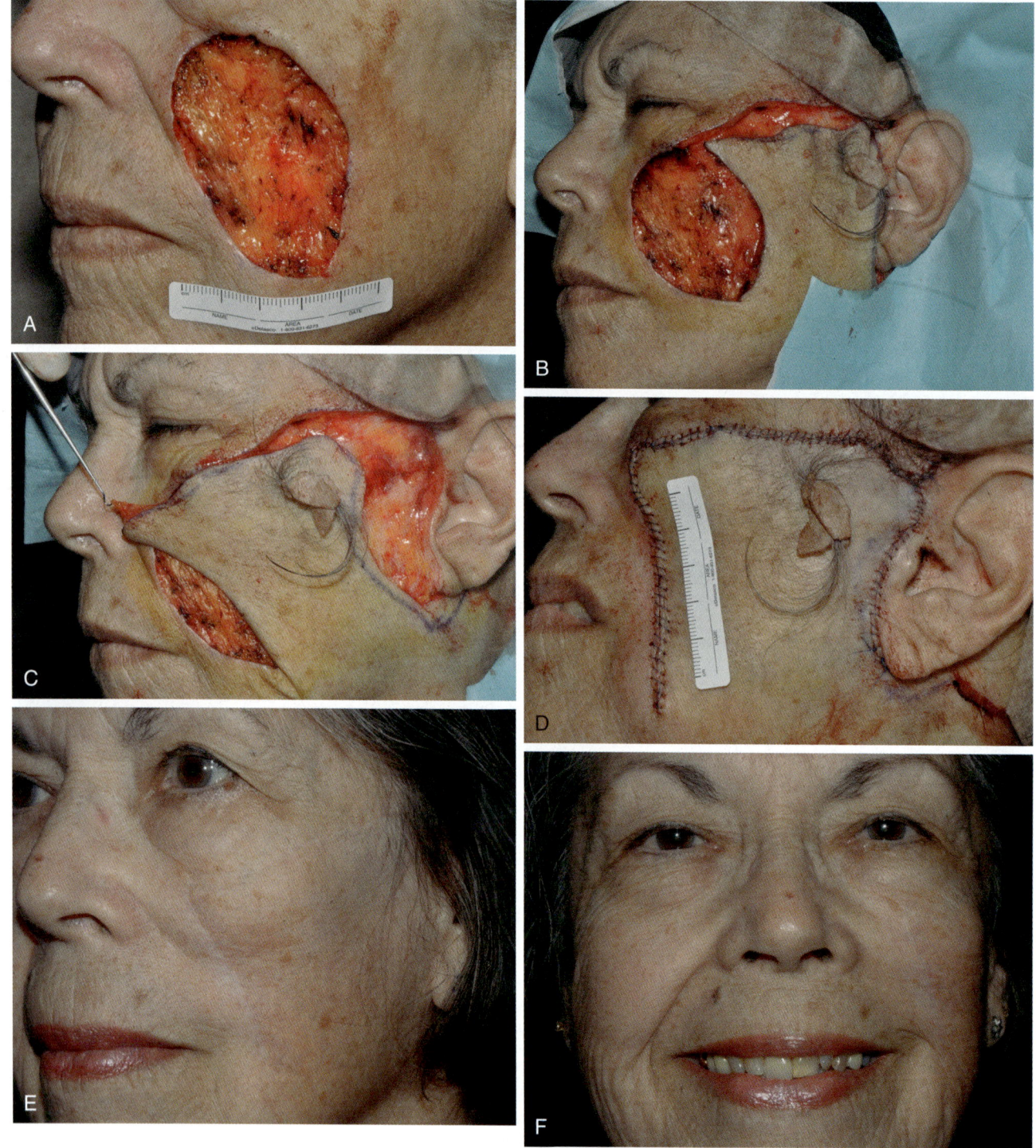

Fig. 13.8 (A) Medial cheek wound with long vertical axis. (B) Lateral cheek flap incised. Note incision carried just above lateral canthus to just above anterior ear then carried inferiorly just in front of ear. A Burow triangle was removed below ear lobule. (C) Flap rotated medially and advanced superiorly. (D) Flap sutured into place. A small standing cone (dog-ear) excised at point just anterior and superior to ear. (E, F) Healed result 1 year postoperatively.

carefully tack the flap superiorly along the orbital rim to prevent ectropion.

Problems that can occur with large advancement rotation flaps on the cheeks include anterior transfer of hair-bearing tissue (see Fig. 13.8C), which may be obvious in men, and ectropion. Therefore it is important to fastidiously tack these flaps to underlying deep tissue in the zygomatic region. Also, if the wound edges are not carefully everted, the scar line may be easily seen.

ANTERIOR CHEEK

A defect on the anterior cheek can be closed with a side-to-side closure if small (Fig. 13.10). For medium-sized defects,

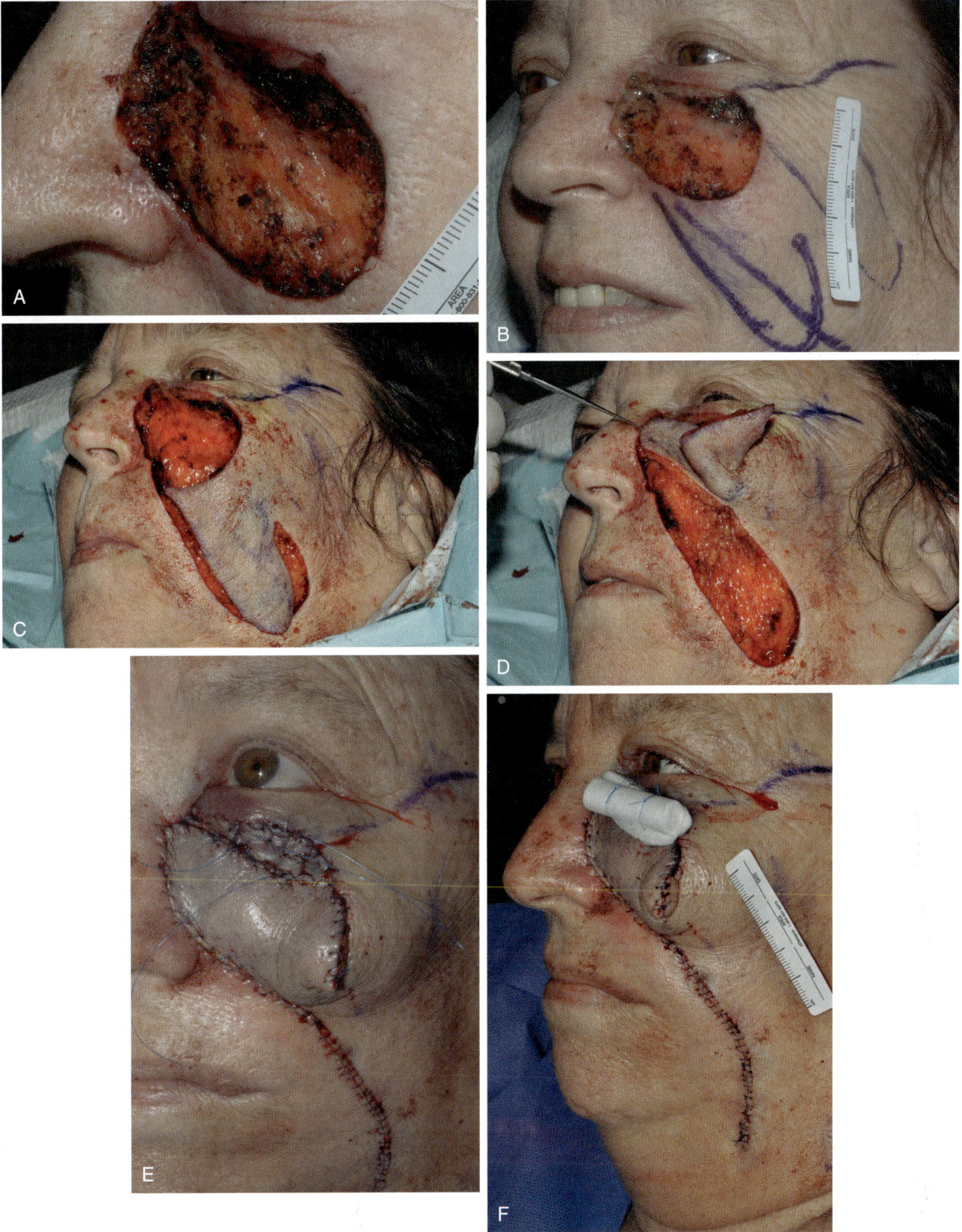

Fig. 13.9 (A) Wound on medial cheek extending onto nose and eyelid. (B) Reconstructive options of lateral cheek. Advancement flap or inferior 180° transposition flap drawn on cheek. (C) 180° transposition flap incised. Note small flap base relative to length. (D) 180° rotated and transposed into wound. Flap base not undermined but remains attached to underlying muscles to provide good blood supply. (E) Flap sutured in place with full-thickness skin graft placed on lower eyelid. (F) Bolster sutured onto full-thickness skin graft. Standing cone (dog-ear) left to ensure blood supply was removed later.

Continued

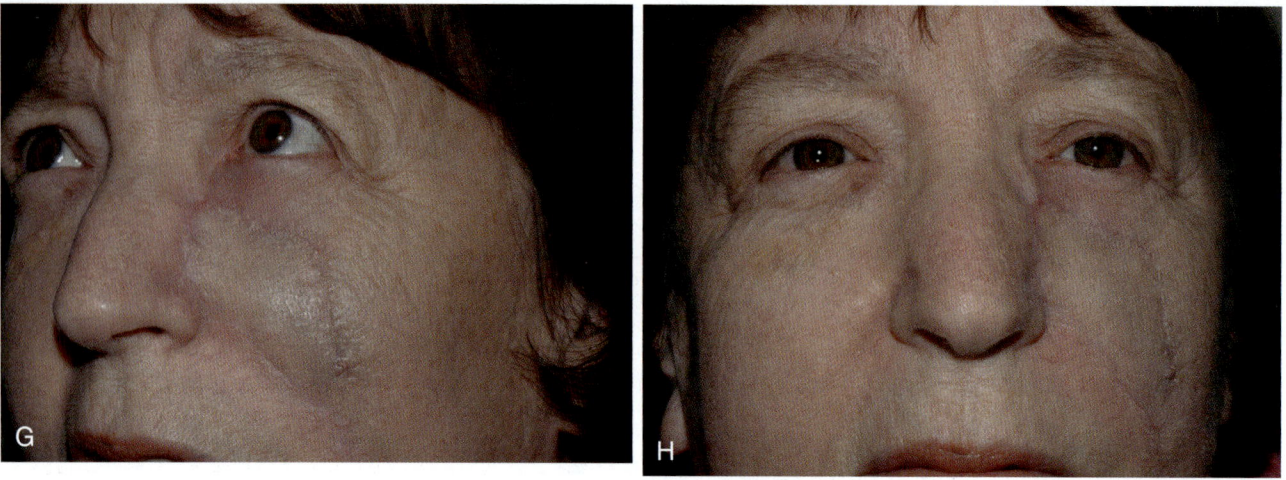

Fig. 13.9, cont'd (G, H) Healed result 6 months postoperatively. (Courtesy of Steven Chow, MD.)

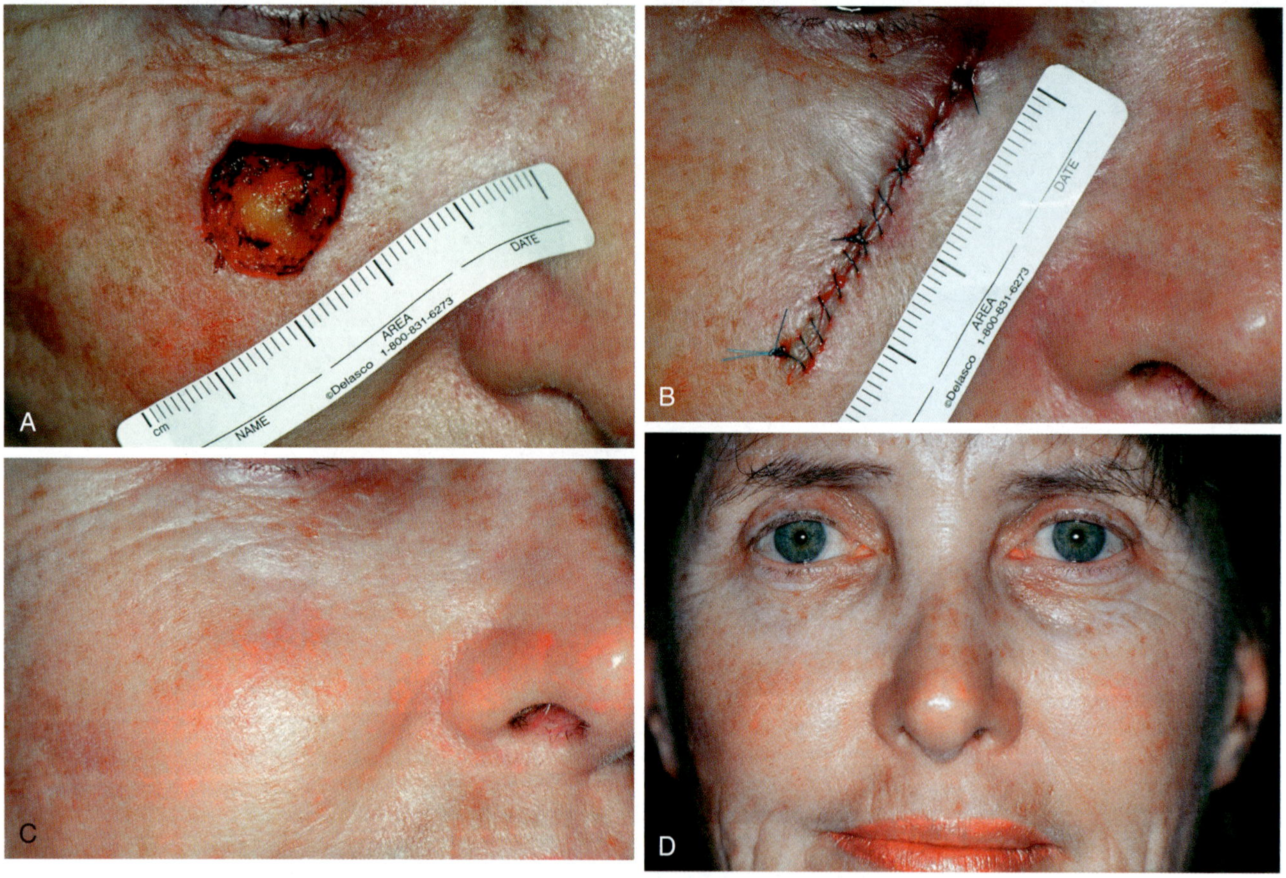

Fig. 13.10 (A) Elliptical wound on anterior cheek with long axis oriented vertically. (B) Side-to-side repair; note running over-and-over sutures. (C, D) Healed result 1 year postoperatively.

the rhombic flap (Fig. 13.11) and the rhombic flap with two Z-plasties is useful (Fig. 13.12). For large defects, a single lobe transposition flap may be considered (Fig. 13.13). The flap may be superiorly based as shown in Fig. 13.13 or inferiorly based.[13,20] Also, as on the medial cheek, a cheek rotation advancement flap may be considered, especially if the defect is large.

INFRAORBITAL CHEEK

This area of the cheek can be a difficult area to repair. It is important to stress that although the transition from the lower eyelid onto the infraorbital cheek seems to be gradual, in many individuals there is a well-defined zone of sebaceous skin on the cheek and smooth skin on the upper

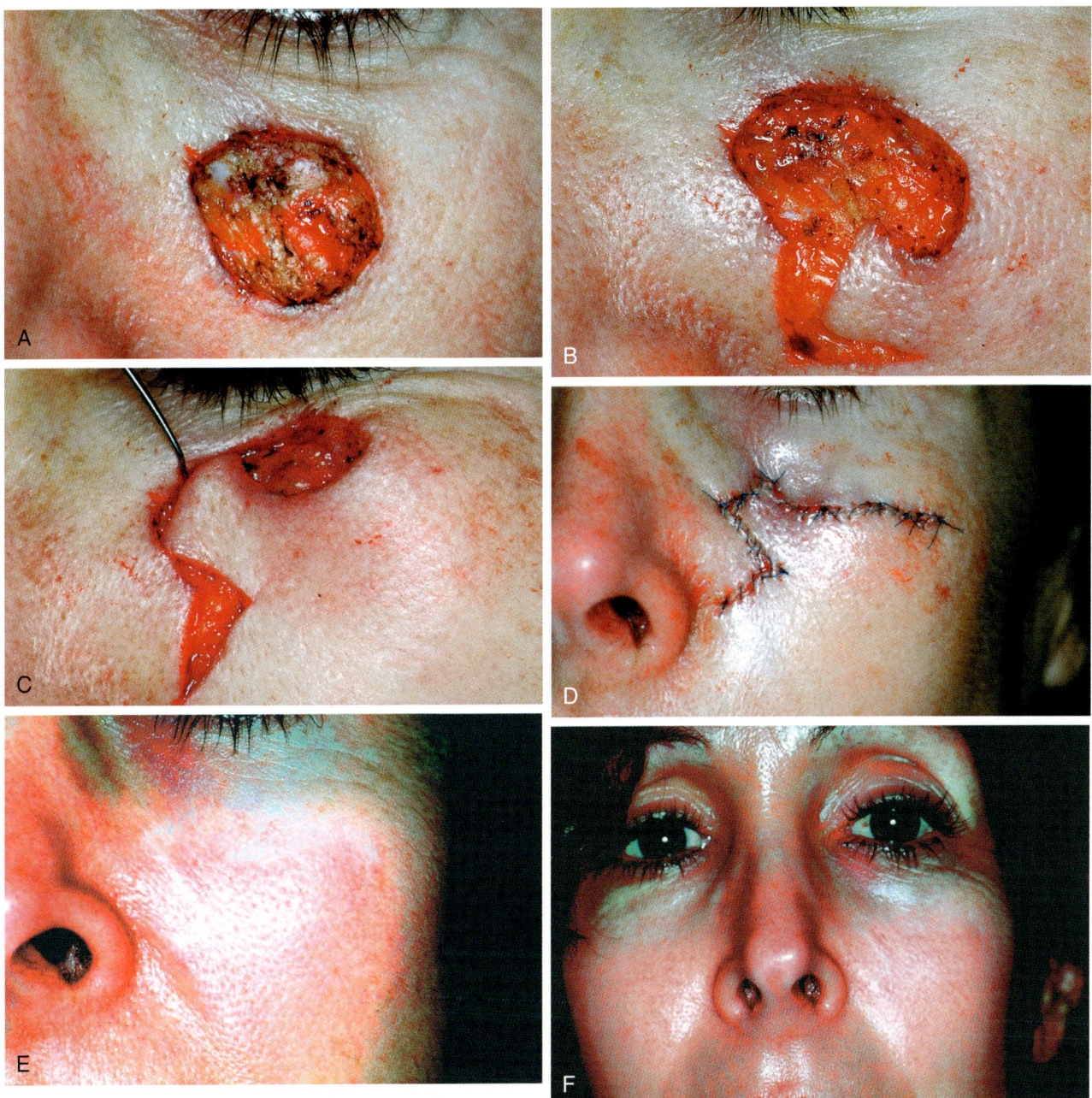

Fig. 13.11 (A) Round wound on anterior cheek. (B) Rhombic flap cut and undermined. (C) Rhombic flap transposed into defect. (D) Rhombic flap sutured into place. (E, F) Healed result 1 year postoperatively. Note slight noticeable scar at leading edge of rhombic flap.

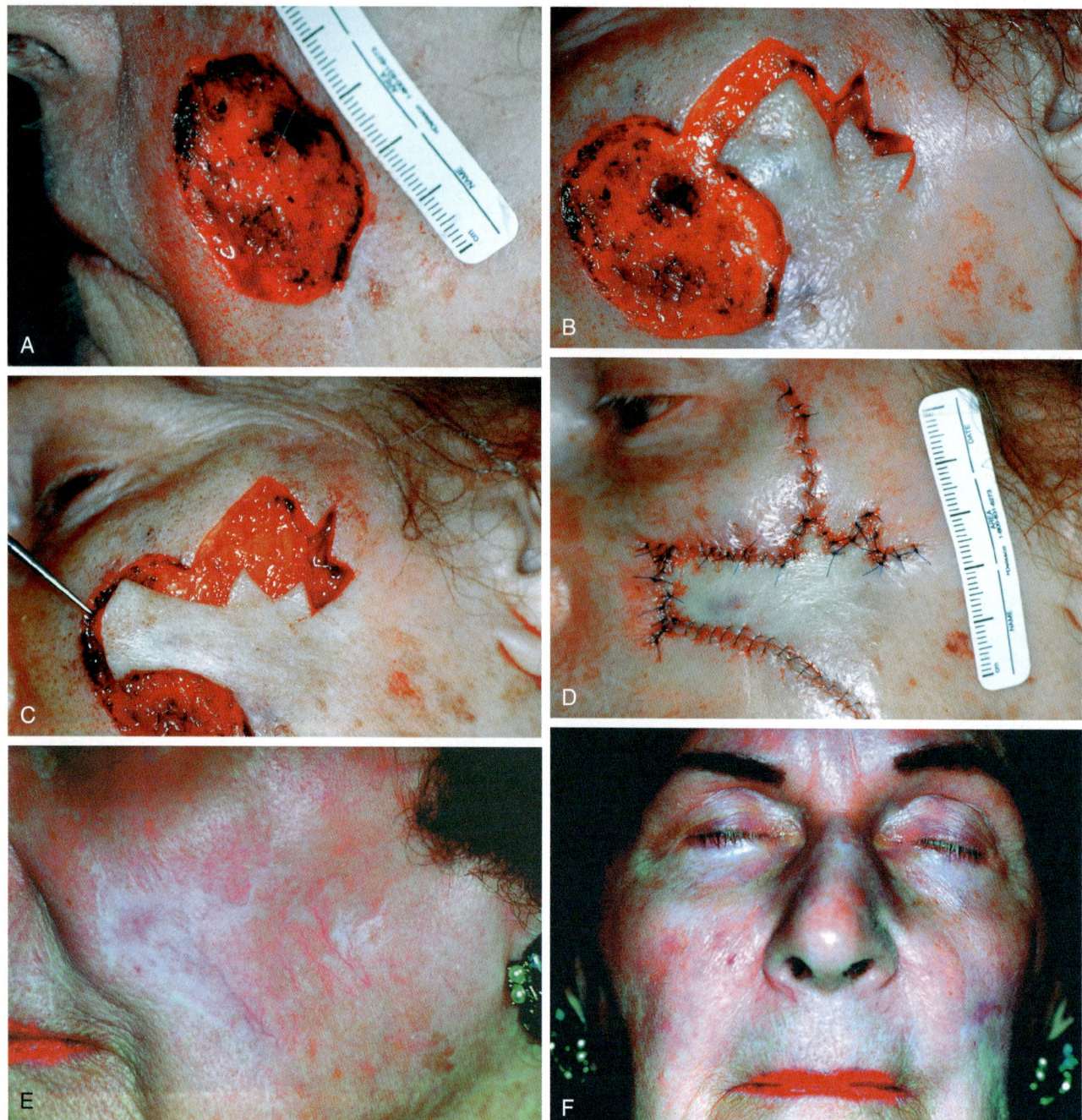

Fig. 13.12 (A) Round wound on anterior cheek. (B) Rhombic flap with double Z-plasty. (C) Rhombic flap transposed into defect. (D) Rhombic flap sutured into place. (E, F) Healed result 1 year postoperatively. Note the telangiectasias on flap.

eyelid. Here it is best to keep the sebaceous skin in one area and the smooth eyelid skin in its area. If a wound includes a significant part of the lower eyelid in addition to the cheek, it is often preferable to use a full-thickness skin graft to repair the eyelid part of a wound and a cheek flap to repair the cheek part of the wound.

MALAR CHEEK

The malar cheek can also be closed linearly or with either a rotation/advancement flap (Fig. 13.14) or a transposition flap (Fig. 13.15). The latter flap type can be combined with a full-thickness skin graft (Fig. 13.16) or a Tripier flap (Fig. 13.17) if the malar wound extends into the lower eyelid. The dynamics of closure in this area are similar to those on the medial cheek. Care needs to be taken to avoid damaging the temporal branch of the facial nerve, which is superficial in this area. When close to the lateral canthus, one should place tacking sutures to prevent distorting the lower lid and creating an ectropion.

Text continued on p. 201

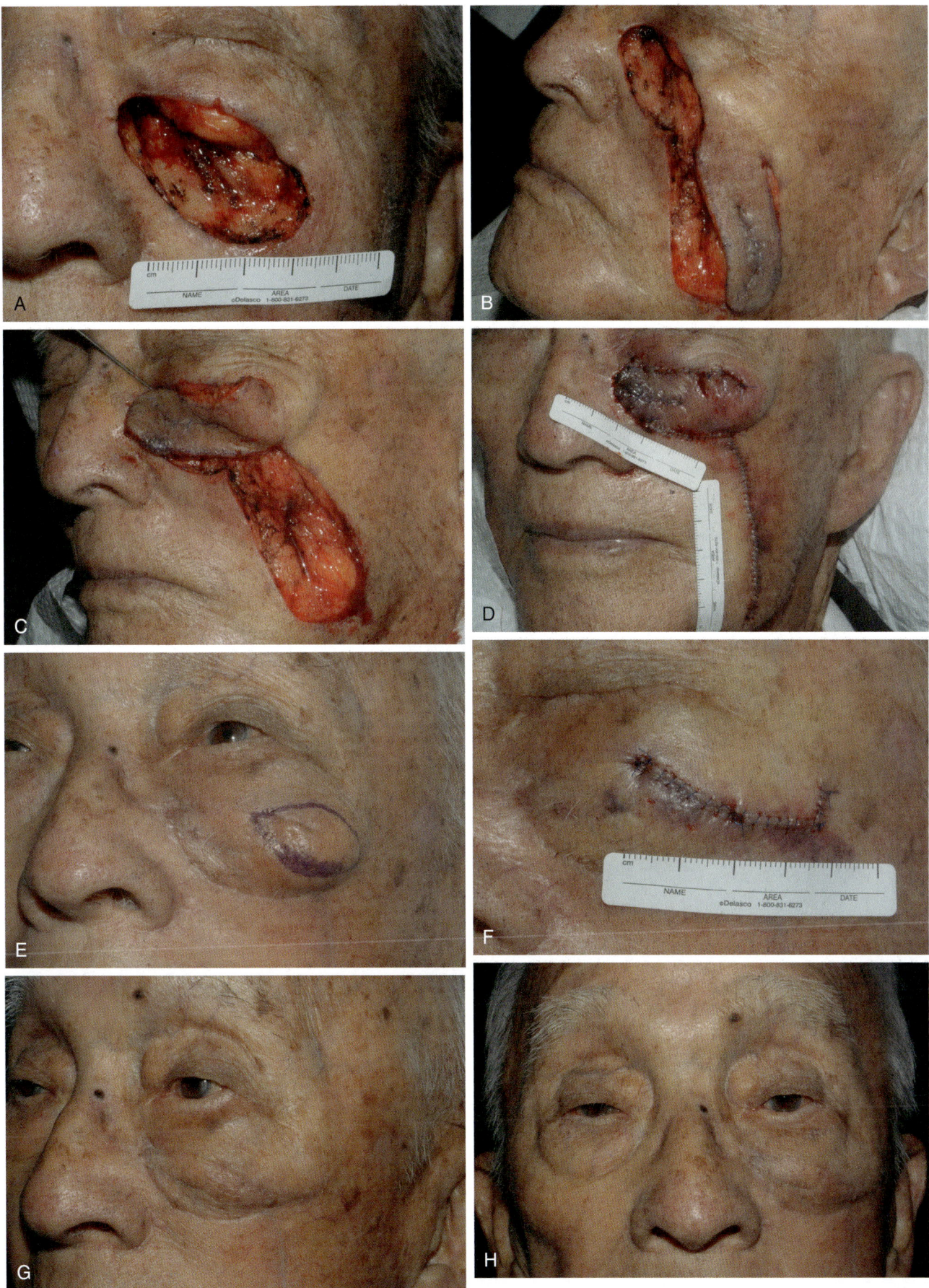

Fig. 13.13 (A) Deep wound on anterior cheek extending to periorbital fat superiorly. (B) Single lobe transposition flap incised and undermined. Note direction of flap along relaxed skin tension lines (RSTLs). Flap cut with adequate amount of underlying fat to support lower eyelid. Base of flap not undermined but left attached to underlying muscles to ensure good blood supply. (C) Flap rotated and transposed. (D) Flap sutured into place. Note large lateral standing cone (dog-ear). (E, F) Standing cone (dog-ear) excised. (G, H) Healed result 3 months after standing cone (dog-ear) excised.

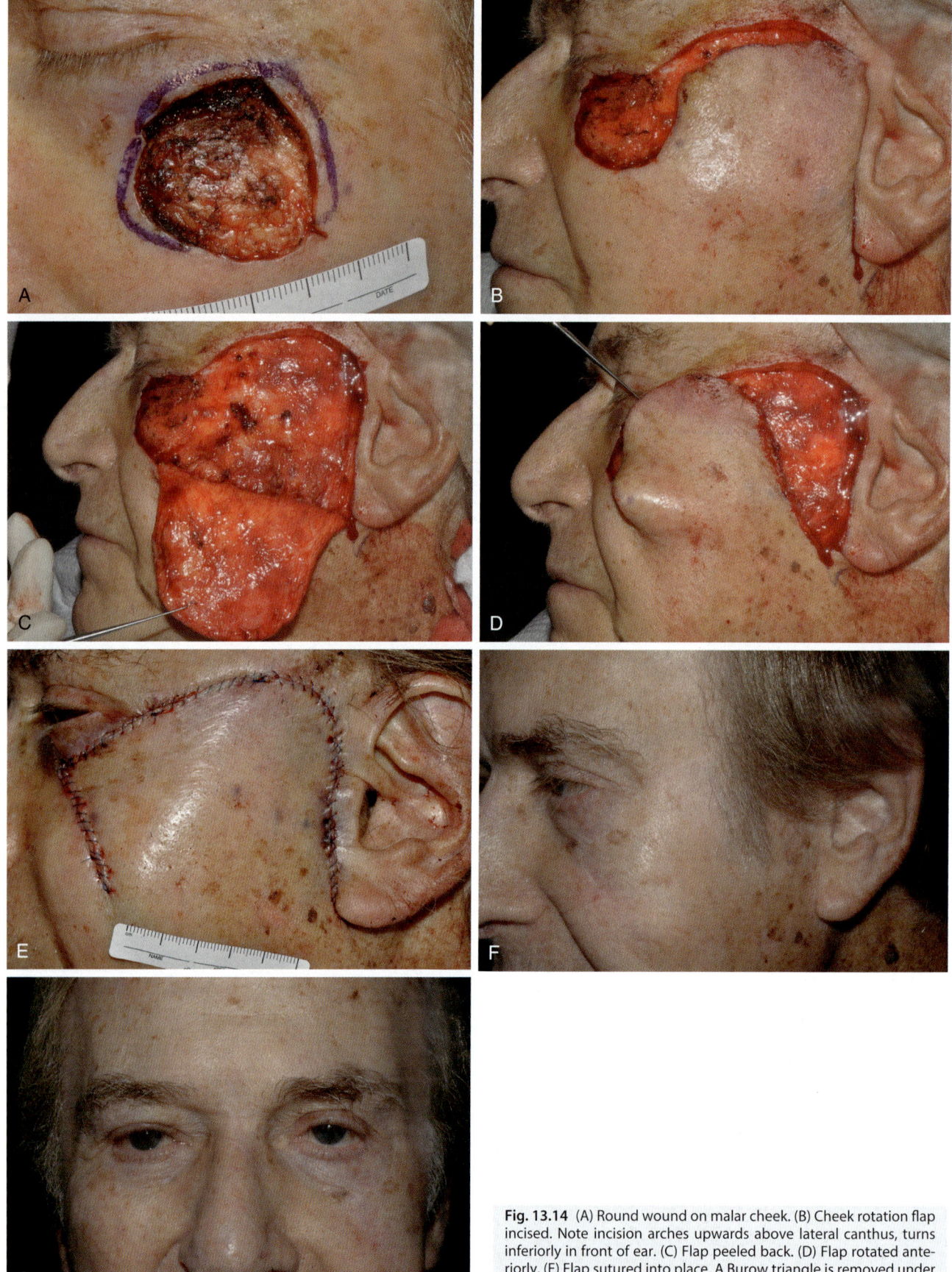

Fig. 13.14 (A) Round wound on malar cheek. (B) Cheek rotation flap incised. Note incision arches upwards above lateral canthus, turns inferiorly in front of ear. (C) Flap peeled back. (D) Flap rotated anteriorly. (E) Flap sutured into place. A Burow triangle is removed under ear lobule. (F, G) Healed result 1 year postoperatively.

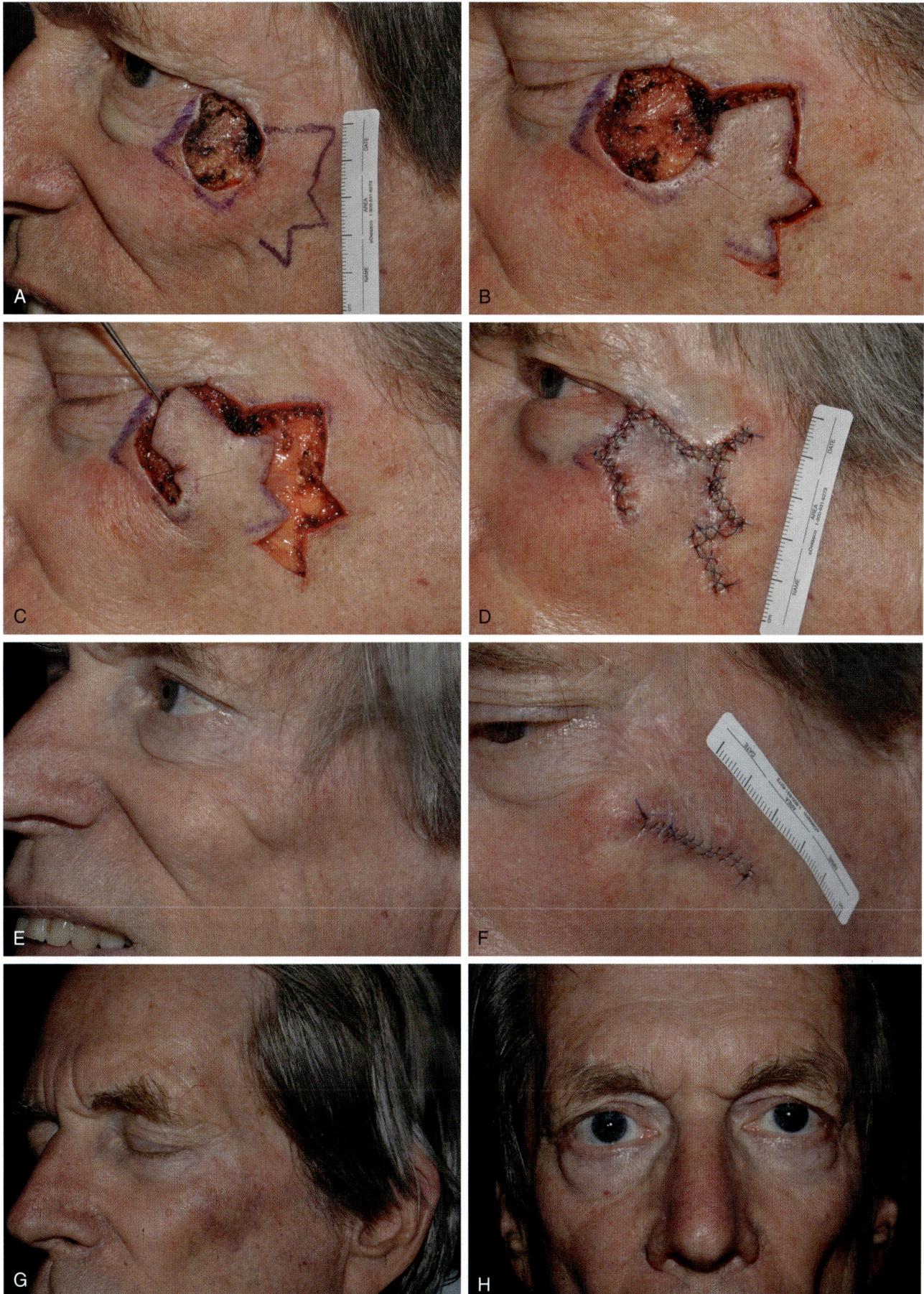

Fig. 13.15 (A) Round wound on malar cheek. (B) Rhombic flap with two Z-plasties incised and undermined. (C) Flap rotated and transposed into wound. (D) Flap sutured into place. (E, F) Standing cone (dog-ear) excised 3 months postoperatively. (G, H) Healed result 3 months after standing cone excision.

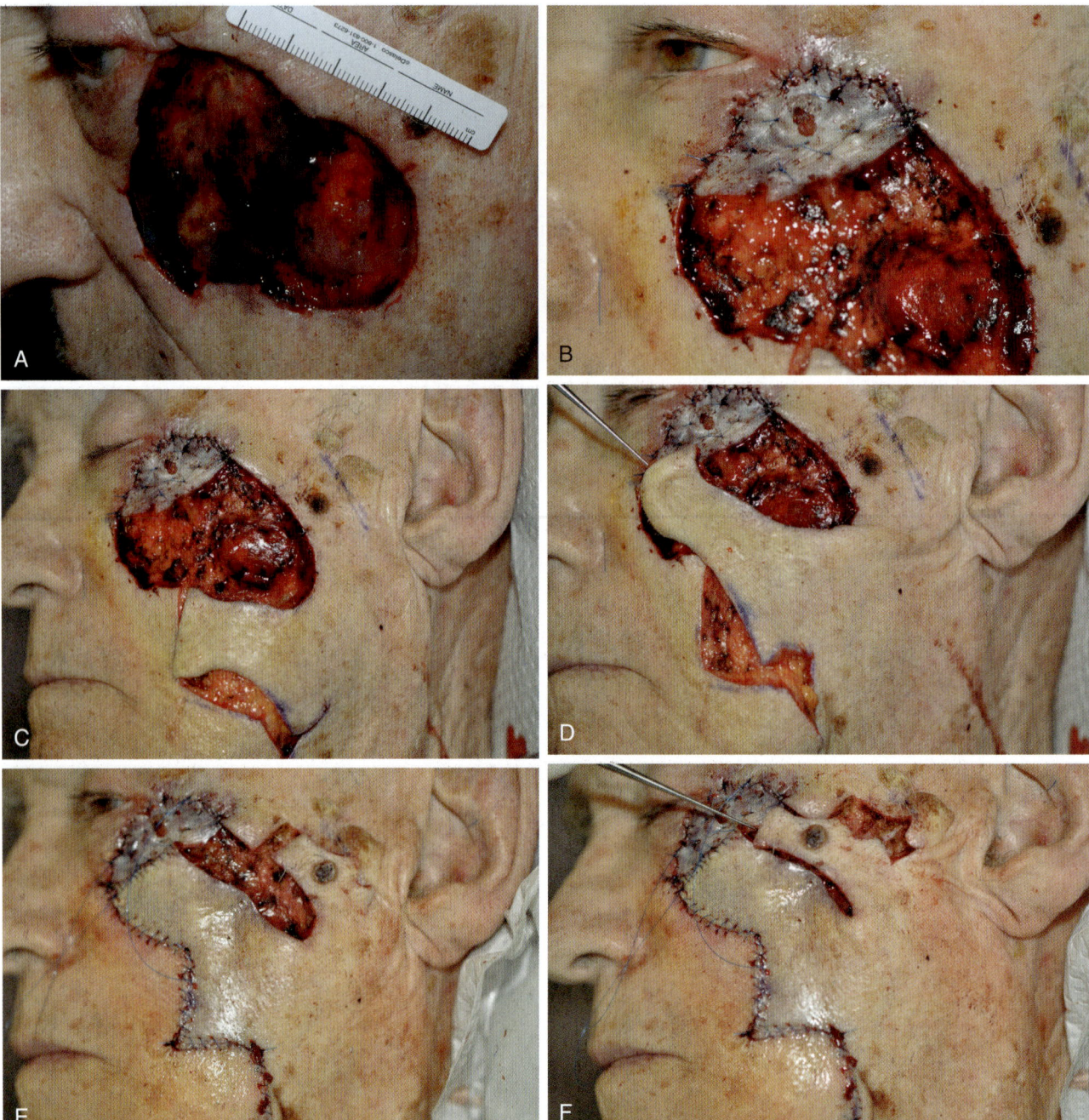

Fig. 13.16 (A) Large wound of malar, anterior, and lateral cheek. In addition, wound extends above orbital rim and includes lateral lower eyelid. (B) Full-thickness supraclavicular skin graft placed on portion of wound above the orbital rim. (C) Rhombic flap with one Z-plasty incised and undermined. (D) Rhombic flap with one Z-plasty transposed into wound. (E) After rhombic flap with one Z-plasty sutured into wound, it was necessary to incise a second flap from above because of tension. Thus a rhombic flap with two Z-plasties was incised and (F) transposed into superior portion of wound.

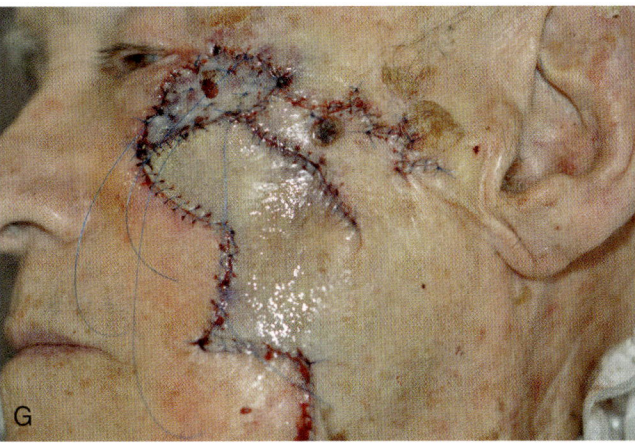
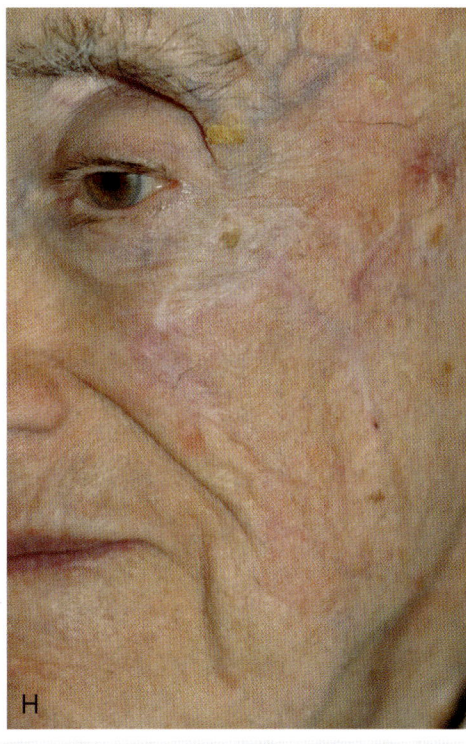

Fig. 13.16, cont'd (G) Second flap sutured into place. (H) Healed result 1 year postoperatively. (Courtesy of Steven Chow, MD.)

If the wound is small in this area, a Burow wedge advancement flap may be done. An incision is made laterally and the Burow triangle taken out lateral to the lateral canthus.[39]

BUCCAL CHEEK

A buccal cheek wound can be repaired linearly if small or if large with a rotation flap, a rhombic flap, a single-lobe transposition flap, or a bilobe transposition flap.

PREAURICULAR CHEEK

Fortunately in this area, even large wounds can often be closed side to side (Fig. 13.18). In this area the SMAS is continuous, and one can take advantage of this by folding (plicating) the SMAS upon itself, as shown in Fig. 13.19.[40] This effectively partially closes the wound (see Fig. 13.19D) and takes tension off the wound edge. The rotation advancement (or the Burow wedge advancement) flap may be useful for small or medium-sized wounds in this area. For the latter flap, an incision is made inferiorly along the preauricular crease and a Burow triangle removed inferior and posterior to the earlobe. The flap is advanced superiorly. The Burow wedge advancement flap helps preserve the cosmetically significant preauricular hairless area in men. Occasionally large preauricular wounds may be closed with a transposition flap. Generally the rhombic flap is inferiorly based.

Very large wounds in the preauricular cheek may be repaired with a cervical neck flap from below or a postauricular banner transposition flap (Fig. 13.20).[41] The posterior auricular transposition flap uses nonhair-bearing skin. An incision is made posterior to the earlobe superiorly along the postauricular sulcus; it is then arched superiorly and descends along the lateral posterior hairline. It utilizes the thin skin overlying the superficial cervical fascia covering the sternocleidomastoid muscles and the posterior auricular muscles. The flap base is posterior to the angle of the mandible and over the sternocleidomastoid muscle. The platysma muscle is present at the inferior and anterior portion of the flap base. The flap is richly vascularized in its subdermal plexus by vessels originating in the thyroid branch of the external carotid artery. Also, there are muscle perforators supplying the flap after coming through the sternocleidomastoid muscle. The dissection is done inferiorly above the platysma so that the cervical and marginal mandibular branches of the facial nerve are not injured. The posterior auricular flap is transposed over the ear to the preauricular cheek.

MANDIBULAR CHEEK

Wounds in this area are generally repaired linearly or with a transposition flap, usually a posterior and inferiorly based rhombic flap. A bilobe flap may also occasionally be useful (Fig. 13.21). Care should be taken to avoid damaging the marginal mandibular nerve when undermining in this area. Advancement/rotation flaps are generally not useful in the mandibular cheek. When closures cross the convex surface at the mandibular cheek–neck border, it helps to incorporate an S-plasty into the closure. This redirects wound contracture tension from going across the convexity and reduces the risk of having an indented (tethered) scar across the convex mandibular area.

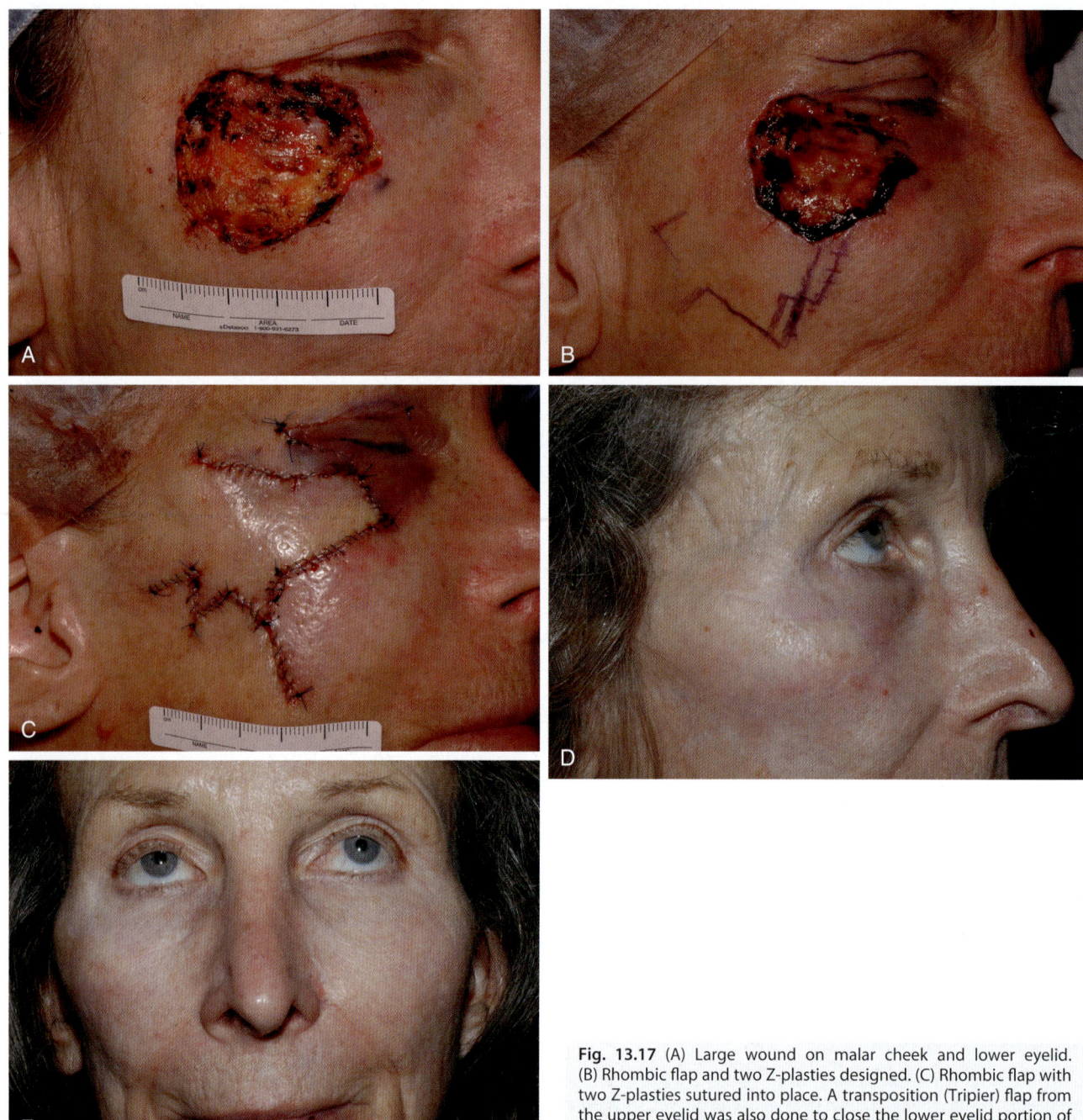

Fig. 13.17 (A) Large wound on malar cheek and lower eyelid. (B) Rhombic flap and two Z-plasties designed. (C) Rhombic flap with two Z-plasties sutured into place. A transposition (Tripier) flap from the upper eyelid was also done to close the lower eyelid portion of the wound. (D, E) Healed result 2 years postoperatively.

Complications

HEMATOMA

Generally bleeding is minimal in the cheek area after flaps. However, for patients on anticoagulants or aspirin, excessive purpura may occur and the skin may turn purple all the way into the neck. Although this event may look scary, patients should be reassured that the discoloration will go away in a week or so; this persistent swelling may take many months to resolve.

EYELID SWELLING

Perhaps the most common problem after cheek repairs, especially on the anterior and medial cheek, is eyelid swelling. This problem occurs particularly in the elderly. The lymphatic drainage occurs laterally and inferiorly on the cheek. As the cheek is pulled tight to close a wound, the tension creates a temporary damming effect and the eyelid lymphatics cannot drain normally. Usually the patient will first notice eyelid swelling the morning after surgery. It will be worse on the second morning after surgery and then

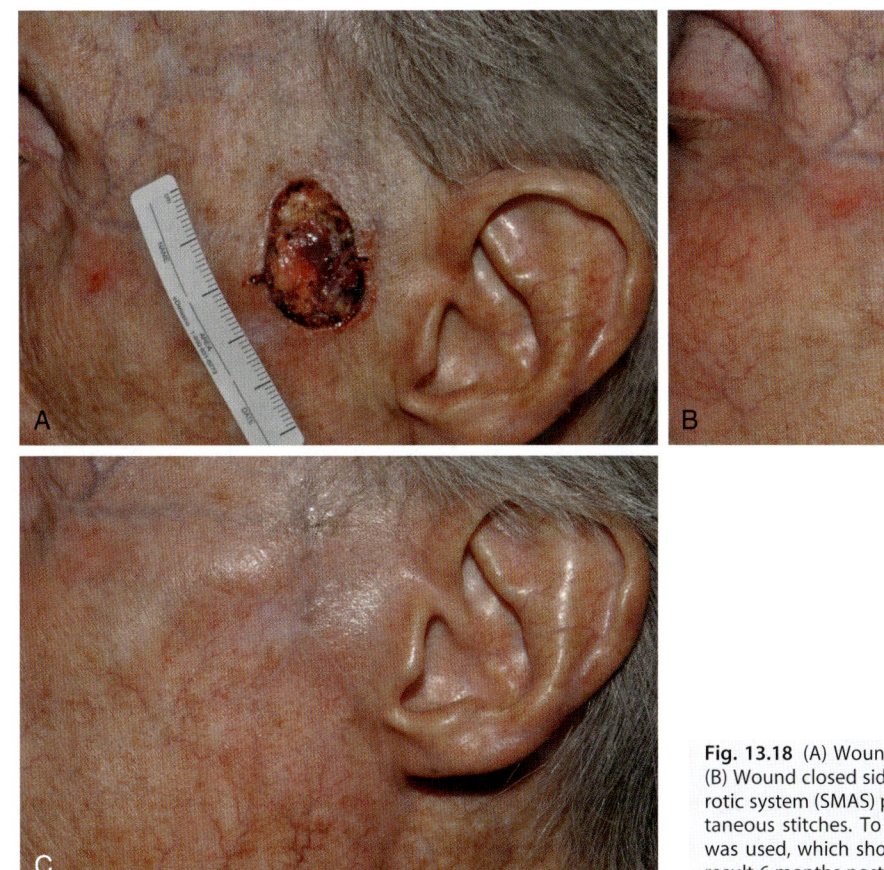

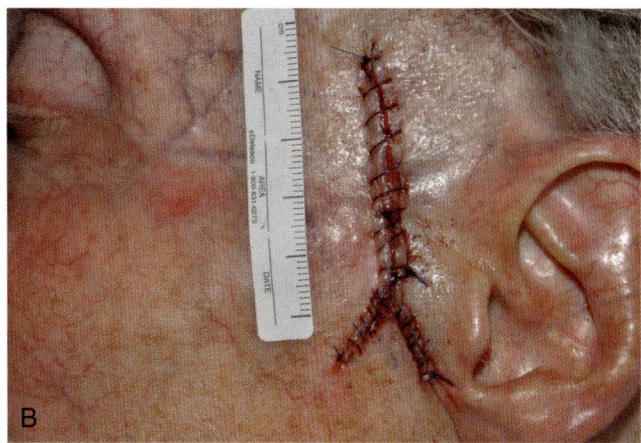

Fig. 13.18 (A) Wound in preauricular cheek with vertical long axis. (B) Wound closed side-to-side in three layers: submuscular aponeurotic system (SMAS) plication, dermal-subcutaneous stitches, percutaneous stitches. To remove standing cone inferiorly, an M-plasty was used, which shortens the incision in that direction. (C) Healed result 6 months postoperatively.

generally regresses thereafter so that the swelling is gone by the time of suture removal. It is wise to inform patients of the likelihood of eyelid swelling. Whether it can be diminished by use of a cold pack has not been shown, but some physicians believe this to be true. Occasionally some eyelid edema may be long-standing following incisions made along the cosmetic unit junction between the lower eyelid and cheek.

FLAP NECROSIS

This problem occurs usually because of inadequate vascularization and/or excessive flap tension. Deep plane dissection on large flaps may help avoid this problem. When flap necrosis occurs, it is important to keep the necrotic tissue moist. It is very difficult to ascertain the depth of the necrosis when it first appears. If there is only partial-thickness necrosis (down to the upper reticular dermis) and the wound is kept moist, the flap will heal almost as if there had been no necrosis. However, if the necrotic area is allowed to dry out, more tissue loss will occur and noticeable scar tissue will result. Patients on warfarin (Coumadin) are more likely to show flap necrosis. Smoking is also commonly thought to contribute to flap necrosis. However, it is only high levels of smoking (greater than one pack/day) that have been shown to have a significant effect.[42]

ECTROPION

Lid displacement may occur because of edema, lid ptosis, flap tension, and denervation of the orbicularis oculi muscle. This is generally prevented by using tacking sutures and by ensuring a high arc lateral to the lateral canthus for cheek rotation flaps. The lateral superior border should be above the lateral canthal-helical plane.[11] If an ectropion persists after cheek surgery, it may be necessary to perform a canthopexy or place a full-thickness skin graft into the lower eyelid between the flap and lid margin to correct the problem.

INFECTION

As with other areas of the face, infection in cheek flaps is quite rare. Should this problem occur, a culture should be done and appropriate antibiotics given. Two organisms that might be overlooked are methicillin-resistant *Staphylococcus aureus* (MRSA) and atypical mycobacterium.

DEHISCENCE

If a flap is well designed and executed, dehiscence generally does not occur. However, if a flap is sutured in very sebaceous skin, the percutaneous sutures may tear through the

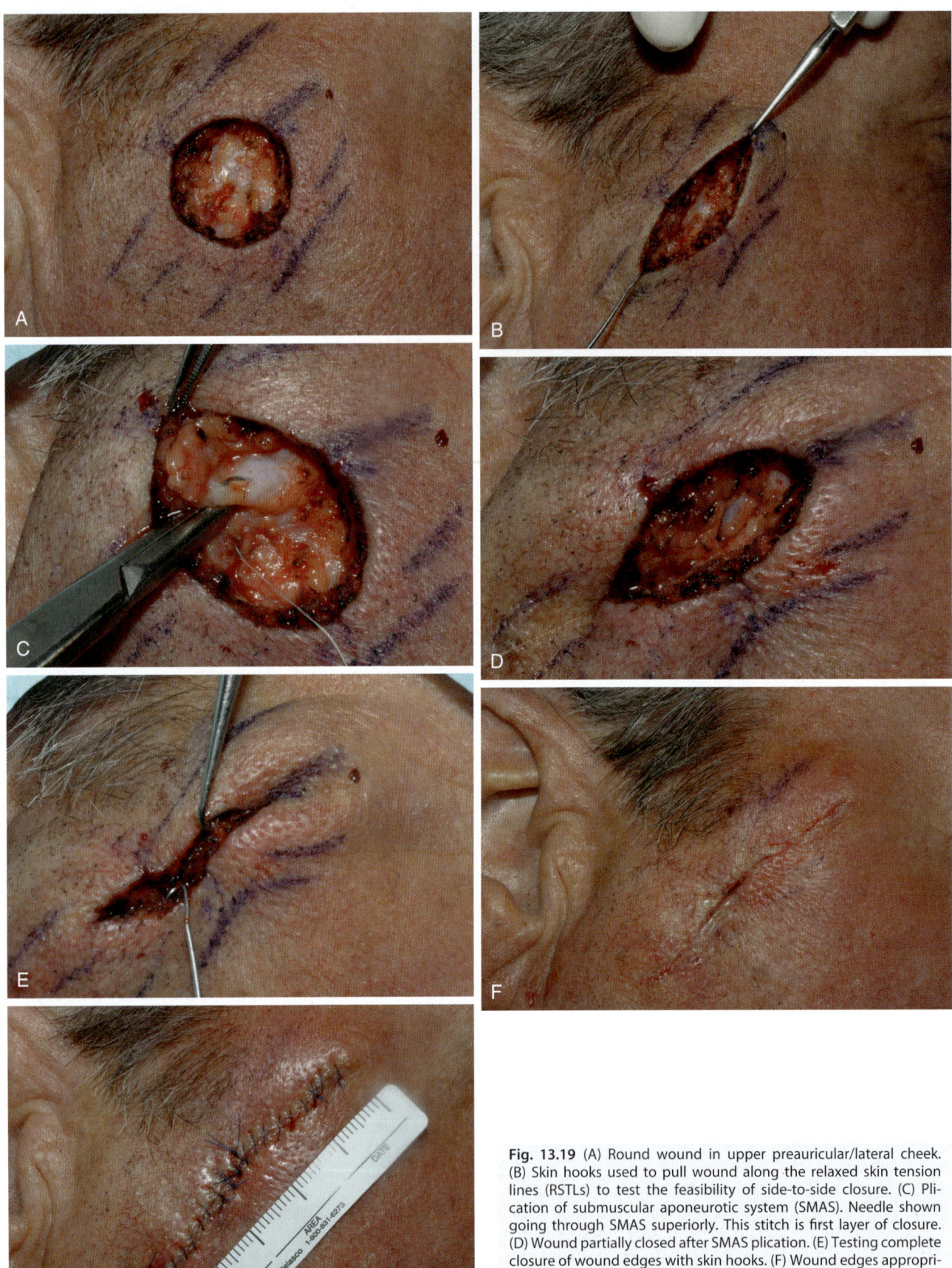

Fig. 13.19 (A) Round wound in upper preauricular/lateral cheek. (B) Skin hooks used to pull wound along the relaxed skin tension lines (RSTLs) to test the feasibility of side-to-side closure. (C) Plication of submuscular aponeurotic system (SMAS). Needle shown going through SMAS superiorly. This stitch is first layer of closure. (D) Wound partially closed after SMAS plication. (E) Testing complete closure of wound edges with skin hooks. (F) Wound edges appropriated with second layer of stitches (dermal-subcutaneous suture). Standing cones have been removed. (G) Wound completely closed with third layer of stitches (percutaneous stitches).

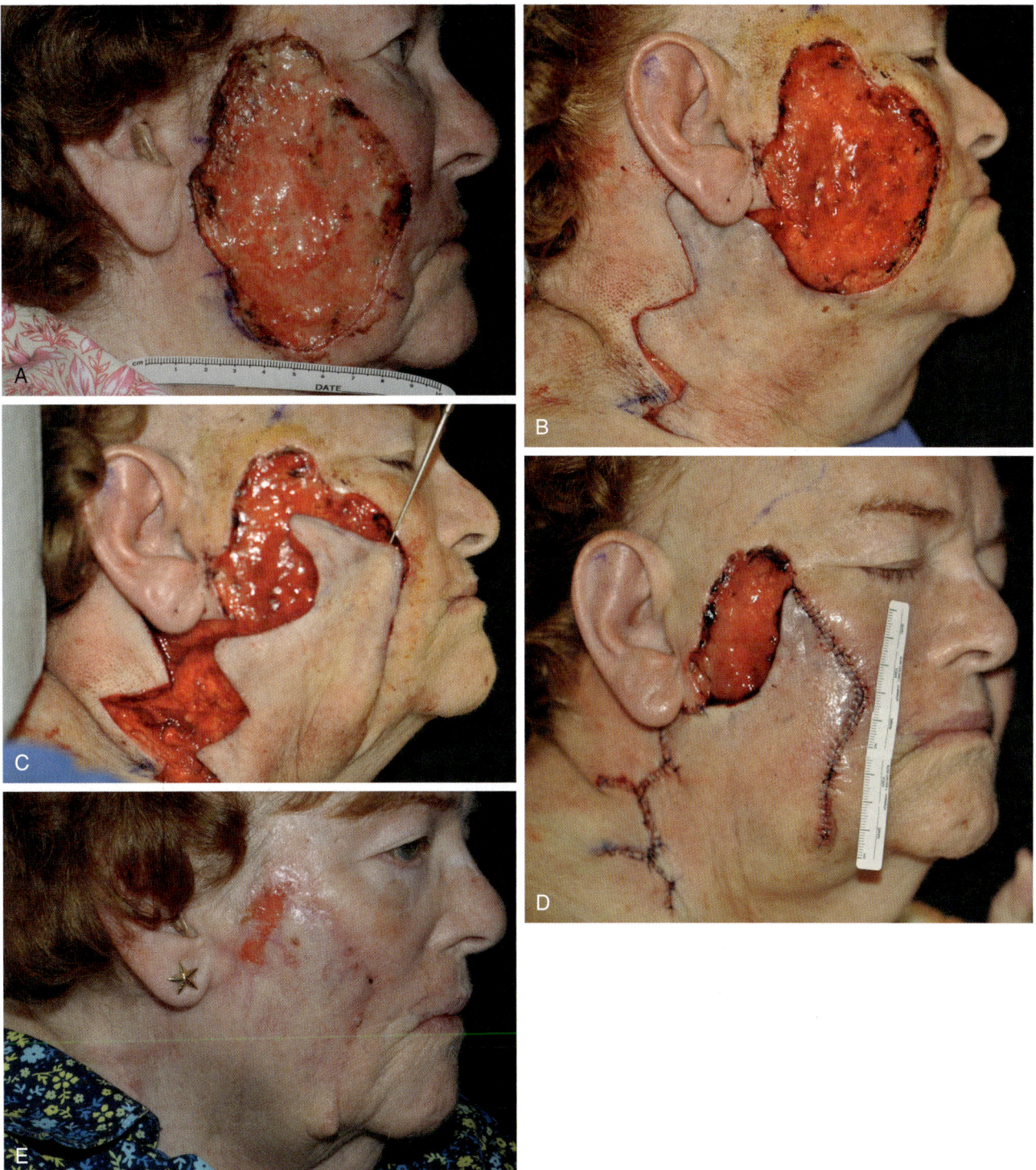

Fig. 13.20 (A) Large wound on lateral anterior and mandibular cheek. (B) Rhombic flap incised from behind ear with two Z-plasties added to enhance from movement. This flap could be considered a trilobe flap or trirhombic flap. (C) Flap rotated and transposed into wound. (D) Flap sutured into place. Note preauricular portion of wound still open. It will be left to heal by granulation. Note that had greater tissue from the postauricular area been incorporated into the flap in (B), the whole cheek wound could have been closed and granulation would have been unnecessary. (E) Preauricular wound almost healed 6 weeks postoperatively. Note standing cone on mandibular cheek that will be excised.

Continued

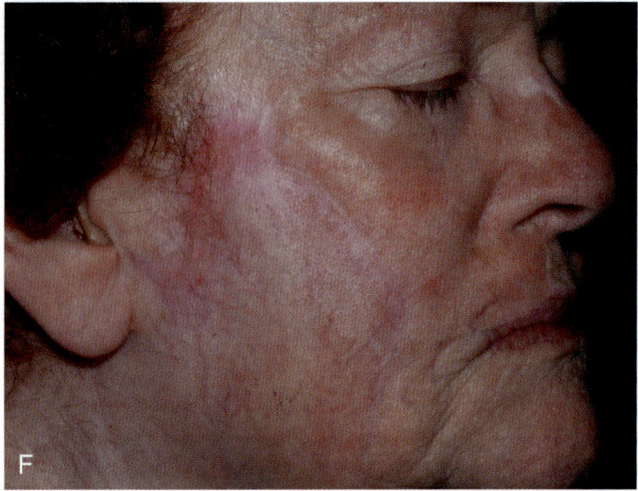
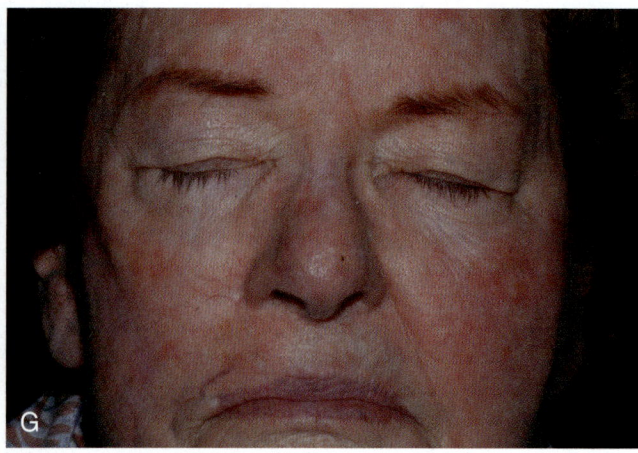

Fig. 13.20, cont'd (F, G) Healed result 1 year postoperatively.

skin easily. This problem can usually be avoided by placing good buried vertical mattress sutures, as well as some cutaneous vertical mattress sutures in this type of skin.

PAROTID FISTULA

Occasionally when operating beneath the parotid fascia, the parotid duct may be nicked or transected. If this occurs, salivary gland leakage occurs, especially when the patient eats or drinks. There are several possible treatment options, which include cannulation with parotid duct repair, duct ligation, tympanic neurectomy with or without chordi tympani section, irradiation of the gland, and even superficial parotidectomy. However, the best course of action is often to wait. In a series of cases of parotid duct and gland injury with salivary leakage, all cases treated conservatively dried up within a short period of time, usually in 3 to 5 weeks.[6] Use of a Jackson-Pratt drain under the flap will lessen accumulation of drainage and make the patient more comfortable (Fig. 13.22). It may be possible to prevent a parotid fistula by suturing SMAS over a parotid defect.[43]

HYPERTROPHIC SCARRING AND KELOID FORMATION

These problems are rare on the cheek. However, when this occurs, usually one or two injections of 10 mg of triamcinolone acetonide (Kenalog) given a month apart generally resolves the problem. Intralesional 5-Fluorouracil injections and pulsed-dye laser treatments have also been shown to be effective in the treatment of hypertrophic scars.

ANESTHESIA

Because of the abundant nerve interconnections in the cheek, anesthesia is rarely seen after flap surgery. Furthermore, if some anesthesia does occur, it generally recedes fairly quickly.

MOTOR NERVE DEFICITS

Motor nerves are generally located deep on the cheek and are rarely injured during surgery in this area. The two possible motor nerves that may be injured are the marginal mandibular branch and the temporal branch of the facial nerve. If one is careful in undermining, these nerves are unlikely to be damaged.

TELANGIECTASIA

Flap tension tends to induce persistent noticeable telangiectasias over and around skin flaps, which occur particularly in those who have rosacea or in women taking exogenous estrogen. Vascular lasers, such as the pulsed-dye laser (PDL) (595 nm) (Vbeam; Candela Corp, Wayland, Massachusetts) and the potassium titanyl phosphate (KTP) laser (532 nm) (Aura; Laserscope, San Jose, California), which treat telangiectasia, can be very useful in eliminating these vessels.

INNER CANTHUS TENTING

Occasionally cheek flaps result in inner canthus tenting. This results from tension in the vertical plane from poor flap design or excessive scar contraction in a downward direction. Although this may improve or even resolve with time, massage and injection of triamcinolone acetonide into the contracted scar tissue may speed the resolution. However, if after a judicious period of waiting the ectropion does not resolve, further surgery may be indicated. Either a V-to-Y-plasty or a Z-plasty is most frequently performed to correct canthal tenting.

Conclusion

Optimal closure of cheek defects requires knowledge of the various flaps types available and where best to place incisions so that the patient will have the fewest number of incisions possible and the least noticeable scar. Fortunately,

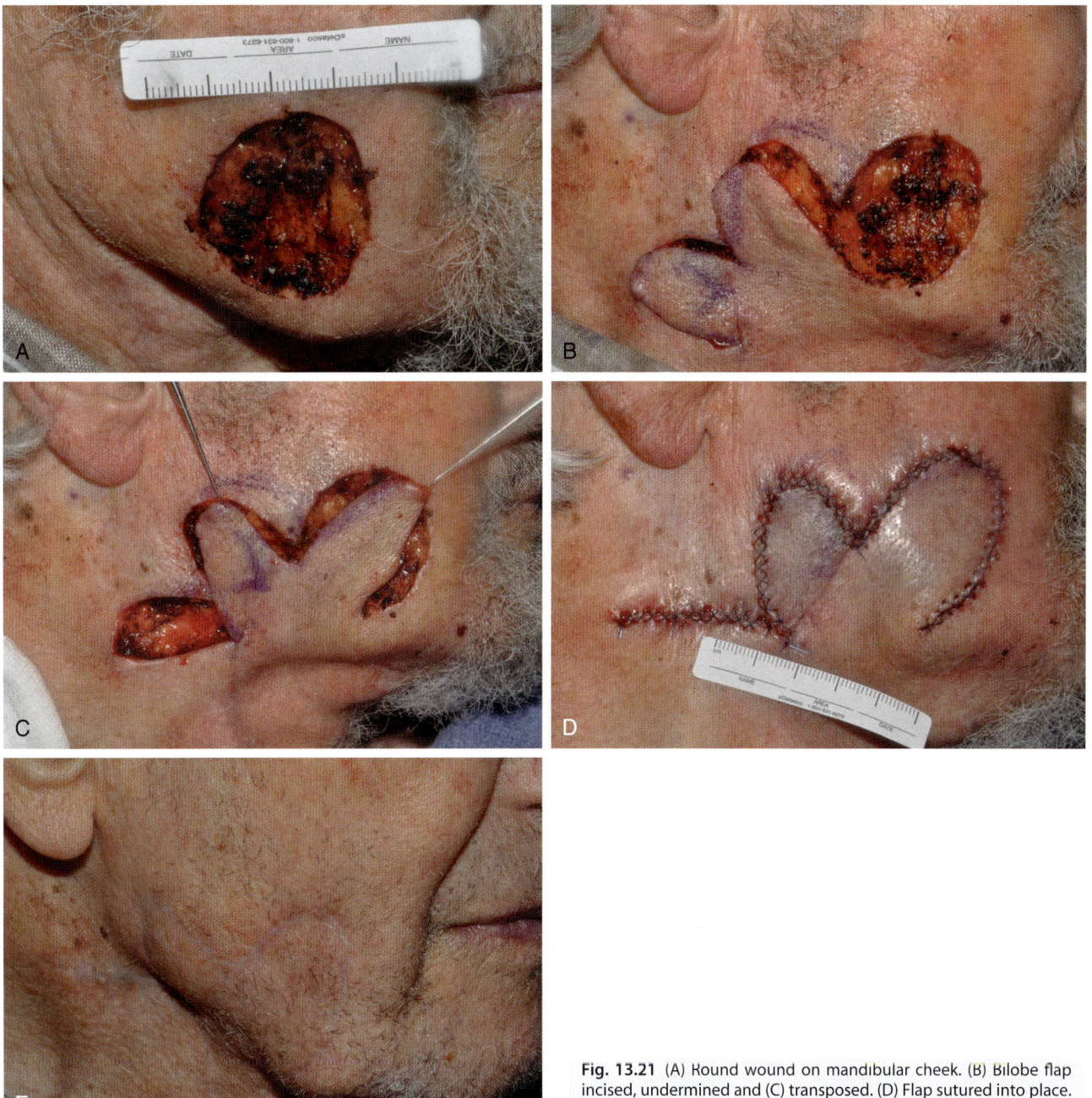

Fig. 13.21 (A) Round wound on mandibular cheek. (B) Bilobe flap incised, undermined and (C) transposed. (D) Flap sutured into place. (E) Healed result 6 months postoperatively.

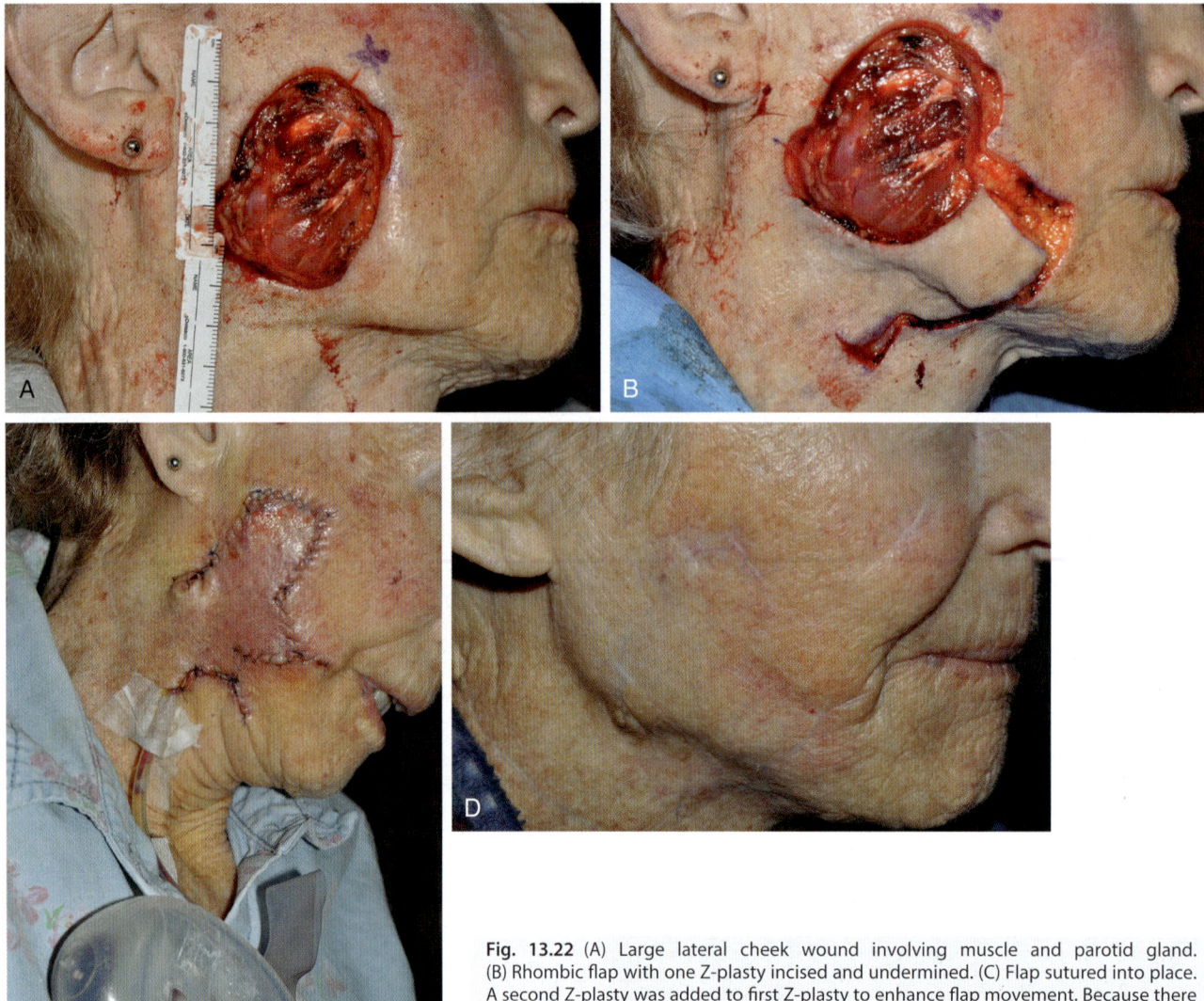

Fig. 13.22 (A) Large lateral cheek wound involving muscle and parotid gland. (B) Rhombic flap with one Z-plasty incised and undermined. (C) Flap sutured into place. A second Z-plasty was added to first Z-plasty to enhance flap movement. Because there was salivary gland leakage at the time of closure, a Jackson-Pratt drain was inserted under flap to prevent accumulation of salivary gland fluid under the flap. The drain was pulled in 1 week. (D) Healed result 6 months postoperatively. (Courtesy of Steven Chow, MD.)

the abundance of mobile cheek tissue allows for most defects to be repaired with excellent cosmetic outcomes. As with all cosmetic units, understanding the regional anatomy and the various repair options available allows the physician to make the appropriate choice for the individual patient.

References

1. Dzubow LM, Zack L. The principle of cosmetic junctions as applied to reconstruction of defects following Mohs surgery. *J Dermatol Surg Oncol.* 1990;16:353-355.
2. Gonzalez-Ulloa M, Castillo A, Stevens E, Alvarez Fuertes G, Leonelli F, Ubaldo F. Preliminary study of the total restoration of facial skin. *Plast Reconstr Surg.* 1954;13:151-161.
3. Burget GC, Menick FJ. The subunit principle in nasal reconstruction. *Plast Reconst Surg.* 1985;76:239-247.
4. Thaller SR, Kim S, Patterson H, Wildman M, Daniller A. The submuscular aponeurotic system (SMAS): a histologic and comparative anatomy evaluation. *Plast Reconst Surg.* 1990;86:690-696.
5. Hollinshead WH. *Anatomy for Surgeons.* Vol 1. 3rd ed. *The Head and Neck.* Philadelphia: Harper and Row Publishers; 1982.
6. Landau R, Stewart M. Conservative management of post-traumatic parotid fistulae and sialoceles: a prospective study. *Brit J Surg.* 1985;72:42-44.
7. Ebrahimi A, Ashaveri M, Rasouli HR. Comparison of local flaps and skin grafts to repair cheek skin defects. *J Cutan Aesthet Surg.* 2015;8(2):92-96.
8. Smith F. Collective review. Flaps utilized in facial and cervical reconstruction. *Plast Reconstr Surg.* 1951;7:415-455.
9. New GB, Figi FA. The repair of postoperative defects involving the lips and cheeks secondary to malignant tumors. *Surg Gynecol Obstet.* 1936;62:182-190.
10. Menick FJ. Discussion: simplifying cheek reconstruction: a review of over 400 cases. *Plast Reconstr Surg.* 2012;129:1300-1303.
11. Menick FJ. Reconstruction of the cheek. *Plast Reconst Surg.* 2001;108:496-504.
12. Larrabee WF Jr, Sherris DA. *Principles of Facial Reconstruction.* Philadelphia: Lippincott-Raven; 1995.
13. Jackson IT. *Local Flaps in Head and Neck Reconstruction.* St Louis, MO: Quality Medical; 2002.
14. Sugg KB, Cederna PS, Brown DL. The V-Y advancement flap is equivalent to the Mustardé flap for ectropion prevention in the reconstruction of moderate-size lid-cheek junction defects. *J Plast Reconstr Surg.* 2013;131:28e-36e.

15. Rappstein ED, Kraus WJ II, Thornton JF. Simplifying cheek reconstruction: a review of over 400 cases. *Plast Reconstr Surg.* 2012;129: 1291-1299.
16. Johnson SC, Bennett RG. Double Z-plasty to enhance rhombic flap mobility. *J Dermatol Surg Oncol.* 1994;20:128-132.
17. Borges AF. Choosing the correct Limberg flap. *Plast Reconstruct Surg.* 1978;62:542-545.
18. Borges AF. The rhombic flap. *Plast Reconst Surg.* 1981;67:458-466.
19. Becker FF. Rhomboid flap in facial reconstruction: new concept of tension lines. *Arch Otolaryngol.* 1979;105:569-573.
20. Cabrera RC, Zide BM. Cheek reconstruction. In: Aston SJ, Beasley RW, Thorne CHM, eds. *Grabb and Smith's Plastic Surgery.* 5th ed. Philadelphia: Lippincott-Raven; 1997:501-512.
21. Lewin JM, Sclafani AP, Carucci JA. An inferiorly based rotation flap for defects based on the lower eyelid and medial cheek. *Facial Plast Surg.* 2015;31:411-416.
22. Metzger JT. Joseph Imre and the Imre flap. *Plast Reconstr Surg.* 1959; 23:501-509.
23. Hussain W, Tan E, Salmon PJM. Inferiorly based crescentic sliding cheek flaps for the reconstruction of perinasal surgical defects. *Derm Surg.* 2012;38:249-255.
24. Jelks GW, Jelks EB. Prevention of ectropion in reconstruction of facial defects. *Clin Plast Surg.* 2001;28:297-302.
25. Regula CG, Liu A, Lawrence N. Versatility of the O-Z flap in the reconstruction of facial defects. *Derm Surg.* 2016;42:109-114.
26. Guerrerosantos J, Lopez-Luque J. Basal cell carcinoma of the cheek, malar region, and lower eyelid: the role of large cheek-neck flaps. *Ann Plast Surg.* 1988;20:304-312.
27. Mustardé JD. The use of flaps in the orbital region. *Plast Reconst Surg.* 1970;45:146-150.
28. de Cholnoky T. The repair of extensive soft tissue losses of the cheek. *Plast Reconst Surg.* 1955;16:288-291.
29. Cook TA, Israel JM, Wang TD, Murakami CS, Brownrigg PJ. Cervical rotation flaps for midface resurfacing. *Arch Otolaryngol Head Neck Surg.* 1991;117:77-82.
30. Juri J, Juri C. Advancement and rotation of a large cervicofacial flap for cheek repairs. *Plast Reconstr Surg.* 1979;64:692-696.
31. Patterson HC, Anonson C, Weymuller EA, Webster RC. The cheek-neck rotation flap for closure of temporo-zygomatic cheek wounds. *Arch Otolaryngol.* 1984;110:388-398.
32. Crow ML, Crow FJ. Resurfacing large cheek defects with rotation flaps from the neck. *Plast Reconstr Surg.* 1976;58:196-200.
33. Stark RB, Kaplan JM. Rotation flaps, neck to cheek. *Plast Reconst Surg.* 1972;50:230-233.
34. Katz AE, Grande DJ. Cheek-neck advancement-rotation flaps following Mohs excision of skin malignancies. *J Dermatol Surg Oncol.* 1986; 12:949-955.
35. Al-Shunnar B, Manson PN. Cheek reconstruction with laterally based flaps. *Clin Plast Surg.* 2001;28:283-296.
36. Garrett WS, Giblin TR, Hoffman GW. Closure of skin defects of the face and neck by rotation and advancement of cervicopectoral flaps. *Plast Reconst Surg.* 1966;38:342-346.
37. Kaplan I, Goldwyn RM. The versatility of the laterally based cervicofacial flap for cheek repairs. *Plast Reconst Surg.* 1978;61:390-393.
38. Kroll SS, Reece GP, Robb G, Black J. Deep-plane cervicofacial rotation-advancement flap for reconstruction of large cheek defects. *Plast Reconst Surg.* 1994;94:88-93.
39. Kouba DJ, Miller SJ. The J-plasty advancement flap for reconstruction of malar cheek defects. *Dermatol Surg.* 2004;30:78-80.
40. Pontes LT, Aluma-Tenorio MS, Firoz BF, Goldberg LH, Jih MH, Kimyai-Asadi A. Plication of the superficial musculoaponeurotic system in reconstruction of cheek defects. *Dermatol Surg.* 2009; 35(11):1822-1825.
41. Dingman RO, Derman GH. Lateral cheek and posterior auricular transposition flap. In: Strauch B, Vasconez LO, Hall-Frindlay EJ, eds. *Grabb's Encyclopedia of Flaps.* Boston: Little, Brown; 1990:395-398.
42. Goldminz D, Bennett RG. Cigarette smoking and flaps and full-thickness graft necrosis. *Arch Dermatol.* 1991;177:1012-1015.
43. Marrero G, Eliezri Y. The use of the SMAS to close Mohs defects invading into the parotid gland. *Dermatol Surg.* 1998;24:1335-1337.

14 Ear Reconstruction

HAYES B. GLADSTONE, MD, and GREG S. MORGANROTH, MD

Introduction

Repair of the auricle can be traced back to India (600 BCE), with subsequent contributions by the Egyptians, Renaissance Italians, 19th-century surgeons, and finally German surgeons such as Diffenbach, who played a major role in refining auricle reconstruction.[1] Much of the literature has focused on providing a reliable framework either after trauma or for microtia repair. These techniques range from harvesting costal cartilage buried in the abdomen to using porous polyethylene.[2]

Because the auricle framework gives the ear its characteristic shape and orientation, until recently little emphasis has been placed on the cutaneous defects of this cosmetic unit. With the increased incidence of skin cancer, these defects have become commonplace. Reconstructive technique that does not restore the natural shape and curvature of the ear will invariably be noticed, particularly when compared with the contralateral ear.

Ear Aesthetics

Although auricle length is somewhat dependent on ethnicity (with African being the shortest and Asian being the longest), the length to width of the auricle should be slightly less than 2:1. Generally, the auricle protrudes from the scalp at a 20- to 30-degree angle.[3] A smooth contour outlined by the helical rim and bilateral symmetry are important universal aesthetic norms (Fig. 14.1).

The superior aspect of the helical rim, defined by a horizontal line from its attachment to the scalp, needs to maintain a gentle curve without any acute angles. As the rim descends it almost approaches a 90-degree angle through its midportion. The lower third of the auricle curves at approximately a 45-degree angle as it descends into the earlobe. The lobule has great variability in its length and curvature. In general, its width is one-third to one-half of the width of the superior portion of the helix. Earlobe length depends on ethnicity but is approximately 2 cm on average.[4] Earlobe thickness or "fleshiness" also varies from barely discernable from the helical rim to a very defined and separate structure. Earlobes tend to be asymmetrical and elongate with age.[5] Aesthetically, the most important aspect of the earlobe is its independence as a separate cosmetic unit while maintaining the curved continuity of the helical rim.

Embryology

Embryologically, the ear develops from the first and second branchial arches. These arches arise as hillocks from the neck.[6] During the early gestational period, they migrate cephalad. The outline of the ear is apparent early in the fetus at approximately the sixth week. Following birth, the external auricle grows quickly. By the age of 6 years, it has attained nearly adult size and proportions.

Topography

With its numerous ridges and valleys designed to improve acoustic reception, the external ear possesses the most complex topography of any cosmetic unit of the head and neck. The auricular framework is formed by cartilage. The earlobe like the nasal alar lobule is made of fibrofatty tissue. The medial-anterior facet of the auricle is characterized by perichondrium and thin skin tightly adherent to cartilage. The posterior-medial aspect has looser skin and some subcutaneous fat overlying the cartilaginous framework (Fig. 14.2).

The major anterior landmarks of the external ear are the helix, scapha, antihelix, concha, and tragus and antitragus. Posteriorly, there are eminences that correspond to these anterior landmarks. Laterally, the helix actually begins with the crus, which originates at the superior aspect of the conchal bowl. The helix extends superiorly in a gentle curve. As it descends, there is a slight prominence known as the Darwinian tubercle. The helix continues its descent uninterrupted to the lobule. Proceeding medially from the helical rim is the scaphoid fossa. This is bounded by superior and inferior crura of the antihelix. As these two limbs of the antihelix stretch to meet the helical rim, a depression known as the triangular fossa bounded by these two limbs and the rim is created. Medially, these ridges bound the concha. This bowl-like structure can be divided into the cymba, which is bounded superiorly by the anterior crus of the antihelix and inferiorly by the crus of the helical rim. Inferior to the crus is the cavum, which has a more concave nature. Although the recessed nature of the concha makes it appear less important to the structure of the auricle, it actually acts as a brace between the mastoid and the remainder of the auricle. Medial-posteriorly, the concha leads to the external auditory canal. Lateral to the canal is the tragus, a roundish prominence. Opposing the tragus, across the conchal valley, is the antitragus, a linear prominence at the origin of the antihelix. The posterior aspect of the ear is marked by various ridges and named prominences known as eminences, which correspond to the anterior anatomic landmarks. Aside from the intrinsic rigidity produced by the cartilaginous framework, the auricle is held in placed by small muscles and ligaments. The musculature can be divided into three extrinsic and three intrinsic bands.

VASCULATURE

The blood supply is mainly supplied by the superficial temporal and the posterior auricular arteries. Both are branches of the external carotid. The superficial temporal artery and its branches, including the direct auricular, supply the anterior (lateral) surface of the ear, particularly the superior half. The posterior auricular artery supplies the entire medial (posterior) surface and has branches that perforate to the opposing surface, mainly supplying the lower half of the ear including the conchal bowl (Fig. 14.3).[6] The postauricular region is also supplied by the occipital artery. A recent cadaver study demonstrated the robust anastomoses in the mastoid and postauricular space. This study is particularly relevant to staged retroauricular flaps because it appears that flaps up to 5 cm from the external auditory canal would have a sufficient vascular supply.[7] Venous drainage occurs via corresponding named veins in addition to the retromandibular vein. These three veins flow into the external jugular vein.

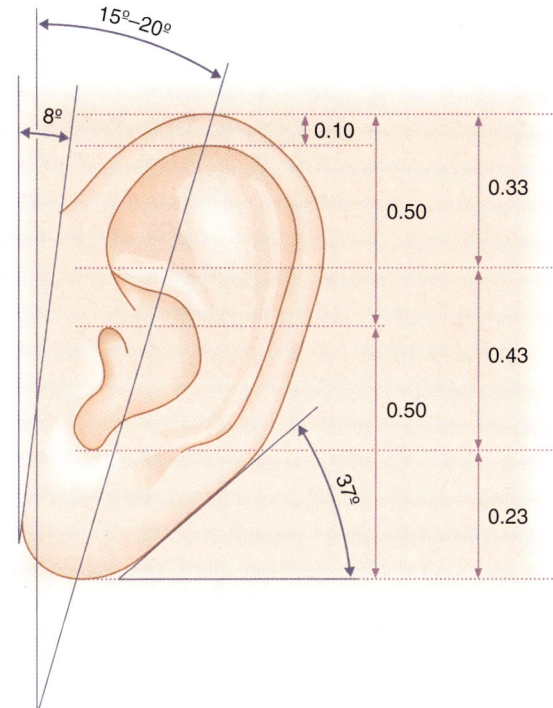

Fig. 14.1 The aesthetic proportions of the ear.

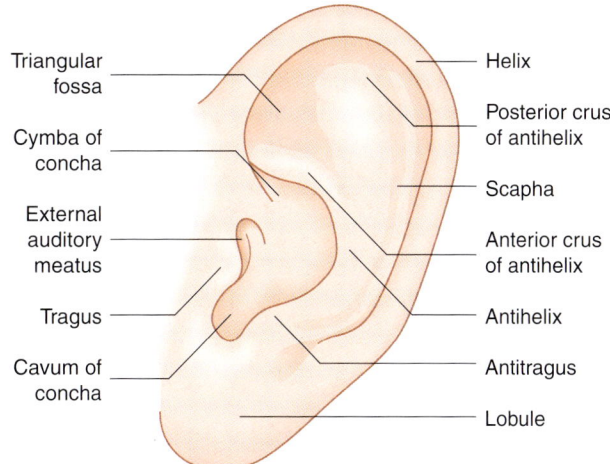

Fig. 14.2 The topography of the ear.

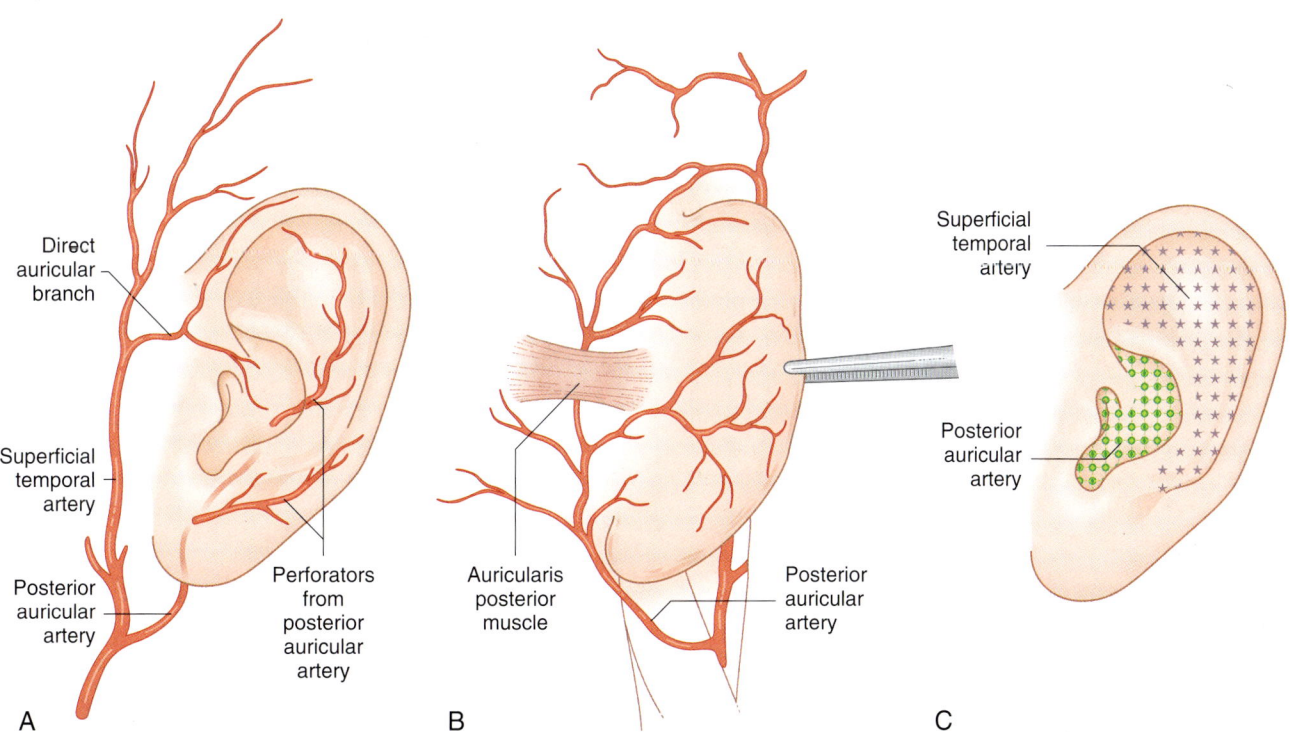

Fig. 14.3 The vasculature of the ear. (A) Superficial temporal artery and branches. (B) Posterior auricular artery and branches. (C) Regions of the auricle supplied by these two arteries.

INNERVATION

The external ear possesses an intricate sensory supply. The innervation is supplied by branches of the cervical nerve, 10th cranial nerve, trigeminal nerve, and lesser occipital nerve. The greater auricular nerve, which originates from C_2 and C_3, extensively innervates the cranial aspect of the ear, including the earlobe. It also branches out to the anterior surface and innervates most of the upper half of the auricle. The auriculotemporal nerve, a branch of V_3, supplies the lateral aspect of the superior portion of the helix. The posterior surface of the helix and the eminences of the scapha and fossa triangularis are innervated by the mastoid branch of the lesser occipital nerve. Finally, the Arnold nerve, a branch of the vagus (CN_{10}), supplies sensory nerves to the concha.[7]

General Principles

The most important principle of reconstructing the ear is to maintain the natural contour and shape as defined by the helical rim. The auricle should appear within the range of expected shapes, be in close approximation to the scalp, and be symmetrical to the contralateral ear. Although not as important as the shape, the height of the auricles should be similar. Unlike the shape, a minor discrepancy in height will be imperceptible to the casual observer. If the shape, particularly the curve of the helical rim, is not smooth, it will be instantly noticeable.

As with other regions of the head and neck, second intent healing is a viable option for many wounds. It is particularly useful in concavities such as the conchal bowl and scaphoid fossa. Because of the robust blood supply, the healing is usually rapid with excellent cosmetic results. If there is exposed cartilage, it may be prudent to provide coverage rather than allowing second intent healing. The coverage will reduce pain, minimize distortion due to wound contraction, and lessen the risk of chondritis.

Tumor extirpation with Mohs micrographic surgery is the treatment of choice in this area for providing the highest possible cure rate and minimal sacrifice of normal tissue. In tumors that are well defined, wedge excisions may be acceptable with proper en face examination of the margin. Unlike the lip, a simple wedge excision may lead to an uneven closure and notching of the helical rim because of the complex topography of the ear cartilaginous framework. The addition of two perpendicular Burow triangles will facilitate a wedge excision closure by removing the redundant cartilage. Another important reconstruction pearl to maintain the smooth curve of the helix is the use of the Z-plasty to prevent retraction of the wound edge and notching.

Reconstructive Options

SKIN GRAFTS

Full-thickness skin grafts have a wide application in resurfacing small to medium auricular defects. Grafts will have the highest chance of surviving if there is intact perichondrium. If the wound base consists of cartilage, multiple full-

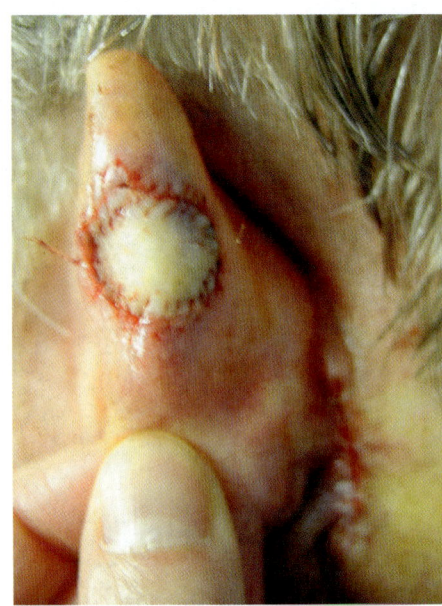

Fig. 14.4 A common donor site for full-thickness skin grafts: the postauricular region.

thickness perforations of the cartilage with a 2-mm punch can be used to facilitate the blood supply.[8] Common donor areas include the preauricular and postauricular sulci. The postauricular region is desirable because the scar will be hidden and it can heal by second intent or be closed primarily (Fig. 14.4). The preauricular region may provide a slightly thicker graft. This site is a good choice when there are significant creases in which to hide the scar. It is rare that this donor site is left to heal by second intention. In general, the donor site is from the ipsilateral side because this will decrease the need for patient repositioning.

For helical rim defects that do not involve cartilage, a full-thickness skin graft will restore the contour without placing tension on the delicate cartilaginous framework. For medium-sized defects of the scaphoid fossa or conchal bowl in which second intent healing may require several weeks, a full-thickness skin graft will minimize wound care and possible chondritis. These grafts can be sewn in with 6-0 absorbable or nonabsorbable sutures. Sutures can be placed through the center of the graft to secure it to the underlying tissue to obliterate a potential space for a hematoma or seroma. The postoperative dressing is as important to a good outcome as securing the graft. It can take the form of a bolster dressing and be stabilized with sutures. The use of a dental roll to maintain well-distributed pressure may improve graft survivability. Alternatively, a secure pressure dressing will most likely be as effective as the most complex bolster. It can also be more easily removed to inspect the graft should that be necessary. The variability in skin graft healing and inosculation may alter how long a dressing is kept in place. However, it is usually prudent to leave a dressing undisturbed for 1 week.

ADJACENT TISSUE TRANSFER

As in other head and neck defects, well-vascularized flaps with bulk that can be contoured are excellent reconstruction options for auricular defects. Random vascular pattern

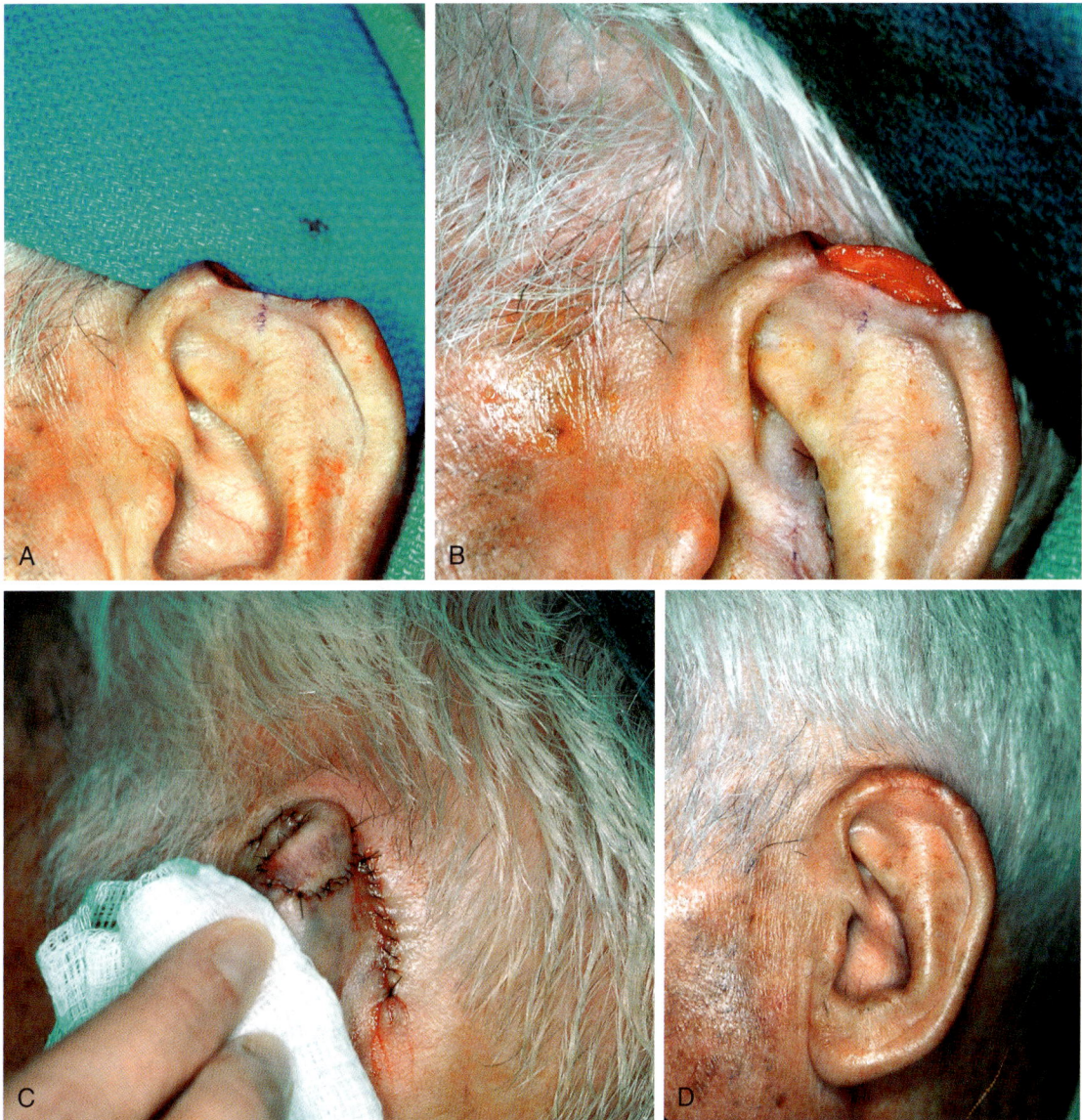

Fig. 14.5 A postauricular staged flap for reconstruction of the superior helical rim. (A) Post-Mohs micrographic surgery. (B) Cartilage attached. (C) Postauricular flap attached. (D) Long-term postoperative result. The helix is smooth and retains its original shape.

flaps based on the generous and redundant blood supply of the ear have a high survival rate. For larger defects, flaps may be staged, either from the preauricular or postauricular regions (Fig. 14.5) or from the temporal scalp. Wide undermining is necessary on the ear because there is minimal skin laxity, particularly on the lateral aspect of the external ear. Flaps may include cartilage, such as the chondrocutaneous helical advancement flap and the conchal bowl transposition flap for partial helical defects. Flaps may also be "tubed" to rebuild the helical rim from the preauricular or postauricular sulci (Fig. 14.6). For full-thickness conchal bowl or antihelix defects, posterior-based flaps may be bivalved to resurface both the lateral and medial side of the defect (Figs. 14.7 and 14.8).[9,10]

CARTILAGE

Because the cartilage framework defines the characteristic shape of this cosmetic subunit, it is necessary to replace "like with like." Using a staged flap without any subsurface support will result in a folded, floppy ear. The donor cartilage should be excised from a location where it will match the missing framework. The choice of donor site also needs to take into account the overall stability of the ear's framework. Donor sites include the ipsilateral or contralateral conchal bowl, antihelix, and scapha (Fig. 14.9). Grafts from the scapha or antihelix are more flexible and may be scored to provide a gentle curve. Harvesting a cartilage graft does not require skin excision. A skin flap can be elevated, the graft removed, and the flap sutured back into place with interrupted sutures and through-and-through sutures to minimize hematoma formation. In the conchal bowl, a firm pressure dressing will be needed because of excellent vasculature and the increased risk of a hematoma. Costal cartilage is another donor source; however, it is usually reserved for near-total or total ear reconstruction because of its rigidity.[11] There is also increased risk for adverse effects in this donor site. For small skin-cartilage defects, a composite

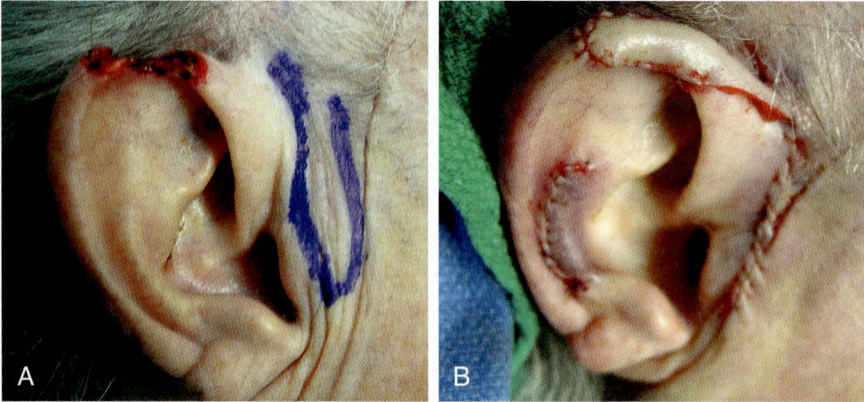

Fig. 14.6 A "finger" or banner transposition flap for helical reconstruction. (A) Mohs defect and marking for superior-based finger transposition flap. (B) Flap attached.

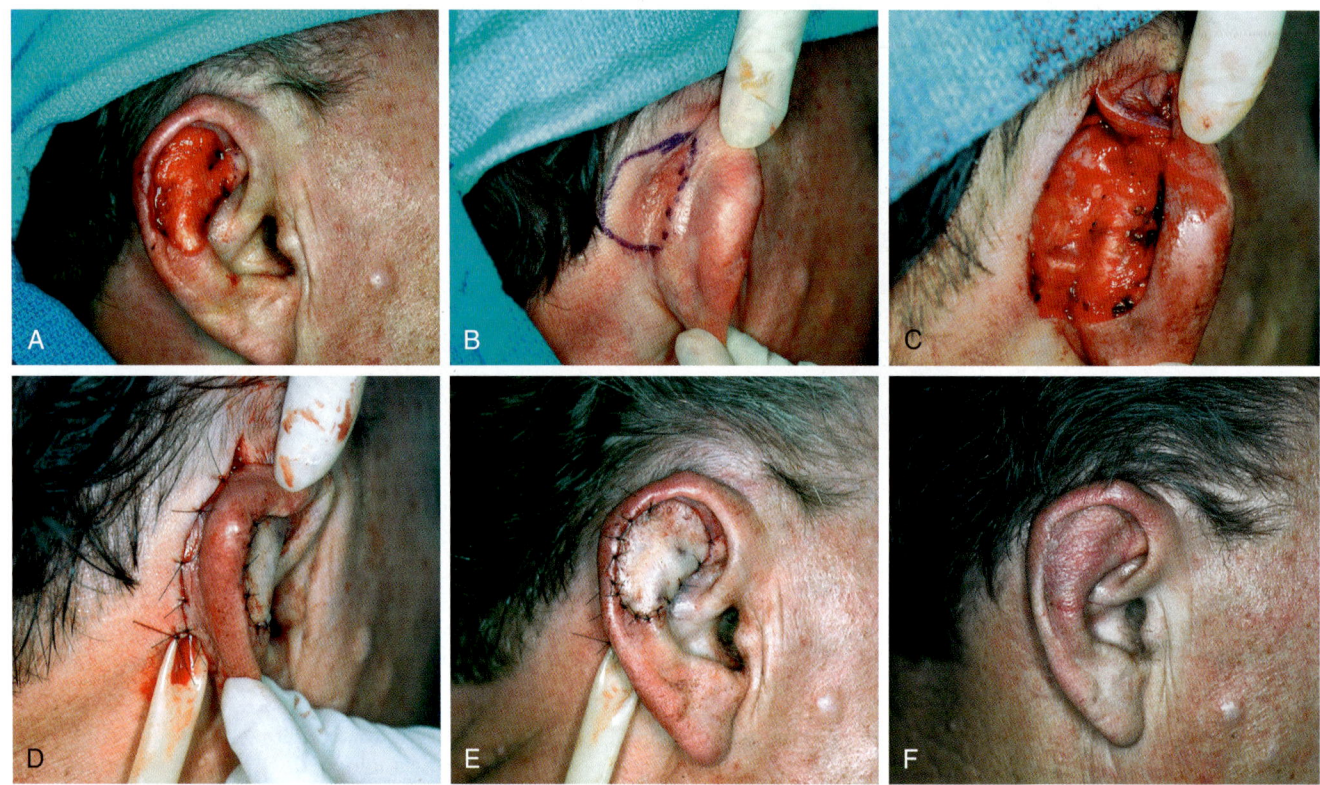

Fig. 14.7 A posterior ear-based island pedicle "pull-through" flap. (A) Defect after Mohs surgery. (B) Marking for island pedicle flap. (C) Raising flap. (D) Flap attached, posterior view. (E) Flap attached, anterior view. (F) Long-term results.

graft taken from the root of the helix is another alternative. However, in smokers, or those with vascular compromise, the composite graft will have a significantly decreased survival rate.

REGIONAL RECONSTRUCTION

As with other cosmetic units of the head and neck, reconstruction of the ear is based on tissue reservoirs and mobility. The greatest tissue mobility is located along the middle portion of the helical rim, resulting in a wide variety of reconstruction options. In contrast, the superior aspect of the helix lacks adjacent tissue laxity and fewer reconstruction choices exist. Because the auricle as a whole generally lacks tissue mobility, distant donor sites including the postauricular region, the temporal scalp, and the preauricular region must be considered. With full-thickness defects or repairs involving cartilage manipulation, the auricle should be reconstructed in multiple layers to prevent buckling of the cartilage framework. Large, composite defects of the concha require some imagination because of the lack of available mobile tissue, often necessitating a posterior donor site. The lobule must be reconstructed with extreme precision because it is another defining characteristic of the ear

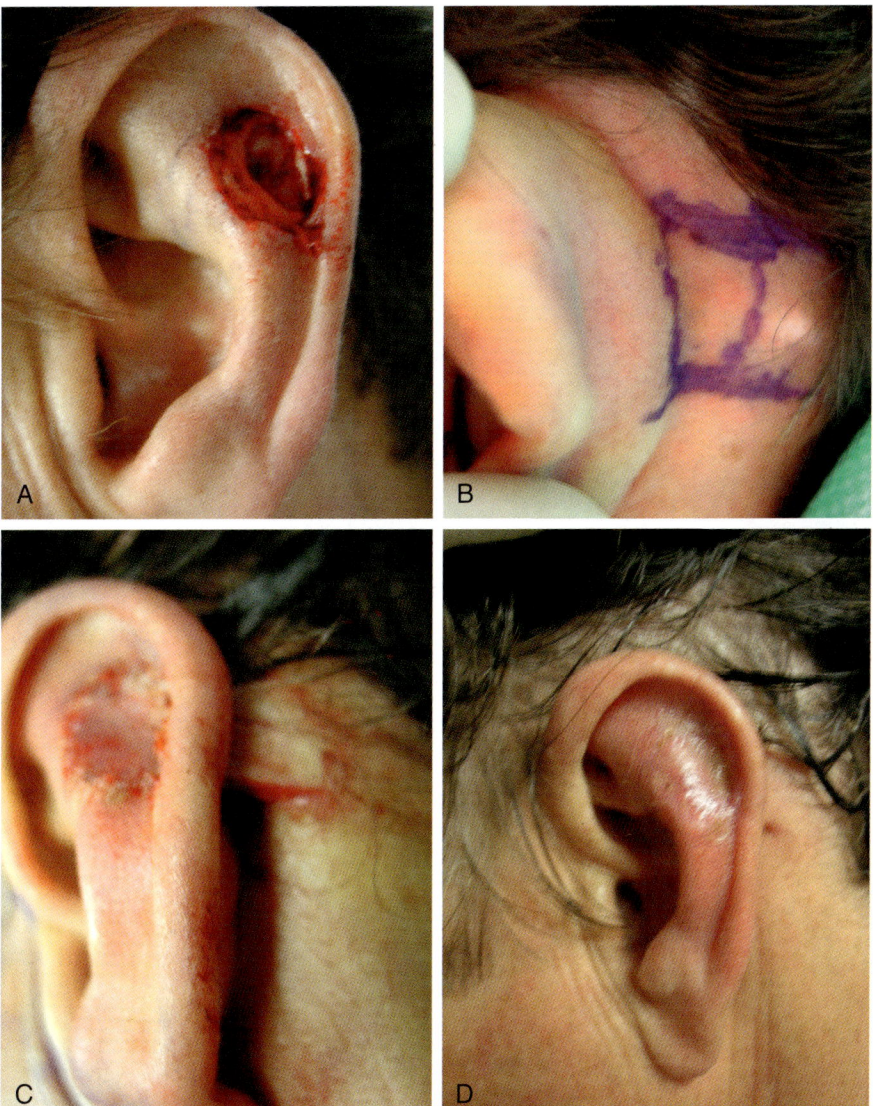

Fig. 14.8 A postauricular staged bivalved flap. (A) Defect after Mohs surgery. (B) Marking the postauricular flap. (C) Flap attached. (D) Long-term results.

and can be viewed in its entirety from an anterior perspective. Recreating a natural shape for the earlobe is particularly important for those who wear earrings.

Upper Auricle

Small defects of the superior helix can be closed primarily. If this option is chosen, wide undermining is necessary to minimize tension on the suture line. A tight closure will invariably result in a flattened rim contour. More commonly, small to medium defects of this region with intact cartilage can be repaired by a full-thickness skin graft. This graft can be harvested from the postauricular or preauricular regions and sutured in place with either 6-0 fast-absorbing gut or nylon sutures. Through-and-through sutures or a secure pressure dressing or bolster is needed for up to 1 week to prevent hematoma and seroma formation. A dental roll and head wrap dressing will provide the necessary compression postoperatively. Although the survival rate of these grafts is good, subtle flattening of the superior helix may occur.

Tubed Flap. More extensive defects of the superior aspect of the helical rim can be repaired using a tubed pedicle flap.[12] This can be a one- or two-stage flap transposed from the adjacent preauricular or postauricular skin. When measuring the length of the flap, it should be at least 20% longer than the rim defect to take into account the transposition as well as the curvature of the helix. The tubed flap is typically superiorly based with its distal aspect sewn into the defect (Fig. 14.10). A two-stage flap is used if there is intact skin that separates the donor site from the defect. If a two-stage flap is necessary, the pedicle is divided centrally after 3 weeks. The proximal pedicle is excised in a circular manner and repaired in a linear fashion. The distal pedicle, now replacing the defect, is thinned and inset with interrupted sutures. Careful sculpting of the distal flap tissue will provide a smooth and natural helical contour.

Composite Chondrocutaneous Flap

For defects that include the superior helical rim and the antihelix and are not amenable to a wedge excision, the chondrocutaneous flap from the conchal bowl is an elegant one-stage repair (Fig. 14.11).[13] The curved inferior border of the concha closely approximates that of the helical rim. A majority of the bowl composed of the skin and cartilage can be incised and transposed to fill the superior-oriented defect. The pedicle extends to the root of the ear and should be kept thin. Although it may be tempting to increase the width of the pedicle to ensure an adequate vascular supply, this may inhibit the mobility of the flap and actually compromise the blood supply. If extra length is needed, then the pedicle may be extended into the preauricular creases. The remainder of the conchal bowl is resurfaced with a full-thickness skin graft or allowed to heal by second intent.

Temporoparietal Flap. For large, complete defects of the superior helix and antihelix, the temporoparietal flap used in microtia repair and facial plastic surgery is an option.[14,15] This flap is based on the superficial temporal artery traveling between the galea and the areolar tissue. It is a superiorly based, staged advancement flap. A skin graft is used to resurface this flap.

Although this flap is a significant addition to the armamentarium for repairing this area, it does possess several challenges. Because this area is not inherently mobile, the flap needs to be approximately 6 cm in length. This can result in extensive scarring and alopecia in the temporal region. This layer is extremely vascular, and hemostasis sometimes can be an issue. In addition, when elevating this flap anteriorly, it is important to be aware of the frontal branches of the facial nerve. One alternative is to incise a flap down to muscle and advance it over the defect. If the leading edge of the flap is in the sulcus at the border of the auricle, then hair growth will not be a factor, and a skin graft is not necessary (Fig. 14.12). This flap is divided and contoured at 3 weeks.

For isolated scaphoid defects, as described previously, a posterior-based tunneled flap can be performed. In addition, a preauricular-based tunneled transposition flap has been described. In both cases, it is important to deepithelialize the flap.[16] These flaps will maintain the topography of this complex region.

Middle Auricle

Because maintaining the outline of the ear is critical, it is rare to allow the middle portion of the helix to heal by second intent. Small superficial defects can be resurfaced with a full-thickness skin graft. Defects less than 1 cm that involve both the helix and antihelix can be converted into a wedge and then closed in a multilayered fashion. Larger defects of the central portion of the helix can be repaired with a chondrocutaneous advancement flap.[17] Anita and Buch first described this technique, which involved a bilateral advancement flap leaving the posterior skin intact.[18] Calhoun definitively showed that this technique was superior to wedge excisions because there was less risk of cupping of the ear. The authors demonstrated that this flap was useful for defects less than 2 cm.[19] Depending on the

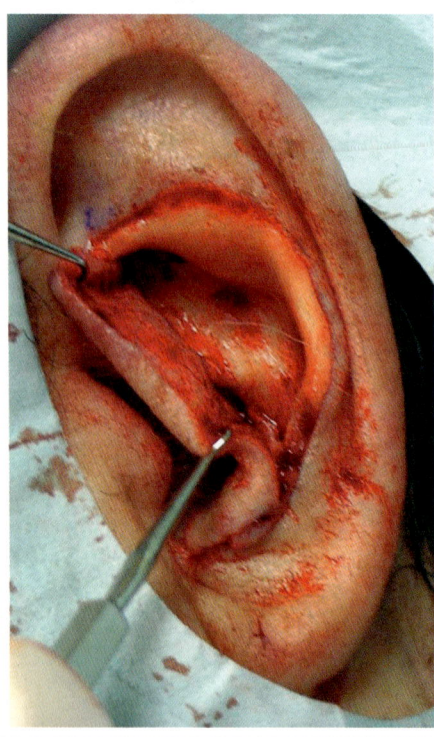

Fig. 14.9 Raising a conchal bowl graft. The conchal bowl approximates the curve of the superior helix.

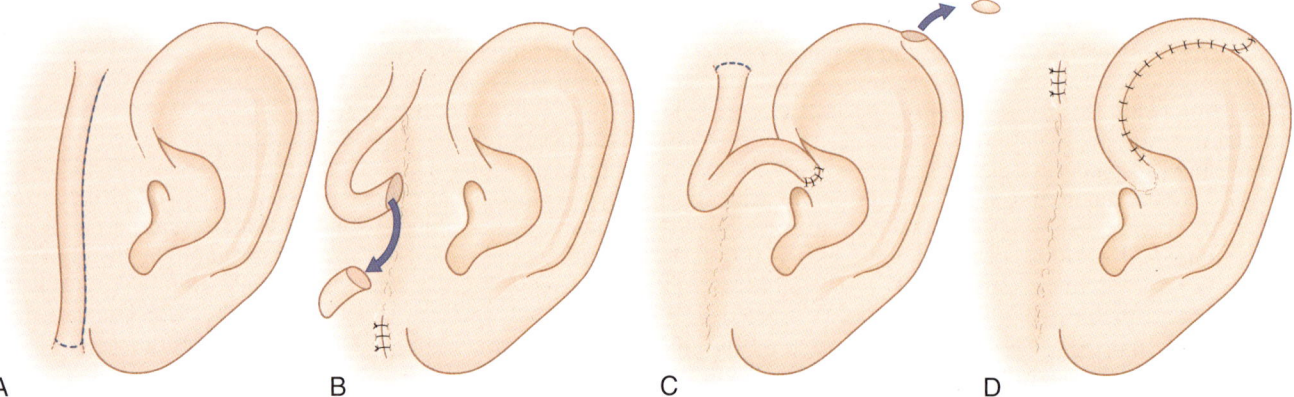

Fig. 14.10 Diagram of a tubed flap. (A) The preauricular donor site. (B) Detachment of the flap. (C) Mobilization of the flap. (D) Insetting the flap to repair the superior helical rim.

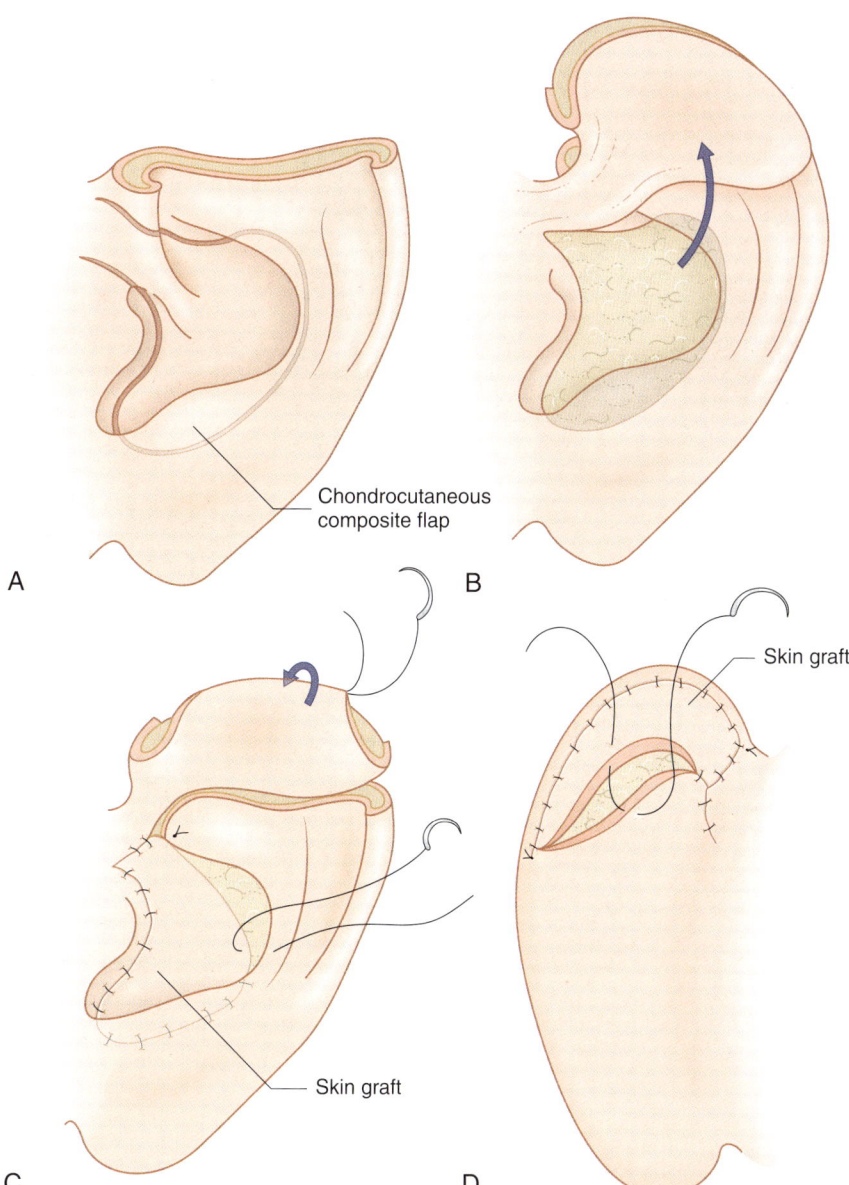

Fig. 14.11 Diagram of a one-stage chondrocutaneous flap for helical reconstruction. (A) Incising the flap. (B) Mobilizing the flap to the superior helical defect. (C) Insetting the flap and resurfacing the donor site with a full-thickness skin graft. (D) Attaching a full-thickness skin graft on the posterior cartilage exposed side of the flap.

size of the defect, a single full-thickness advancement flap can be mobilized. Because the skin laxity is more pronounced in the inferior rim including the earlobe, the advancement is typically inferiorly based. For larger defects, a bilateral flap may be necessary. The chondrocutaneous flap can be a full-thickness flap (Fig. 14.13). When suturing, it is important to approximate the cartilage with 4.0 absorbable interrupted sutures to prevent buckling of the helix. The anterior and posterior aspects of the skin are sutured with interrupted or running nylon for fast-absorbing gut sutures. When aligning the newly created helical rim, a vertical mattress suture to evert the skin edges may reduce the risk of notching. Alternatively, a Z-plasty may be used to prevent notching.

Similar to the fossa triangularis, shallow defects of the antihelix may be left to heal by second intent. Deeper defects can be repaired with full-thickness skin grafts. Perforations of the cartilage will facilitate graft survival in this area. However, if the surgeon wants to preserve the elegant topography of the antihelix, then either a single or a double island pedicle flap can be performed. In these techniques, the posterior skin is left intact. Because of the lack of mobility in these island pedicles, these flaps are a good solution for only small to medium defects.[20] As with the superior portion of the helix, a postauricular pedicle flap can be used to fill full-thickness defects.

For full-thickness defects involving the middle helix and antihelix, a staged retroauricular flap is usually the best option (Figs. 14.14 and 14.15).[21,22] This reconstruction advances postauricular skin and has a robust random blood supply. Although in select cases it may be used alone to recreate the helix, it most often is used in conjunction with a cartilage graft harvested from the contralateral conchal bowl or the antihelix. Without the restoration of the cartilage framework, the helical rim may fold on itself or appear unnaturally flattened.

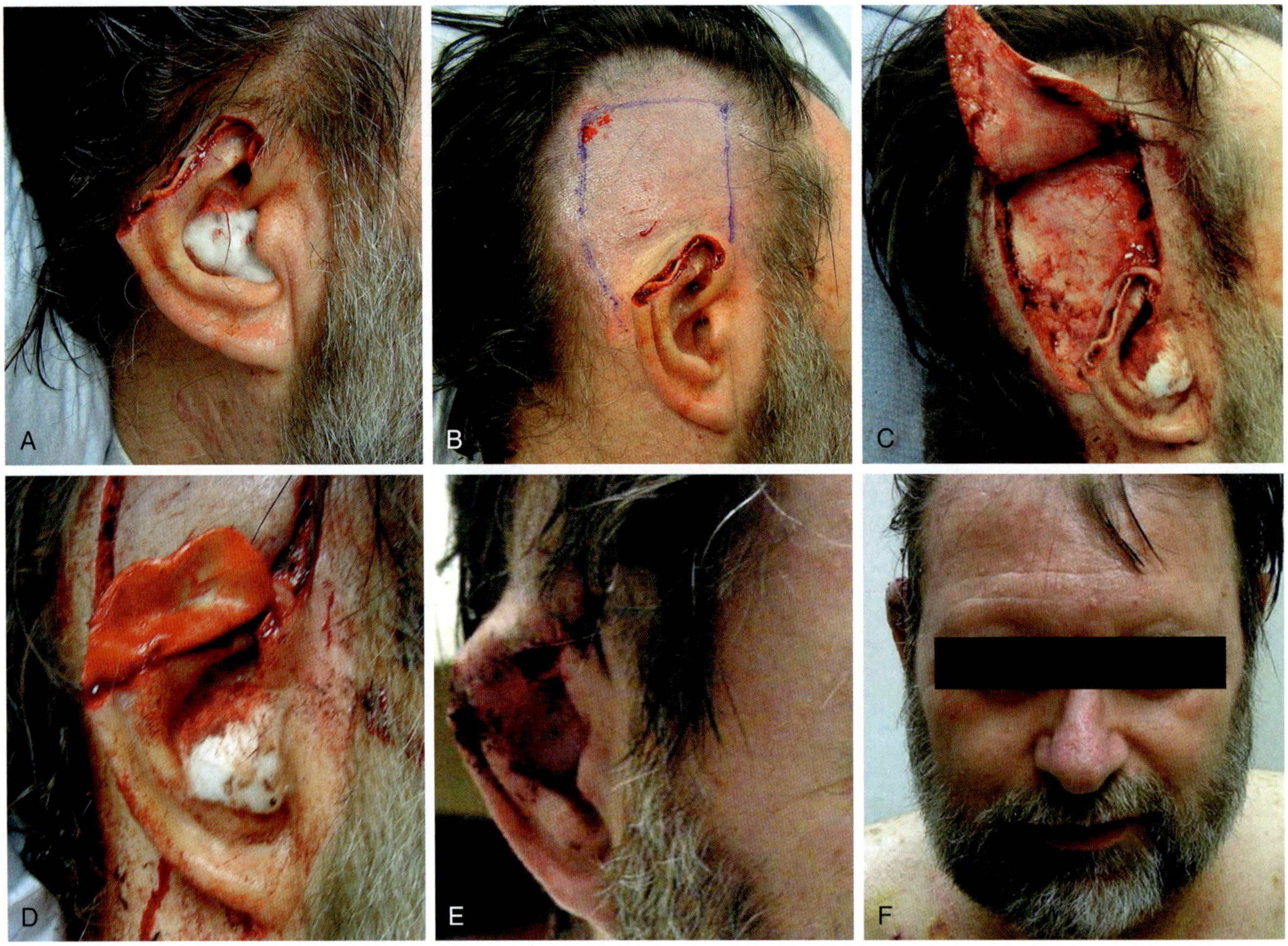

Fig. 14.12 The temporoparietal flap for repair of combined helix and antihelix defects. (A) Defect after Mohs surgery. (B) Flap marked. (C) Raising flap. (D) Cartilage attached. (E) Flap attached. (F) Long-term results. Helical symmetry is retained.

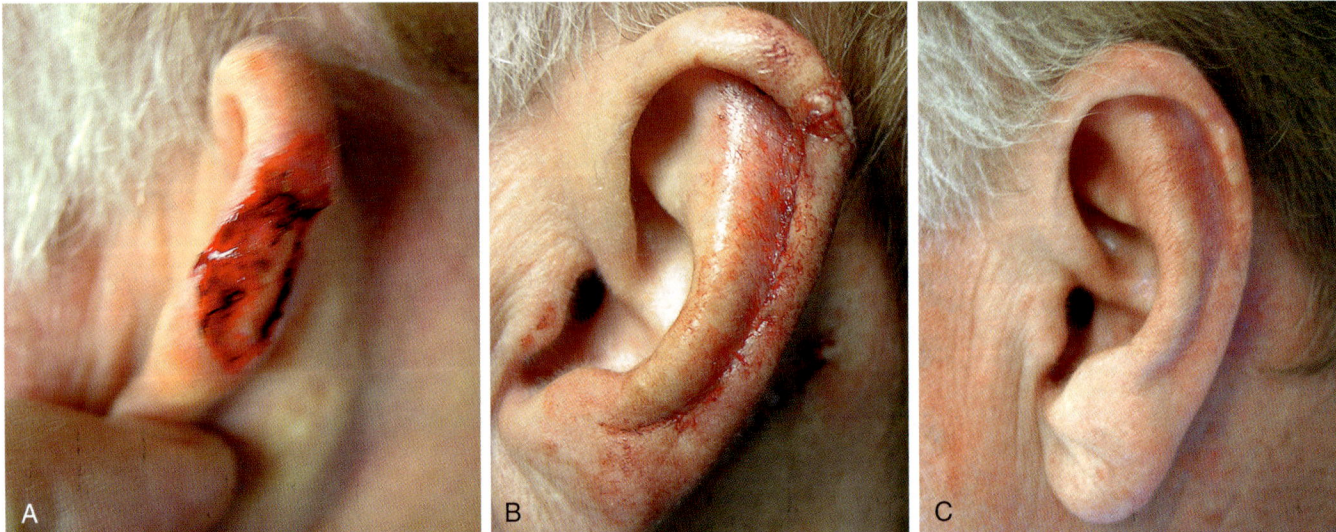

Fig. 14.13 The bilateral chondrocutaneous advancement flap for repair of helical defects. (A) Defect after Mohs surgery. (B) Bilateral flap inset. Because of the size of the defect (>2 cm), a bridge graft (from the postauricular sulcus) was used at the superior aspect. (C) Long-term results.

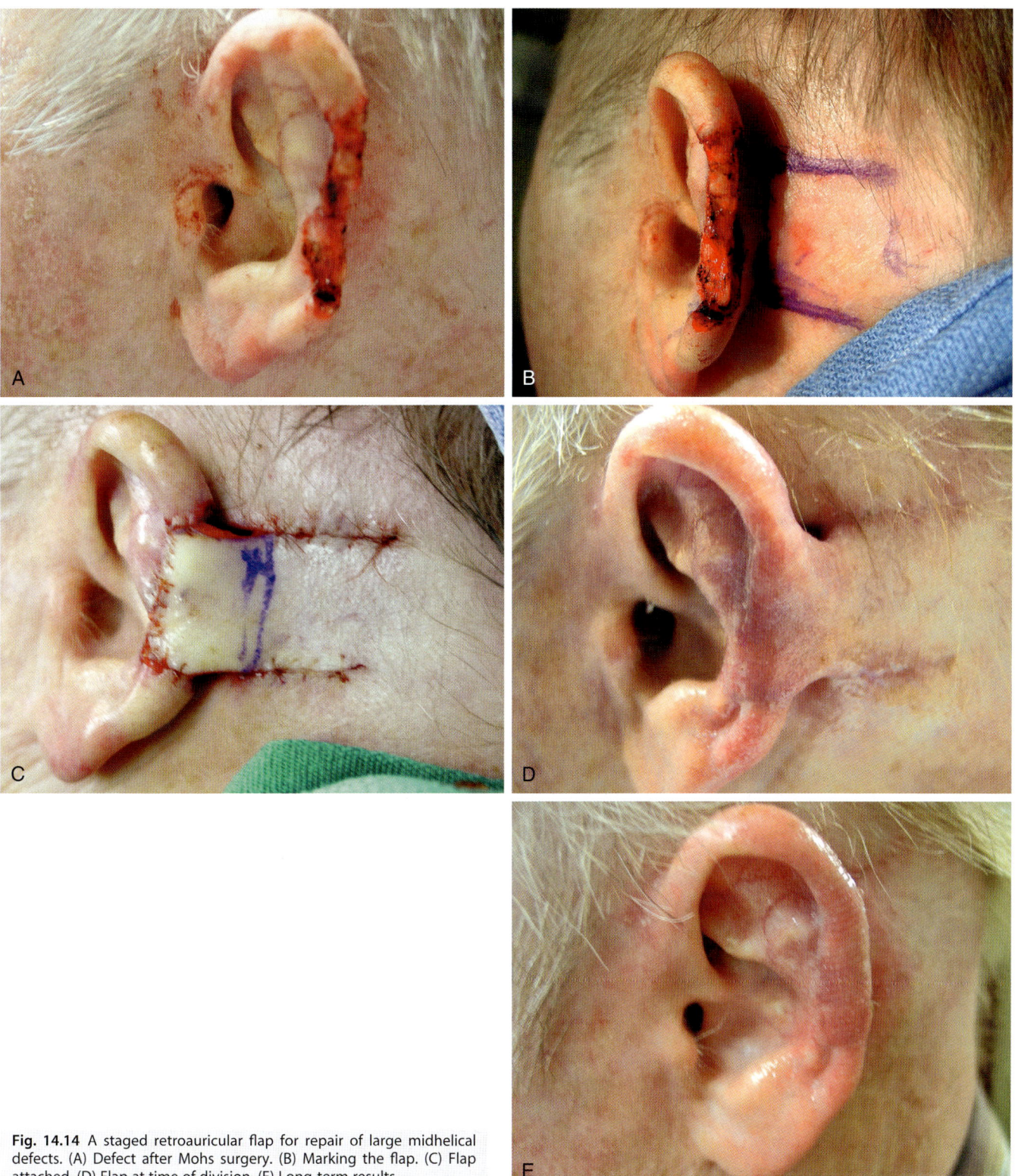

Fig. 14.14 A staged retroauricular flap for repair of large midhelical defects. (A) Defect after Mohs surgery. (B) Marking the flap. (C) Flap attached. (D) Flap at time of division. (E) Long-term results.

When marking, it is important to extend the flap into the postauricular sulcus. The length of the flap should be outlined so that it does not excessively pin the auricle and has a 3:1 to 4:1 length-to-width ratio. The flap width should be slightly greater than the defect width to compensate for the helical curvature. The flap is inset with a layered closure.

Vaseline gauze is placed in the postauricular sulcus. The flap is divided and contoured at 3 weeks. Division of the flap may be performed in two manners. Traditionally, the flap is marked so that there is enough length to wrap around the posterior aspect of the auricle. In patients with thin and delicate ears, this method may provide too much bulk.

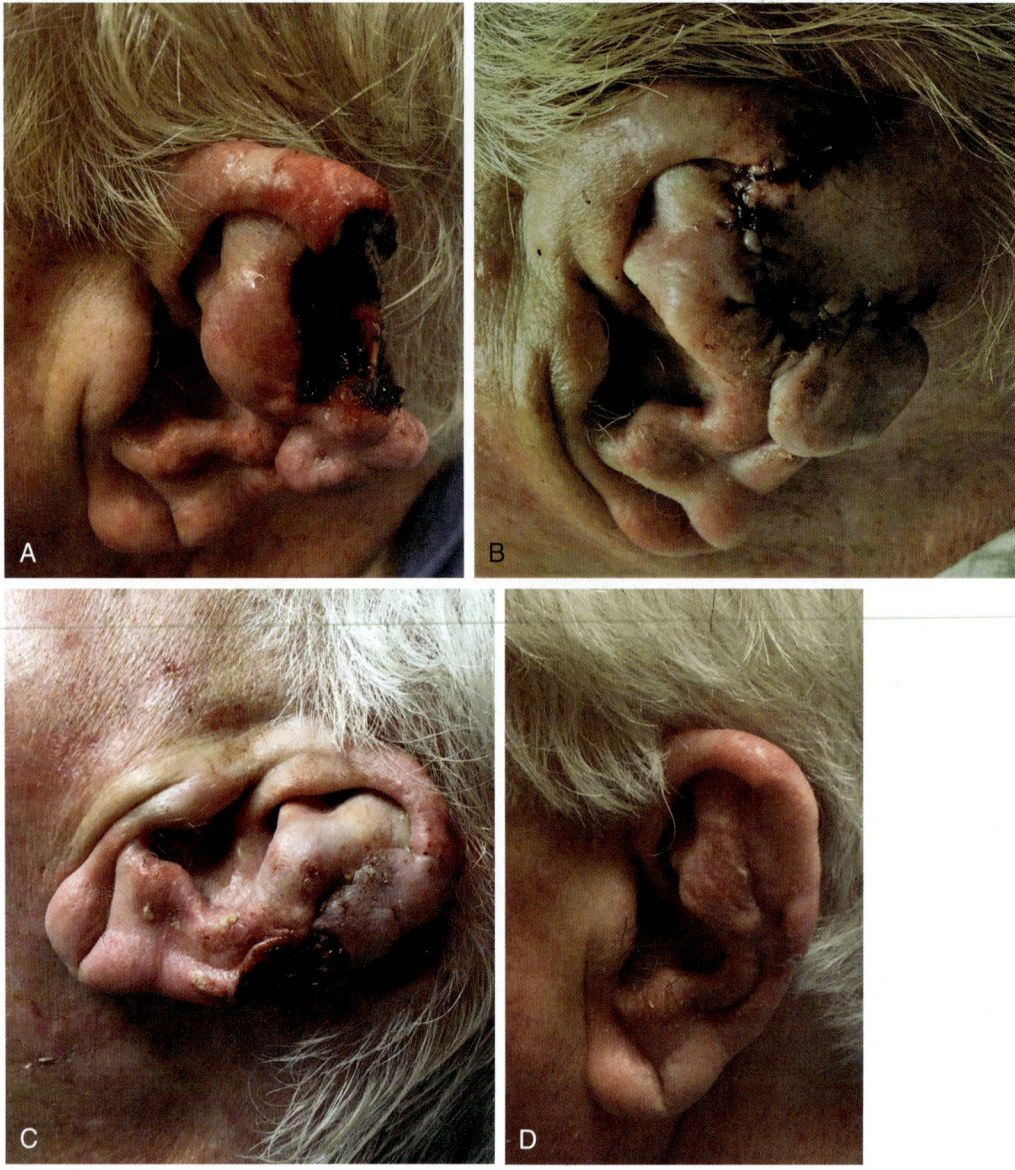

Fig. 14.15 A staged retroauricular flap for a Mohs defect that also required a cartilage graft from the contral lateral antihelix. (A) Defect after Mohs surgery. (B) Cartilage and flap inset into defect. (C) Division and contouring. (D) Two months post division.

Alternatively, the posterior aspect may then be covered with a full-thickness skin graft. In patients in whom there is not a cartilage graft, the posterior aspect of the flap may be left to granulate. The remainder of the flap is sewn into the retroauricular space, and the sulcus may be left to granulate.

Lower Auricle

Defects of the lower third of the auricle can be repaired in much the same manner as those of the middle third. Because this portion of the auricle is fleshier and widens into the lobule, there are more closure options for medial defects. To maximize tissue movement, it is important to include the earlobe to take advantage of its laxity.

Lobule

In many ways, the lobule is a continuation of the helical rim and requires a reconstructive technique for restoring the smooth edge, curve, and symmetry. Lack of attention in restoring the lobule to its preoperative proportions will almost always be noticeable. In deciding whether to sacrifice shape or size, the latter has more room for compromise. For small lesions a wedge excision with a primary closure designed to evert the wound edges will retain the natural shape. Alternatively, a Z-plasty will minimize notching. A small decrease in lobule size resulting from a small wedge excision is unlikely to draw attention. Because of the laxity of the lobule, primary closure is possible for sizable defects. Should these repairs create a noticeable disparity in earlobe size, then the contralateral earlobe can be reduced by a simultaneous or delayed wedge excision.[23] In patients who wear earrings, care must be taken to minimize tension on the lobule. If a primary closure will distort the lobule or impact the patient's ability to wear an earring, flaps or grafts should be considered to minimize distortion. A popular method of restoring the earlobe is the transposition

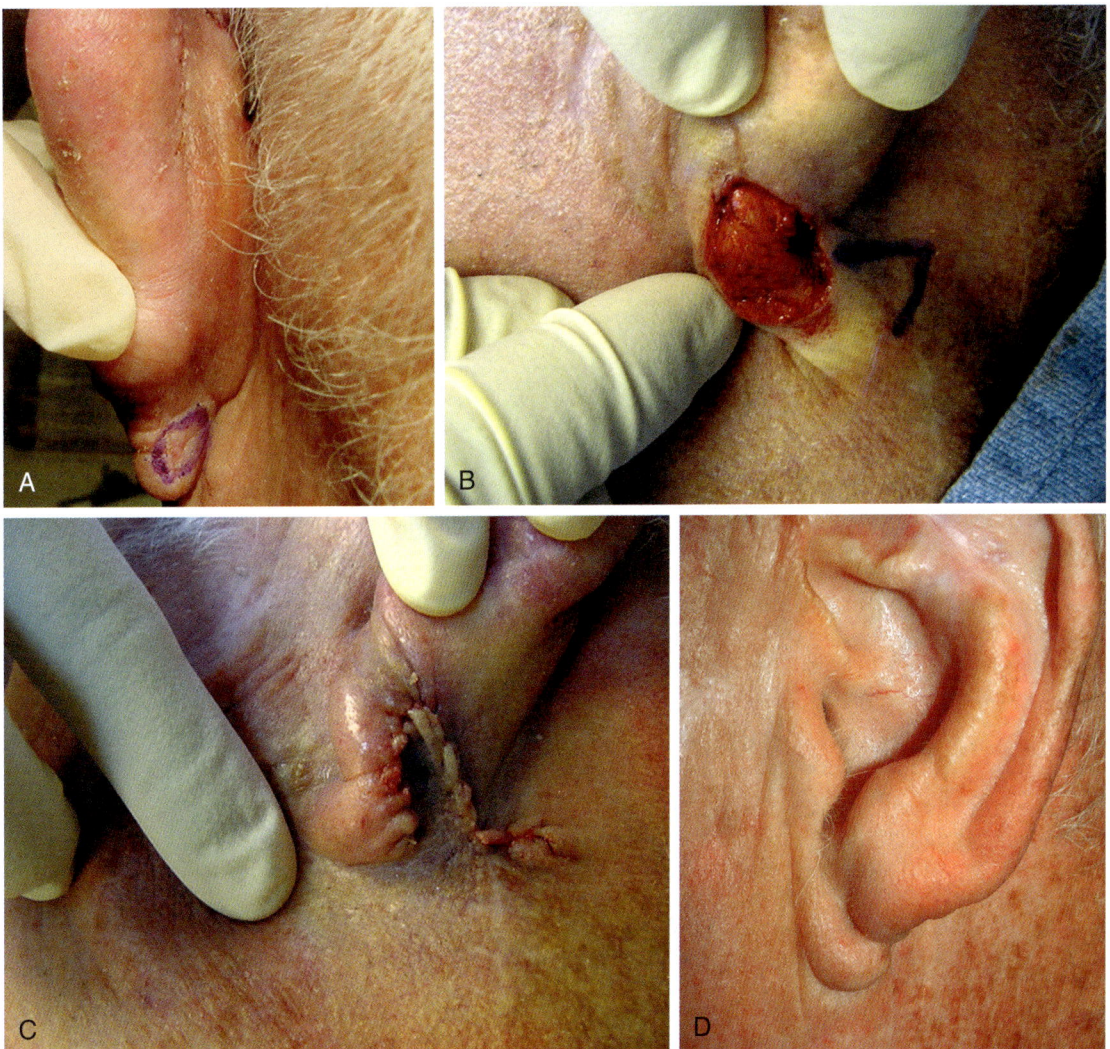

Fig. 14.16 A transposition flap for repair of a posterior lobule defect. (A) Note the pendulous earlobe. (B) Post-Mohs and marking the posterior-based transposition flap. (C) Flap inset. (D) Long-term retention of pendulous earlobe shape.

flap (Fig. 14.16).[24] A one- or two-stage transposition flap can be designed from the preauricular or postauricular crease. The secondary defect scars can be hidden with the crease and will be less visible in the postauricular crease. The preauricular skin is thicker and may be a better thickness and color match for the lobule. A staged infraauricle flap can be used to repair inferior lobular defects. It possesses the advantage of a camouflaged scar, but it lacks mobility. For those individuals with a naturally shortened lobule, the helical rim may be advanced for coverage. Care should be taken not to distort the rim with this repair.

Concha

In many instances, defects in the conchal bowl can heal by second intent. An exception would be those defects directly adjacent to or including the external ear canal. In these areas, a wound allowed to heal by granulation has an increased risk of canal stenosis. Full-thickness skin grafts will minimize wound contraction and decrease the likelihood of this complication. For outer concha defects for which some skin mobility exists, an advancement flap may be a reasonable option (Fig. 14.17). For full-thickness defects, a postauricular island flap similar to that for the antihelix can be used, although the position of this flap will enter at the level of the concha. Pinning of the auricle may occasionally occur. This condition may be corrected by a subsequent Z-plasty to lengthen the postauricular scar line. Mellette has described a preauricular transposition flap that will also provide excellent coverage for large conchal bowl defects.[25]

Posterior Auricle

The posterior auricle is characterized by thin skin coverage overlying the cartilage eminences. The skin is bound down superiorly but possesses moderate laxity as one proceeds inferiorly. Shallow defects can heal by second intent. Although many defects can be closed primarily, it is important to assess the amount of pinning that may result. Because of the mid and inferior skin mobility, advancement, rotation, and transposition flaps are options. In some cases, these advancement flaps may be mobilized to resurface helical rim defects—although this is more successful in the

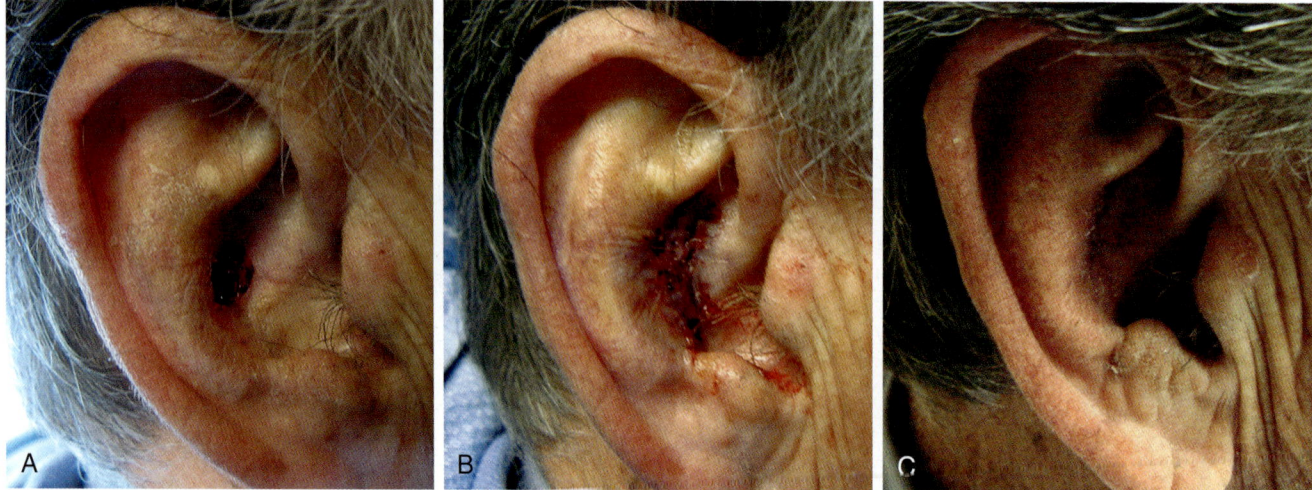

Fig. 14.17 An outer conchal advancement flap. (A) Defect after Mohs surgery. (B) Flap inset. (C) Long-term results.

midhelical region rather than superiorly, where this could lead to flattening of the rim. For larger posterior ear defects, postauricular skin can be transposed.

Prosthetics and When to Refer

Although it is within the skill set of dermasurgeons to reconstruct complex ear defects, there are circumstances in which it would be better to consider a prosthesis or to refer to a facial plastic surgeon or plastic surgeon who specializes in total ear reconstruction. For the infirm patient or one who truly does not desire further surgery, a prosthetic is a viable option.[26] This alternative will lessen the patient's potential morbidity and be functionally viable because many patients' primary concern is the ability to wear glasses. If an individual has two-thirds or more of his or her auricle excised after Mohs surgery and still desires reconstruction, it may be wise to refer to a surgeon specializing in microtia or full ear reconstruction because they will have greater experience in using costal cartilage and fascial flaps; however, this is a decision that needs to be made on a case-by-case basis. If one attempts to repair a defect of this size, an alloplastic material such as Medpor to replace the cartilage framework may be a reasonable option. A temporoparietal flap can provide adequate coverage.

References

1. Berghaus A, Toplak F. Surgical concepts for reconstruction of the auricle. *Arch Otolaryngol Head Neck Surg.* 1986;112:388-397.
2. Berghaus A. Porous polyethylene in reconstructive head and neck surgery. *Arch Otolaryngol Head Neck Surg.* 1985;111:154-160.
3. Park SS, Hood RJ. Auricular reconstruction. *Otolaryngol Clin North Am.* 2001;34:713-738.
4. Azaria R, Adler N, Silfen R, Regev D, Hauben DJ. Morphometry of the adult human earlobe: a study of 547 subjects and clinical application. *Plast Reconstr Surg.* 2003;111:2398-2402.
5. Mowlavi A, Meldrum DG, Wilhelmi BJ, Zook EG. Incidence of earlobe ptosis and psuedoptosis in patients seeking facial rejuvenation surgery and effects of aging. *Plast Reconstr Surg.* 2004;113:712-717.
6. Larrabee WF, Makielski KH. *Surgical Anatomy of the Face.* New York: Raven Press; 1993:177-185.
7. Lohasammakul S, Turbpaiboon C, Chompoopong S, Ratanalekha R, Aojanepong C. Vascular nature and existence of anastomoses of extrinsic postauricular fascia: application for staged auricular reconstruction. *Ann Plast Surg.* 2017;doi:10.1097/SAP.0000000000000947. [epub ahead of print].
8. Vital JM, Grenier F, Dautheribes M, Baspeyre H, Lavignolle B, Sénégas J. An anatomic and dynamic study of the greater occipital nerve (n. of Arnold). *Surg Radiol Anat.* 1989;11:205-210.
9. Ceilley RI, Bumstead RM, Paige WR. Delayed skin grafting. *J Dermatol Surg Oncol.* 1983;9:288-293.
10. Krespi YP, Ries WR, Shugar JMA, Sison GA. Auricular reconstruction with postauricular myocutaneous flap. *Otolaryngol Head Neck Surg.* 1983;91:193-196.
11. Ellabban MG, Maamoun MI, Elsharkawi M. The bi-pedicle postauricular tube flap for reconstruction of partial ear defects. *Br J Plast Surg.* 2003;56:593-598.
12. Brent B. Ear reconstruction with an expansile framework of autogenous rib cartilage. *Plast Reconstr Surg.* 1974;53:619-628.
13. DiMascio D, Castagnetti F. Tubed flap interpolation in reconstruction of helical and earlobe defects. *Dermatol Surg.* 2004;30:572-578.
14. Park SS, Wang TD. Temporoparietal fascial flap in auricular reconstruction. *Facial Plast Surg.* 1995;11:330-337.
15. Brent B, Byrd HS. Secondary ear reconstruction with cartilage grafts covered by axial, random, and free flaps of temporoparietal fascia. *Plast Reconstr Surg.* 1983;72:141-152.
16. Pereira N, Brinca A, Vieira R, Figueiredo A. Tunnelized preauricular transposition flap for reconstruction of auricular defect. *J Dermatolog Treat.* 2014;5:441-443.
17. Ramirez OM, Heckler FR. Reconstruction of nonmarginal defects of the ear with chondrocutaneous advancement flaps. *Plast Reconstr Surg.* 1989;84:32-40.
18. Antia NH, Buch VI. Chondrocutaneous advancement flap for the marginal defect of the ear. *Plast Reconstr Surg.* 1967;39(5):472-477.
19. Calhoun KH, Slaughter D, Kassir R, Seikaly H, Hokanson JA. Biomechanics of the helical rim advancement flap. *Arch Otolaryngol Head Neck Surg.* 1996;122(10):1119-1123.
20. Kueder Pajares T, Cocunubo Blanco HA, Rodriguez Prieto MA. Reconstruction of the central antihelix using a novel double chondrocutaneous island flap. *J Amer Acad Dermatol.* 2016;74:e65-e66.
21. Brent B. The acquired auricular deformity. A systematic approach to its analysis and reconstruction. *Plast Reconstr Surg.* 1977;59:475-485.
22. Renard A. Postauricular flap based on a dermal pedicle for ear reconstruction. *Plast Reconstr Surg.* 1981;68:159-165.
23. Johnson TM, Fader DJ. The staged retroauricular to auricular direct pedicle (interpolation) flap for helical ear reconstruction. *J Am Acad Dermatol.* 1997;37:975-978.
24. Mellette JR. Reconstruction of the ear. In: *Principles and Techniques of Cutaneous Surgery.* New York: McGraw-Hill; 1996:363-380.
25. Griffiths RW. Earlobe reconstruction using a Limburg flap in six ears. *Br J Plast Surg.* 2003;56:620.
26. Renner G, Lane RV. Auricular reconstruction: an update. *Curr Opin Otolaryngol Head Neck Surg.* 2004;12:277-280.

15 Nasal Reconstruction

JONATHAN L. COOK, MD

Skin cancer wounds commonly occur on the nose, and the nose's unique aesthetic prominence presents particular reconstructive challenges. Although early nasal reconstructive procedures sought simply to cover the exposed wound, modern nasal reconstruction strives to restore a nearly perfect appearance to the nose following tumor extirpative procedures. Given the nose's highly complex visual construction, where areas of deeply shadowed concavities abut areas of light-reflecting convexities, exact restoration of the nose's delicate appearance can be one of the most demanding, yet gratifying, operative interventions that the dermatologic surgeon can undertake. Although the entire spectrum of nasal reconstructive alternatives cannot be described within this constraint of space, the principles of nasal reconstruction, with particular attention placed on procedures available to most surgically oriented dermatologists, can be suitably examined.

The nose occupies a prominent position of visual attention in the central face. In examining a face, observers spend a large amount of gaze time on the eyes and on the nose.[1] The visual scrutiny applied to the nose emphasizes the obvious need to offer nasal reconstructive procedures that do more than simply "fill a hole." The normal nose is a pyramidal structure with its apex in the glabella and its broad, freely mobile base between the eyes and mouth. Although anchored proximally to the face through rigid bony connections, at its distal aspects, the nose is a malleable soft tissue construct comprising mucosa, cartilage, muscle, subcutaneous tissue, and skin. The underlying architectural support for the distal nose is characterized by an interconnecting arrangement of flat and curved cartilages, and the particular size and shape of these cartilages is what is chiefly responsible for the wide diversity of noses that can still be appreciated as "normal." When skin is draped over the underlying bony and cartilaginous framework of the nose, a visually complicated facial feature begins to emerge.

To succeed in nasal reconstruction, the surgeon must first realize how the various visually distinct areas of the nose contribute to the nose's overall appearance. In general, the face can be divided into aesthetic units—areas in which the skin has its own unique color, texture, porosity, and surface contour. On the face, these aesthetic units are often broad areas of tissue bounded by naturally occurring landmarks. For example, the forehead—as defined by the anterior hairline, the brows, and the bilateral zygomatic arches—is a single visual unit. On the nose, however, the arrangement of aesthetic units becomes much more complicated. Although on casual inspection the nose might seem to represent a single prominent feature, the nose is more properly conceived to represent an intricate arrangement of concave and convex surfaces that are separated by predictable ridges and depressions. These aesthetic units of the nose are exactly symmetrical, and any surgical introduction of asymmetry has dramatic influence on the nose's final appearance. The division of the nose into aesthetic subunits (Fig. 15.1) has great relevance to the success of all nasal repairs, since surgical procedures that attempt to recreate the proper nasal topography and strive to place incision lines along naturally occurring boundaries are generally much more aesthetically successful than procedures that simply cover a wound without attention suitably placed on the aesthetic subtleties that define the normal nose's topography (Figs. 15.2–15.4).[2]

In addition to realizing that the nose is a facial feature with great topographic visual complexity, the dermatologic surgeon should also understand that the nose, in distinction to many other areas of the face, has areas in which the thickness, malleability, and sebaceous gland density of the skin varies tremendously. The nose is typically divided into areas in which the skin is thin, loose, forgiving, compliant, and relatively less sebaceous (the areas of the dorsum, sidewalls, soft triangles, and columella) and areas in which the skin is more adherent, less flexible, thicker, and more sebaceous (the areas of the nasal supratip, tip, and alae).[3] Unfortunately the distribution of these varying skin types (Fig. 15.5) is not nearly as predictable as the arrangement of the nasal aesthetic subunits; the surgeon therefore needs to assess the locations of these varying skin types prior to designing an operative procedure. That is, thick, sebaceous skin can have a great tendency to distort alar symmetry as it is moved distally. Additionally, if deeper distal defects are filled with the thinner skin of the proximal nose, volume replenishment will be insufficient and the important contours of the nose will not be appropriately restored.

After critically assessing the nose's normal topography and tissue availability, the physician should be well prepared to begin conceptualizing nasal reconstructive procedures. Nasal wounds can vary tremendously in size, depth, and location. Extensive nasal wounds should be approached with great caution, as the deeper architectural support elements of the nose serve to protect its important roles in olfaction, phonation, and respiration. If full-thickness nasal wounds are produced upon tumor removal, the complexity of the operative procedures required to repair the wound dramatically increases because internal nasal lining, rigid structural support, and aesthetically proper skin coverage must all be supplied in order to reconstruct the nose

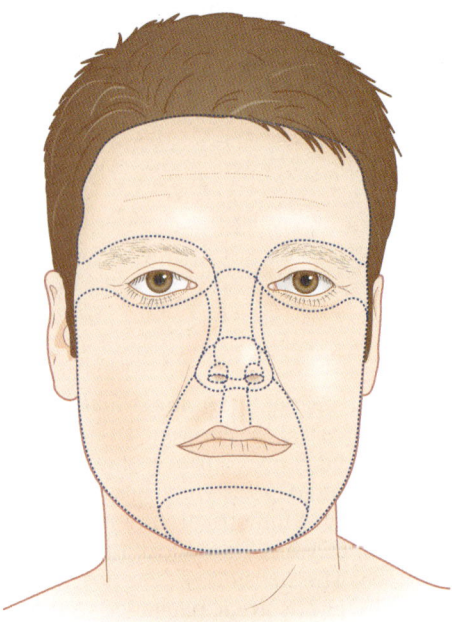

Fig. 15.1 The nose is divided into distinct visual areas (aesthetic subunits) that are separated by a predictable arrangement of ridges and valleys.

functionally and aesthetically. Prior to considering the aesthetic coverage of nasal wounds, the surgeon should be prepared to address the functional losses that tumor extirpation might have introduced. The nose must have protected patency for proper functioning; the distal nasal margins must therefore be appropriately braced with rigid cartilage grafts if the depth of tumor excision has been great enough to produce alar flaccidity (Fig. 15.6). If the rigidity of the alae is not restored prior to covering the wound, the weight of any flap will simply exacerbate alar collapse, and the inevitable contraction that accompanies any wound healing will add further distortion to the unsupported alar margin as the flap matures.

The proper selection of nasal reconstructive techniques begins, then, with an assessment of the wound's characteristics. One of the most important variables in categorizing the nasal wound is the wound's location. In the shadowed areas of the alar grooves and the medial canthus, select wounds can be allowed to heal by second intention (Fig. 15.7). In general, wounds amenable to such healing are small (less than 1 cm in diameter), shallow, within concave areas of shadowing, and at a significant distance (0.5 cm or greater) from the mobile alar margin.[4] In other areas of the nose (particularly in convex areas), the selection of second intention healing as a wound management strategy

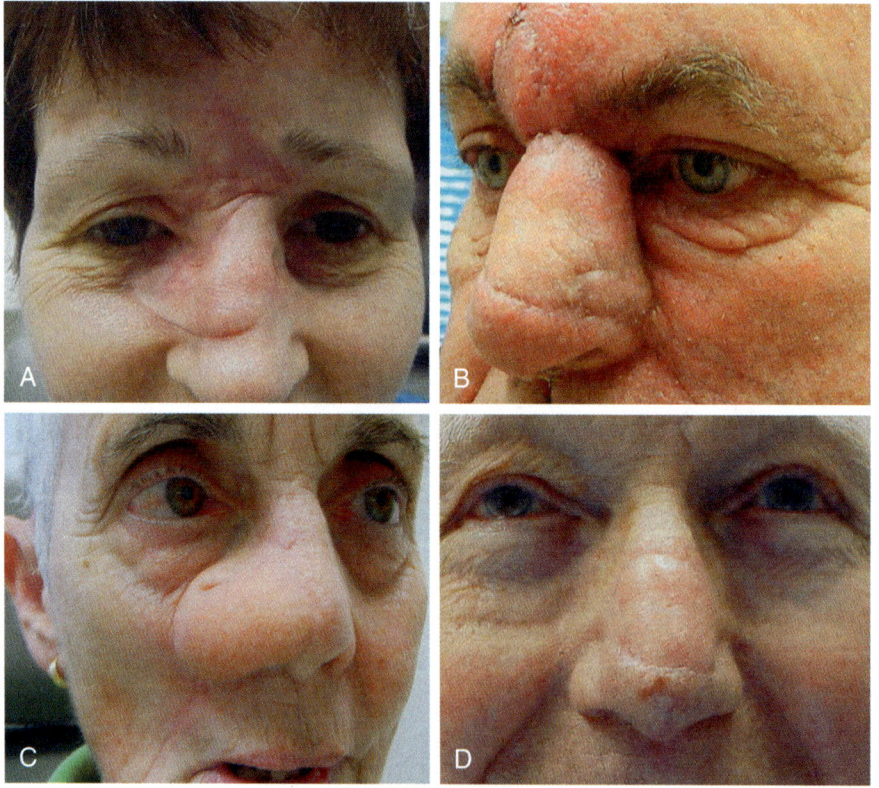

Fig. 15.2 In general the nose is ideally reconstructed using subunit principles. In these photos of reconstructive procedures done by physicians other than the author, the aesthetic results have been significantly hindered by a failure to adhere to the concept of reconstructing the nose by subunits. (A) A broad wound encompassing aesthetic units of the nose and the medial cheek/canthus has been repaired with a single large flap. Because aesthetic units have been crossed, the flap resulted in an unnatural appearance. (B) A less than ideal forehead flap, too redundant and extending onto the separate aesthetic units of the cheek and medial canthus, resulted in a poor reconstructive outcome in this case. (C) A tremendously oversized cheek-based flap was used to repair a deep alar wound. Because the flap was too large and it crossed the normally shadowed nose-cheek-lip junction, the flap looks like a cosmetically inappropriate "blob." (D) A forehead flap was used to cover a central dorsal nasal wound. When the flap failed to conform to the aesthetic subunits, a "patch-like" appearance resulted.

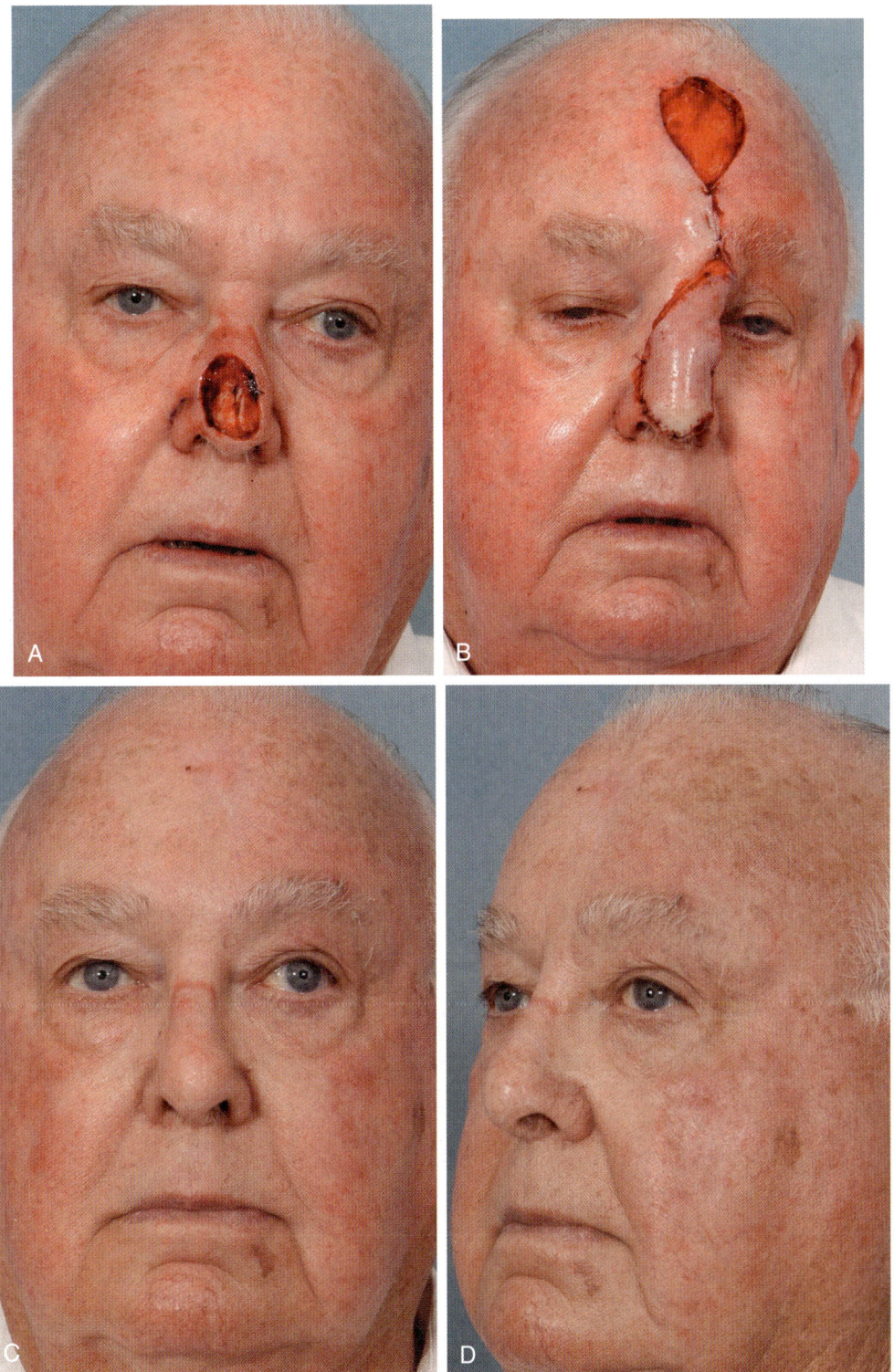

Fig. 15.3 (A) Following a Mohs excision, a large, deep nasal wound is present on the nasal tip. (B) To reconstruct the nose using the subunit concept, the wound's borders were extended to meet the boundaries of the aesthetic subunits before covering the wound with a paramedian forehead flap (note the flap's extension onto the junction of the infratip lobule and the columella). (C, D) At only 4 months following flap completion, the flap is not particularly apparent because the wound has been repaired with incision lines placed in areas of low aesthetic vulnerability, and the contour of the distal nose has been appropriately restored.

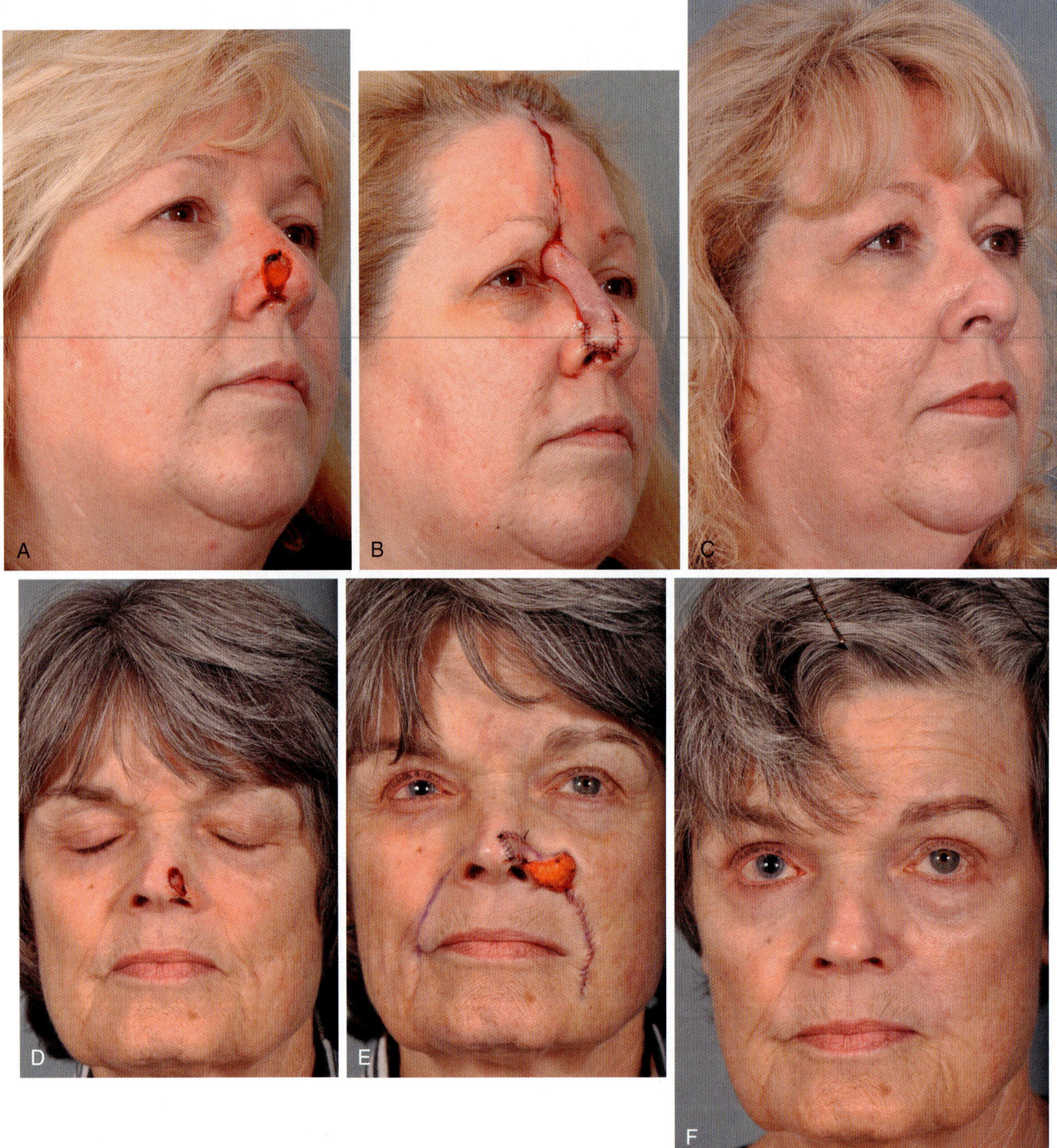

Fig. 15.4 Although it is often suggested that the nose should be repaired using the aesthetic subunit concept, these case examples of a paramedian forehead flap (A–C) and a pedicled nasolabial flap (D–F) illustrate that, with proper surgical technique, even complicated surgical techniques that repair wounds without strict adherence to the subunit concept can be successful.

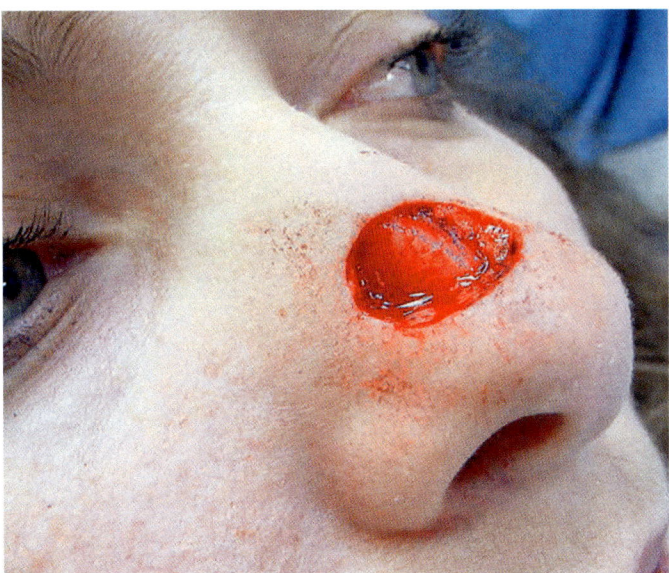

Fig. 15.5 In this patient with a Mohs surgical wound, note the difference between the thin skin of the nasal dorsum and the much thicker, more sebaceous skin in the area of the supratip.

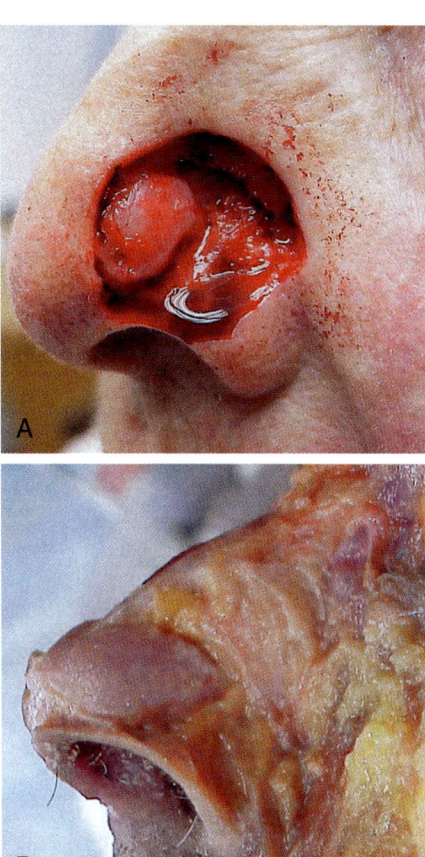

Fig. 15.6 After a Mohs excision (A), the abrupt termination of the lower lateral (alar) cartilage is visualized in the wound bed. A more extensive cadaveric dissection (B) in the same anatomic location demonstrates that the lateral ala is supported only by soft tissue, the resiliency of which varies tremendously from patient to patient. If deep wounds in the area of the lateral alae are not supported by appropriate cartilage grafts, alar collapse or distortion will result.

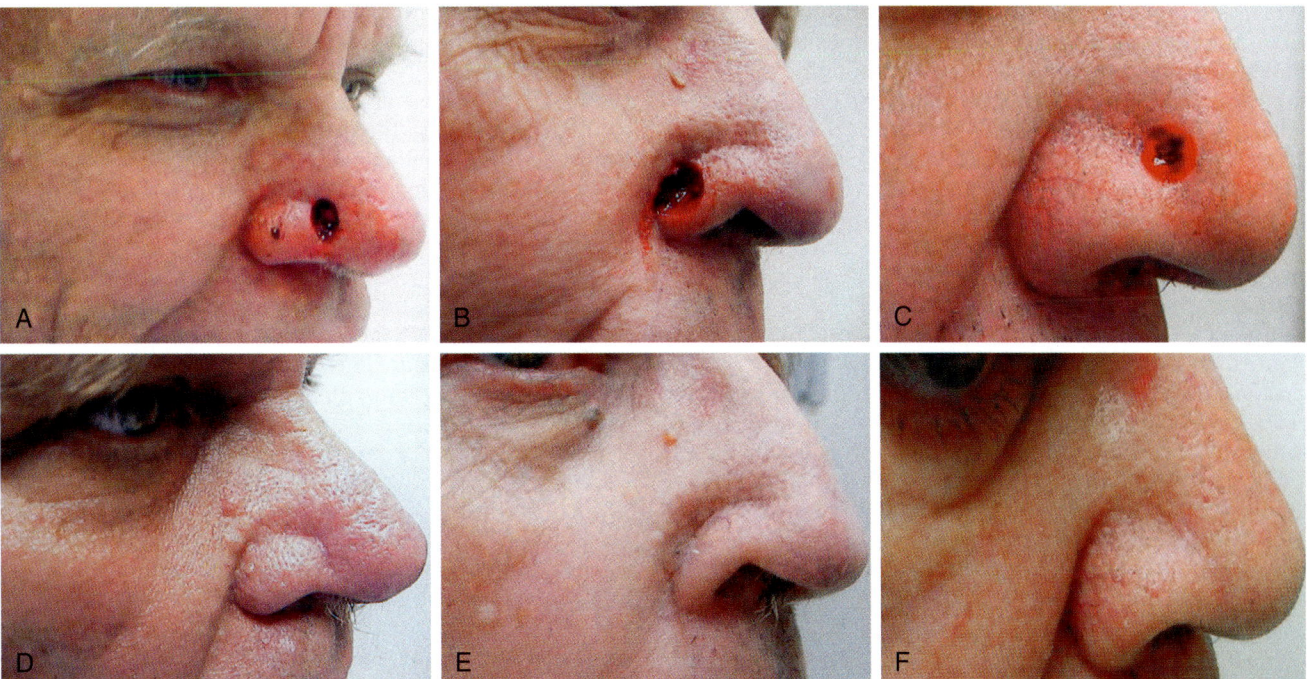

Fig. 15.7 Small shallow wounds that are present in areas of shadowed concavities can occasionally heal appropriately by second intention (A/B, C/D, E/F). Note, however, that several of these examples (A/D and B/E) demonstrate that the contraction associated with second intention healing can introduce a slight degree of alar elevation. Nonetheless, the aesthetic results of this type of healing in the cases shown here likely exceed the results seen with alternative reconstructive procedures.

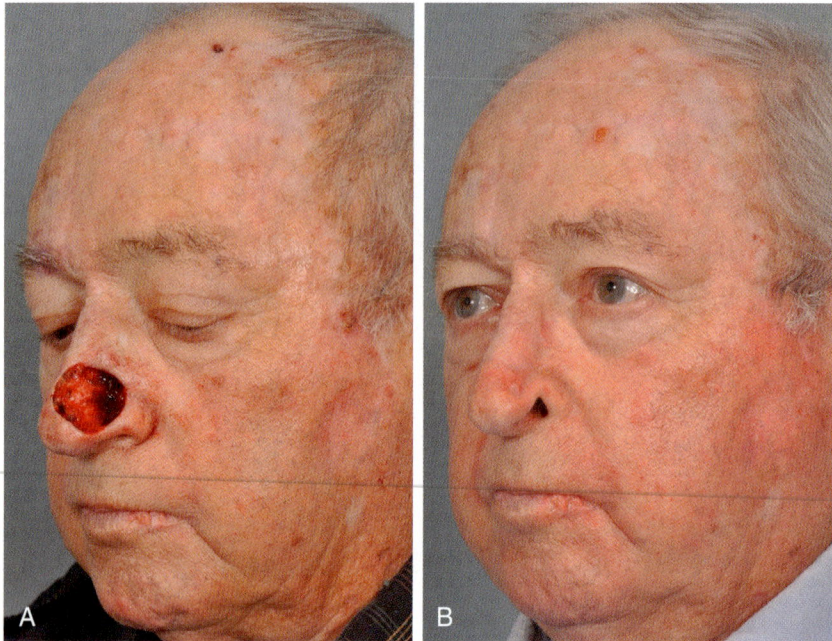

Fig. 15.8 This patient declined a reconstructive procedure. Although his nasal wound was very shallow (A), the inevitable contraction associated with healing by second intention produced alar elevation and distortion that would be difficult to revise successfully (B).

often produces anatomic distortion, contour irregularities, and aesthetically inferior scars (Fig. 15.8). If the nasal wound is not located within the shadowed alar groove or medial canthus, it is likely poorly suited for healing by second intention (unless it is very small). To begin selecting a nasal repair alternative, the location of the wound should be noted in reference to the quality and availability of the surrounding nasal skin. There is often sufficient laxity on the proximal nasal dorsum and sidewalls to allow primary closure of small wounds. Because of the compliance of the relatively nonsebaceous skin in these areas, small local flaps can also be created from adjacent tissues. If wounds located along the proximal nasal dorsum or sidewalls are broader, skin grafts can occasionally be useful. Although, in general, skin grafts are a poor aesthetic match for nasal skin, the relatively nonsebaceous skin of the more proximal nose is better suited for a graft repair than the sebaceous skin of the nasal alae and tip.

Distal nasal wounds offer more significant reconstructive challenges. The distal skin of the nose is thick and sebaceous, and wounds in such skin are very difficult to manage without relying upon more complicated reconstructive techniques. Second intention healing over the thickly skinned areas of convexity on the distal nose produces scars that are rarely cosmetically ideal. Additionally, the sebaceous quality of the skin of the nasal tip tends to make even the most appropriately selected skin graft repair look like a shiny, slick, frequently hypopigmented patch that also commonly fails to offer sufficient volume replenishment (Fig. 15.9). For that reason, if the surgeon wishes to restore the nose's delicate contour, wounds in the distal thickly skinned areas of the nose frequently demand flap repairs. Distal nasal wounds can often be repaired with flaps that harvest the looser, available nasal skin located immediately proximal to the wound. This allows the unique skin of the nose to be rearranged appropriately. If, however, the surgical wound on the nose is too broad or anatomically complicated to cover with donated skin from the areas of remaining nasal skin proximal to the wound, flaps from the adjacent forehead or cheek can be designed.

The size of the surgical wound also has important ramifications in terms of the success of any nasal reconstructive procedure. As previously mentioned, many small nasal wounds can be allowed to granulate. Wounds up to 1 cm in diameter can also be closed primarily, even when they are located in difficult areas, such as the nasal tip (provided that there is sufficient adjacent tissue laxity). More complicated wounds understandably require larger reconstructive efforts. If the large wound is shallow (well-perfused soft tissue remains in the wound's bed), a skin graft is sometimes the best repair alternative. If the larger nasal wound has significant depth (to the deeper subcutaneous tissue or to the underlying cartilage or bone), a flap repair will be a more suitable reconstructive alternative. Regardless of the size of the wound, the wound should be examined from the aesthetic subunit perspective. If the wound already involves a significant proportion of any aesthetic subunit of the nose, consideration should be given to expanding the wound (sacrificing adjacent normal skin) until the aesthetic subunit boundaries are encountered,[2] which will favorably place the incision lines along areas of lowest cosmetic burden.

After the surgical wound has been adequately characterized, repair alternatives can be considered. Of course, no surgical reconstructive procedure should be contemplated before an absolute determination of the adequacy of tumor removal, as persistent tumor buried under a graft or flap may be clinically unrecognizable for several disastrous years. The Mohs micrographic surgical technique offers unrivaled success in the treatment of many cutaneous tumors,[5] and the Mohs technique also has important tissue conservation abilities.[6] For these reasons, many primary

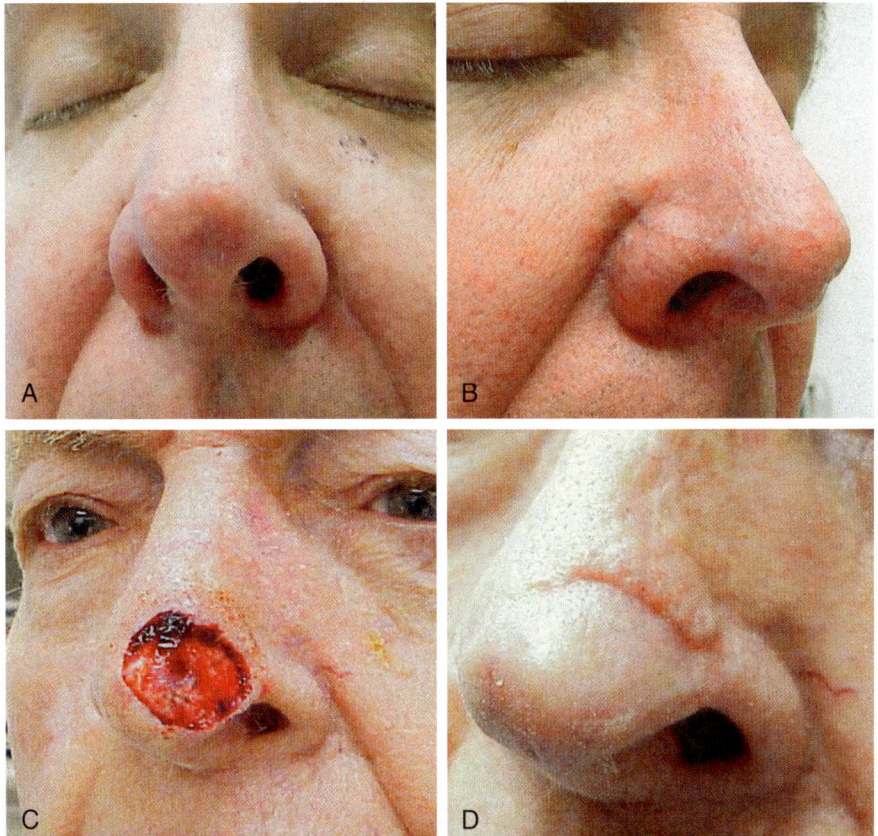

Fig. 15.9 A full-thickness skin graft has offered a reasonable color and texture match to the distal nasal tip (A). On lateral view (B), however, it is apparent that the graft has failed to offer sufficient volume replenishment. A skin graft has been used to repair a wound in a patient who refused to undergo a more involved flap repair (C). Although the skin graft survived, the color and texture do not match the sebaceous skin of the nasal tip. Additionally, the graft offers no contour restoration to the nasal tip's convexity (D).

and recurrent/persistent nasal tumors are ideally excised with the Mohs technique before the resulting wounds are repaired.

Following adequate tumor removal, as already noted, repair alternatives are considered based on the size, complexity, and location of the operative wound. Simple wound management strategies such as healing by second intention or primary closure are selected if the characteristics of the wound predict success with these uncomplicated techniques. If sufficient tissue is available on the nose, the use of random-pattern flaps is often considered to be the ideal repair alternative. If a local flap cannot be created without introducing anatomic distortion/asymmetry, a more complicated pedicled flap from the adjacent cheek or forehead can be useful. Skin grafts, because of their very frequent visibility, are generally thought to represent appropriate choices only when a flap repair is judged to be undesirable or unavailable.

Repair Alternatives

PRIMARY CLOSURE

The layered linear repair (primary closure) is occasionally an ideal reconstructive solution for smaller nasal wounds located along the nasal sidewalls, within the alar groove, or directly centered on the nasal tip (Fig. 15.10). All linear closures have wound closure tensions that are oriented perpendicularly to the long axis of the wound; on the nose, these wound closure tensions can introduce dramatic nasal distortion if broader nasal wounds are selected for closure, particularly on thickly skinned sebaceous noses with little tissue laxity. For that reason, only small (<1 cm) and shallow (no disruption of the underlying architectural framework of the nose) wounds are appropriately selected for primary closure.

Along the proximal nasal sidewalls, a properly oriented linear closure will point toward the medial canthus, as the relaxed skin tension lines in this area are obliquely oriented. If wounds greater than 1 cm in diameter along the proximal sidewalls are closed linearly, however, the obliquely oriented wound closure tensions will typically result in undesirable ipsilateral alar elevation. In the area of the central nasal tip, small wounds can be directly closed in a vertically oriented linear manner.[7] In order to prevent the introduction of very distracting alar asymmetry, the surgical defect must be exactly located in the midline. Before excising the dog-ear redundancies that accompany the closure of any circular defect, the surgeon should make certain that the thick, adherent skin of the distal nose has sufficient laxity to allow closure of the distal nasal wound

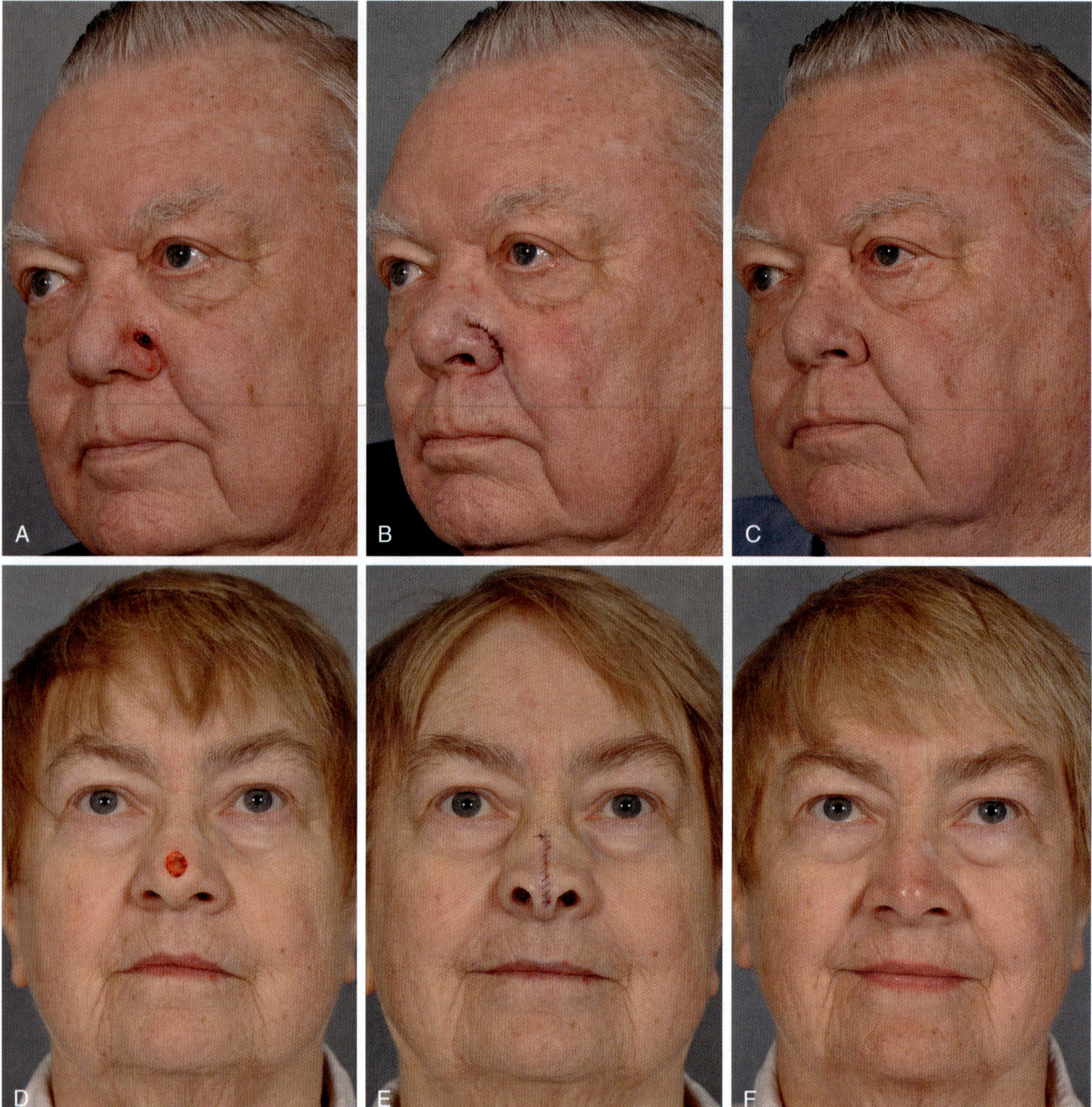

Fig. 15.10 Linear closures in various areas of the nose are demonstrated. Because the wounds (A, D) were relatively small and there was sufficient adjacent tissue laxity, lasting undesirable anatomic distortion seen with the wound closure tensions was avoided (B, C, E). In figures (D) through (F), note that the closure of the nasal tip wound with modestly elevated wound closure tensions produced a slight alar "flare." Because the alar lift was minimal, there was no permanent deformity.

under minimal wound closure tensions. If the wound is closed under inappropriately elevated tension, wound edge ischemia (and the resulting unaesthetic scarring) can result. If wound closure tensions are too high, significant deformity of the nasal dorsum will also be apparent on a profile view. These elevated wound closure tensions will result in an anatomically incorrect indentation, often in the area of the nasal supratip. Higher wound closure tensions also produce an artificial "flared" appearance to the nasal alae. If the degree of alar lift associated with the vertical closure of nasal tip wounds is minor and symmetric, the cosmetic penalty will be small. Greater degrees of alar distortion can produce an acutely angled, sharp, "beak-like" distal nasal deformity.

In performing any linear closure on the nose, care should be taken to avoid producing dog-ear redundancies at the ends of the elliptical closure, as the shadowing that such redundancies produce can be particularly distracting on the nose. For that reason, the length-to-width ratio of linear closures on the nose should be at least 4:1.[7] After the dog-ear redundancies adjacent to the wound are excised, the wound is widely undermined in the plane immediately above the paired nasal cartilages. Undermining at this plane ensures that the nasalis musculature (an important source of perfusion to the skin) is preserved. Wide undermining is required in order to minimize wound closure tensions, and the wound should be subsequently closed in a layered manner in order to produce a less apparent scar. Wound-edge eversion is particularly important on the distal nose, where the bulky sebaceous lobules tend to produce invagination of the wound's edges.

FULL-THICKNESS SKIN GRAFTS

Because there is a general lack of abundant available donor tissue on the nose, the temptation to cover many nasal wounds with skin grafts can be quite high. Skin grafting techniques, described in great detail elsewhere in this text, are certainly inherently less complicated endeavors than the design and execution of many nasal flaps, where tissue motion and wound tensions need to be very accurately predicted if anatomic distortion is to be avoided. To be certain, skin grafts have an important role in the reconstruction of select nasal defects. In general, though, the grafts' inability to offer significant volume replenishment limits their utility to exquisitely shallow nasal wounds. Skin grafts are also more unpredictable in their eventual aesthetic outcomes than properly executed flaps, and it is common to notice that grafts do not share similar color and texture characteristics with the surrounding nasal skin.

Split-thickness skin grafts are very thin grafts that lack the density of adnexal appendages sufficient to offer any hope of an aesthetically proper outcome when the grafts are used in facial reconstructive surgery. In nasal reconstruction, these grafts serve little aesthetic purpose. Occasionally, split-thickness skin grafts are used to cover deep nasal wounds in anticipation of a prosthetic rehabilitation, but such grafts should not be considered to be anything other than purely functional repairs. On the other hand, full-thickness skin grafts can offer appropriate aesthetic outcomes if the proper patients, wounds, and donor sites are selected. Patients with significant peripheral vascular disease, a history of radiation therapy to the recipient site, or with current heavy tobacco abuse are at greater risk of ischemic graft failure. Indeed, such patients are at greater operative risk for surgical complications with any nasal reconstructive procedure.

Not surprisingly, skin grafts are less apparent on the thinner, less sebaceous skin of the nose. As such, skin grafts are acceptable reconstructive options for relatively shallow wounds located in the thinned skin zones of the columella, soft triangles, and along the nasal dorsum and sidewalls (where greater tissue abundance typically allows more appropriate flap repair options). On occasion, skin grafts can be viable repair options for very small and shallow wounds in the more sebaceous areas of the nasal alae and tip (Figs. 15.11 and 15.12), although the textural mismatch of any skin graft when applied to such thicker nasal skin is often glaringly apparent. To minimize the size of the skin graft, Burow grafts (where the superior portion of the wound is closed in a linear manner and the redundancy that is removed upon closure of this area is donated to the distal aspect of the wound as a full-thickness skin graft) are occasionally useful (Fig. 15.13).[8] Because of potential textural mismatches and the limited ability of skin grafts to offer sufficient volume replenishment for many deeper nasal wounds, flaps are generally far superior reconstructive alternatives for a considerable number of more significant nasal defects.

Donor sites for full-thickness skin grafts used in nasal reconstruction could possibly include any hairless area of skin. An ideal skin graft site would offer skin that is a similar color, texture, and thickness to the skin of the nose. Additionally, the desirable skin graft donor site would be located in an area of low aesthetic attention. Common donor sites for skin grafts used in nasal reconstruction include the preauricular cheek, the postauricular sulcus, the clavicular area of the chest, and the cavum concha. All skin graft donor sites have advantages and disadvantages. Preauricular grafts have been historically championed as ideal nasal repair options, but the scars at preauricular donor sites can occasionally be quite apparent. Despite expert surgical technique, some degree of facial asymmetry can also be introduced when the graft is harvested from the lateral cheek. Additionally, in male patients, the harvesting of skin grafts from the preauricular area moves hair-bearing skin much closer to the ear, and the tragus can be frustratingly cut during shaving. Postauricular skin can be used as a skin graft donor site, but the photo-protected, less sebaceous skin in this area is uncommonly an ideal match for the exposed, thick skin of the nose. Skin of the supraclavicular chest can also be very useful for larger wounds on the nose, but this skin's quality is particularly variable. In some patients, this skin is quite atrophic and inappropriate for the repair of nasal wounds; in some patients, the thick dermis of the skin in this area makes grafting challenging. Skin grafts harvested from this area also demonstrate a common tendency to heal with distracting hyperpigmentation. The skin of the conchal bowl is often an ideal site for the harvesting of smaller skin grafts used in nasal repairs. Because the skin of the concha has been shown to have sebaceous lobules with similar densities and sizes compared to the thicker skin of the distal nose,[9] this skin offers superior donor possibilities. Conchal grafts of up to 2 cm in diameter can be quickly harvested from the cavum and cymba concha, and the perichondrium underlying the skin can be retained in order to offer thicker grafts that nonetheless routinely survive. The donor site of the conchal graft is allowed to heal by second intention, and the cartilage is routinely perforated in order to allow the postauricular skin to more easily cover the exposed conchal cartilage. Such manipulation of the conchal cartilage, though traditionally feared to increase the likelihood of potentially disastrous infectious chondritis, has not been shown to increase the probabilities of concerning postoperative complications.[10] Nonetheless, conchal donor sites frequently develop an inflammatory perichondritis following graft harvesting, and patients often complain of significant donor-site pain that can last several weeks until the donor wound has completely reepithelialized. Therefore other donor sites may be preferable.

Regardless of the graft's donor site, the success of skin grafting techniques actually depends more on the qualities of the recipient bed than on the characteristics of the donor tissue. Recipient sites that have predictably poor perfusion (due to the patient's exposed cartilage or bone,

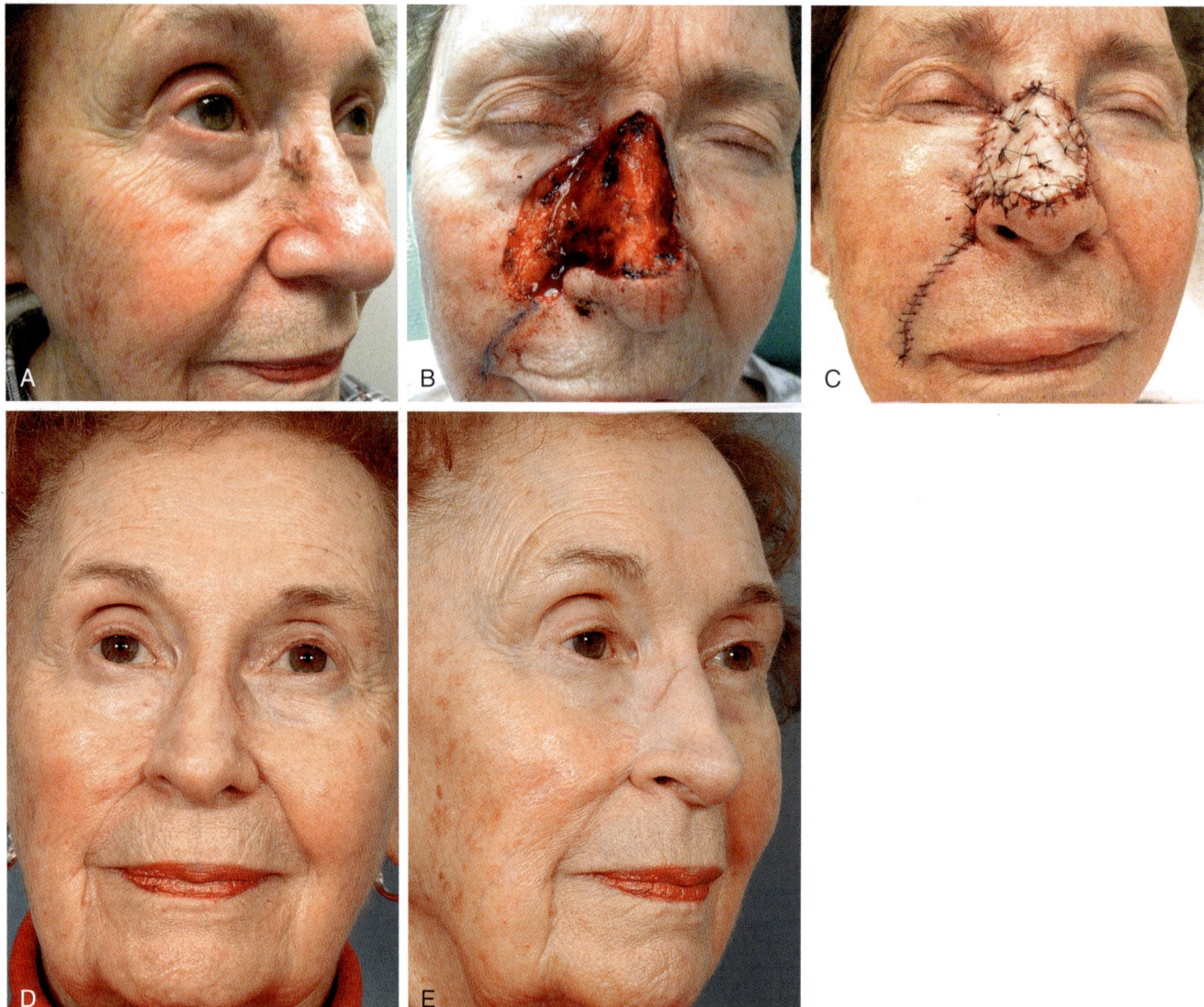

Fig. 15.11 (A) An ill-defined melanoma in situ of the nose and medial cheek is well suited for excision using the Mohs surgical technique. (B) Significant subclinical tumor extension was noted upon tumor removal, and the resulting wound spanned several aesthetic subunits on the nose and medial cheek. (C) In order to minimize the visibility of the planned skin graft on the nose, the cheek was advanced medially. Because the underlying well-vascularized perichondrium was intact, a full-thickness skin graft was used to reconstruct the nasal portion of the wound in a patient unwilling to consider a pedicled flap repair. (D, E) Anterior and lateral views at postoperative month 4 reveal acceptable aesthetic results for this difficult wound. Note that the erythematous depression along the proximal nasal dorsum reflects compression from the patient's spectacle frames.

associated vascular disease, tobacco abuse,[11] previous radiation therapy, anemia, or a host of other concomitant medical issues) rarely promote ideal graft results. Even if the graft survives, the relatively poor initial perfusion rarely allows the graft to offer an aesthetically ideal repair. Despite the inherently poor perfusion of cartilage, small cartilage batten grafts can be used to support the alar margin prior to covering the exposed wound with a skin graft if care is taken to appropriately tack the skin graft around the cartilage graft and to ensure that the majority of the graft is in direct contact with a well-perfused wound bed.[3] Care should be taken to debride the graft's recipient site of any detritus (including electrocautery char), and the graft should be secured with peripheral and basting sutures. Because tie-over bolster sutures have been shown to offer no significant benefit to smaller grafts,[12] they are not typically required for the relatively small grafts used in nasal repair. For larger grafts, immobilization has important benefits, and bolster dressing may improve the graft's survival and final appearance. With significant grafts on the distal nose, intranasal immobilization with an appropriate technique can also be beneficial (Fig. 15.14).

In addition to split- and full-thickness skin grafts, composite grafts are occasionally useful in nasal reconstruction. Composite grafts are grafts that contain an element other than skin and subcutaneous tissue. On the nose, the most commonly used composite grafts are cartilage-containing grafts harvested from various donor sites on the ear. Although the composite graft has an opportunity to restore contour to deeper surgical wounds, particularly along the

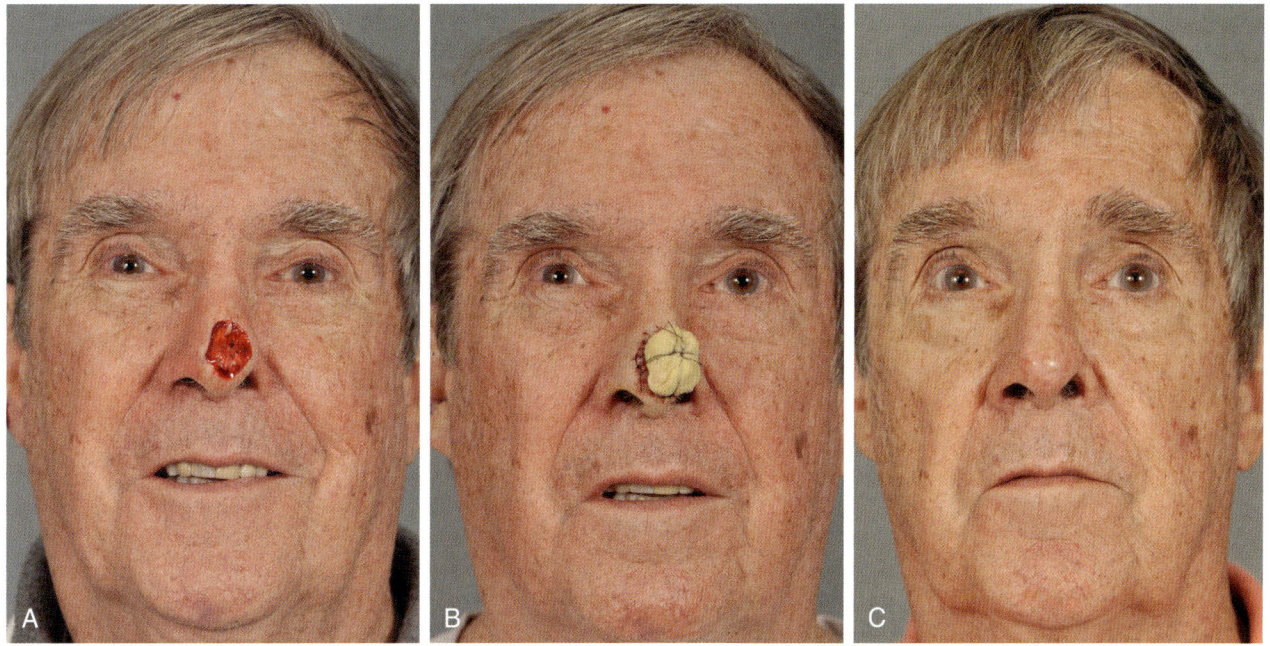

Fig. 15.12 A basal cell carcinoma of the nose was excised (A); the shallow wound along the sebaceous nasal tip was repaired with a full-thickness skin graft harvested from the postauricular sulcus. A tie-over bolster dressing was used to immobilize the graft and improve the likelihood of graft survival (B). Because the defect was shallow, the graft offered an appropriate tip restoration (C).

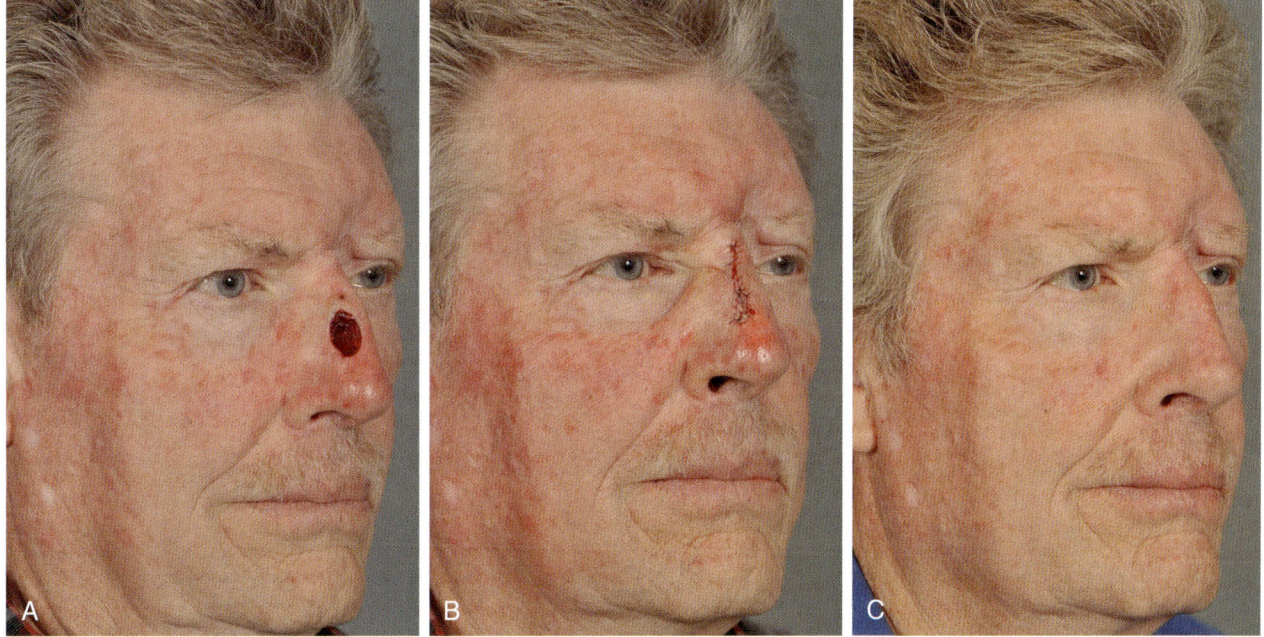

Fig. 15.13 (A) A basal cell carcinoma defect on the nasal sidewall was apparent. (B) A larger full-thickness skin graft was thought to be less than ideal, given the patient's sebaceous skin, so a Burow graft harvested from the looser skin of the proximal nose was used to repair the wound. (C) At postoperative month 3, the linear component of the wound was not particularly apparent, and the diminished size of the patch-like skin graft improved the final aesthetic result.

alar rim (Fig. 15.15), composite grafts are often less than ideal reconstructive options than suitably designed flaps. The harvesting of inherently thick composite grafts can cause aesthetic concerns at the donor site if the ear is not repaired properly,[13] and the presence of cartilage within the graft increases the graft's metabolic demands and the likelihood of ischemic failure. In addition, composite grafts are subject to significant shrinkage in the later postoperative period, and it is not uncommon for a composite graft along the alar margin to heal with a noticeable "notch" deformity if care is not taken to size the graft appropriately at the time of harvesting.

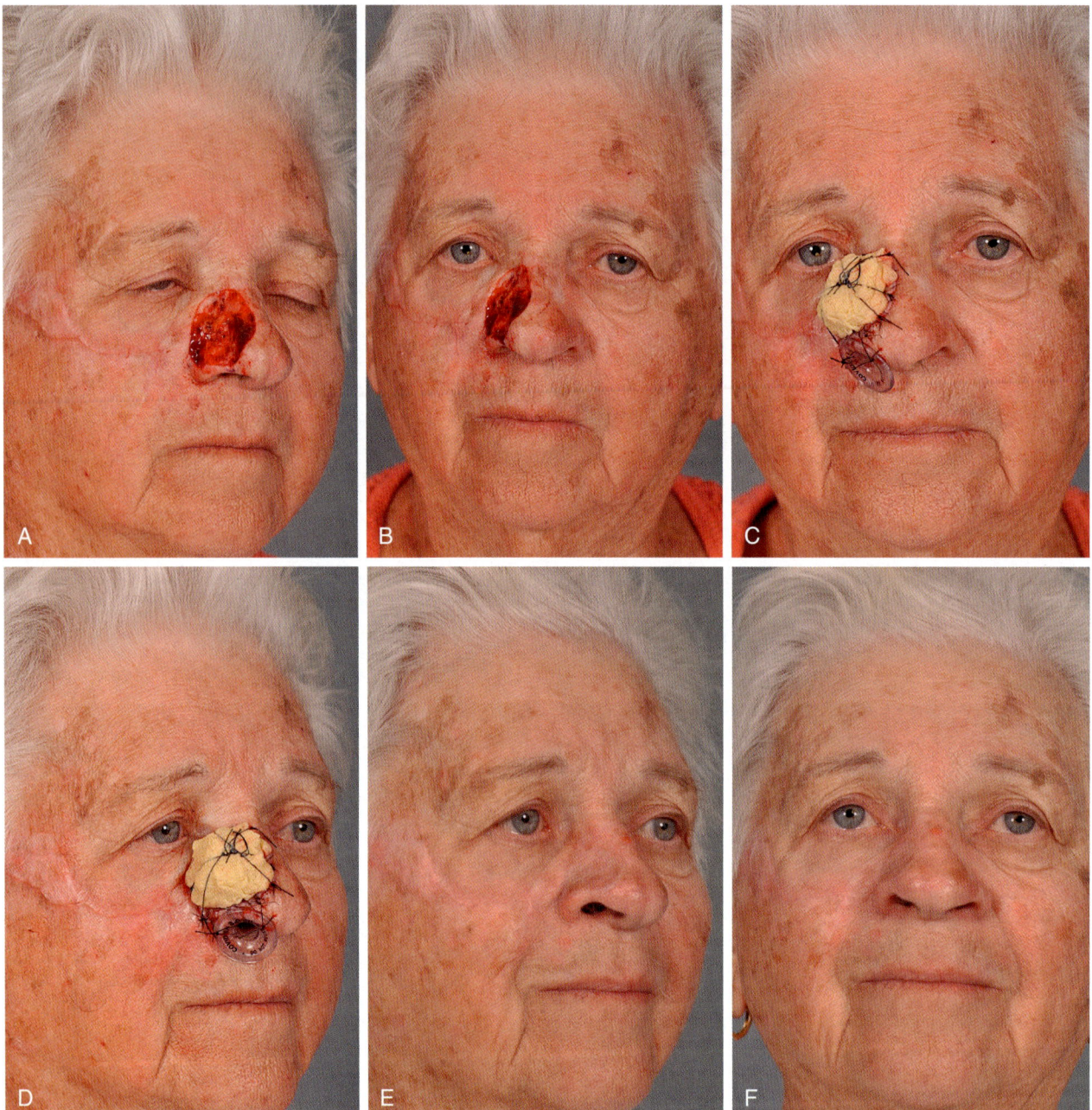

Fig. 15.14 (A, B) A large defect was produced upon removal of an anatomically complicated basal cell carcinoma. (C, D) Because this patient was not willing to consider a pedicled flap repair, the wound was repaired with a large full-thickness skin graft harvested from the supraclavicular chest. In order to improve the probability of graft survival and to "brace" the functionally important alar rim during the important initial days of wound healing, the graft was immobilized with a tie-over bolster dressing and a nasopharyngeal airway, which was sutured to the adjacent remaining nose and allowed to remain in place for 1 week. (E, F) Oblique and anterior reviews reveal very reasonable aesthetic results with preservation of alar patency.

FLAP RECONSTRUCTION OF THE NOSE

Cutaneous flaps are constructs of skin and soft tissue that are harvested from anatomic sites adjacent or near to the primary surgical defect. Created from adjacent skin, flaps retain a connection to a protected vascular supply, thus dramatically lowering the risk of ischemic failure seen with skin grafts, where the skin is initially entirely severed from its underlying vascular supply. Flaps offer multiple advantages in the reconstruction of nasal wounds. When properly designed and executed, flaps are safe and predictable reconstructive options for wounds that should not be allowed to heal by second intention or cannot be closed in a simpler linear manner. In distinction to skin grafts, cutaneous flaps offer abilities to cover deeper and more complicated nasal wounds with tissue that has a similar color, texture, and thickness to the adjacent nasal skin. Because the perfusion of a well-designed flap is protected, the survival rates of flaps typically exceed the survival rates of both split- and full-thickness skin grafts.[14] The protected perfusion of a flap also allows the survival of integrated reconstructive elements such as autologous cartilage grafts.

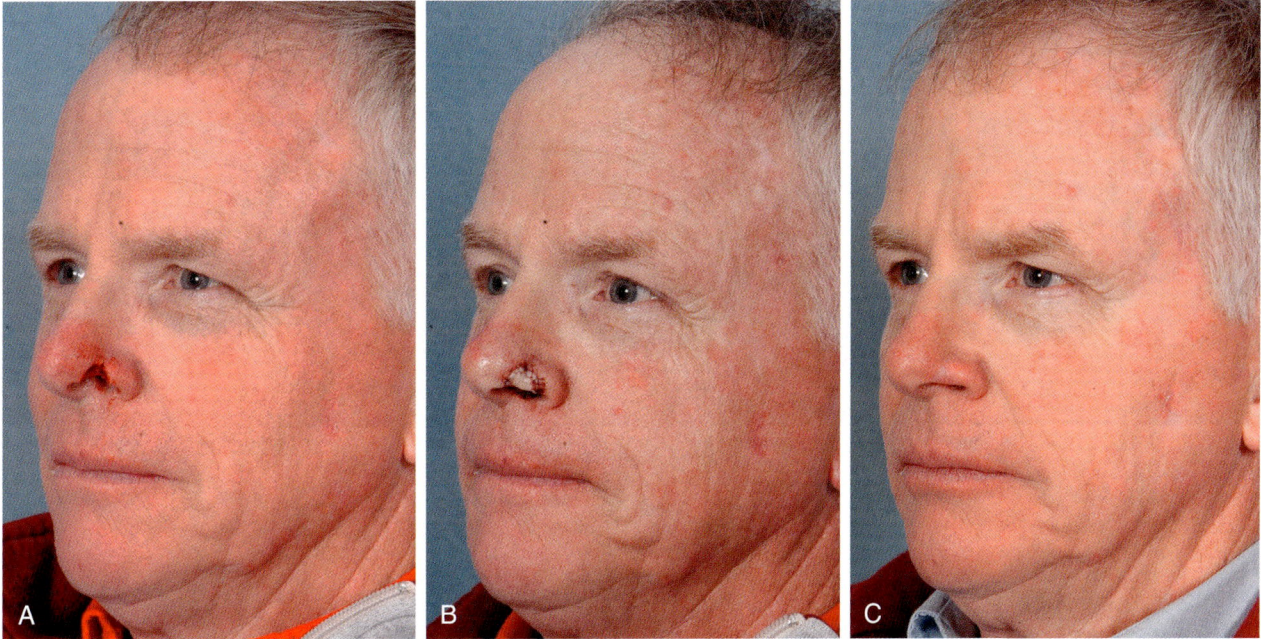

Fig. 15.15 (A) Excision of a basal cell carcinoma at the distal nose produced a small but full-thickness defect along the alar rim. (B) A composite graft harvested from the root of the helix was used to restore the thickness and stability of the rim. (C) Aesthetically and functionally appropriate restoration of the alar rim was accomplished.

Despite their impressive utility, cutaneous flaps possess several distinct disadvantages. The geometric design of nasal flaps demands an intricate knowledge of the biomechanical properties of skin and the principles of tissue movement. Flaps created without attention to proper design have great ability to introduce nasal distortion that can be difficult (and frequently impossible) to correct. Additionally, the creation of nasal flaps demands the introduction of longer incision lines on the face, and unless expert surgical technique is used, the aesthetic appearance of the flap's lengthy scars can be more distracting than the appearance of a wound that has healed by second intention or has been reconstructed with a skin graft. Finally, because nasal flaps frequently require large amounts of undermining, the potential for introducing surgical morbidity is greater than that seen with simpler reconstructive alternatives.

Flaps have been historically classified by many different means: by blood supply (random, axial), by location (local, regional), by eponymous name (Rieger, Tenzel, etc.), and by primary motion (advancement, rotation, transposition). The majority of smaller nasal wounds can be reconstructed with random-patterned cutaneous flaps, flaps that rely on the highly anastomotic dermal vasculature for perfusion but that lack a larger-caliber named artery in their bases. Such flaps can be created from the somewhat sebaceous skin of the nose or the adjacent cheek or forehead. Larger or more anatomically complicated nasal wounds can require the use of a pedicled flap for most appropriate repair. These pedicled flaps can rely on the unnamed, luxurious perfusion of the underlying muscle (the pedicled melo-labial flap) or on the presence of a named artery in the flap's base (the paramedian forehead flap). The primary challenge in nasal reconstruction, therefore, is to select a flap that offers low donor morbidity, predictable perfusion, operative simplicity, and aesthetic success.

Advancement Flaps

Traditional U-shaped advancement flaps have little utility on the nose. The mobilization of such flaps requires long linear incisions that would be unlikely to be aesthetically successful on the nose.

Additionally, such traditional advancement flaps nearly always also depend upon secondary motion around the primary defect's location in order to close the wound. Such secondary motion typically causes undesirable distal nasal deformation and asymmetry. Advancement flaps can be quite successful, however, in the repair of nasal wounds of medium size (1 to 2 cm) when the wounds are located on the lateral nasal sidewall and supratip. Such flaps, based on the richly perfused nasalis musculature that covers the entire lateral nose, are viable and uncomplicated repair alternatives (Figs. 15.16 and 15.17). The incision lines of these advancement flaps are favorably placed along the alar grove and the proximal melo-labial crease. As the flaps are advanced medially, care must be taken to accurately excise the superior dog-ear redundancies that inevitably result from flap motion, to excise a crescent of tissue along the alar groove to prevent ipsilateral alar depression, and to place tacking sutures in the area of the nasofacial groove in order to prevent an unaesthetic "bridging" of this normally shadowed concavity. Like all tacking sutures placed in facial flaps in this anatomic area, the deep bite of the suture should attempt to capture the underlying tissue in the area of the piriform aperture, and the superficial bite of the tacking suture should be placed longitudinally along the axis of the flap in order to prevent the introduction of unnecessary ischemia. Additionally, tacking sutures should be placed deeply enough within the leading edge of the flap so that an unaesthetic (though temporary) "dimple" in the skin's surface is not created. When there is insufficient

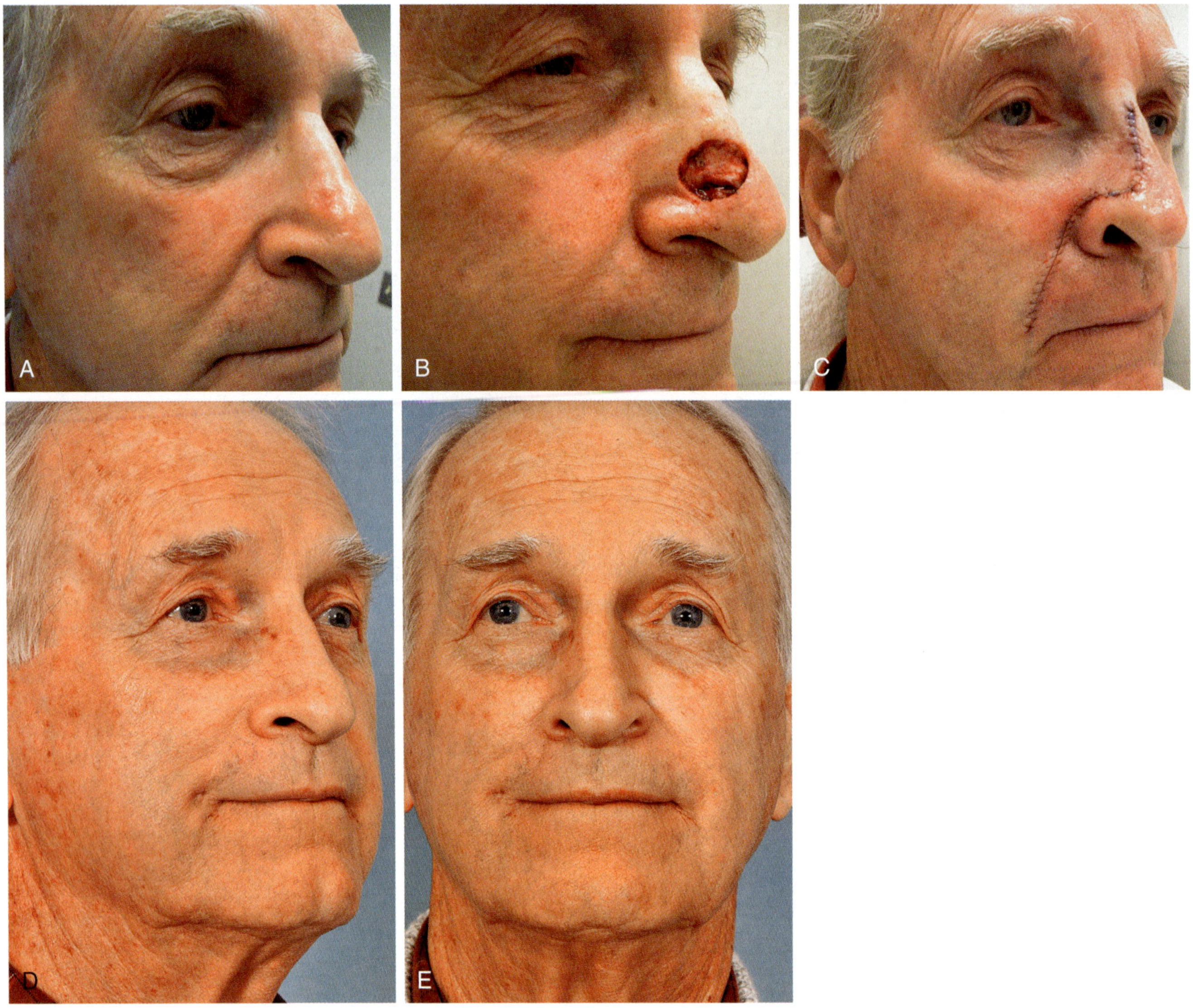

Fig. 15.16 A basal cell carcinoma of nasal sidewall (A) was excised using the Mohs technique (B), and the wound's location near the alar groove allowed the harvesting of an advancement flap based on the underlying nasalis musculature (C). Critical to the aesthetic success of this flap (D, E) was the placement of deep tacking sutures to preserve the shadowed nasofacial sulcus and the excision of a curved redundancy along the flap's inferior margin to prevent the depression of the ipsilateral alar margin.

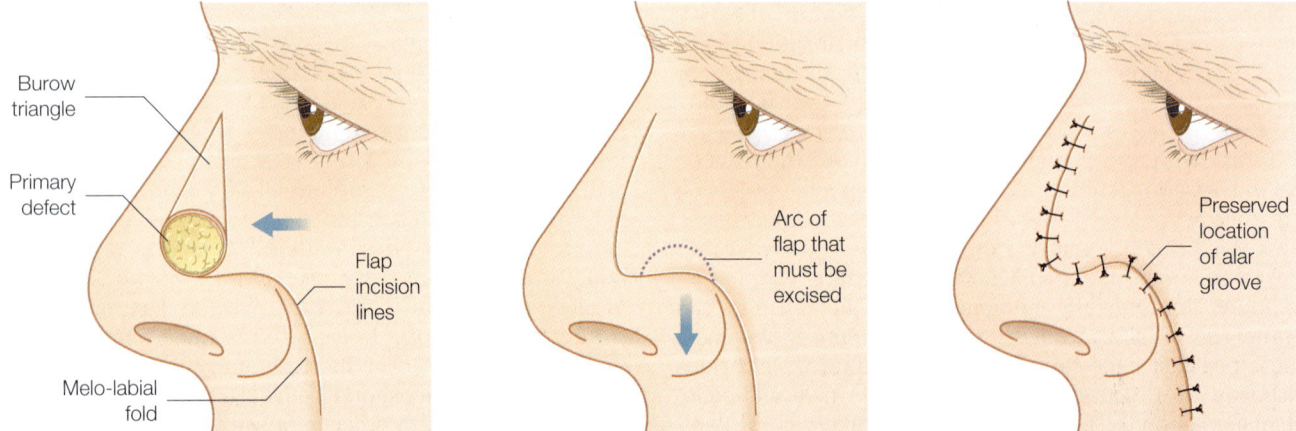

Fig. 15.17 This schematic drawing illustrates the type of advancement flap depicted in Fig. 15.14. Although the inferior incision line of the flap is logically placed within the alar groove, as the flap is advanced, simple suturing of the flap to the existing secondary defect would result in predictable depression of the lateral aspect of the ipsilateral ala. Instead, a curved redundancy is removed along the flap's edge, and the location of the entire alar groove remains protected. Because the flap is richly perfused, this excision along the flap's margin does not compromise the flap's viability.

laxity to allow for the reconstruction of a nasal dorsum defect with a single advancement flap, bilateral advancement flaps can also be designed in order to harvest available tissue on both sides of the wound (Fig. 15.18).

A Burow advancement flap is useful in the reconstruction of small wounds in the areas of the nasal tip and supratip.[15,16] This flap is particularly helpful because its design allows for the repair of wounds that are slightly off center of the nasal midline, where linear repairs can be preferentially used. The flap is a variation of the linear repair where the inferior dog-ear redundancy is relocated to the exact nasal midline, removing any possibility of introducing alar asymmetry (Fig. 15.19).

The V-Y flap is an attractive repair option for deeper wounds of the face because the flap's centrally located thick, muscular pedicle produces a flap that is nearly

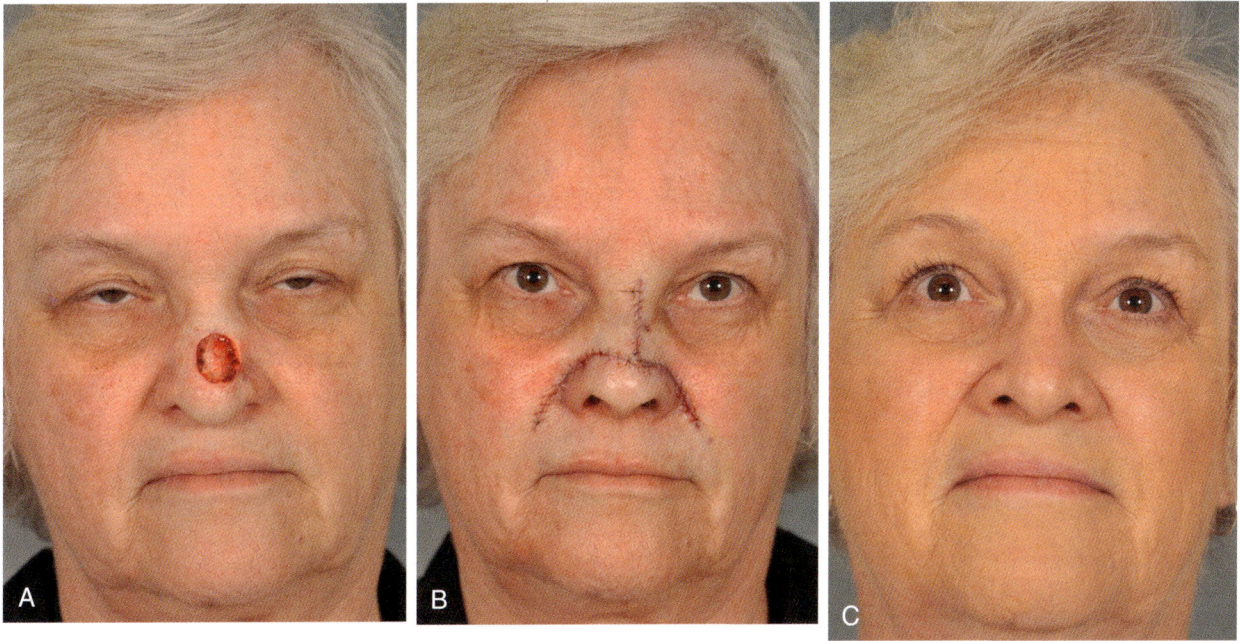

Fig. 15.18 (A) A moderately deep nasal wound was noted in a patient with relatively immobile nasal dorsal skin. (B) Because there was insufficient laxity to allow for repair with unilateral tissue advancement, the distal defect was repaired with bilateral advancement flaps incised within the bilateral alar grooves and undermined widely into the paranasal cheek. (C) Acceptable contour restoration and preserved alar symmetry were noted at a 4-month follow-up examination.

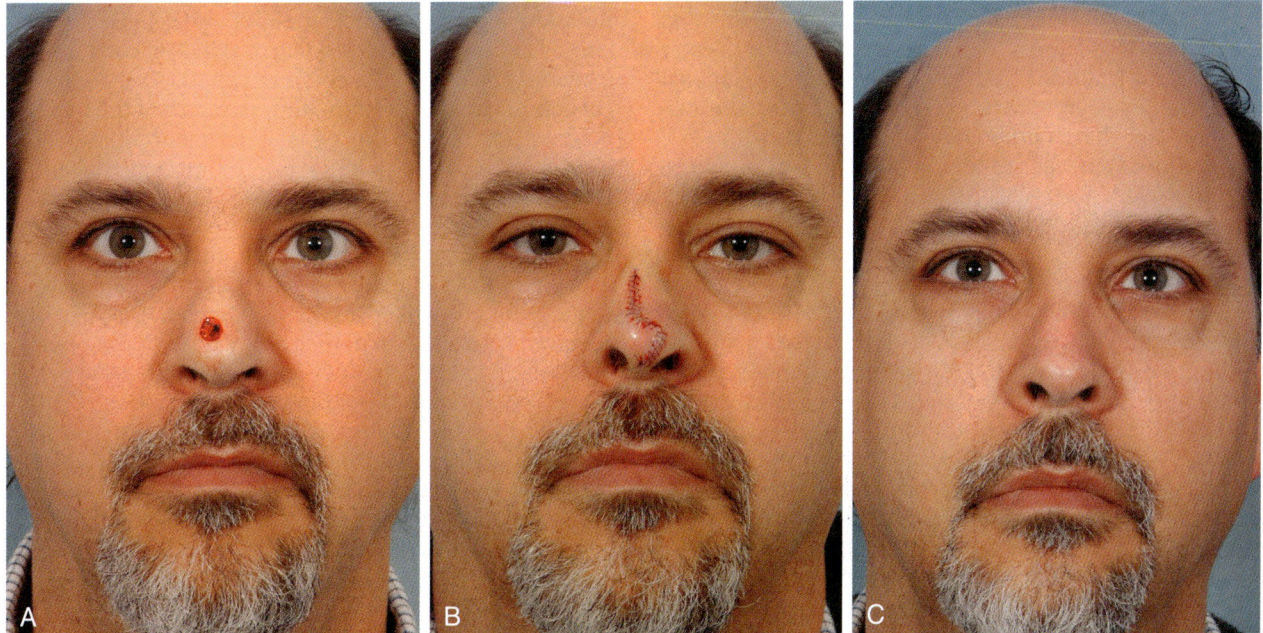

Fig. 15.19 (A) A small Mohs surgical defect was noted in the area of the nasal supratip. A linear repair was considered to be undesirable because the wound was not located precisely in the nasal midline. (B) A small Burow flap was used to relocate the excision of the inferior dog-ear redundancy towards the midline nasal tip. (C) Minimal incision line visibility and preserved distal symmetry were accomplished with this small flap repair.

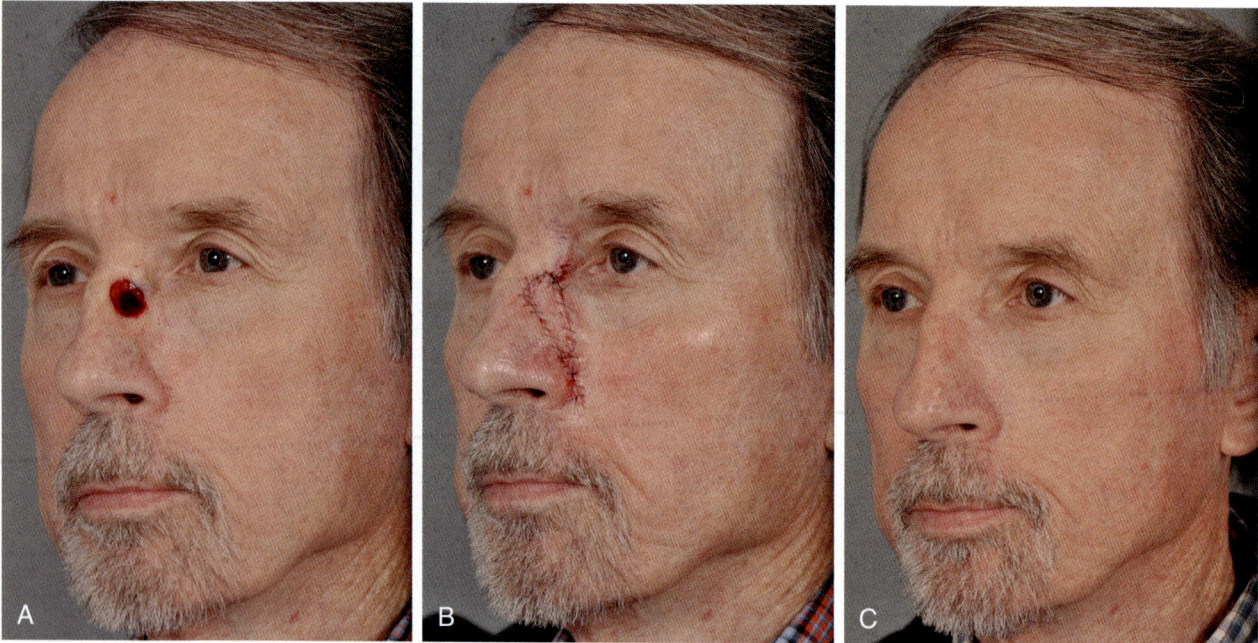

Fig. 15.20 (A) A relatively deep Mohs defect was located along the superior lateral nasal sidewall. (B) A laterally based V-Y advancement flap was used to repair the defect. Note that the flap has been slightly undersized and inserted under moderate tension, which causes the central flap concavity. This is a requirement for preventing the development of the unsightly trap-door deformity. (C) Acceptable nasal contour and minimally visible incision lines were observed at postoperative follow-up.

impervious to ischemia. For this reason, the V-Y flap is useful for critically located facial wounds, particularly when factors such as exposed cartilage/bone or a history of previous radiation therapy would predict potential ischemia with alternative reconstructive alternatives. For nasal reconstruction, the V-Y flap has potential utility for deeper wounds located along the lateral nasal sidewalls (Fig. 15.20) and for select wounds along the lateral nasal tip. The flap is particularly useful when the inferior limb of the flap can be placed along the alar groove.[17] Although this flap has been touted as a reconstructive option for a far greater range of nasal wounds,[18] particularly if the flap is created along a "sling" of preserved nasalis musculature, the secondary motion that is inherently associated with the V-Y flap's creation often leads to unacceptable distortion of the nasal tip or ala.[19] Regardless of the undermining strategy that is used to provide flap motion, care must be taken with the V-Y flap to anticipate secondary motion at the flap's recipient site (the primary defect) and to also account for the secondary motion that is required to close the flap's donor site as the flap advances. Along the nose, motion at the primary defect can produce distracting asymmetry, and the motion at the flap's donor site can often create additional deformity. The utility of the V-Y flap is also occasionally limited by the fact that distal nasal skin is thick and sebaceous, and this skin, especially when used to create the inherently bulky V-Y flap, can depress the alar tip or ala as the flap advances into place.

In addition to the traditional V-Y flap, in which a central, muscle containing pedicle nourishes the overlying skin, there are also many variants of these advancement flaps (including bipedicle flaps with central undermining[20] and even flaps that move along a single lateral muscular "hinge")[21] that have been described. A particularly valuable variant of the island flap is the buried or tunneled flap that is useful in reconstructing deeper wounds near the nasal vestibule. The flap originates in the sebaceous skin along the melo-labial fold, and the flap, once adequately mobilized, is tunneled under the cutaneous portion of the upper lip, where it is brought into the surgical defect under minimal tension (Fig. 15.21).

Rotation Flaps

Rotation flaps are conceptually simple flaps that use a curved incision to liberate a flap of skin that rotates to cover a primary defect. As the rotation flap moves into the surgical defect, a dog-ear redundancy develops at the flap's pivot point. Additionally, the typically circular primary defect also develops a redundancy on flap motion that must be properly addressed if appropriate flap contour is to be achieved. In order to minimize the tension on the rotation flap and to reduce the secondary motion that is inevitably associated with the flap's creation, rotation flaps typically require much longer incisions than would usually be required with the creation of many other types of cutaneous flaps. Because long incision lines on the nose are often undesirable and because the secondary motion required to close the flap's donor site can be associated with the production of significant nasal distortion, traditional rotation flaps are useful for only a small percentage of nasal defects. Wounds located distally near the alar groove can occasionally be repaired with a heminasal rotation flap, where the dog-ear redundancy near the primary defect can be excised along the alar groove (Fig. 15.22).

The rotation flap that has the greatest utility in nasal reconstruction is the dorsal nasal rotation flap, a flap originally conceptualized by Rieger in 1967.[22] The proper use of the flap depends entirely upon the mastering of rotation flap

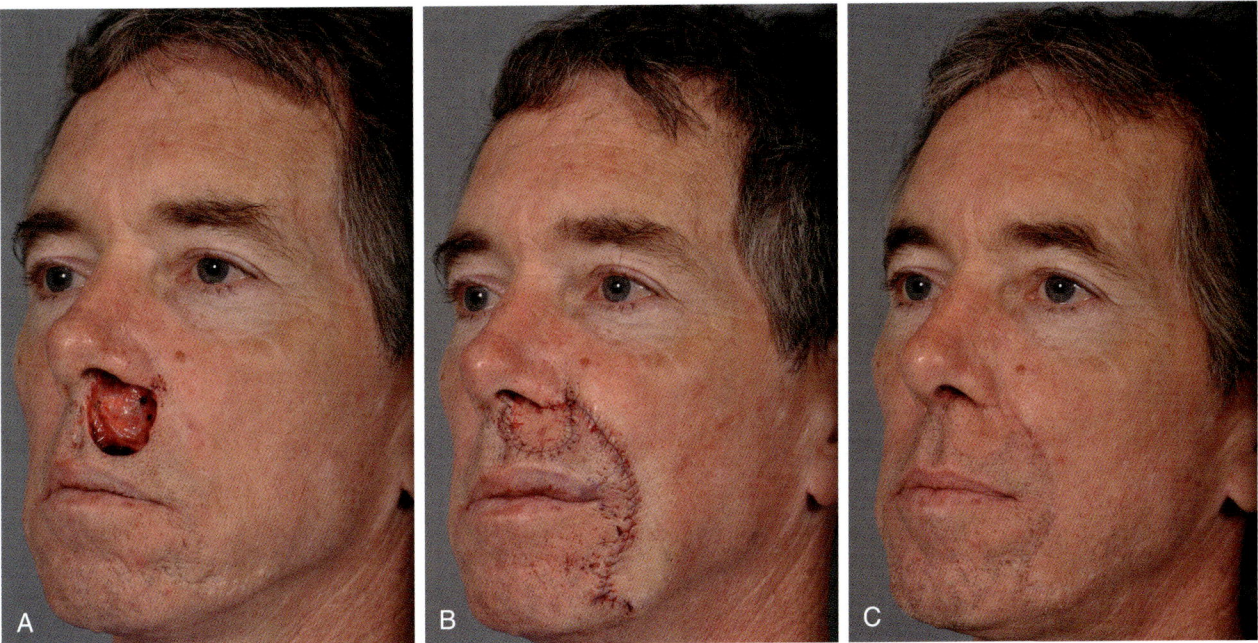

Fig. 15.21 (A) The excision of a basal cell carcinoma located on the upper lip at the nasal vestibule resulted in a relatively deep surgical defect in an area where local tissue availability is low. (B) An island flap originating in the melo-labial fold (an area where the skin is quite sebaceous and similar in appearance to the nose) was tunneled under the upper lip remnant and brought into the wound while maintaining an intact buried pedicle. (C) The flap effectively restored the volume of the nasal sill by the 12th postoperative week.

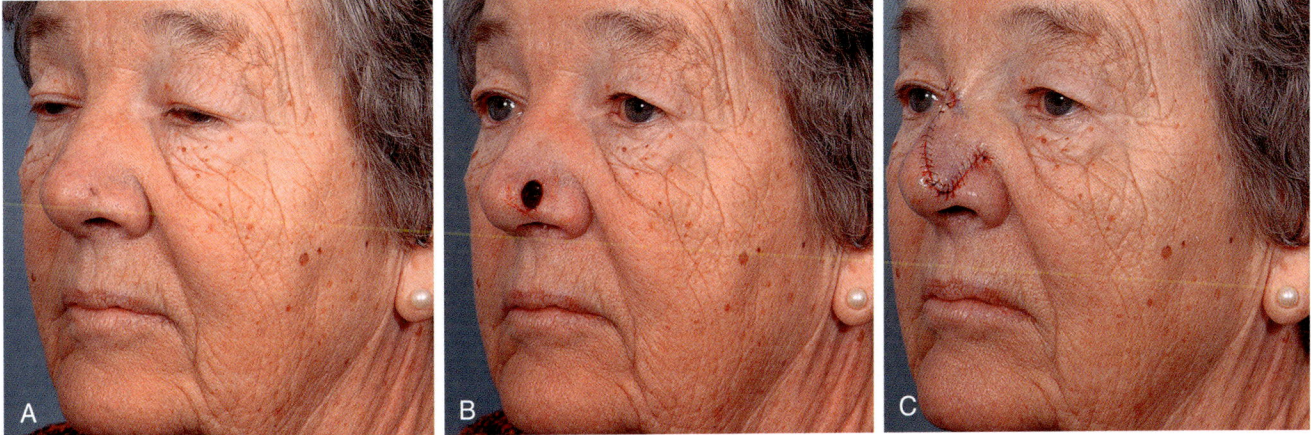

Fig. 15.22 A basal cell carcinoma (A) located within a very sebaceous, deeply shadowed alar groove has been excised using the Mohs technique (B). A superiorly based rotation flap has been used to cover the defect (C), and the dog-ear redundancy produced by flap rotation has been placed as much as possible within the alar groove.

concepts, and the utility of the flap has been traditionally underestimated due to a failure to modify the flap's design appropriately in order to reflect the nuances of proper rotation flap creation. The dorsal nasal flap is typically used for deeper distal nasal defects that are greater than 1.5 cm in diameter (Fig. 15.23). For smaller nasal wounds, there are typically other flap reconstructive options that require shorter incision lines, less complicated operative designs, and fewer undermining requirements. The wound ideally suited for the dorsal nasal flap is a moderately sized wound located on the central nasal tip or supratip. Wounds that are distally located (along the alar rim, for example) are more difficult to repair with the flap without introducing alar asymmetry, but, on occasion, the dorsal nasal flap can even be used to repair defects along the alar rim (Fig. 15.24). To minimize the tension on the flap and to reduce the likelihood that the secondary motion around the flap's donor site along the nasal sidewall will be associated with significant distortion, the arc of the flap must be generous. As a result the flap is nearly always required to extend into the area of the glabella. Of course, long incision lines create the possibility of undesirable visibility if improper surgical technique is used.

In addition to a lengthy arc, the dorsal nasal flap should have an extended leading edge in order to reduce the possibility of nasal distortion that is produced when the flap

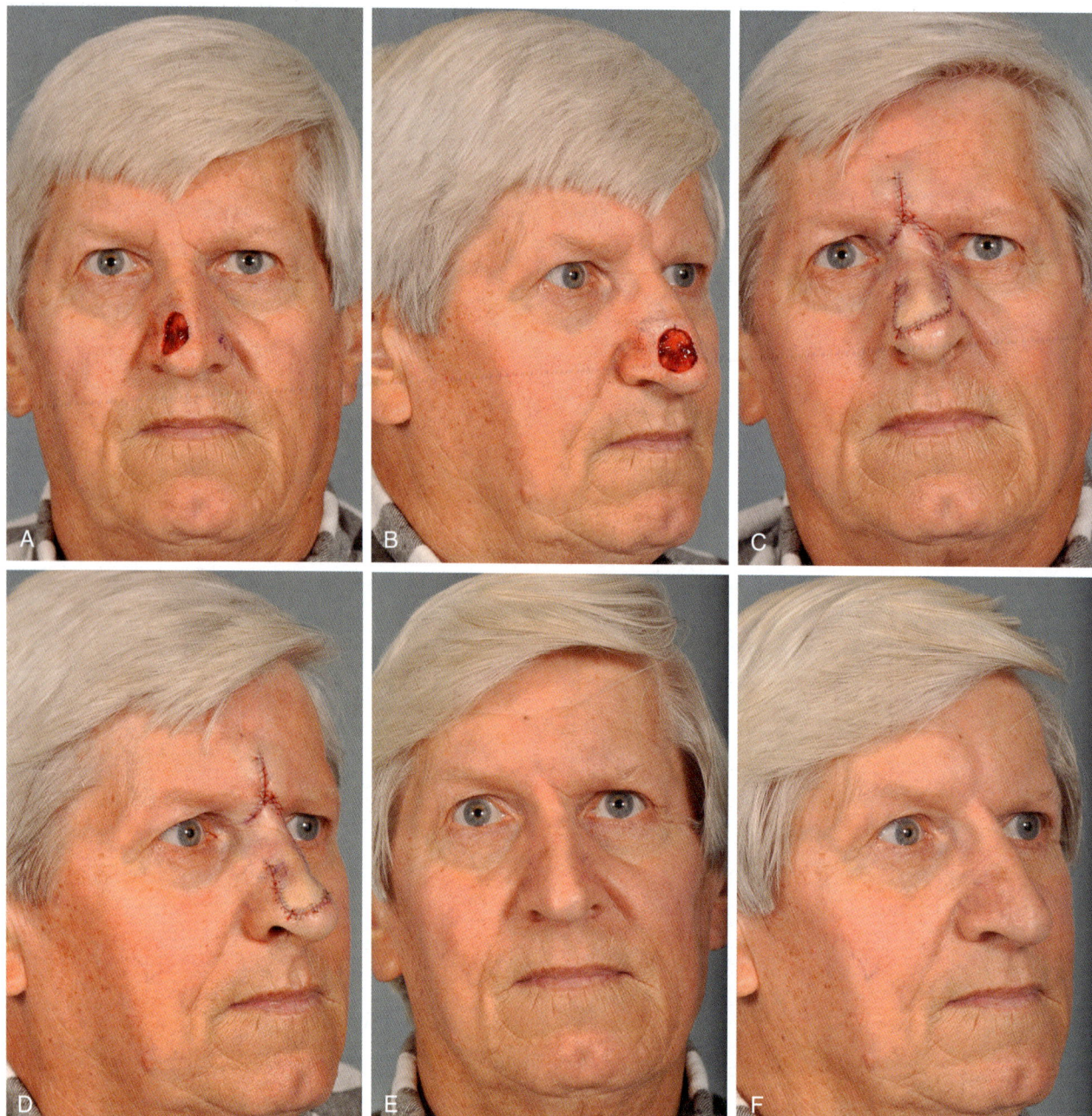

Fig. 15.23 A basal cell carcinoma on the nasal tip of a man with thick, sebaceous, inelastic nasal skin is a particular challenge. The surgical defect following tumor removal extended to the depth of the underlying perichondrium (A, B), and the patient was not interested in a staged, pedicled flap repair. A dorsal nasal flap using the sebaceous skin of the entire nasal dorsum was created (C, D). Note that the tension of the flap has produced alar asymmetry, and that the flap has placed the lateral incision line at the favorable junction of the lateral nasal sidewall and cheek. For proper flap length and to minimize the chance of deformation along the secondary defect, the flap has significantly been extended into the glabella. Four months after the reconstructive procedure (E, F), the dorsal nasal flap has offered an appropriate restoration of the nasal tip while introducing essentially no nasal asymmetry.

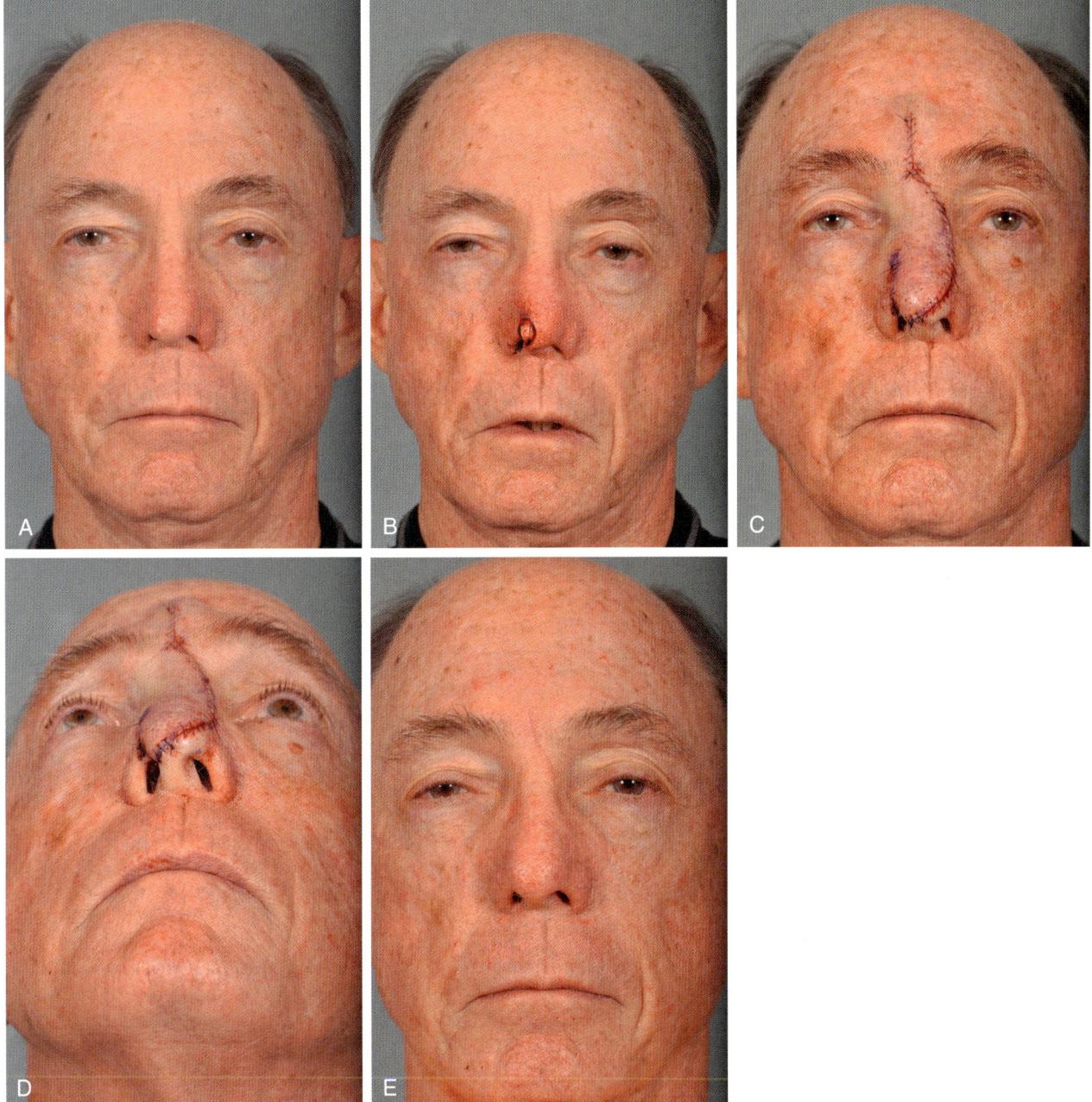

Fig. 15.24 A recurrent basal cell carcinoma of the right soft triangle area of the distal (A) was referred for a Mohs surgical excision. Note the preexisting alar asymmetry and slight vestibular stenosis—the result of a prior surgical excision. The defect following tumor removal (B) was repaired with a modified dorsal nasal rotation flap (C, D). The flap relied on significant flap advancement rather than pure rotation, and the flap was folded upon itself to restore the alar rim where a full-thickness wound was apparent. The excision of the dog-ear redundancy produced by flap motion was extended almost vertically into the body of the flap with no deleterious effect on flap perfusion. Postoperatively, the flap offered restored stability to the alar rim, introduced no additional alar asymmetry, and a slightly widened the right nasal vestibule (E).

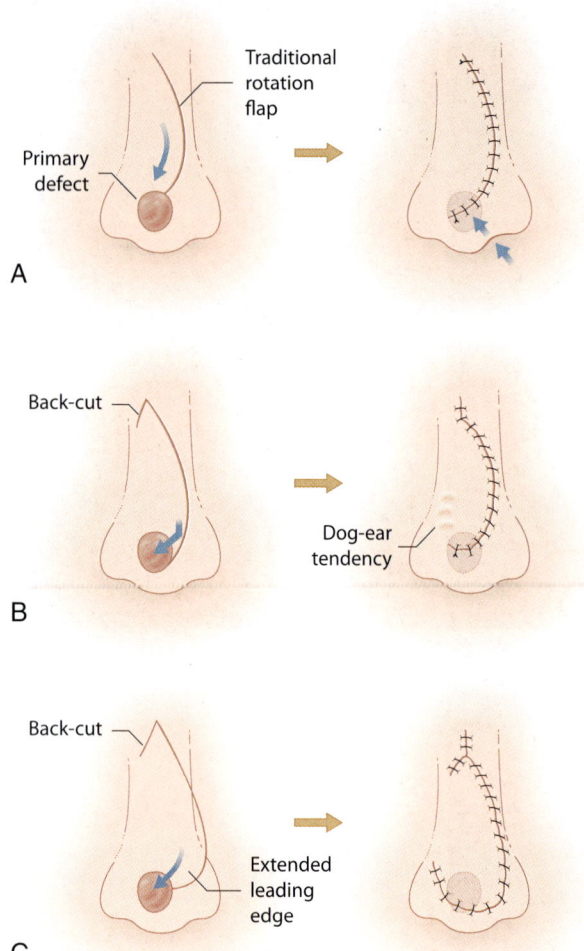

Fig. 15.25 (A) A traditional rotation flap is designed to cover a distal nasal defect. Because the rotation flap lacks a back-cut, it cannot easily turn, given the stiff nature of sebaceous nasal skin. Also, because the flap's leading edge has not been extended, the flap will "fall short" on rotation, and ipsilateral alar elevation will be produced by the secondary motion required to close the wound. (B) A back-cut on the flap will allow more motion. However, because the flap originates near the inferior border of the defect, the flap will rely on a large component of tissue advancement in addition to rotation. This advancement will propel the Burow triangle too superiorly, where its excision may threaten the distal flap's perfusion. (C) The proper dorsal nasal flap design: a back-cut again allows proper flap rotation. Because the flap originates at the superior border of the wound, the dog-ear redundancy that will be created with flap motion will be more laterally located. Additionally, the extended leading edge of the flap will compensate for pivotal restraint, and the flap will close the defect without relying upon secondary motion at the mobile alar rim.

undergoes some degree of relative "shortening" as the flap rotates distally (Fig. 15.25).[23] If unaccounted for, this shortening (associated with the flap's pivotal restraint)[24] will produce elevation of the ipsilateral alar margin, and this design problem, frequently visible in examples in reconstructive texts, accounts for the traditional admonitions that the flap produces less than aesthetically ideal results. If the dorsal nasal flap has sufficient length and an extended leading edge to compensate for the inevitable flap tethering that occurs around its pivot point, the flap can extend to even very distal nasal defects without producing significant tip asymmetry.

In addition to proper design, the dorsal nasal flap must also be skillfully executed in order to achieve acceptable results. Like all nasal flaps, the dorsal nasal flap should be carefully incised, liberally undermined, and closed in a layered manner to ensure success. Because the Rieger flap requires that the entire skin and subcutaneous tissue of the nose rotate under minimal tension to reach a distal surgical defect, the proper undermining of the flap is essential. The flap and the surrounding tissue should be generously undermined for the entire length of the nose. When undermining and thinning the flap, the surgeon should take care to preserve the dorsal nasal flap's perfusion, which is largely based on the highly anastomotic network of vessels that are present in the area of the medial canthus. Undermining all nasal flaps at the level of the perichondrium minimizes bleeding, liberates the flaps by releasing the fascial connections of the subcutaneous tissue to the underlying cartilage, and promotes more aesthetically pleasing scars.[25] Additionally, because the skin of the glabella is typically thick and relatively sebaceous, this area of the flap must be thinned, as the medial canthal skin that receives this portion of the flap is typically very thin skinned.

Transposition Flaps

There are several transposition flaps that serve as reliable alternatives to reconstruct even complicated nasal wounds. The prototypical transposition flap is the rhombic flap, a simple design in which a triangulated flap is used to cover an adjacent wound.[26] Although transposition flaps are conceptually more difficult to envision than simpler advancement and rotation flaps, their use on the nose can be very appropriate when proper cases are selected. The rhombic flap has its greatest utility in the repair of surgical wounds located on the proximal nose (Fig. 15.26). The flap is an ideal choice to harvest the looser skin of the proximal sidewall and dorsum to cover wounds located more distally, where the tissue immediately adjacent to the wound might not be sufficiently mobile. Because the incision lines of the single-lobe transposition flap are shorter and less complicated than the incision lines of other transposition flaps, such as the bilobed flap, there is a tendency to attempt to use the simple rhombic flap for very distal nasal tip or alar wounds. This is nearly always unsuccessful, as the thick skin of the more proximal nasal tip tends to depress the alar margin as it moves inferiorly. Also, the donor site of these distally located flaps, within thickly sebaceous nasal skin, cannot be closed without dramatically increasing the likelihood of producing significant deformity. For these reasons, the use of the simple rhombic flap is nearly always limited to the repair of wounds located along the nasal dorsum or sidewalls or in the area of the glabella.[27]

The bilobed flap, a modification of the traditional transposition flap that uses one flap to cover the distal primary nasal defect and a second flap to cover the first flap's donor area, is a conceptually more difficult nasal flap that has emerged as a particularly valuable option for the reconstruction of small to moderately sized distal nasal defects. The flap is well suited for deeper nasal wounds located in the areas of the nasal supratip and tip. Because the tertiary defect of the flap (the defect that results from harvesting the

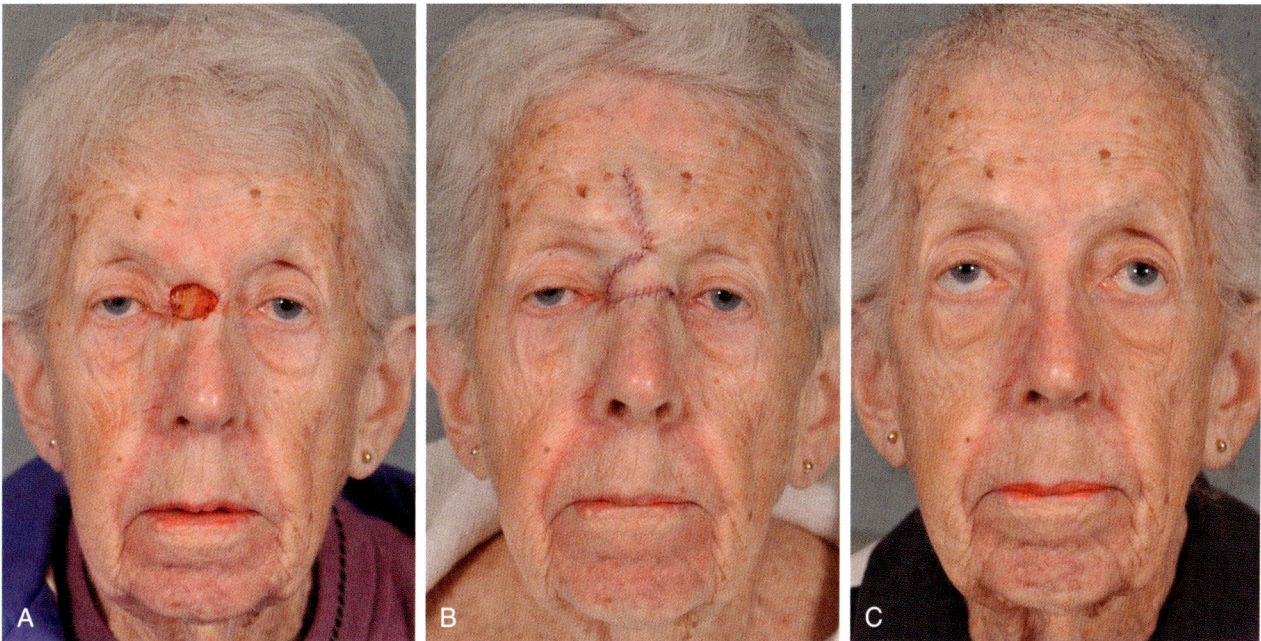

Fig. 15.26 A basal cell carcinoma of the proximal nasal dorsum was excised (A). The broad nature of the wound precluded a linear repair, and abundant loose donor tissue was noted in the adjacent glabella. A superiorly based traditional rhombic flap was used to use the loose donor tissue in the glabella (B), producing ideal postoperative results (C).

flap's secondary lobe) must be closed in a direct manner, the bilobed flap is limited to the reconstruction of nasal wounds that are less than approximately 1.5 cm in diameter. If the bilobed flap is used to close larger nasal wounds, particularly on even moderately sebaceous skin, the distortion created to close the flap's donor sites precludes any opportunity for aesthetic success. The bilobed flap can also be used to repair wounds located more proximally along the dorsum or sidewalls, but the aesthetic results of the flap tend to be most ideal when all of the flap's incision lines are kept on the nasal surface; extension of the flap's incision lines onto the medial cheek or glabella typically produces less optimal results. Although the flap has longer incision lines that could be assumed to increase the possibility of postoperative visibility, the flap, when properly designed and executed, offers nearly unrivaled opportunities to restore the convexity of the nasal tip in a single operative procedure.

The bilobed flap, initially described by Esser in 1918,[28] was of limited use until Zitelli introduced significant improvements in the flap's design in 1989 (Fig. 15.27).[29] Even though the bilobed flap does not follow relaxed skin tension lines and does not repair the nose using the subunit principle, the flap does offer an ability to transpose thicker sebaceous skin onto the nasal tip without producing alar asymmetry if the proper flap technique is used (Fig. 15.28). The design of the bilobed flap is an intricate arrangement of adjacent rounded flaps that rely upon the availability of tissue along the nasal dorsum. In order to prevent alar distortion, careful attention should be placed on the magnitude and direction of the flap's Burow triangle excision, on the location and sizing of the primary and secondary lobes, and on the utilization of meticulous operative technique.

In order to prevent unwanted secondary motion around the primary defect along the distal nose, the flap's primary lobe should be roughly equal in size to the primary defect. Similarly, the secondary lobe of the flap should be almost equally sized with the primary lobe in order to reduce the likelihood of unaesthetic alar elevation.[30] Attention should also be given to the exact arrangement of the lobes' origination points, as small amounts of secondary motion required to close the operative defects can produce significant amounts of nasal distortion. Despite the complexity of the bilobed flap's design, the flap, once mastered, is an impressively predictable reconstructive choice for many tip defects.

A trilobed flap, in which an additional lobe is added to the traditional bilobed flap design, can occasionally be very helpful in the reconstruction of distal nasal defects.[31] Many patients lack sufficient dorsal nasal skin laxity to allow the execution of a bilobed flap without the introduction of significant alar asymmetry, and very distal defects near the soft triangle and infratip lobule are not easily repaired using the conventional bilobed flap design. By adding an additional lobe the flap's design, the trilobed flap recruits looser tissue in the area of the more proximal nasal dorsum, and the flap can have great utility in the repair of difficult small to medium-sized distal nasal wounds (Fig. 15.29).

The nasolabial (or, more properly, the melo-labial) transposition flap is another traditional flap used to repair nasal defects (Fig. 15.30). This flap relies on the color and textural similarities between the sebaceous skin of the lateral nasal ala and the available skin of the melo-labial crease. The flap offers a one-step reconstruction of surgical defects in the areas of the nasal alae and the very lateral portions of the nasal tip.[32] The donor site visibility of the flap can be minimal given the flap's origination directly within the

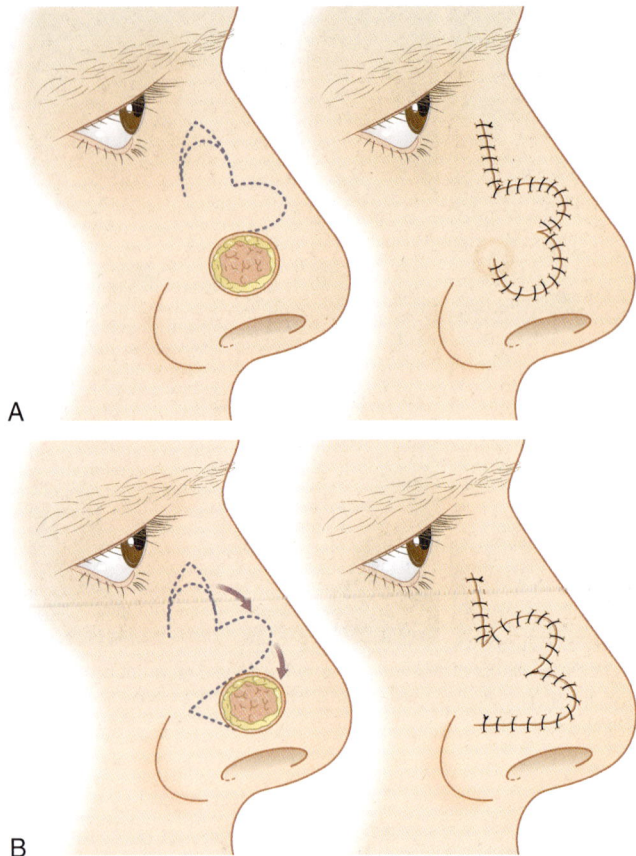

Fig. 15.27 In Esser's original bilobed flap design (A), both lobes of the flap move through 90 degrees to cover distal defects. Because the flaps are located within thicker nasal skin, such movement is occasionally difficult. Additionally, the flap's motion around the primary defect inevitably produces a tissue redundancy near the primary defect. This redundancy cannot be excised at the time or the original procedure, since doing so would effectively sever the primary lobe's perfusion. In Zitelli's design modification (B), both lobes of the flap move through smaller angles of transposition, and the prospective removal of the dog-ear at the lateral edge of the primary defect prevents the development of an unnatural contour deformity and eliminates the need to do a revision procedure.

melo-labial crease. Additionally, the thickness of the flap can be easily manipulated, and the flap can be used to cover even deeper wounds along the distal nose (Fig. 15.31). Because the flap relies upon the redundancy of vasculature in the areas of the medial cheek and medial canthus, the flap is uncommonly subject to ischemia.[33]

Despite the melo-labial flap's advantages, it is one of the more difficult flaps with which to achieve predictably excellent results. The disadvantages of the flap are readily apparent: it always blunts the shadowed concavity of the alar groove to some degree, can displace the lateral alar base, and does not reconstruct the nose using the subunit principle. The flap is also much more likely than many other nasal flaps to undergo the pin-cushioning deformation, causing aesthetically poor results. Although the donor scar can be quite hidden within the melo-labial crease, the soft tissue harvesting from the cheek that the flap requires can occasionally introduce significant medial cheek asymmetry.

Because the melo-labial flap is particularly prone to developing the trap-door deformity, careful attention should be given to strategies to prevent this complication, which frequently turns the flap into a fingerlike protuberance along the distal nose (Fig. 15.32).[34] The most important strategy to avoid the production of flap redundancy is to avoid oversizing the flap—both in width and in thickness.[35] Additionally, deep tacking sutures should anchor the flap at the flap's pivot point near the junction of the cheek and nose and along the flap's undersurface in the area of the former alar groove.

In addition to the traditional version of the melo-labial flap, the flap can also be modified to reconstruct even full-thickness wounds along the lateral alar margin. One particularly valuable variation of the melo-labial flap involves folding the flap onto itself in order to provide both internal lining and external coverage in the repair of challenging full-thickness alar wounds (Fig. 15.33).[36,37]

Interpolation Flaps

Interpolation flaps are pedicled flaps that cover nasal wounds by transferring tissue from areas not immediately adjacent to the primary defect across relatively large expanses of intervening normal skin. These flaps offer unparalleled opportunities to repair difficult nasal wounds, but their use is limited by the fact that the flaps require at least two surgical procedures (initial flap creation and later flap separation/insertion) that are typically separated by a several-week period of flap attachment, during which the patient must contend with an unsightly, clumsy flap appearance. Despite this obvious disadvantage, pedicled flaps offer great utility in the repair of larger and more anatomically complicated nasal wounds, especially when local tissue is insufficient to create single-staged random pattern cutaneous flaps from the remaining adjacent nasal or cheek skin.

The pedicled melo-labial (nasolabial) flap is a particularly valuable flap to reconstruct difficult wounds of the distal nose (Fig. 15.34). Similar to the traditional (single step) melo-labial flap, this flap's donor site is relatively hidden within the melo-labial crease on the medial cheek. Wounds that are particularly well suited for this interpolated flap repair are deeper wounds of the ala. Because the pedicled melo-labial flap remains temporarily attached to its donor site on the medial cheek, the flap is not required to transpose over the remaining alar groove in order to cover the wound. Thus, the pedicled melo-labial flap is particularly useful in reconstructing alar wounds in which the alar groove has been largely spared. This pedicled flap is also very useful in reconstructing difficult-to-reach areas of the nose, such as the very medial aspect of the alar rim or the area of the soft triangle (Fig. 15.35).

The advantages of the pedicled melo-labial flap include its predictable vascular supply, its ability to reach wounds even involving the nasal tip, its opportunity to repair the distal nose using aesthetic subunit concepts, its relatively well-hidden donor site along the melo-labial crease, and the flap's ability to prevent blunting of the alar crease and the nose-lip-cheek junction that can be seen with a number of other random-patterned flaps. The flap can also be used to repair the nasal portion of a complicated wound also involving the medial cheek (Fig. 15.36). The interpolated nasolabial flap does, however, have several relative disadvantages:

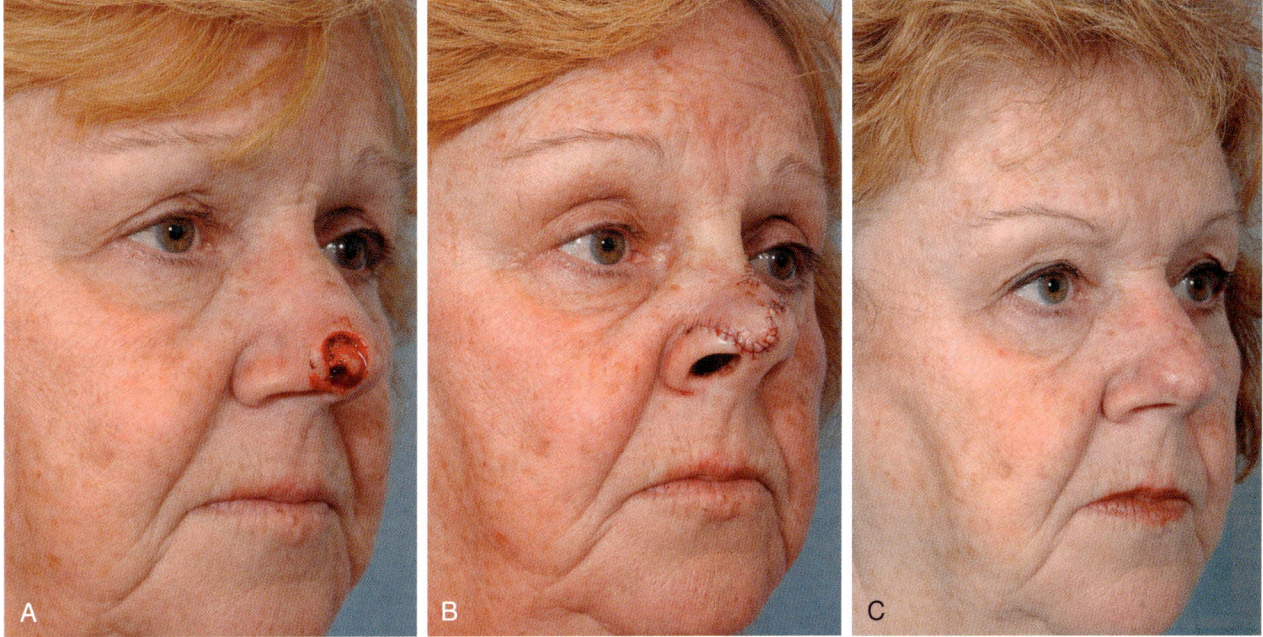

Fig. 15.28 A basal cell carcinoma was located in a difficult area of the very sebaceous nasal tip, and the defect that resulted from tumor removal extended to the depth of the underlying alar cartilage (A). A bilobed flap, even though it was created from the very thick, sebaceous skin of the nasal tip, was used to cover the wound (B), as second intention healing or a skin graft repair would have been associated with an unacceptable contour deformity. Note that the primary lobe of the flap was roughly equal in size to the primary defect; this prevented the secondary motion that would elevated the patient's left alar rim. Note also that the Burow triangle that was created when the primary lobe covered the primary defect has been very superiorly oriented so that the thickly sebaceous skin of the moving primary lobe of the flap did not depress the patient's right alar rim. Several months after the repair, the flap's complicated incision lines had faded very nicely (C), and the very sebaceous skin of the nasal tip had restored the appropriate convexity of this area adequately.

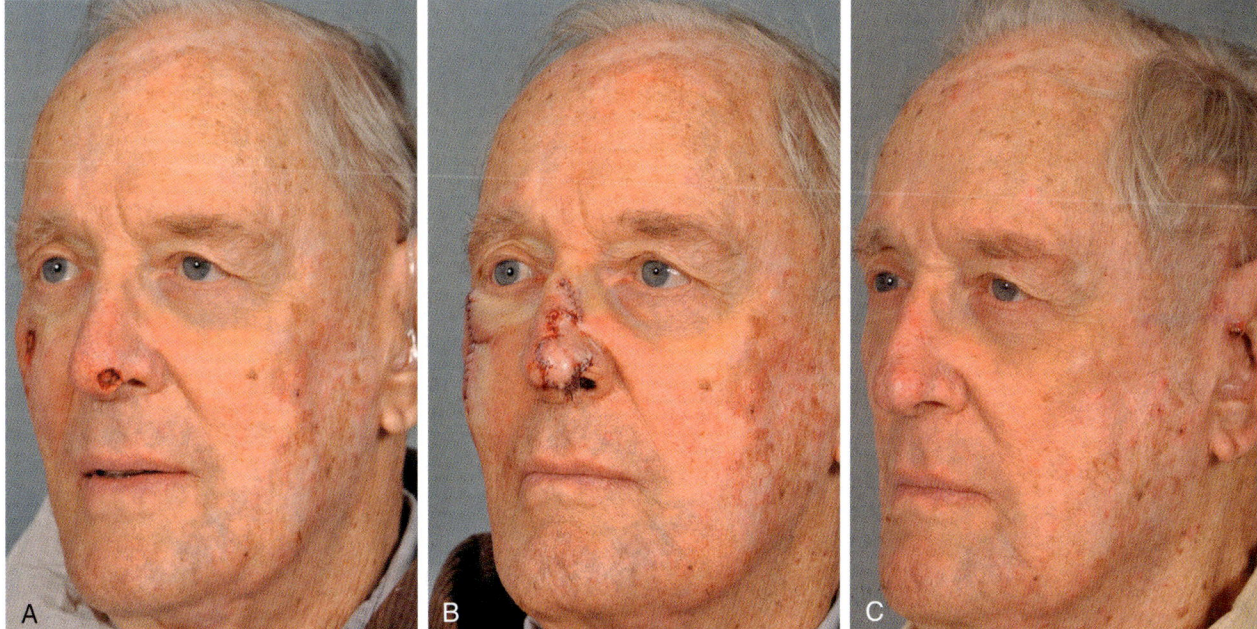

Fig. 15.29 (A) A basal cell carcinoma was excised on the distal nose, and the patient's thickly sebaceous nasal skin type predicted alar asymmetry if many traditional flaps were used for repair of the wound. A trilobed flap was used (B) to extend the flap's origination into the looser areas of the more proximal nasal dorsum, producing appropriate aesthetic results with restoration of the convexity of the distal nasal tip without the introduction of alar asymmetry (C).

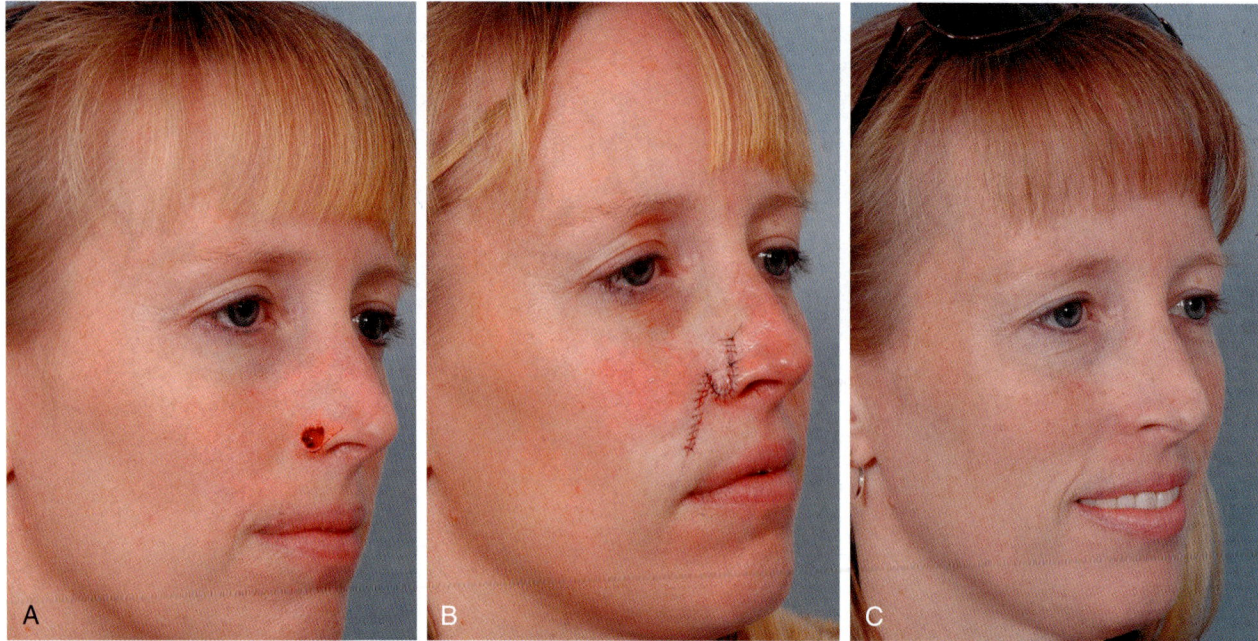

Fig. 15.30 (A) A small defect was apparent on the lateral aspect of the ala. (B) A traditional melo-labial/nasolabial flap was used to repair the wound. (C) The aesthetic results were pleasing, as the flap restored the convexity of the lateral ala. Tacking sutures to secure the flap at its base minimized the degree of inevitable blunting of the shadowed concavity of the lateral alar crease.

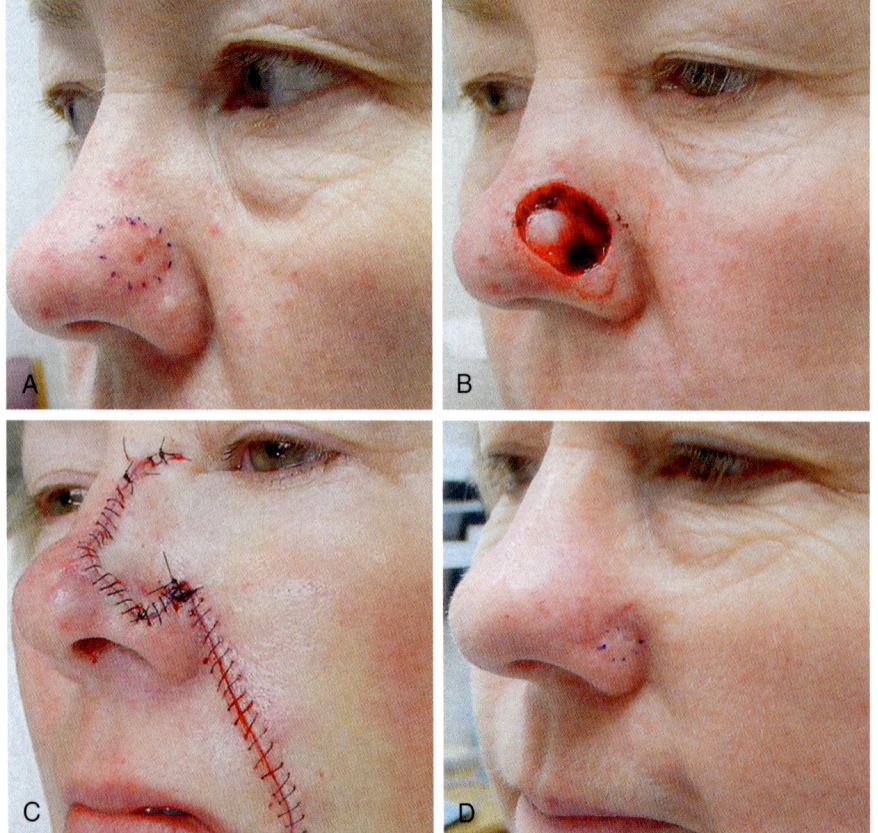

Fig. 15.31 An ill-defined basal cell carcinoma of the distal nose (A) was excised using the Mohs technique (B). The depth of the wound (note the exposed alar cartilage) precluded the likelihood of success with a graft repair. A traditional melo-labial flap was harvested from the ipsilateral cheek and transposed across the remaining lateral ala to cover the surgical wound (C). In an effort to prevent the flap from undergoing a trap-door deformation, the flap was thinned to nearly dermis, which revealed the structure of the underlying nasal cartilage through the distal flap. Deep tacking sutures have also been placed, and these sutures helped to achieve the proper flap contour. At 4 months after the reconstructive procedure, the flap had nicely restored the nose's contour (D). Although all nasolabial flaps blunt the alar groove, the aesthetic penalty of such blunting was minimal in this case because the patient had an alar groove that was shallow and largely visible only in the lateral-most areas of the nose. The gentian violet circle notes a papule that was of concern to the patient on a follow-up visit.

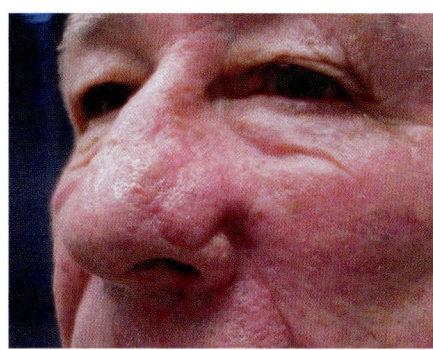

Fig. 15.32 A melo-labial flap was appropriately used to reconstruct a deep alar wound. Despite a thoughtful flap design and meticulous operative technique, the flap underwent a trap-door deformation (in addition to predictably obliterating the alar groove). A different reconstructive alternative could have avoided these complications to a large degree.

it can be used only for smaller nasal wounds unless significant donor site asymmetry can be tolerated, it can place terminal hair onto the nose in male patients, and it can be more technically challenging than many simpler flap alternatives.

The donor site of the flap is placed within the melo-labial fold, and a cotton sponge is used to ensure that the flap will reach the nasal defect as the flap undergoes predictable "shortening" in rotating into the surgical defect. Although the flap is distally thinned to nearly dermis in order to prevent a globular appearance, the proximal portion of the pedicled flap is deeply undermined so that the highly perfused medial cheek musculature supports the vascular demands of the flap.[38] The flap is sutured under minimal tension. If minor degrees of alar or columellar distortion are apparent, they typically resolve when the flap is separated. At the time of flap separation, traditionally performed

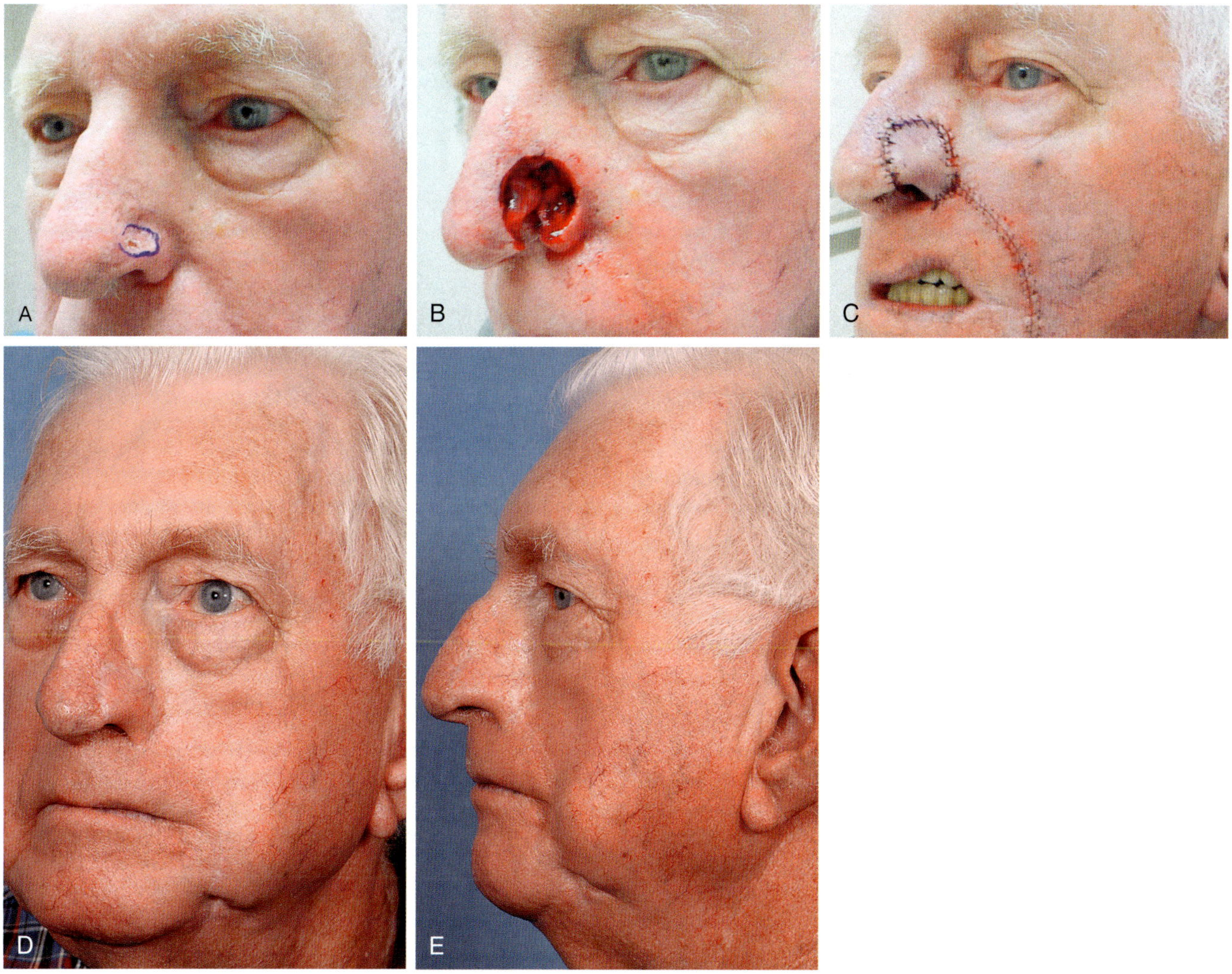

Fig. 15.33 A recurrent basal cell carcinoma of the left ala (A) was excised with the Mohs technique, creating a full-thickness alar wound (B). Traditional nasal reconstructive surgery dictates that any nasal wound should be repaired with tissue designed to closely replace missing tissue, and a repair of this wound would typically involve mucosal lining flaps for internal nasal coverage, cartilage grafts for structural support, and a pedicled flap for cutaneous coverage. Because the patient was not interested in a staged repair, a turnover nasolabial flap, in which the medial cheek skin serves as both the internal nasal lining and the external coverage, was used for a single-step repair (C). Note that the width of the required flap has produced a slight eclabium, which quickly resolved. At 3 months after the repair (D, E), the turnover flap offers an appropriate repair of the aesthetic unit of the ala. Note also that the delicate curve of the alar margin and the lateral ala's insertion point onto the lip have been restored.

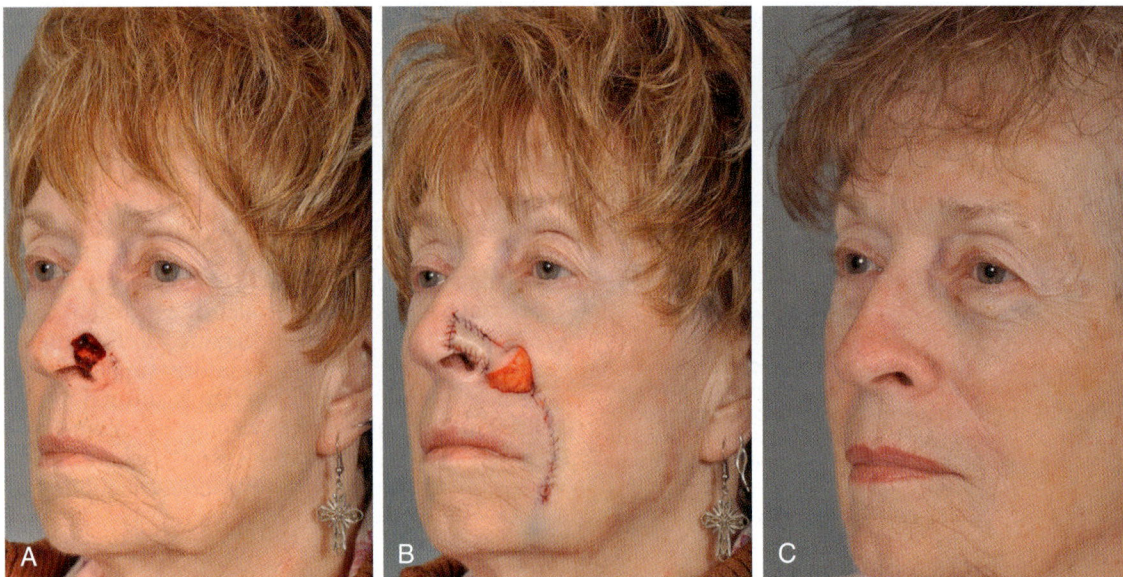

Fig. 15.34 (A) A basal cell carcinoma excision defect was limited to the central nasal ala. (B) The wound was repaired with a pedicled flap from the ipsilateral medial cheek. The donor site was directly within the melo-labial crease, and the defect was enlarged so that the entire ala was repaired as a single aesthetic unit. A cartilage batten graft harvested from the antehelix was also used to ensure architectural stability of the nascent alar rim and to preserve nasal function. (C) The slight and predictable contraction of the flap has rounded the construct into a form mimicking the convexity of the native ala, and the flap's incision lines have been hidden within normal anatomic boundaries.

at 3 weeks after the flap's creation, the flap is severed and thinned to match to the contour of the nose. At the time of flap separation, the flap can be aggressively thinned to promote a more appropriate alar contour.[39] The donor site in the medial cheek can be linearly inserted as a continuation of the newly created melo-labial fold.

Perhaps the most versatile of the pedicled flaps used to reconstruct more challenging wounds of the nose is the paramedian forehead flap, an axial patterned flap designed around the predictable location of the supratrochlear artery. Because the visual significance of the forehead is miniscule compared with the aesthetic prominence of the nose, even large areas of the forehead can be sacrificed to cover complicated nasal wounds (Fig. 15.37). The forehead flap's advantages include its ability to reach nearly any area of the nose (regardless of the size of the wound), its luxurious vascular supply and relative immunity to ischemia, and the similarity in color and texture between forehead and nasal skin. The forehead flap, a viable reconstructive alternative for most larger nasal wounds, has several potential disadvantages. Besides the obvious need to place a relatively large donor wound on the forehead and the need to perform a second surgical procedure to separate and insert the flap, the forehead flap is also limited by the tendency of the flap to undergo trap-door deformation as the flap matures. For that reason, the design and execution of the forehead flap are particularly important. If proper design and technique are not used, it is quite possible for the forehead flap to appear as an undefined spherical "blob" rather than as a normal nasal tip.

The forehead flap is ideal for nasal wounds that lack suitable random pattern nasal flap solutions. Because the forehead flap's perfusion is predictably protected, the flap is particularly appropriate for deeper wounds that also require the introduction of relatively avascular structural elements such as cartilage. If alar flaccidity has introduced functional concerns, plans should obviously be made to reconstruct the rigidity and flexibility of the distal nose in addition to designing skin coverage. If the wound involves a majority of any aesthetic subunit of the nose, consideration should be given to enlarging the size of the primary defect until the borders of the adjacent aesthetic subunits have been reached (Fig. 15.37).[2] Placing the incision lines of the flap along theses boundaries will often improve the aesthetic subtlety of the flap's final appearance. Even if the flap does not replace the entire aesthetic subunit, aesthetically appropriate results can be achieved if the color and texture of the flap offer a suitable match to the adjacent skin (Fig. 15.38).[40]

After the defect has been evaluated, a three-dimensional model of the missing nasal tissue is constructed from the foil of a suture package, using the contralateral nose as a model in the case of unilateral nasal wounds. The approximate location of the supratrochlear artery is located using the corrugator fold near the medial brow. Although a Doppler device can confirm the location of the artery, the artery's location is so predictable that an exact confirmation of the artery's location is typically unnecessary. The flap should be constructed with a width of 1.2 to 1.5 cm, taking care to ensure that the arterial input to the flap is located within the flap's base. Larger widths would seemingly offer assurance that the surgeon has appropriately included the nourishing artery within the flap's base, but this greater pedicle width actually causes difficulty in rotating the flap under minimal tension, paradoxically reducing flap perfusion. The flap should extend far enough superiorly on the forehead so that the flap can reach the nasal defect under essentially no wound closure tension. Rather than extend the flap into the hair-bearing scalp, the surgeon can gain additional flap length by safely extending the flap's origin below the bony orbital margin. At the origin of the

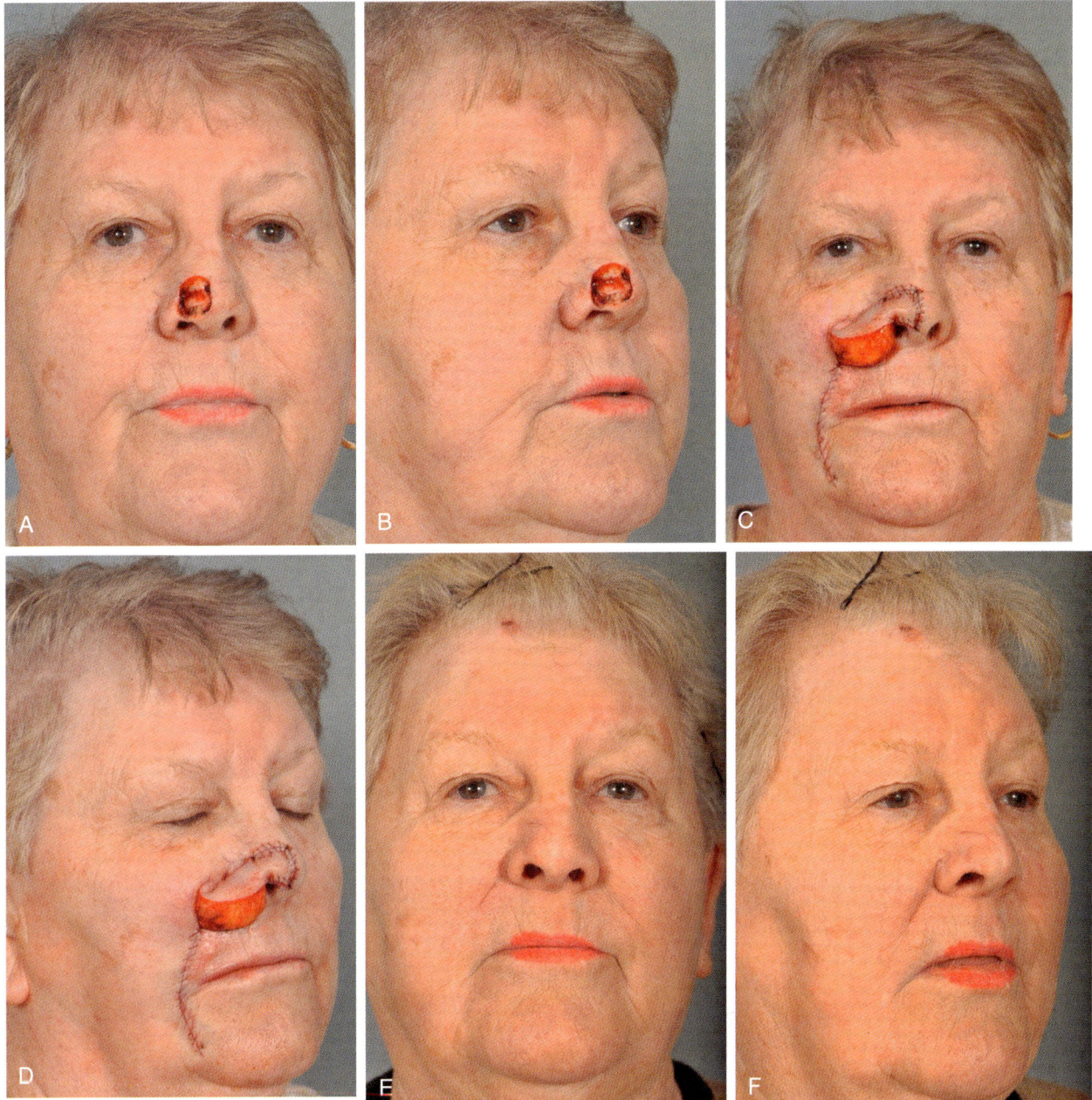

Fig. 15.35 (A, B) A basal cell carcinoma was excised on the nasal tip and supratip. (C, D) A pedicled flap from the cheek was used for repair of the wound in an effort to avoid the introduction of a vertical scar on the forehead. (E, F) The flap offered aesthetically appropriate restoration of the nasal tip convexity despite the fact that the wound was not repaired using the traditional subunit principle. Note the minimal donor site morbidity associated with the use of this reconstructive alternative.

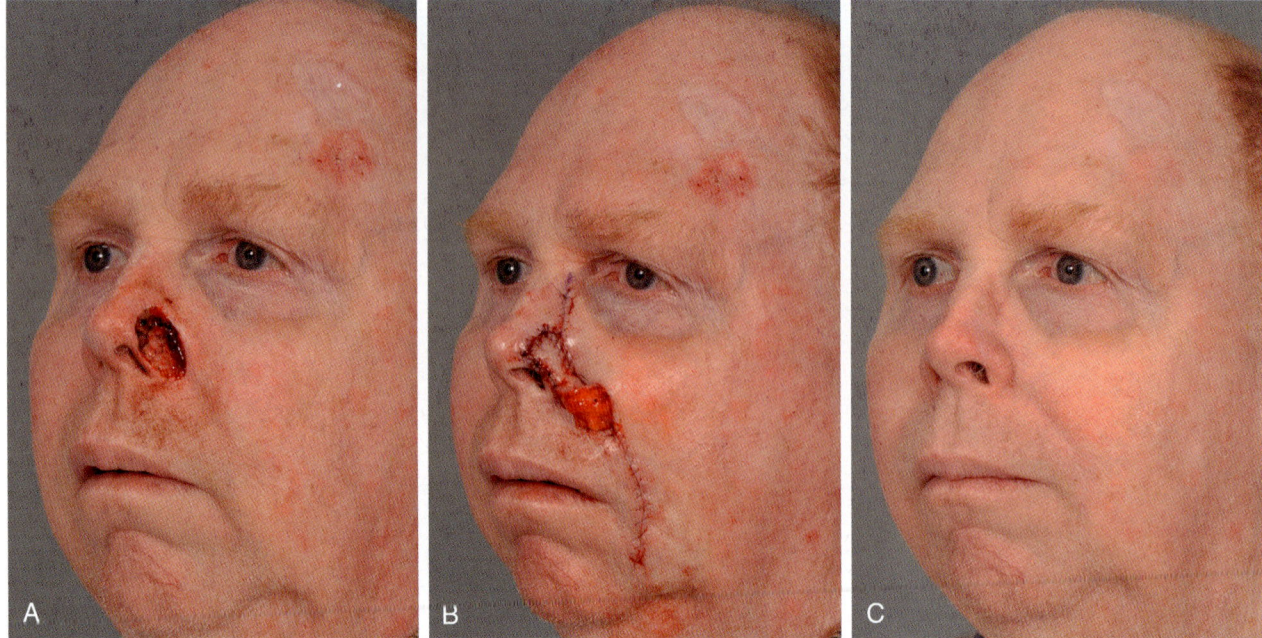

Fig. 15.36 (A) A squamous cell carcinoma excision produced a wound that involved the disparate aesthetic units of the ala and medial cheek in the area superior to the alar groove. (B) A pedicled flap from the medial cheek was used to repair the nasal portion of the wound. Advancement of the medial cheek was also used to address the extranasal component of the wound. This flap's advancement required a vertical dog-ear excision along the nasal sidewall. Failure to address the cheek portion of the wound with this additional flap would have entirely obliterated the shadowed junction of nose and cheek. (C) Postoperatively, the ala has been restored to its proper form, and the junction between nose and cheek has been appropriately recreated.

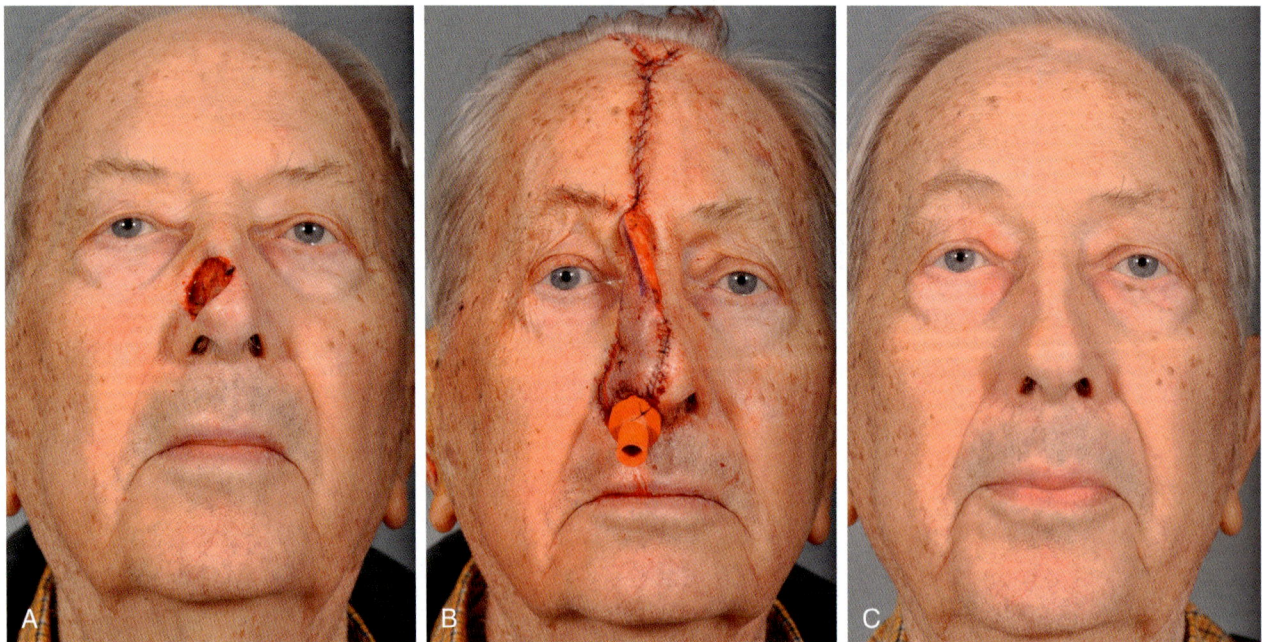

Fig. 15.37 (A) A basal cell carcinoma defect involved several aesthetic subunits of the nose. Because the patient desired to have his appearance restored as much as possible, a pedicled flap from the forehead was selected as the most appropriate reconstructive alternative. (B) The surgical defect was enlarged to allow reconstruction of the distal nose using the subunit principle. A cartilage graft was used to restore stability of the alar rim, and a nasopharyngeal airway was allowed to remain in place for several days in an effort to "splint" the ala. The flap's donor site was closed primarily given this patient's desirable degree of tissue laxity. (C) Postoperatively the reconstructive results were ideal, given the minimal degree of donor site visibility, the restoration of the ala's position and volume, and the placement of all nasal incision lines along normal anatomic boundaries.

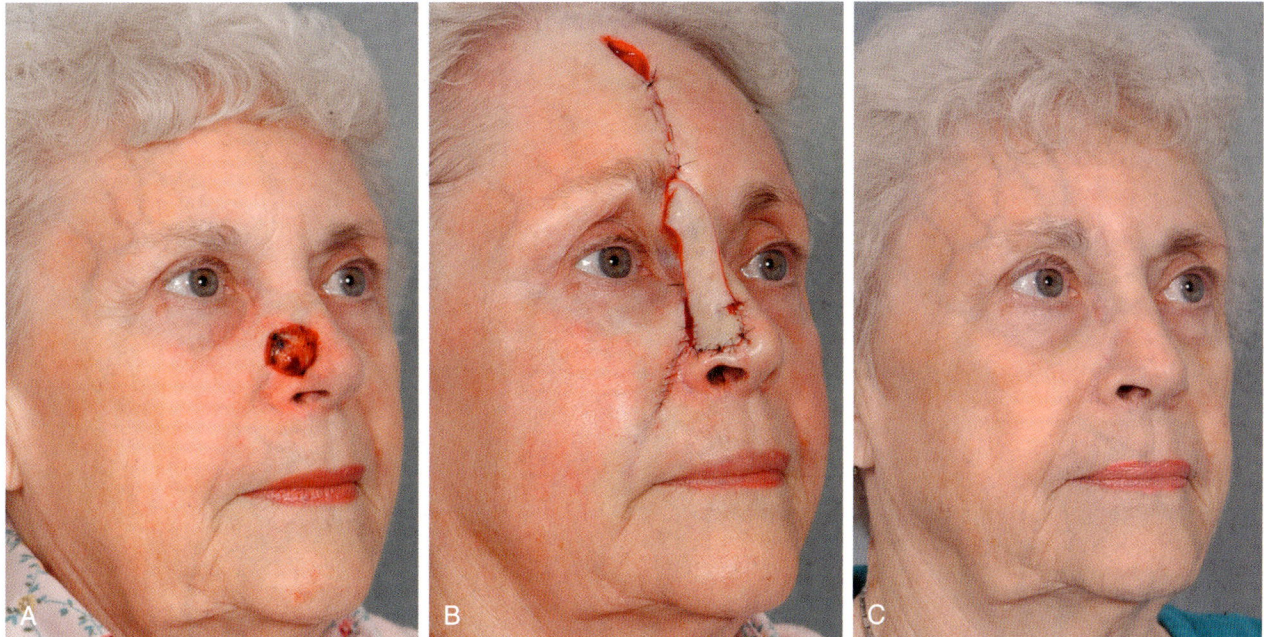

Fig. 15.38 (A) A basal cell carcinoma excision defect involves the lateral nose and medial cheek. (B) Initially, the cheek was advanced medially to restore the normal boundary between nose and cheek. A nonsubunit forehead flap was used to repair the nasal portion of the wound. (C) Although the nasal component of the wound was not repaired using the subunit principle, the aesthetic success of the repair was achieved with the restoration of appropriate contour and the attention to meticulous operative technique.

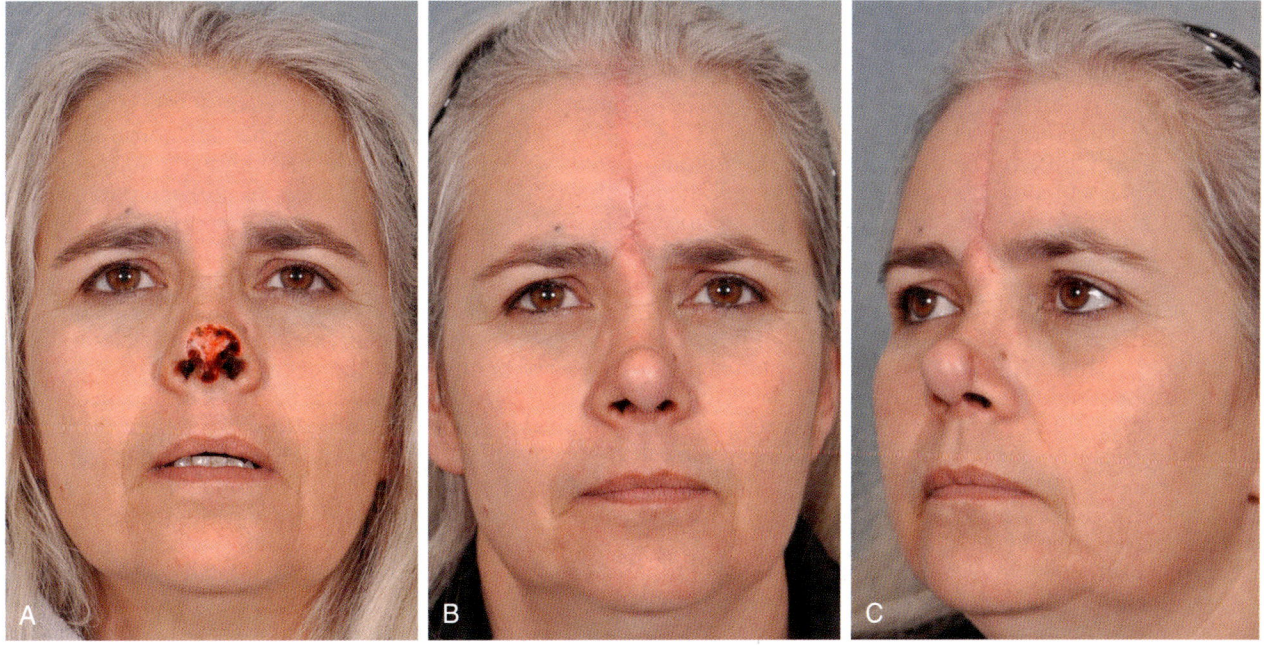

Fig. 15.39 (A) A basal cell carcinoma was excised using the Mohs technique. (B, C) The wound was repaired by a surgeon other than the author using a forehead flap. Because the flap was likely oversized and not appropriately contoured, the distal nasal tip looks like an unaesthetic "blob," and revision procedures are likely to be difficult and largely unsuccessful.

flap, the supratrochlear artery is located between the frontalis and the corrugator musculature, and care should be taken with flap undermining to preserve the narrow artery's integrity. As the supratrochlear artery courses up the forehead, the artery becomes nearly subdermal in location.[38]

If the forehead flap is not thinned at its distal margin, the skin of the forehead will nearly always be thicker than the missing skin and soft tissue of the distal nose. Placing this untrimmed flap onto the nose will therefore result in a globular, amorphous mass rather than the delicate arrangement of convexities and concavities that defines the appearance of the normal nose (Fig. 15.39). Thinning of the flap, however, introduces some operative risk; such thinning inevitably threatens the flap's perfusion to some degree.

Flap thinning should therefore be undertaken with great care, particularly in smokers, for whom the risks of flap necrosis are higher. During the initial flap transfer, the distal 1.5 to 2 cm of the forehead flap can typically be thinned to nearly the underlying dermis, leaving only a thin layer (2 to 3 mm) of residual subcutaneous fat. This produces a flap whose thickness is very close to that of the distal nasal skin, and the thinning produces a flap that is essentially random-patterned at its insertion point. After a period of delay (traditionally 3 weeks), the flap is separated from its glabellar attachment and inserted onto the nose. At this time the more superior aspects of the flap that were not aggressively thinned during the original flap creation can be now appropriately sculpted. Because the skin of the proximal nose is thinner than the sebaceous skin of the nasal tip, thinning of the flap along the nasal dorsum and sidewalls is especially important.

To create better nasal contour, an interim third surgical stage can be added to the traditional two-staged forehead flap repair. As with the traditional two-staged forehead flap repair, the flap is initially created and secured on the nose. After 3 weeks of traditional flap delay, the flap can then be thinned while preserving the flap's perfusion with an intact arterial source. Preservation of the flap's named larger-caliber arterial input offers an unrivaled opportunity to thin the flap, which can lead to the reintroduction of much more anatomically correct nasal contours. On occasion, the pedicle of the forehead flap is allowed to remain attached, and the flap is lifted off of the wound bed while keeping both the proximal pedicle and the distal insertion intact. The flap can be very aggressively thinned at this point, since the perfusion is quite redundant; the flap is subsequently separated at 3 weeks after this interim revision procedure.[41] This interim thinning procedure can eliminate the occasional need to perform a sculpting procedure 6 to 12 months after the original reconstructive procedure in order to restore proper contour to the nose.

More frequently, the second stage of flap contouring involves the incision of the entire forehead flap along its distal insertion, completely elevating the flap off of its nasal recipient site.[42] While the arterial input of the flap is preserved with retention of the flap's pedicle, the flap can be aggressively thinned in order to promote a more suitable final contour (Fig. 15.40). Such thinning can even allow the introduction of the shadowed alar crease, and tacking sutures are also important to promote better nasal flap contour. After an additional period of several weeks of flap delay, the flap is then separated and inserted (Fig. 15.41).

A three-staged forehead flap also allows for the reconstruction of more challenging full-thickness distal nasal wounds. Full-thickness nasal wounds require restoration of nasal lining, introduction of architecturally stable cartilage elements, and replacement of an aesthetically proper skin covering. Traditionally, the replacement of nasal lining has been the most demanding element of nasal reconstruction, and a number of highly vascular—but technically challenging—nasal lining flaps from the septum have been used to line the nascent alae. Because of the predictable perfusion of the forehead flap, however, more contemporary alternatives to replace nasal lining rely on a folded forehead flap, in which the donor site's forehead skin is used both as internal nasal lining and as external nasal coverage

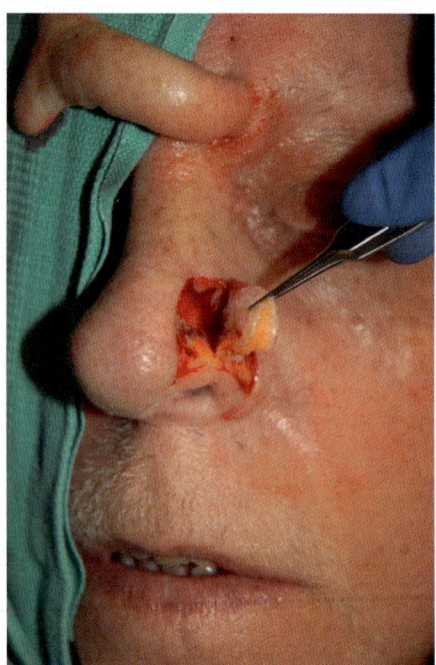

Fig. 15.40 The interim procedure of a three-staged forehead flap is illustrated in this case. The forehead flap has been entirely incised along its distal insertion point, allowing the flap to maintain its proximal pedicle. The previously placed cartilage batten graft is noted along the alar rim at the inferior aspect of the nasal wound. Redundant fibrous and subcutaneous tissue is excised so that a more delicate alar contour can be created.

after the flap has been folded upon itself. This technique eliminates the need for more demanding intranasal manipulations required to harvest septal lining flaps, and nonetheless allows for restoration of an appropriately thin, highly vascular, and functionally proper nasal lining (Fig. 15.42). After the flap has matured for several weeks, an interim procedure in performed to thin the flap and to introduce any needed cartilaginous support elements. This interim procedure maintains the flap's pedicle in order to preserve perfusion of the distal flap, and because of this protected vascular input and because the flap has been conditioned to relative ischemia, the surgeon has an unrivaled opportunity in this interim step to thin the flap aggressively, allowing for the production of a much more nuanced flap appearance. In a third procedure performed several weeks later, the forehead flap is definitively separated and inserted (Fig. 15.43). This three-staged forehead flap repair can also be used as one component of several procedures used to address difficult wounds involving several aesthetic units (Fig. 15.44).

Complications

All surgical procedures have risks, and nasal reconstructive procedures are certainly fraught with potential complications if appropriate reconstructive alternatives are not carefully selected, designed, and executed. As with any cutaneous surgical procedure, nasal repairs can be occasionally complicated by bleeding and wound infection. These complications can usually be minimized or avoided if proper

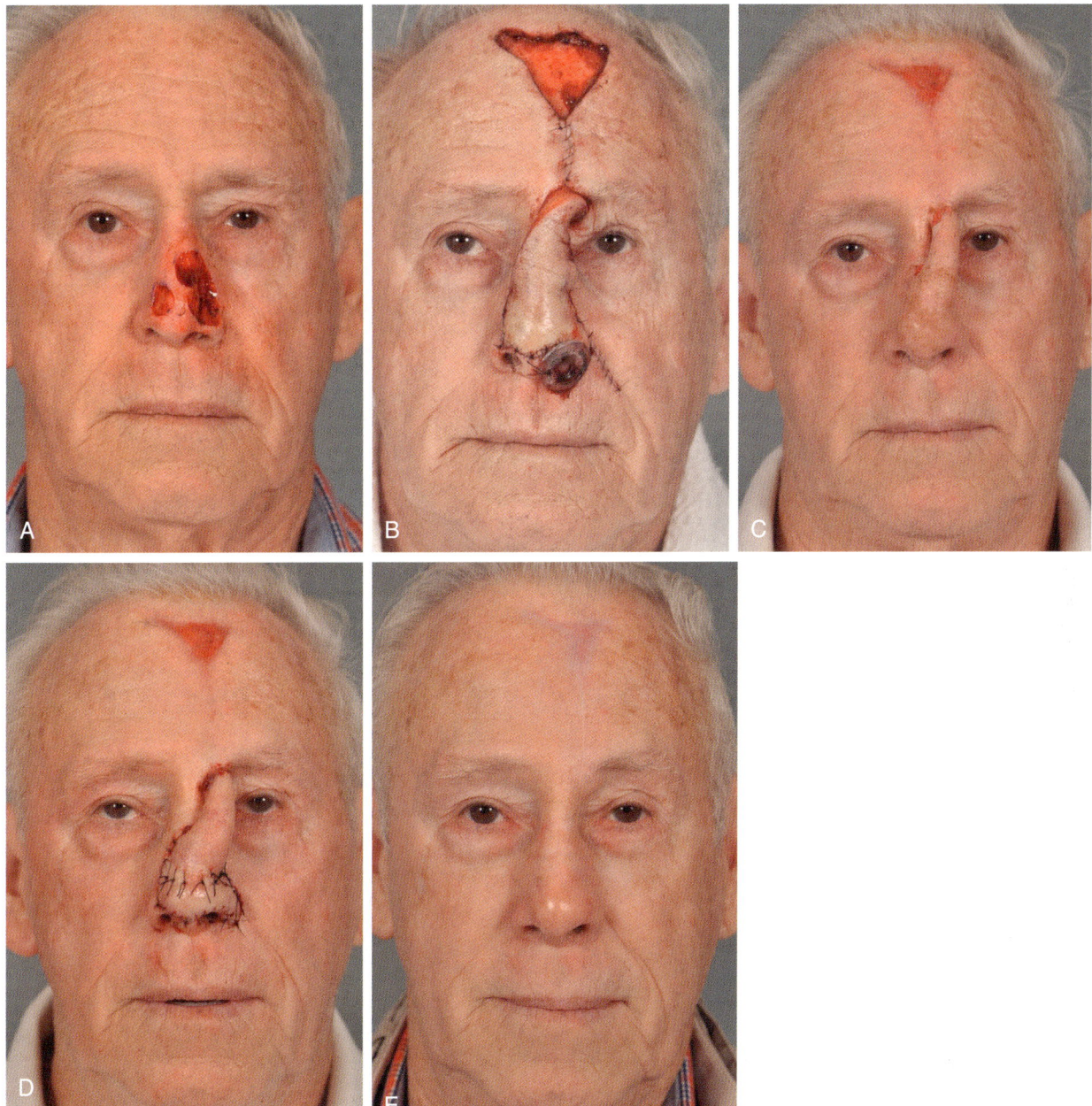

Fig. 15.41 (A) Difficult recurrent basal cell carcinomas were excised from the distal nose. (B) A paramedian forehead flap was used to cover the nasal defects. A small advancement of the medial cheek was also used to reposition the border between the cheek and nose more accurately. A nasopharyngeal airway was used to "splint" the nascent alar rim for the initial week of healing. Note that the broad donor area on the forehead was allowed to heal by second intention when a primary repair was not possible owing to very high wound closure tensions. (C) At 3 weeks, the flap was doing well, and it was decided that an interim procedure would allow for a more appropriate restoration of contour, particularly in the area of the shadowed alar crease. (D) The flap was incised along its prior distal insertion points and thinned aggressively, allowing the flap to maintain its arterial input from the area of the medial brow. After the flap was thinned and reinserted, transmural tacking sutures were used to apposition the flap to its wound bed and reintroduce contour. The sutures were removed after 48 hours. (E) Reconstructive success was apparent because nasal function was preserved, incision lines were placed along normal anatomic boundaries, and important convexities and concavities were restored.

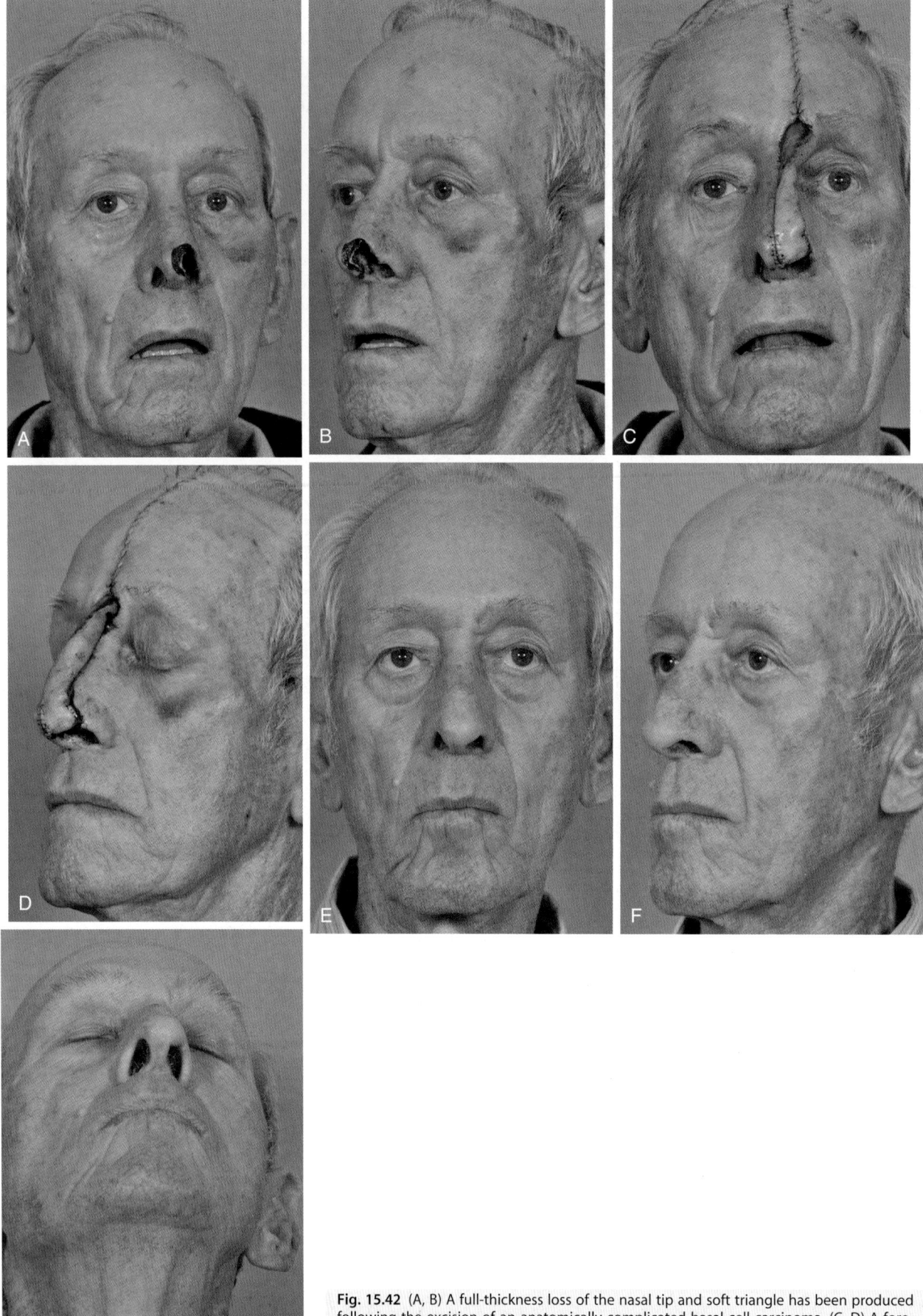

Fig. 15.42 (A, B) A full-thickness loss of the nasal tip and soft triangle has been produced following the excision of an anatomically complicated basal cell carcinoma. (C, D) A forehead flap is folded upon itself to serve as both nasal lining and external nasal coverage. (E–G) Cartilage support was not required in this case given the inherent stiffness of this patient's donor tissue on the forehead, and the flap has allowed for aesthetic and functional success.

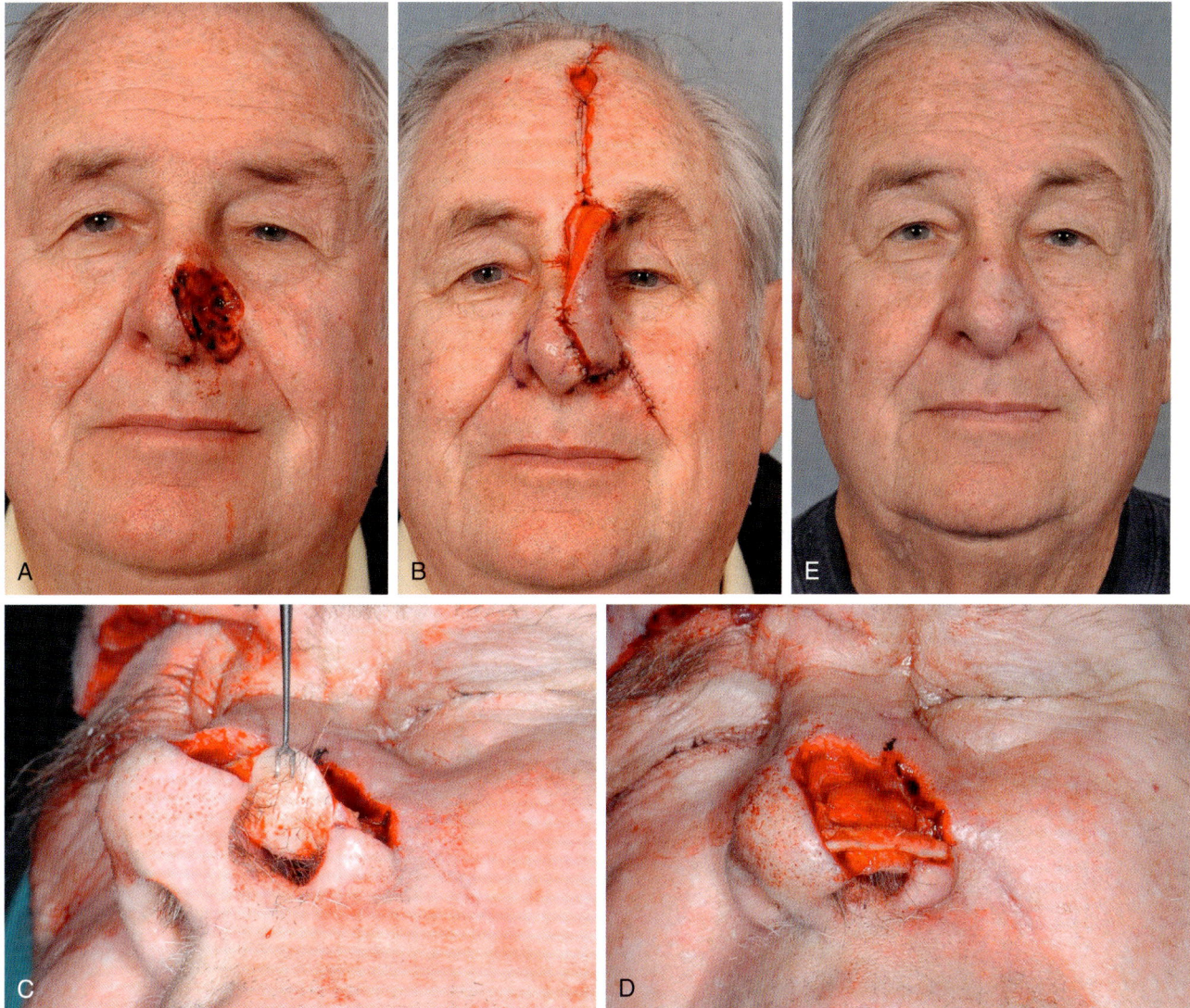

Fig. 15.43 (A) Excision of a recurrent/persistent basal cell carcinoma has introduced a challenging wound of the distal nose and cheek. (B) A small cheek advancement was initially used to place the border between cheek and nose at an anatomically appropriate position. A forehead flap was then folded upon itself to replace the full-thickness loss of the ala and sidewall. (C, D) At an interim procedure, the flap was incised from its distal insertion point and entirely elevated off the wound bed, allowing preservation of the flap's arterial source. The recipient bed was then thinned until the contour of the bed approached the contour of the normal, flexible nasal lining. Cartilage grafts from both the antehelix and cavum concha were used to reintroduce architectural stability and functional preservation. (E) Appropriate form was noted several months after repair.

operative care is used. Functional complications such as alar collapse can occur if the reconstructive procedure addresses only the nose's skin coverage and not its underlying structural support. For this reason, it is imperative to properly assess the need to reintroduce structural rigidity (with the use of cartilage grafts)[43] prior to repairing deeper nasal wounds with bulky flaps. In addition to functional difficulties, many nasal repairs, particularly flap procedures, can introduce significant alar asymmetry if the nuances of flap motion are not fully understood. Flap and skin graft necrosis can also occur with many nasal repair options (Fig. 15.45), but tissue necrosis does not seem to be apparent with greater frequency on the nose than at any other facial location. Indeed, the liberally perfused underlying musculature of the nose nourishes both skin grafts and flaps quite readily, and ischemic complications in nasal reconstructive surgery are quite uncommon if expert technique is used.

Two complications that are seen in nasal reconstructive surgery with a greater frequency than at other facial sites include the presence of very visible incision lines and the development of the trap-door (or pin-cushioned) deformity.

The presence of visible incision lines with nasal repairs is simply a reflection of the nose's aesthetic prominence in the central face and the fact that sebaceous, thick skin, regardless of site, tends to heal with more inverted, visible incision lines. For this reason, particular attention should be given to placing nasal incision lines along aesthetic boundaries, using layered closures to minimize the tension on the overlying epidermis and promoting appropriate wound edge eversion with proper suture technique.[44] Elective dermabrasion of nasal repairs can often minimize the appearance of prominent incision lines,[45] but even gently performed dermabrasion procedures can introduce undesirable pigmentary and textural changes to the skin.

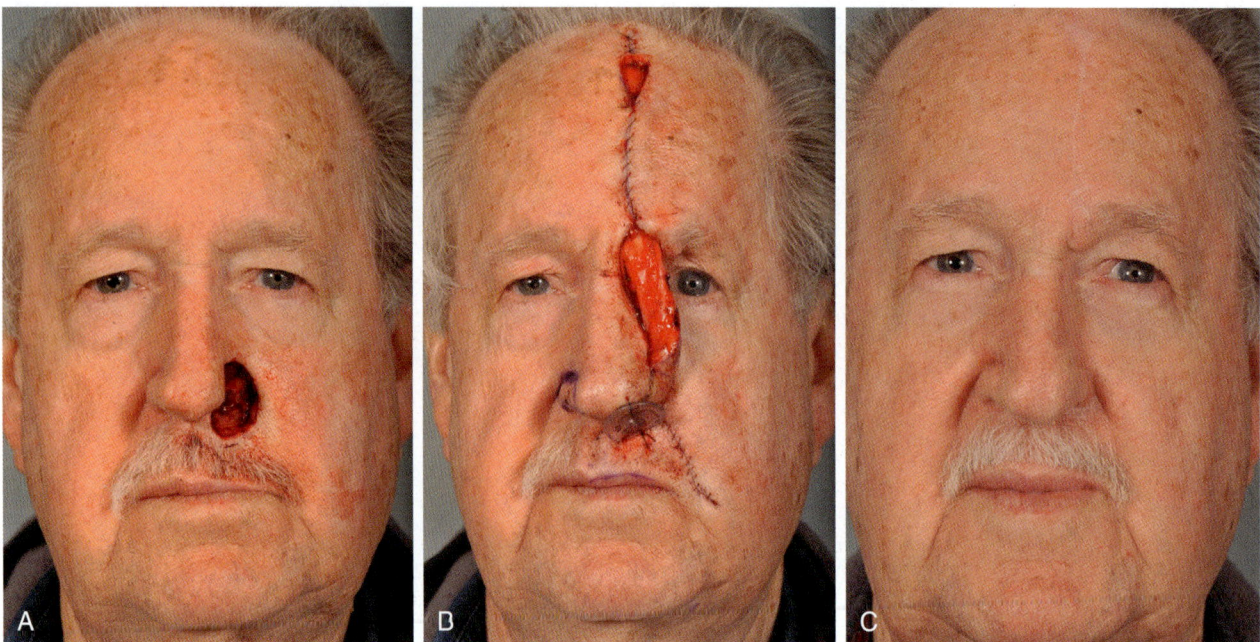

Fig. 15.44 (A) A difficult Mohs surgical excision produced a full-thickness loss of the entire ala and a deep wound involving the apical corner of the upper lip and the medial paranasal cheek. (B) A folded forehead flap was used to address only the alar component of the wound. The lip and cheek portions of the wound were repaired with flap rotation and advancement, respectively. (C) The complex visual relationship between the alar base, upper lip, and medial cheek has been reasonably restored with this series of repair procedures.

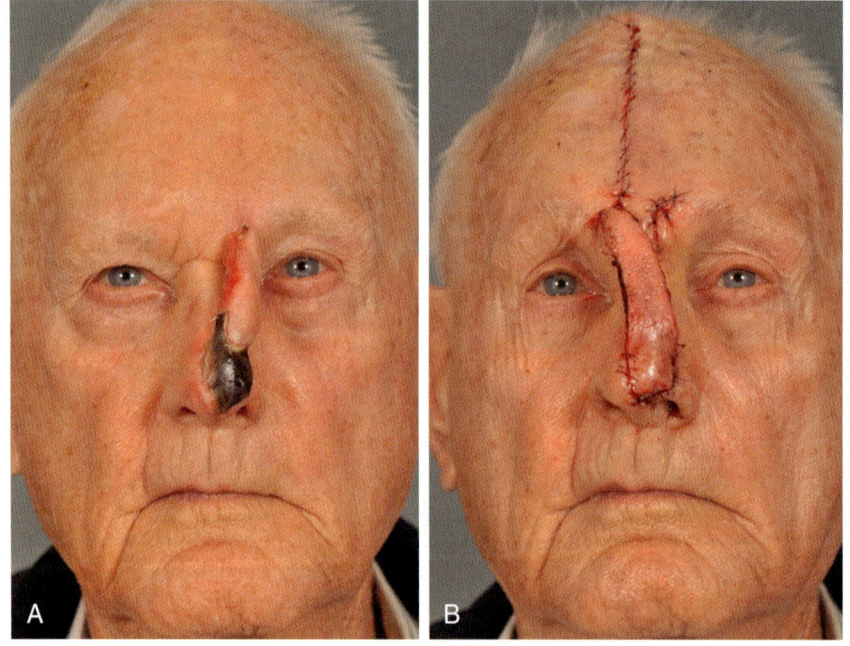

Fig. 15.45 (A) A distal nasal defect was repaired with a forehead flap. At the time of flap separation and insertion, full-thickness ischemic necrosis of the flap was noted. This type of catastrophic flap loss should occur in less than 1% of forehead flap repairs. (B) The necrotic flap was excised and discarded, and the primary surgical defect was repaired with a second flap harvested from the contralateral forehead.

The trap-door deformity typically begins at 3 to 6 weeks after a reconstructive procedure. The deformity is characterized by the development of protuberant, globular-appearing flap. This is likely due to the centrifugal contraction of platelike scar tissue under the nascent flap.[46] To prevent the trap-door deformities on nasal flaps, the cutaneous surgeon should undermine the nasal recipient site liberally,[30] thin flaps cautiously, and, perhaps most importantly, avoid oversizing flaps.[31] If the trap-door deformity develops, intralesional injections of corticosteroids can usually be quite effective. Uncommonly, surgical revision procedures to contour the deformed flap are required.

If nasal reconstructive procedures are aesthetically or functionally unsuccessful, surgical revision procedures can certainly be offered. The most expertly performed revision procedure, however, cannot compare with a proper initial performance of the nasal reconstructive procedure, and the surgeon should therefore be advised to design and perform nasal reconstructive procedures that leave little need for later revision. If the best-intentioned repair nonetheless fails, revision techniques (dermabrasion, flap "sculpting," Z-plasty reorientations of scars, introduction of structural elements such as cartilage, flaps and grafts to correct alar notching, etc.) can certainly be contemplated. The surgeon is cautioned, however, that such repair options can be much more difficult to perform than the original reconstructive procedure and that the results from such repairs are often less than ideal.

Conclusion

The cutaneous surgeon's reconstructive skill is no more apparent than on the nose, where the naturally occurring interweaving of light and shadow create aesthetic subtleties that are critical to the appreciation of both normalcy and beauty. As surgical concepts and techniques have matured over the past several decades, nasal reconstruction has progressed far beyond the ability to simply "fill a hole." With a thorough understanding of facial anatomy and flap biomechanics, the experienced dermatologic surgeon can offer the skin cancer patient a reconstructive procedure that safely and effectively preserves function and restores appearance.

References

1. Burget GC, Menick FJ. Aesthetics, visual perception, and surgical judgment. In: Burget GC, Menick FJ, eds. *Aesthetic Reconstruction of the Nose*. St. Louis: Mosby; 1994:1-55.
2. Burget GC, Menick FJ. The subunit principle in nasal reconstruction. *Plast Reconstr Surg*. 1985;76:239-247.
3. Burget GC, Menick FJ. Repair of small surface defects. In: Burget GC, Menick FJ, eds. *Aesthetic Reconstruction of the Nose*. St. Louis: Mosby; 1994:117-156.
4. Zitelli JA. Wound healing by first and second intention. In: Roenigk RK, Roenigk HH, eds. *Dermatologic Surgery*. New York: Marcel Dekker; 1996:101-130.
5. Rowe DE, Carroll RJ, Day CL. Long-term recurrence rates in previously untreated (primary) basal cell carcinoma: implications for patient follow-up. *J Dermatol Surg Oncol*. 1989;15:315-328.
6. Bumstead RM, Ceilly RI. Auricular malignant neoplasms. *Arch Otolaryngol*. 1982;108:225-231.
7. Cook J, Zitelli JA. Primary closure for midline defects of the nose: a simple approach to reconstruction. *J Am Acad Dermatol*. 2000;43:508-510.
8. Zitelli JA. Burow's grafts. *J Am Acad Dermatol*. 1987;17:271-279.
9. Rohrer TE, Dzubow LM. Conchal bowl skin grafting in nasal tip reconstruction: clinical and histologic evaluation. *J Am Acad Dermatol*. 1995;33:476-481.
10. Kaplan A, Cook JL. The incidences of chondritis and perichondritis associated with the surgical manipulation of auricular cartilage. *Dermatol Surg*. 2004;30:58-62.
11. Goldminz G, Bennett RG. Cigarette smoking and flap and full-thickness graft necrosis. *Arch Dermatol*. 1991;127:1012-1015.
12. Davenport M, Daly J, Harvey I, Griffiths RW. The bolus tie-over "pressure" dressing in the management of full-thickness skin grafts: is it necessary? *Br J Plast Surg*. 1988;41:28-32.
13. Cook JL. An optimal repair of the composite graft donor site at the helical root. *Dermatol Surg*. 2010;36:1588-1591.
14. Cook JL, Perone J. A prospective analysis of complications associated with Mohs' micrographic surgery. *Arch Dermatol*. 2003;139:143-152.
15. Lambert RW, Dzubow LM. A dorsal nasal advancement flap for off-midline defects. *J Am Acad Dermatol*. 2004;50(3):380-383.
16. Goldberg LH, Alam M. Horizontal advancement flap for symmetric reconstruction of small to medium-sized defects of the lateral nasal supratip. *J Am Acad Dermatol*. 2003;49(4):685-689.
17. Rybka FJ. Reconstruction of the nasal tip using nasalis myocutaneous sliding flaps. *Plast Reconstr Surg*. 1983;71:40-48.
18. Papadopoulos DJ, Trinei FA. Superiorly based island pedicle flap with bilevel undermining for nasal tip and supratip reconstruction. *Dermatol Surg*. 1999;25:530-536.
19. Burget GC. Commentary on the bipedicle nasalis musculocutaneous flap. *Dermatol Surg*. 1999;25:916-917.
20. Millman B, Klingensmith M. The island rotation flap: a better alternative for nasal tip repair. *Plast Reconstr Surg*. 1996;98:1293-1297.
21. Hairston BR, Nguyen TH. Innovations in the island pedicle flap for facial reconstruction. *Dermatol Surg*. 2003;29:378-385.
22. Rieger RA. A local flap for repair of the nasal tip. *Plast Reconstr Surg*. 1967;40:147-149.
23. Dzubow LM. Dorsal nasal flaps. In: Baker SR, Swanson NA, eds. *Local Flaps in Facial Reconstruction*. St Louis: Mosby; 1995:225-246.
24. Dzubow LM. The dynamics of flap movement: effect of pivotal restraint on flap rotation and transposition. *J Dermatol Surg Oncol*. 1987;13:1348-1353.
25. Tardy ME. Topographic anatomy and landmarks. In: Tardy ME, ed. *Surgical Anatomy of the Nose*. New York: Raven Press; 1990:1-23.
26. Limberg AA. Design of local flaps. In: Gibson T, ed. *Modern Trends in Plastic Surgery*. London: Butterworth; 1966:38-61.
27. Field LM. The glabellar transposition "banner" flap. *J Dermatol Surg Oncol*. 1988;14:376-379.
28. Esser JSF. Gestielte locale Nasenplastik mit zweiplifgem Lappen, Deckung des sekundaren Defektes vom ersten Zipfel durch den zweiten. *Dtsch Z Chir*. 1918;143:385-390.
29. Zitelli JA. The bilobed flap for nasal reconstruction. *Arch Dermatol*. 1989;125:957-959.
30. Cook JL. A review of the bilobed flap's design with particular emphasis on the minimization of alar displacement. *Dermatol Surg*. 2000;26:354-362.
31. Albertini JG, Hansen JP. Trilobed flap reconstruction for distal nasal defects. *Dermatol Surg*. 2010;36(11):1726-1735.
32. Zitelli JA. The nasolabial flap as a single-stage procedure. *Arch Dermatol*. 1990;126:1445-1448.
33. Lindsey WH. The reliability of the melolabial flap for alar reconstruction. *Arch Facial Plast Surg*. 2001;3:33-37.
34. Koranda FC, Webster RC. Trapdoor effect in nasolabial flaps. Causes and corrections. *Arch Otolaryngol*. 1985;111:421-424.
35. Field LM. The nasolabial flap—a definitive reappraisal. *J Dermatol Surg Oncol*. 1990;16:429-436.
36. Spear SL, Kroll SS, Romm S. A new twist to the nasolabial flap for reconstruction of lateral alar defects. *Plast Reconstr Surg*. 1987;79:915-920.
37. Cook JL. Reconstruction of a full-thickness alar wound with a single operative procedure. *Dermatol Surg*. 2003;29:956-962.
38. Fosko SW, Dzubow LM. Nasal reconstruction with the cheek island pedicle flap. *J Am Acad Dermatol*. 1996;35:580-587.
39. Cook JL. The reconstruction of the ala with interpolated flaps from the cheek and forehead: design and execution modifications to improve surgical outcomes. *Br J Dermatol*. 2014;171:29-36.
40. Singh DJ, Bartlett SP. Aesthetic considerations in nasal reconstruction and the role of modified nasal subunits. *Plast Reconstr Surg*. 2003;111:639-648.
41. Menick FJ. A 10-year experience in nasal reconstruction with the three-staged forehead flap. *Plast Reconstr Surg*. 2002;109:1839-1855.
42. Menick FJ. Practical details of nasal reconstruction. *Plast Reconstr Surg*. 2013;131(4):613e-630e.
43. Byrd DR, Otley CC, Nguyen TH. Alar batten cartilage grafting in nasal reconstruction: functional and cosmetic results. *J Am Acad Dermatol*. 2000;43:833-836.
44. Zitelli JA, Moy RL. Buried vertical mattress suture. *J Dermatol Surg Oncol*. 1989;15:17-19.
45. Yarborough JM Jr. Ablation of facial scars by programmed dermabrasion. *J Dermatol Surg Oncol*. 1988;14:292-294.
46. Hosokawa K, Susuki T, Kikui T, et al. Sheet of scar causes trapdoor deformity: a hypothesis. *Ann Plast Surg*. 1990;25:134-135.

16 Perioral Reconstruction

JOSEPH F. SOBANKO, MD

Introduction

Skin cancer frequently occurs on and around the lips,[1,2] and repairs of perioral surgical defects present numerous unique reconstructive challenges. Asymmetries and visible scars in the centrofacial region are distracting to onlookers,[3] reduce levels of perceived attractiveness,[4] and can create profound psychosocial stigma.[5] In addition to its highly aesthetic positioning, the lip is a mobile subunit that contributes to speaking, facial expressions, mastication, and oral competence. Its sensory capabilities also allow for it to examine the qualities and temperature of food prior to eating. Successful reconstructive efforts recapitulate natural perioral anatomy, hide incisions discreetly, and fully restore function and sensation. As with other anatomic sites, thoughtful surgical planning and meticulous execution facilitate desirable outcomes. Small perioral defects are repaired in a single stage but can sometimes take many weeks for patients to return to their "baseline" appearance and functioning. Larger lip defects may be exquisitely difficult to repair in a single stage and patients should be counseled that certain repairs sometimes benefit from revision or staging to achieve optimal cosmesis and functioning.

Perioral Anatomy

The lips are prominently positioned in the lower central face, bounded by the nose above, cheeks laterally, and chin below. Adult lips are approximately 7 to 8 cm long with 4 to 5 cm between commissures in repose.[6] The upper lip lies slightly anterior to the lower lip and is approximately half the height of the lower lip and chin.[7] Similar to the nose and eyelids, the lips are a trilaminar structure with multiple delicately shaped subunits. From superficial to deep, skin covers a concentrically oriented muscle that is lined posteriorly by buccal mucosa. The bulk of the lip is formed by the orbicularis oris muscle, which consists of four independent quadrants that arise from the modiolus. Each quadrant contains a larger pars peripheralis and a smaller pars marginalis, with the two divisions meeting along the vermilion cutaneous junction (VCJ) to create the bulge of the white roll. Rather than a single collection of encircled muscular fibers, the lip should be considered a collection of eight unique muscular segments that work together for dynamic movement.[8]

SURFACE ANATOMY

The cutaneous skin of the lips is similar in thickness and composition to other centrofacial skin such as the forehead.[9] In men, the terminal hair follicles produce a porous texture, while women have smoother cutaneous skin. Since the orbicularis muscle directly inserts into the undersurface of the perioral skin, dynamic muscular movement creates circumferential radial lines around the lips that are accentuated with pursing. These lines are ideal to hide incisions when reconstructing the lip. Sun damage and chronic smoking ultimately leave these lines etched into the skin and visible at rest.

The perioral region can be divided into five distinct subunits: two upper cutaneous subunits, philtrum, lower lip/chin, and vermilion lip (Fig. 16.1). The upper lip has paired lateral cutaneous subunits that begin laterally at the melolabial fold and end medially at the philtral column. Each superolateral portion of these subunits has a small triangular portion of skin adjacent to the ala that is distinctly lip skin and not cheek or alar skin; these concave apical triangles favor heavily into reconstructive designs and must be preserved for optimal cosmetic outcomes. The philtrum is the medial concave subunit of the upper lip, and it is bounded by the convex philtral columns laterally, the columella superiorly, and the Cupid's bow of the vermilion lip inferiorly.

The lower lip and chin are considered a single aesthetic subunit, and similar to the upper cutaneous subunits, the skin is approximately 8 to 9 mm thick and tethered to the underlying musculature. Of the two lips, the lower lip plays the greater role in oral competence by functioning as barrier to retain intraoral contents such as saliva.[6]

Upper and lower lip skin transitions to specialized mucosa at the VCJ, where there is a marked change in native skin color to a pink–red hue due the thin, nonkeratinizing epithelium and abundant vascularity beneath. The vermilion mucosa is a distinct subunit devoid of salivary glands, and a coronal plane divides it into two components: an internal wet portion and an external dry portion, analogous to the gray line division of the eyelid. The transition from vermilion to cutaneous lip is seamless and forms an ideal location where incisions may be hidden.

NEUROMUSCULAR ANATOMY

The muscles of facial expression attach radially along the outer margin of the orbicularis muscle in bilaterally paired sets to allow for dynamic facial animation and function.[10] These lip elevators and depressors are innervated by the zygomatic, buccal, and marginal mandibular segments of the facial nerve. Many of these muscular fibers intersect at the modiolus, a tissue thickening that can be palpated 1.5 cm lateral to the commissure. The modiolus contributes to dimple formation and can be used as a point of fixation

16 • Perioral Reconstruction

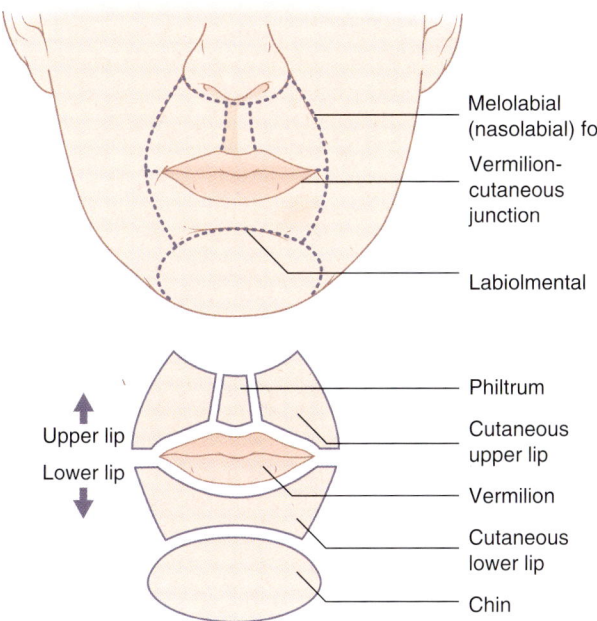

Fig. 16.1 Perioral cosmetic subunits.

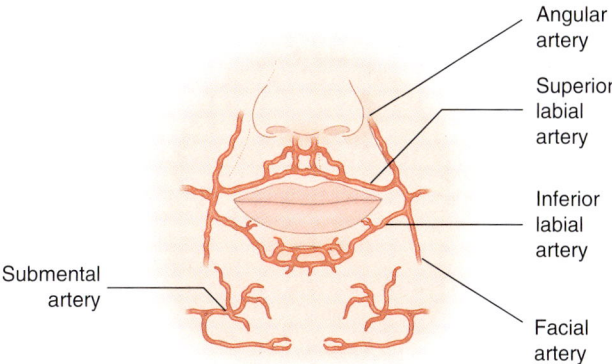

Fig. 16.3 Arterial supply to the lip.

arteries are approximately 10 mm apart from the lip margin then run closer to the surface as they progress medially.[13,14] Additional arteries that perfuse the central lip include the columellar and septal perforators that arise from the superior labial artery and the mental artery that perfuses the chin and lower lip (Fig. 16.3).[14–16]

Evaluation of the Patient and Defect

Perioral reconstruction, similar to other highly mobile and aesthetic facial units such as the eyelids, can be equal parts challenging, humbling, and rewarding. Algorithms for perioral reconstruction abound[17] and may be a useful means early in one's career to develop a conceptual framework. However, each patient's face is unique and each patient's aesthetic goals may vary. When embarking on lip reconstruction three fundamental pieces of information allow for development of an appropriate reconstructive plan:

1. Where upon the lip is the defect located?
   - Defects spanning more than one cosmetic subunit require more attention and effort than defects contained within a single subunit.
   - Upper lip defects have different reservoirs of skin for reconstruction than lower lip defects.
   - Philtral reconstruction is often more challenging than lower lip reconstruction.
2. What is the size and shape of the defect?
   - The width of the lip that the defect spans is often the main determinant of repair type.
   - The percentage of lip missing is a helpful guide for repair selection, but each patient's skin laxity must be tested so as to avoid incisional tension or iatrogenic microstomia.
   - Because of natural relaxed skin tension lines (RSTLs), defects that are greater in the vertical dimension are often less challenging to repair than defects that are greater in the horizontal dimension.
3. What is the defect depth?
   - Dermatologic surgeons most frequently encounter partial-thickness lip defects that extend to the orbicularis muscle. When located on nonvermilion lip, these always benefit from suturing.

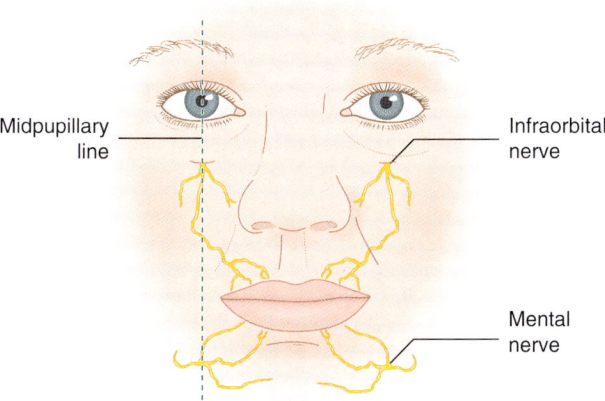

Fig. 16.2 Sensory innervation to the lip.

for certain flaps. Sensation to the upper lip is provided by the infraorbital nerve and sensation to the lower lip is provided by the mental nerve (Fig. 16.2).

VASCULAR ANATOMY

The blood supply to the perioral region is supplied by the facial artery, which is consistently identified in its corkscrew configuration crossing the border of the mandible at the anterior edge of the masseter muscle.[11] As the artery crosses over the buccinator muscle, it runs underneath the depressor anguli oris and orbicularis oris muscles, where it gives off the inferior and superior labial arteries in succession. The labial arteries originate approximately 10 to 12 mm from the oral commissures to encircle the mouth by running within the salivary glands or buccal side of the orbicularis oris muscle.[12] At the lateral portions of the lip, the labial

- Thin defects on mucosa granulate well.
- Full-thickness defects through muscle and mucosa require reapproximation of all three layers of tissue.

General Principles of Perioral Reconstruction (Box 16.1)

> **Box 16.1 General Principles for Perioral Reconstruction**
>
> - Three goals of perioral reconstruction:
>   - Maintain oral competence; preserve mobility and sensation; maximize cosmesis
> - Second intention works well for superficial vermilion defects.
> - Incisions heal well when placed in relaxed skin tension lines (RSTLs) and within or parallel to aesthetic subunit boundaries.
> - Oblique scars and skin grafts on the cutaneous lip are often conspicuous.
> - The vermilion cutaneous junction (VCJ) is best marked with indelible ink or a scalpel before anesthetizing.
> - Minimize swelling of local anesthesia by utilizing nerve blocks.
> - Recruitment of skin for flaps is lateral to medial.
> - Scar inversion is a greater risk in men because of a dense supply of folliculosebaceous structures.
> - Muscular activity of the orbicularis oris increases likelihood of scar inversion and patients should be counseled to avoid opening their mouth widely in the postoperative period.
> - Revisions may be necessary to achieve optimal results, especially for larger, composite defects.

Methods of Closure

SECOND INTENTION HEALING

Second intention healing is a reliable approach for partial-thickness upper or lower mucosal lip defects, particularly in patients seeking to avoid additional reconstruction after tumor extirpation. Superficial defects restricted to the mucosal lip are often best managed with granulation alone (Fig. 16.4A–B).[18] Patients are counseled to apply a thin coat of petrolatum after they cleanse their wound one to two times per day. With proper wound care small mucosal defects heal rapidly, and defects spanning the breadth of the entire mucosal lip will reepithelialize in less than 4 weeks because of rich anatomic vascularity (Fig. 16.5A–B). Larger lip defects with partial resection of orbicularis muscle and defects that cross the VCJ onto the cutaneous lip still may heal satisfactorily with second intention (Fig. 16.6A–B).[19] Disadvantages of the second intention healing include visible stellate scarring, which may be more conspicuous when larger sized defects are allowed to granulate. Once fully healed, these smaller scars can be resected and repaired with minimal effort and recovery.

MUCOSAL ADVANCEMENT FLAP

Large mucosal defects, with or without muscle involvement, may be repaired with a mucosal advancement flap. This closure obviates the need for diligent daily wound care that must be performed for second intention healing. Flaps are designed off of the lateral aspect of the defect along the VCJ (Fig. 16.7A). Incisions are often carried from commissure to commissure, and redundant mucosal cones are removed in order to camouflage scarring (see Fig. 16.7B). Undermining is performed posterior to the orbicularis oris by spreading the scissor tips to bluntly release the glistening yellow salivary glands off of the muscle (see Fig. 16.7C). Elevating mucosa down to the gingival sulcus is often not necessary to facilitate stretching of mucosa to the VCJ, and minimizing the extent of undermining reduces postoperative hypoesthesia.

The flap is sutured in place with a single layer of sutures due to the thinness of the mucosa (Fig. 16.7D–E). When performed on the upper lip for philtral mucosal defects, a gull wing design for the mucosal advancement flap can restore the Cupid's bow.[20] Another variation of the mucosal advancement flap incorporates an axial myomucosal design by bluntly dissecting the labial artery and including it in the flap by incising through the orbicularis muscle, elevating the flap below the vessel, and sliding the flap laterally toward the defect.[21]

While advancement of the mucosa provides immediate closure of certain lip defects, it possesses inherent disadvantages. The new lip is prone to cracking, and patients may

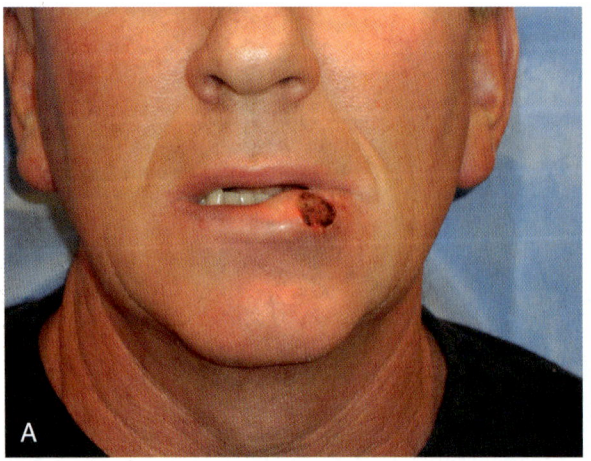 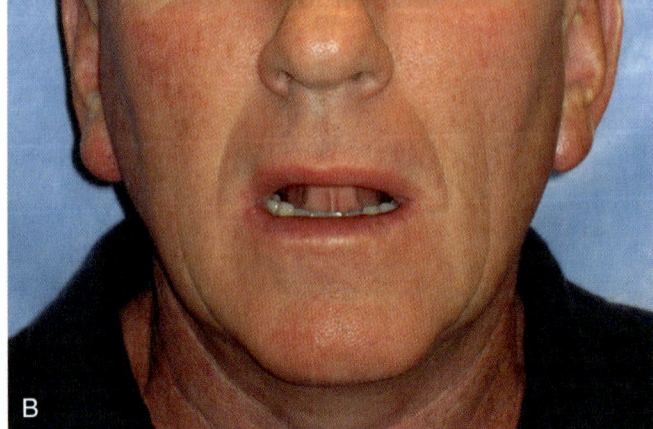

Fig. 16.4 Second intention healing. (A) Mucosal defect. (B) Final result.

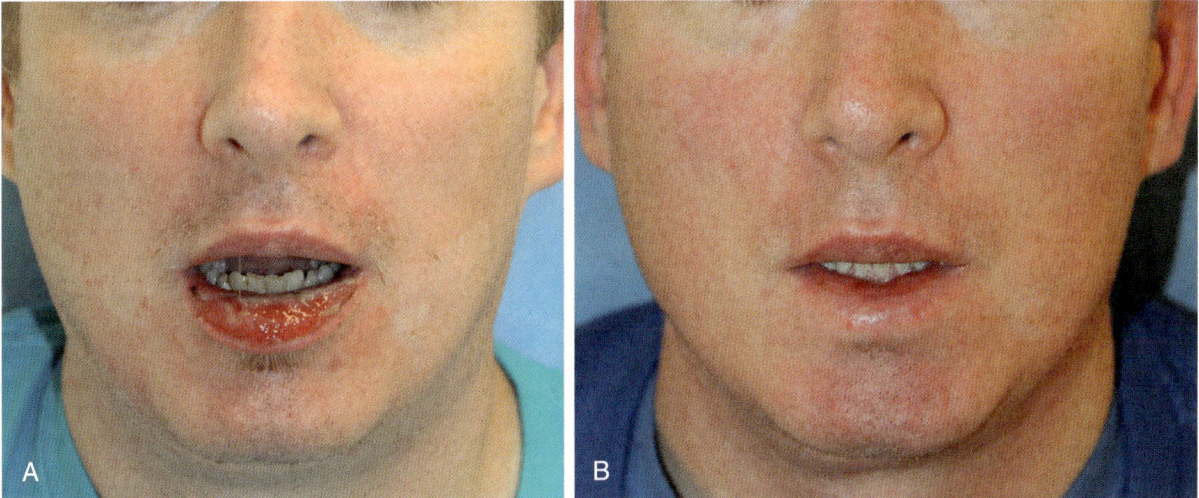

Fig. 16.5 Second intention healing from vermilionectomy. (A) One week postoperative appearance. (B) Final result at 6 weeks.

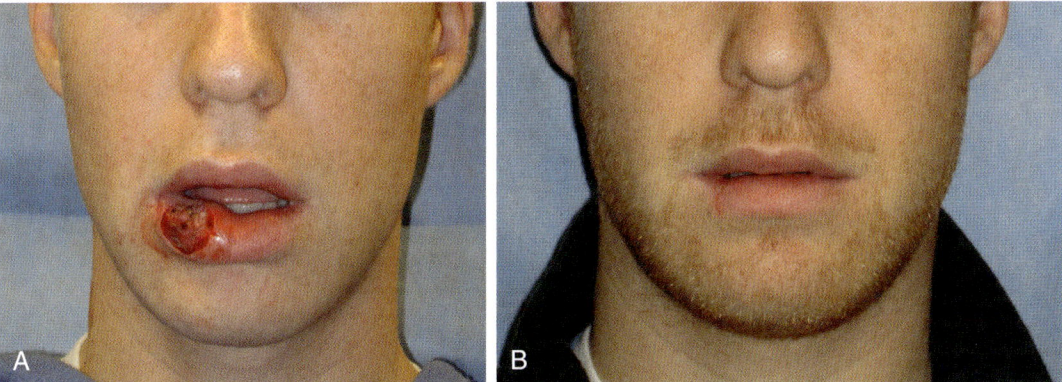

Fig. 16.6 Second intention healing of vermilion-cutaneous defect. (A) Defect extends past vermilion cutaneous junction (VCJ). (B) Final result with small stellate scar on vermilion. Patient declined revision.

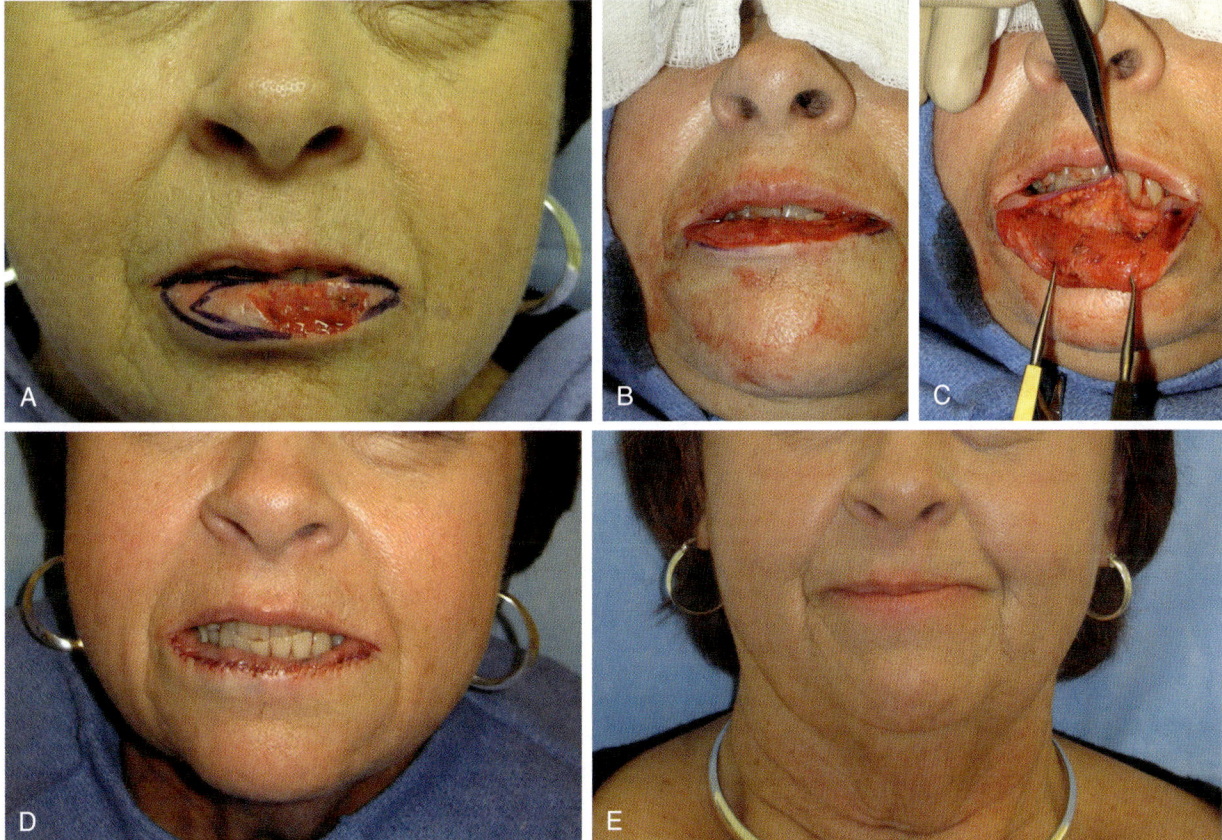

Fig. 16.7 Mucosal advancement flap. (A) Design. (B) Tissue cones removed to subunit border. (C) Flap elevated in submucosal plane. (D) Flap sutured in place. (E) Final result.

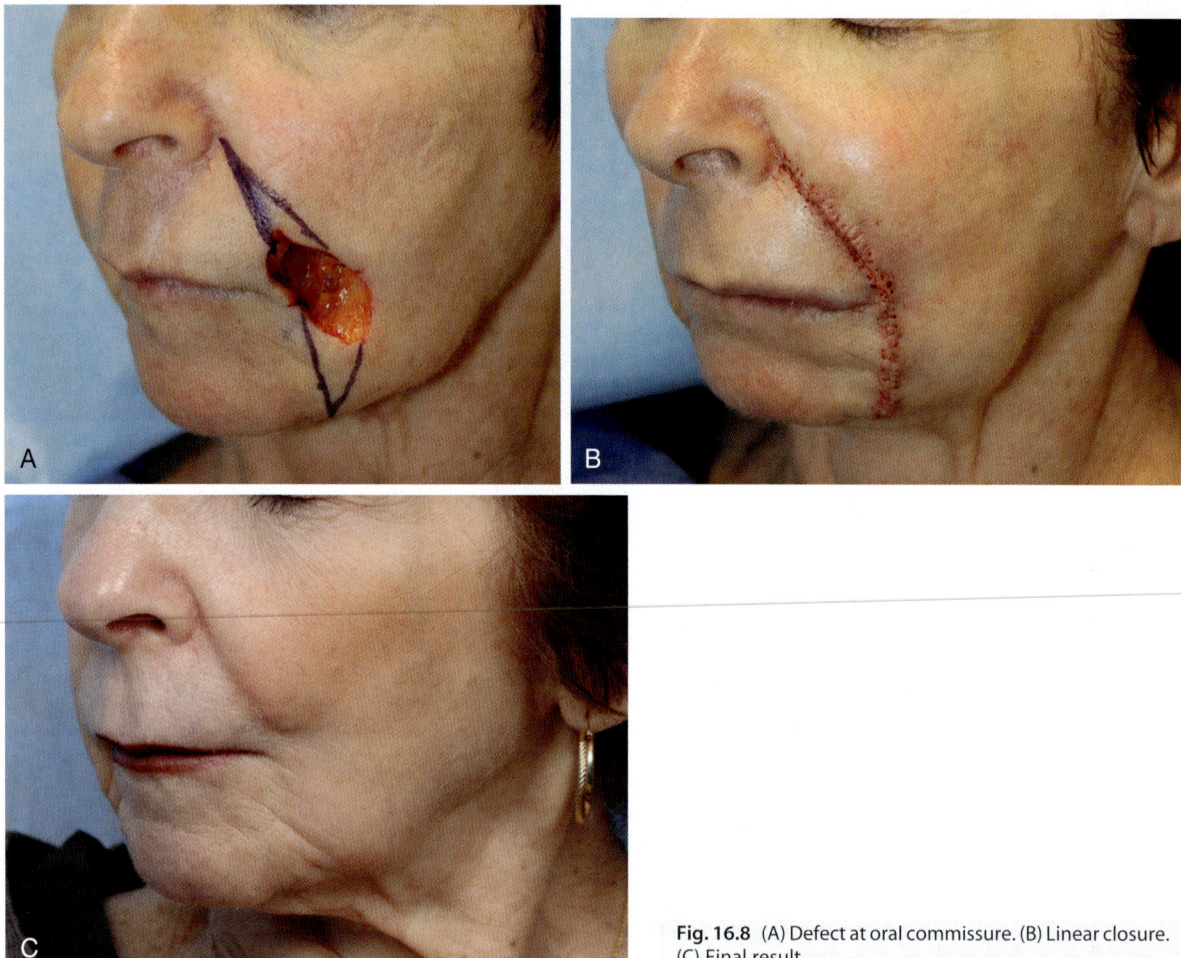

Fig. 16.8 (A) Defect at oral commissure. (B) Linear closure. (C) Final result.

find the need to moisturize with lip balm routinely. Patients frequently report loss of lip sensation, which can impair eating and drinking. Mucosal advancement flaps also decrease the anterior–posterior dimension of the lip, particularly for larger defects, and secondary flap motion can redirect beard hairs in men causing lip irritation.

LINEAR CLOSURE

As with other facial subunits, linear closures (LCs) in the perioral region are a workhorse repair that can produce excellent results. When designed for appropriately sized lip defects within RSTLs or along cosmetic junction borders, scar visibility is reduced and free margin position is preserved.[22] The ideal defect for an LC is partial thickness, situated in the middle of the lateral cutaneous subunit, and is taller than wider. LC of defects greater than one-fourth the width of the upper lip or one-third of the lower lip risks excessive incisional tension, displacement of the philtrum, or extending incisions perpendicularly beyond cosmetic junction borders.

Standard design of the LC creates straight tissue incisions off of the defect that form a rhombus shape with apical angles of 30 degree or less. The final length of most LCs is approximately 3 to 4 times longer than the short axis diameter of the defect. Burow triangles, approximately the same length or slightly larger than the defect diameter, may be designed off of the defect parallel to the lip's radially oriented RSTLs. As defects are positioned more laterally on the subunit, the final design will be drawn more obliquely in order to mimic the RSTLs. Lateral-most defects can mirror the melolabial fold curvature if tissue approximation does not excessively displace the lip or commissure (Fig. 16.8).

Contour of a scar should not be compromised in order to reduce scar length, because persistent tissue redundancies will negatively impact cosmesis. Redundant cones on the upper lip that extend past the VCJ or alar sill are precisely reapproximated to preserve the aesthetic junction lines. Tissue cones may be carried into the apical triangle/alar-facial sulcus with minimal aesthetic penalty if 1 to 2 mm of skin is preserved lateral to the ala (Fig. 16.9). However, if the anticipated LC design extends perpendicularly past the NLF onto the cheek, then an alternative repair is better selected in order to avoid a noticeable step-off scar. Lower lip scar length can be reduced with implementation of an M-plasty (Fig. 16.10).

Execution of LCs on the lip is identical to other locations on the central face. Redundant tissue cones (RTCs) are removed to the SMAS/muscle layer. In order to minimize incisional tension, the wound margins are sharply undermined with scissors to release skin from the tethering of the orbicularis oris. Undermining is performed up to 1 cm from

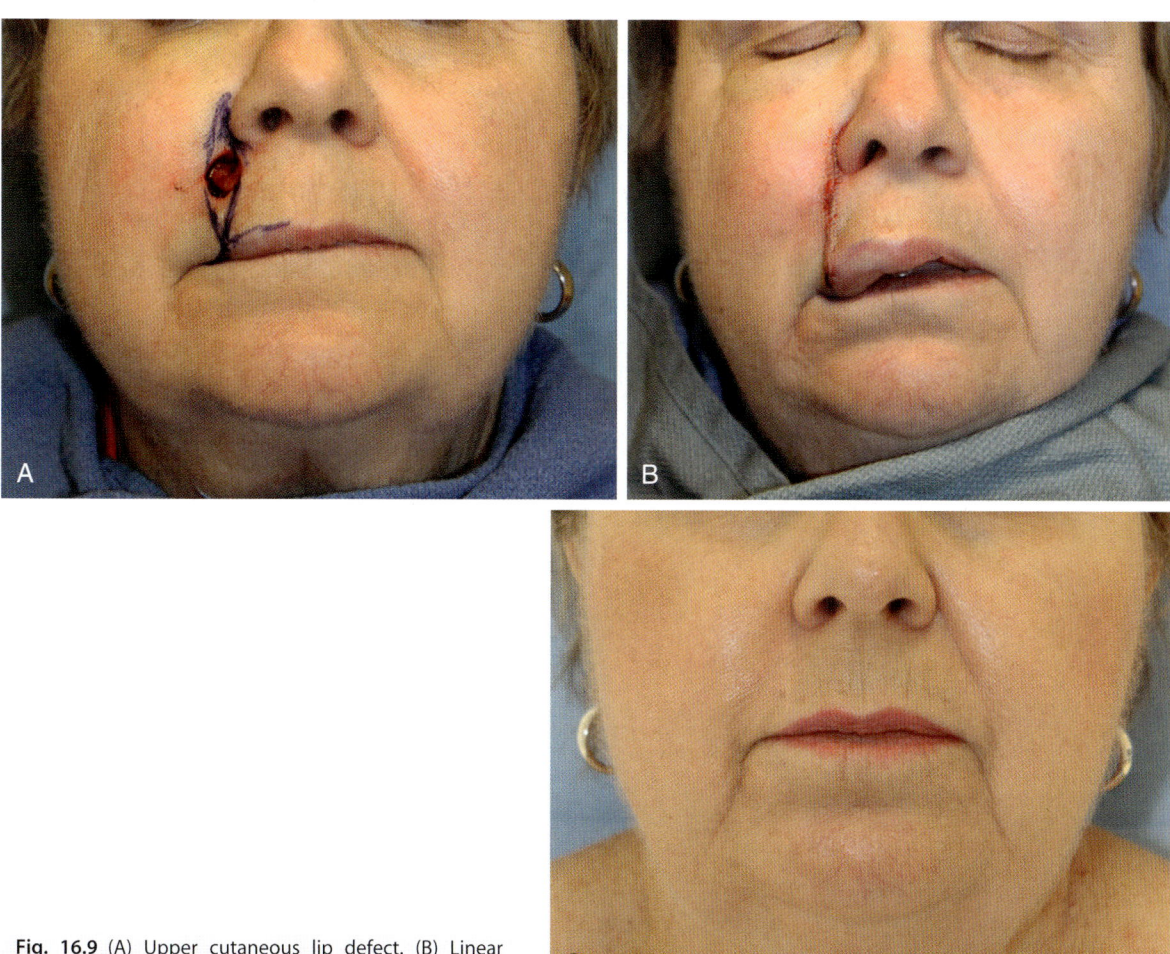

Fig. 16.9 (A) Upper cutaneous lip defect. (B) Linear closure extended into apical triangle. (C) Final result.

the wound margin. Elevating tissue beyond this distance increases the possibility of postoperative bleeding and does not facilitate further tension reduction. Once meticulous hemostasis is achieved, suturing the lip is performed in a bilayered fashion, first with buried vertical mattress sutures and then with a cuticular layer of sutures.[23]

There is little margin of error for suturing the cutaneous lip. Misalignment of the VCJ results in a jarring appearance and can detract from an otherwise seamless scar. In male patients the high density of follicular structures reduces the surface area of collagen gripped with each suture bite, thus increasing the risk of scar inversion (Fig. 16.11). Attempts should be made to take greater bites of dermis in order to accentuate eversion and combat the natural forces that pull the scarline apart. Displacement of the VCJ can occur despite prudent LC design because of "central axis lengthening" that pushes the free margin away from the defect.[24] Direct primary closures on the lip may also result in fullness of the lip due to an external rolling of the labial mucosa or compression of the underlying orbicularis oris muscle (Fig. 16.12).[25] While typically unfavorable, this pushing effect tends to be transient or can be revised with minor tissue resection. Asymmetry from inferomedial displacement of the melolabial fold may also occur if too large a redundant cone is removed from the lip's apical triangle.[26]

Wedge Repair

Lip wedge repairs produce scarlines that mimic LCs and are a more versatile and reliable method of reconstruction. For many patients, defects up to one-fourth the width of the upper lip or up to one-third the width of the lower lip may be repaired with a lip wedge without risking microstomia or subunit distortion. This repair may be used along any position of the lower lip or lateral cutaneous upper lip. However, wedge repair of centrally located upper lip defects will distort or eliminate the Cupid's bow, and alternative methods of reconstruction that preserve this nuanced architecture are recommended.

A traditional wedge repair design begins with creating a triangular cone extending from the defect to the opposing subunit border. On the upper lip, this design usually crescentically curves along the alar-facial sulcus. Lower lip wedge designs may be converted to a W-shape in order to keep the scarline above the mental crease. Full-thickness resection of tissue may span the entire vertical height of the lip or be modified so as to not resect muscle and mucosa all the way to the gingival sulcus. In either scenario, removal of full-thickness tissue at the free margin reduces buckled, protruding tissue frequently encountered with partial-thickness LCs.

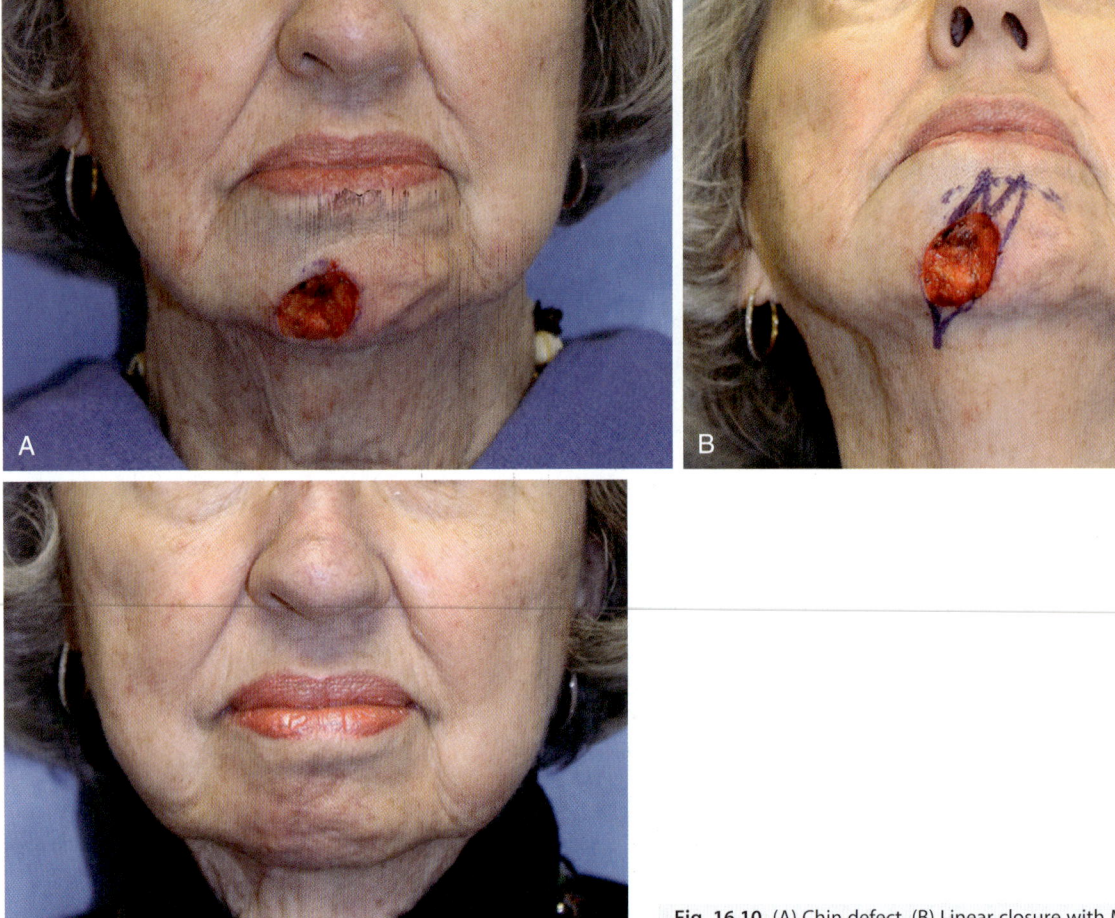

Fig. 16.10 (A) Chin defect. (B) Linear closure with M-plasty. (C) Final result.

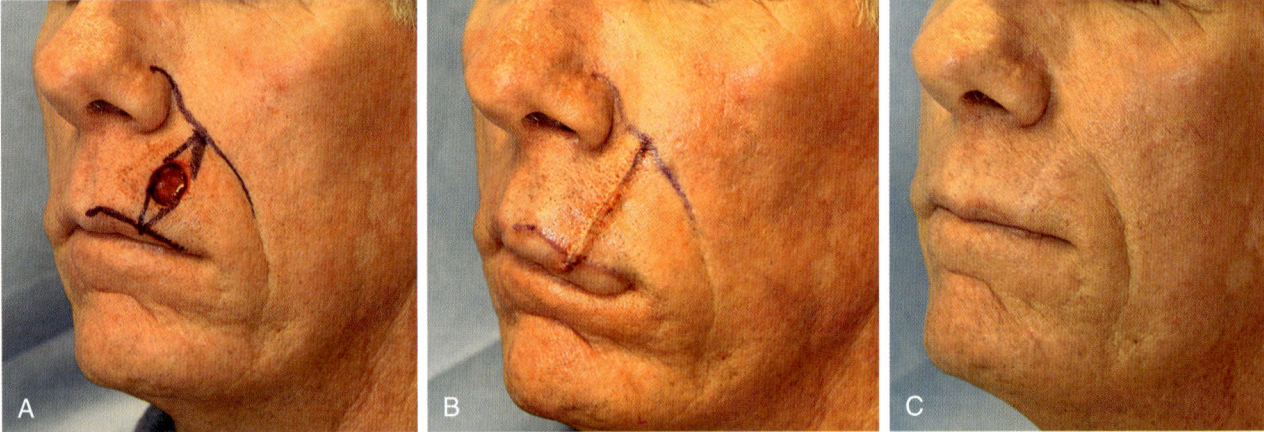

Fig. 16.11 (A) Upper cutaneous lip defect on hair-bearing male lip. (B) Linear closure. (C) Final result with notable scar inversion.

The repair is carried out by resecting a composite columnar piece of mucosa-muscle-skin. Small defects may only require resection of mucosa and muscle to the VCJ (Fig. 16.13), while wider defects necessitate resection of mucosa and muscle to the subunit border (Fig. 16.14). Care should be made when incising through the labial artery on each side. The vessel ends may be ligated with suture or precisely destroyed with indirect electrocoagulation. Undermining of the skin flaps is not necessary because inherent tissue elasticity facilitates easy side-to-side movement. Closure of the resultant wound begins by closing all three layers of tissue with four layers of suture. First the mucosa is repaired with a short-acting dissolving suture (e.g., chromic gut), then muscle with a long-acting dissolvable

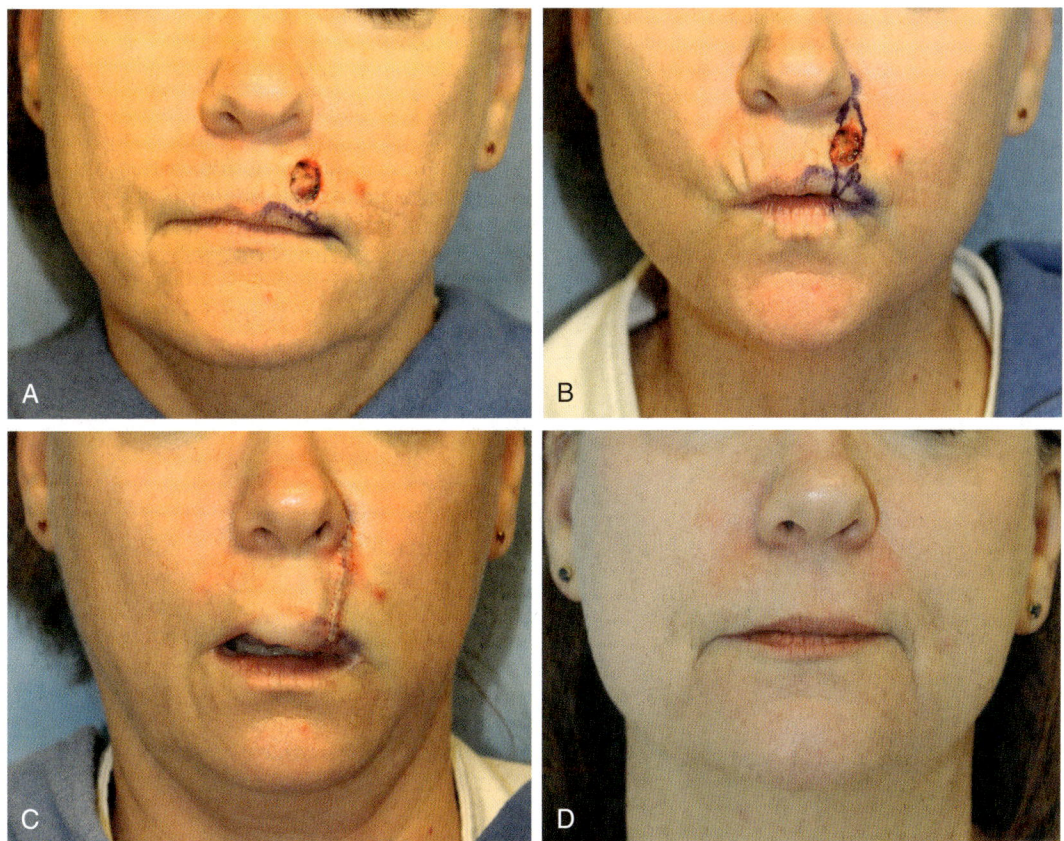

Fig. 16.12 (A) Upper cutaneous lip defect. (B) Linear closure design extending into apical triangle and past vermilion border. (C) Immediate postoperative result. (D) Final result with fullness of left side of upper lip.

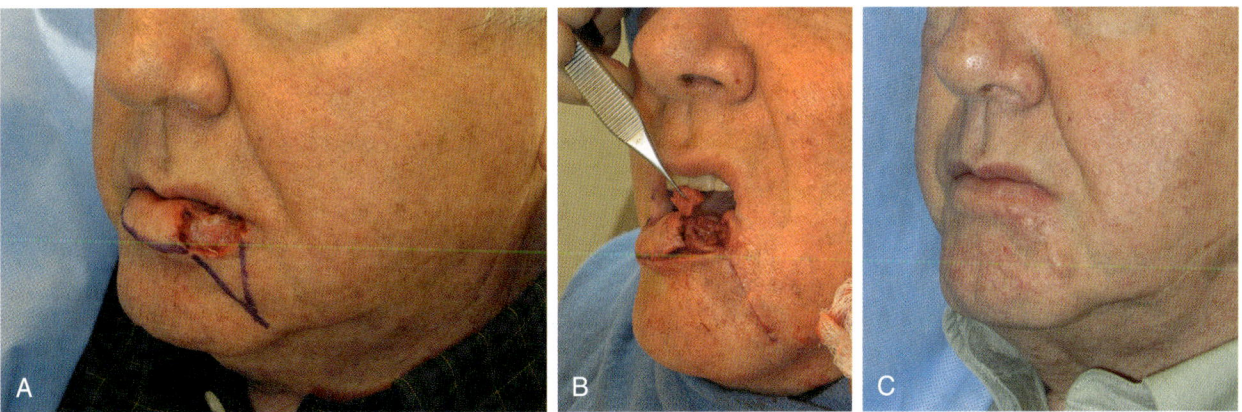

Fig. 16.13 (A) Vermilion-cutaneous lower lip defect. (B) Partial height wedge repair illustrating resection of orbicularis muscle above vermilion-cutaneous junction. (C) Final result.

suture (e.g., polydioxanone, PDS), and then the skin with a bilayered repair of the dermis and epidermis. As with LCs, reapproximation of the VCJ with precisely placed dermal sutures is critical to achieve an appropriate aesthetic result (Fig. 16.15).

Wedge repairs do have disadvantages. The closure's tension vector can laterally displace the philtrum. Furthermore, recruitment of vermilion from the lateral aspects of the lip often fails to fully restore the true vertical height of the vermilion because the medial vermilion lip is taller and thicker. Finally, precise alignment of the VCJ can be difficult if the lip line is not marked prior to infiltration of anesthesia.

Flaps

Although many perioral defects are amenable to repair with primary closure or wedge repair, numerous occasions arise where these methods will displace adjacent free margins or create excessive closure tension. In these instances, repair is best performed with adjacent tissue in the form of local

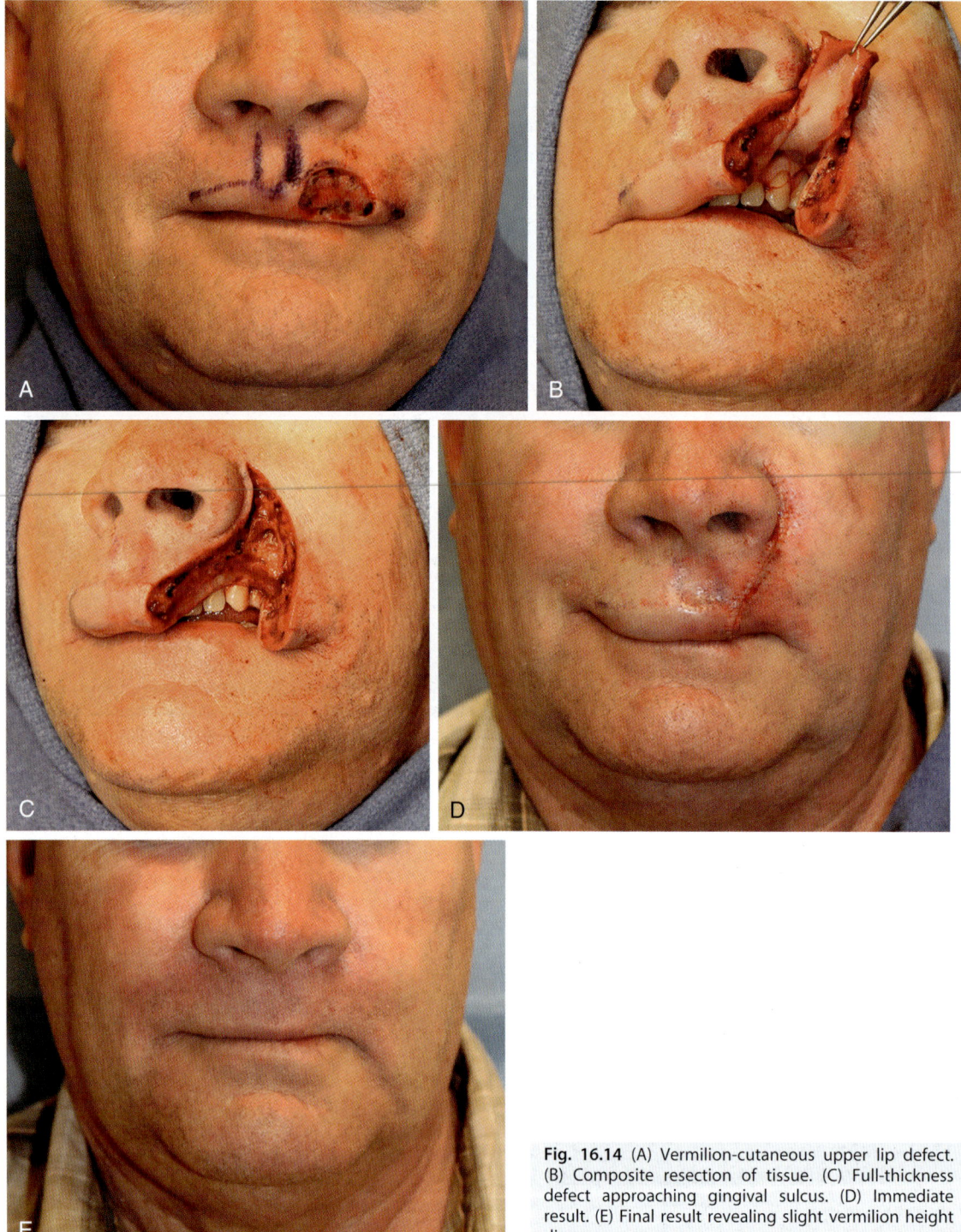

Fig. 16.14 (A) Vermilion-cutaneous upper lip defect. (B) Composite resection of tissue. (C) Full-thickness defect approaching gingival sulcus. (D) Immediate result. (E) Final result revealing slight vermilion height discrepancy.

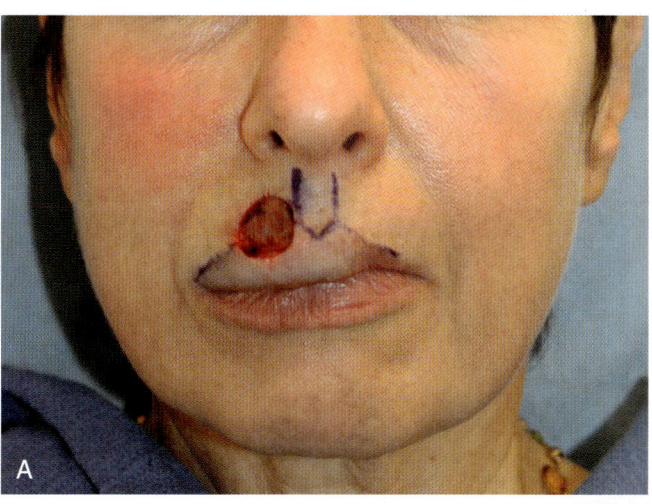
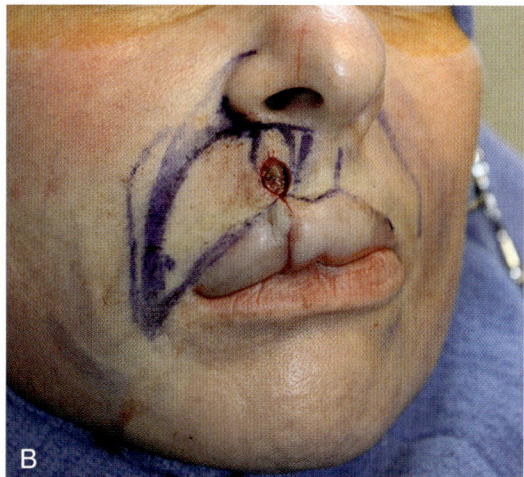
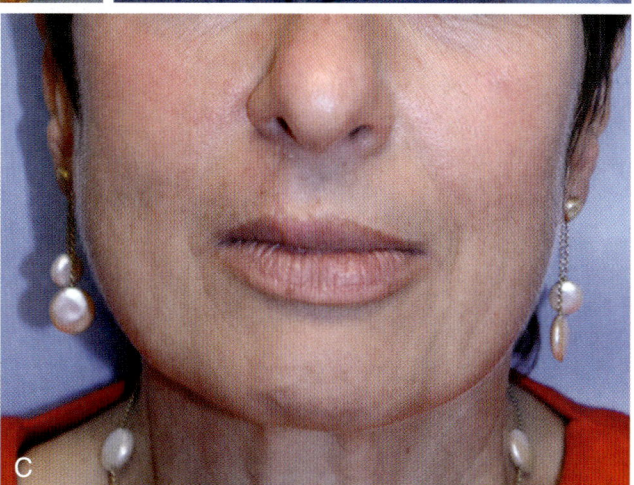

Fig. 16.15 (A) Vermilion-cutaneous upper lip defect. (B) Wedge repair illustrating reapproximation of vermilion cutaneous junction (VCJ). (C) Final result revealing slight lateral displacement of philtral subunit.

flaps. Generally, these flaps are designed from laterally and inferiorly based tissue because of the abundant reservoir and natural motion vectors. Most local perioral flaps are "sliding" flaps that advance or rotate tissue with varied geometric and anatomic nuances. Transposition flaps lift abundant tissue from the neck, ipsilateral cheek, or opposing lip, and allow for closure of larger defects, albeit with higher levels of difficulty. Detailed knowledge of aesthetic boundaries and vascular and muscular anatomy allow for the surgeon to appropriately design and execute flap repairs for perioral defects.

ADVANCEMENT-ROTATION FLAPS

Advancement flaps are sliding flaps that facilitate tissue movement and hide scarlines along cosmetic junction lines and RSTLs. They are best implemented on the upper and lower lip for medium-sized cutaneous defects where free margins such as the VCJ would be susceptible to displacement with an LC or wedge repair. Most advancement flaps are skin-only, elevated above the muscle, and based on a random blood supply. Modifications of advancement flaps by inclusion of muscle and incorporation of vessels directly into the flap will increase vascularity and facilitate closure of larger defects.

Burow Wedge

The Burow wedge closure is considered a cutaneous advancement flap but may also be conceptualized as a variation of an LC.[27] This closure design displaces half of the linear scar into a more desirable location simply by modifying the typical fusiform design. Lateral upper cutaneous lip defects closed with this method produce a superior cone in the RSTLs of the upper lip and an inferior cone along the lower lip's VCJ (Fig. 16.16). Lower cutaneous lip defects produce an inferior cone down the chin and a superior cone in the melolabial fold (Fig. 16.17). In both instances, incisions are made within the VCJ to camouflage scarlines, and the flap is sharply elevated above the orbicularis muscle. The tangential movement that displaces the scar produces a zigzag shape, but the overall outline camouflages well when used for appropriately sized and positioned defects.[28] The length of the laterally released skin can be minimized by creating a medial incision and mobilizing this skin above the muscle. While recruitment of medial-based skin is limited on the lips, this O-T design is feasible for smaller defects and permits the flap to be restricted to only one lip subunit (Fig. 16.18). Another modification that may be used for larger defects is carrying the upper redundant tissue cone into the alar-facial sulcus as a crescent (Fig. 16.19).

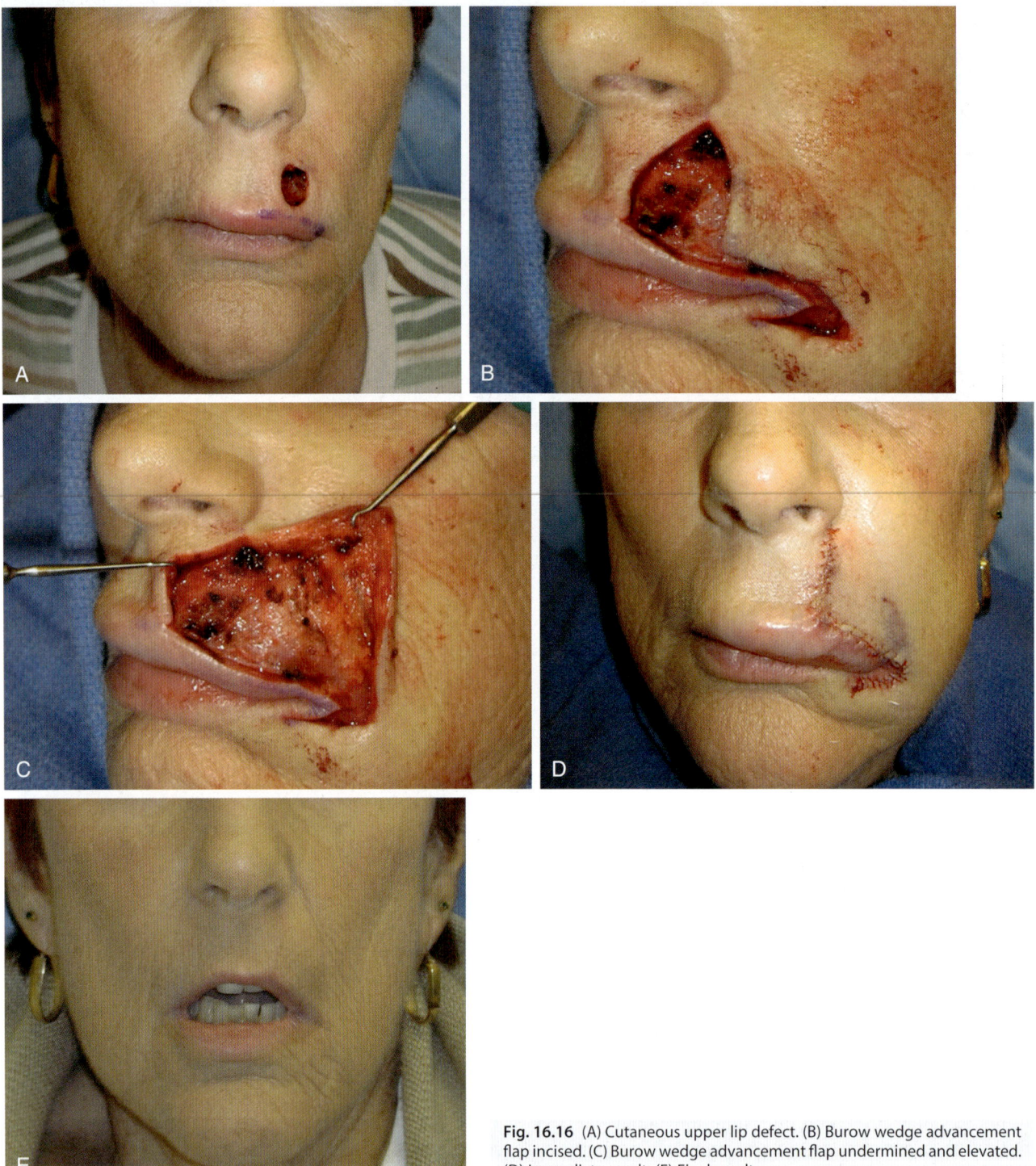

Fig. 16.16 (A) Cutaneous upper lip defect. (B) Burow wedge advancement flap incised. (C) Burow wedge advancement flap undermined and elevated. (D) Immediate result. (E) Final result.

Fig. 16.17 (A) Cutaneous lower lip defect. (B) Burow wedge advancement flap sutured. (C) Final result.

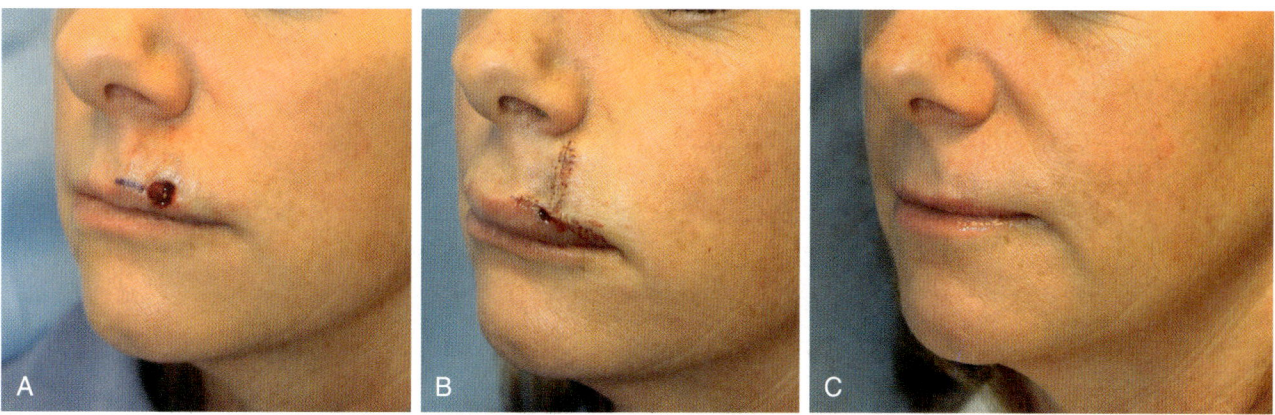

Fig. 16.18 (A) Vermilion-cutaneous upper lip defect. (B) Bilateral O-T advancement flap sutured. (C) Final result.

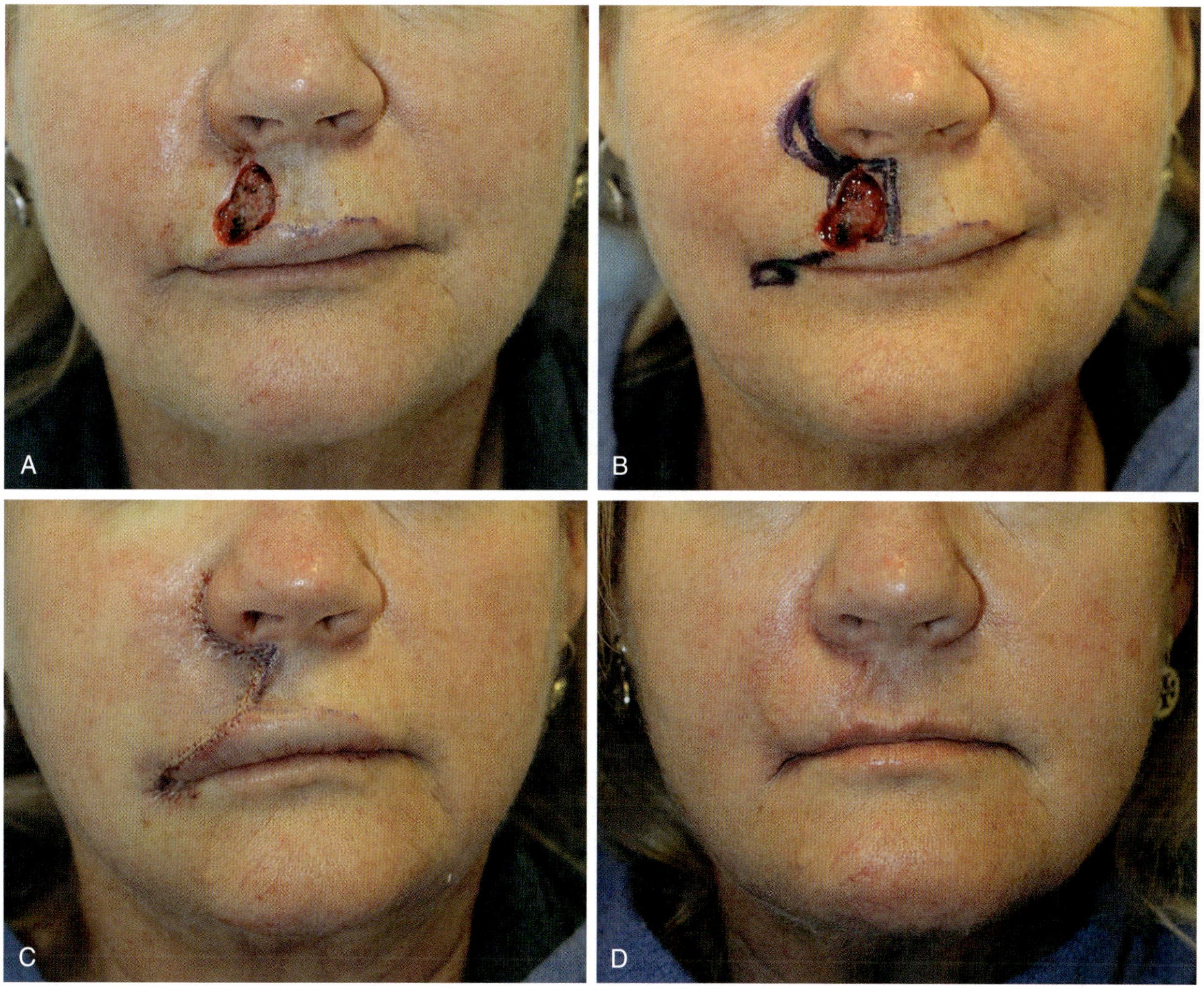

Fig. 16.19 (A) Cutaneous upper lip defect. (B) Crescentic advancement flap design. (C) Flap sutured. (D) Early postoperative result with slight pincushioned appearance.

Rotation Flap

Advancement flaps create horizontal incisions perpendicularly off of a defect and thus do not recruit additionally appreciable amounts of tissue for closure. More tissue can be delivered with rotation flap closure because of the flaps' leading edge curvature. The size, orientation, and location of a defect on the upper or lower lip influence the ideal path of a flap's leading incision. Rotation flaps are a workhorse flap for partial-thickness defects that are situated in the superolateral upper cutaneous quadrant (Fig. 16.20). Ideally, defects are taller than wider, but rotation flaps can

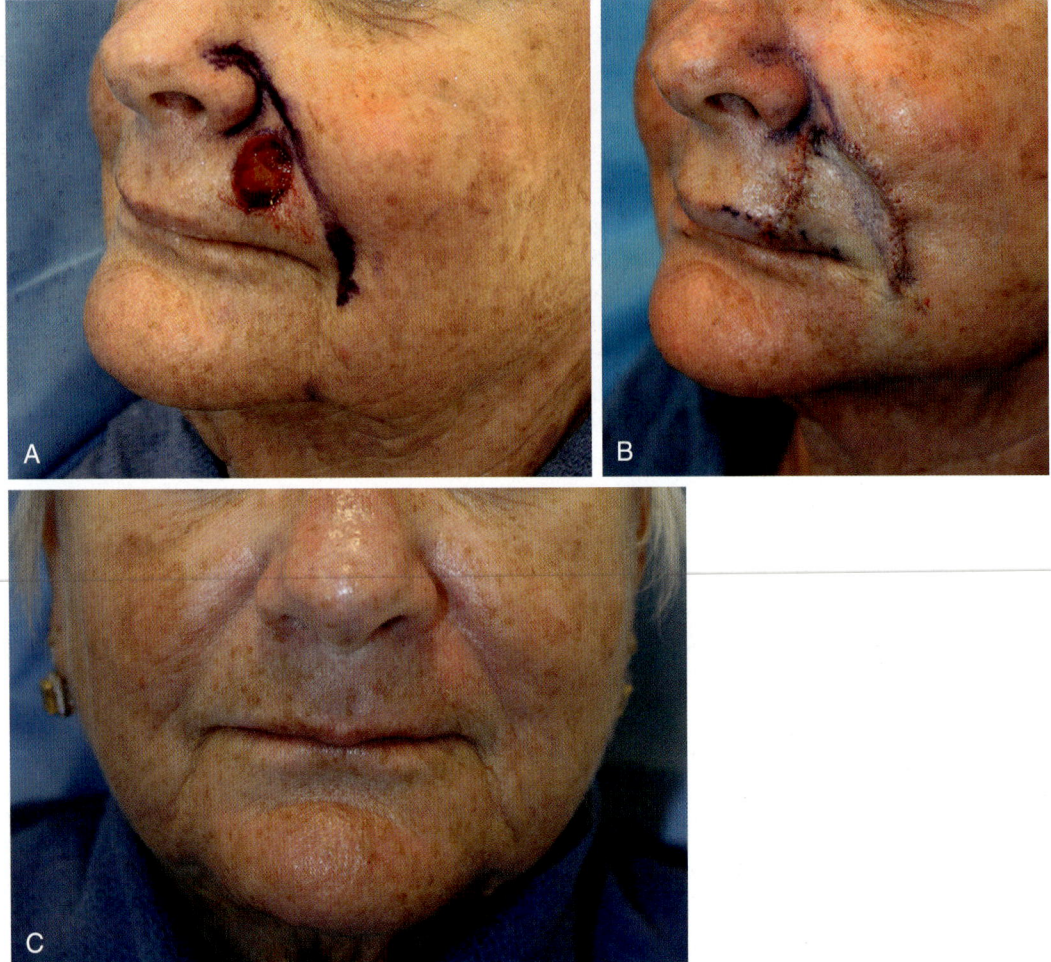

Fig. 16.20 (A) Cutaneous upper lip defect. (B) Rotation flap sutured. (C) Final result.

reduce the risk of eclabian for superolateral defects that are wider than taller (Fig. 16.21). The leading arm of the flap is designed from the cephalic border of the defect extending into and down the melolabial fold, mimicking its curvature. Since the flap rotates medially, the leading edge incision should be designed outside the melolabial fold, anticipating that the lateral arm of the flap will recreate this junction border once the defect is closed. Similar to advancement flaps, random-based rotation flaps are elevated above the orbicularis muscle and, if the secondary defect extends as far, the melolabial fat pad. Redundant tissue cones are removed parallel to the RSTLs of the upper lip. The discrepancy in length between the cheek skin and lateral border of the flap may be "sutured out" by evenly dividing the skin redundancy or by removing a small tissue cone anywhere along the length of the flap. Lower lip defects are also repaired well with rotation flaps as the mental crease provides a suitable border upon which to hide a scarline (Fig. 16.22).

V-Y Advancement Flap

V-Y advancement flaps are another common option to reconstruct medium-sized defects of the upper cutaneous lip located lateral to the philtrum.[29,30] V-to-Y a.k.a. island advancement flaps may also be useful for reconstructing the apical portion of the upper lip between the cheek, lip and ala, and are also useful for reconstruction of defects limited to the philtrum and alar sill. Their triangular design frequently allows flap limbs to be hidden in cosmetic junction borders. (Unlike traditional advancement-rotation flaps, these flaps are not stretched toward the defect but mobilized on a subcutaneous island and pushed toward the primary defect by closure of the secondary defect.)[10] The blood supply to V-Y flaps is centrally located beneath the flap and is more resistant to ischemia than other random-based flaps.

The traditional V-Y advancement flap has limbs that are based off of the cephalic and caudal borders of the defect and extend laterally, often toward to the oral commissure. The flap limbs should meet and form an angle less than or equal to 30 degrees. Depending upon the size and location of the defect, one or both of the flap limbs may be hidden in the melolabial fold or VCJ. The flap is circumferentially incised to the orbicularis muscle, and the peripheral edges are undermined in this plane. The central 30% to 50% of the subcutaneous tissue is preserved, and it is this tissue upon which the flap "rocks" forward. Once careful hemostasis has been achieved, the flap is sutured in place with

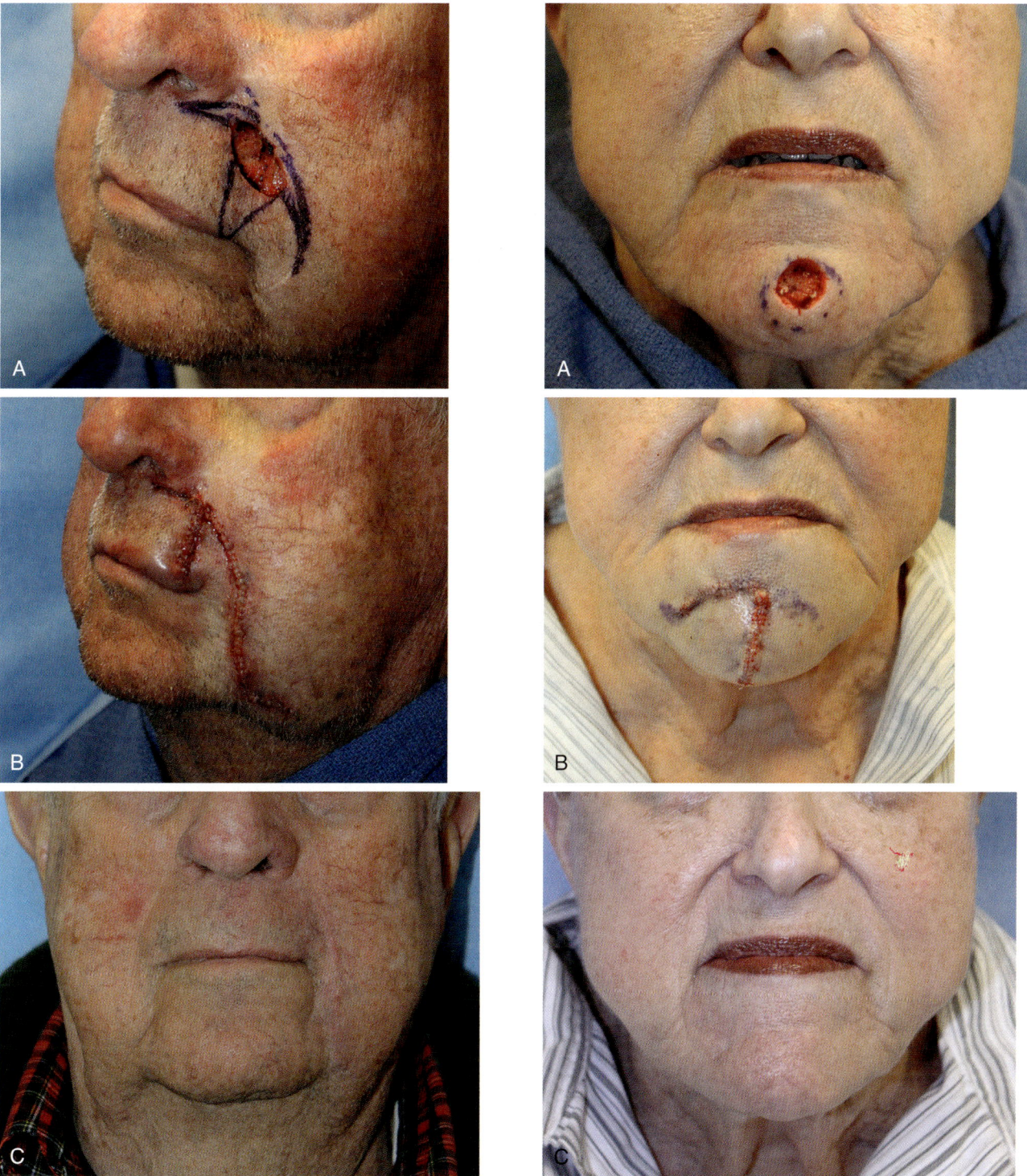

Fig. 16.21 (A) Cutaneous upper lip defect with oval shape approaching melolabial fold. (B) Rotation flap sutured in order to preserve position of fold and vermilion-cutaneous junction (VCJ). (C) Final result.

Fig. 16.22 (A) Chin defect. (B) Rotation flap sutured. (C) Final result.

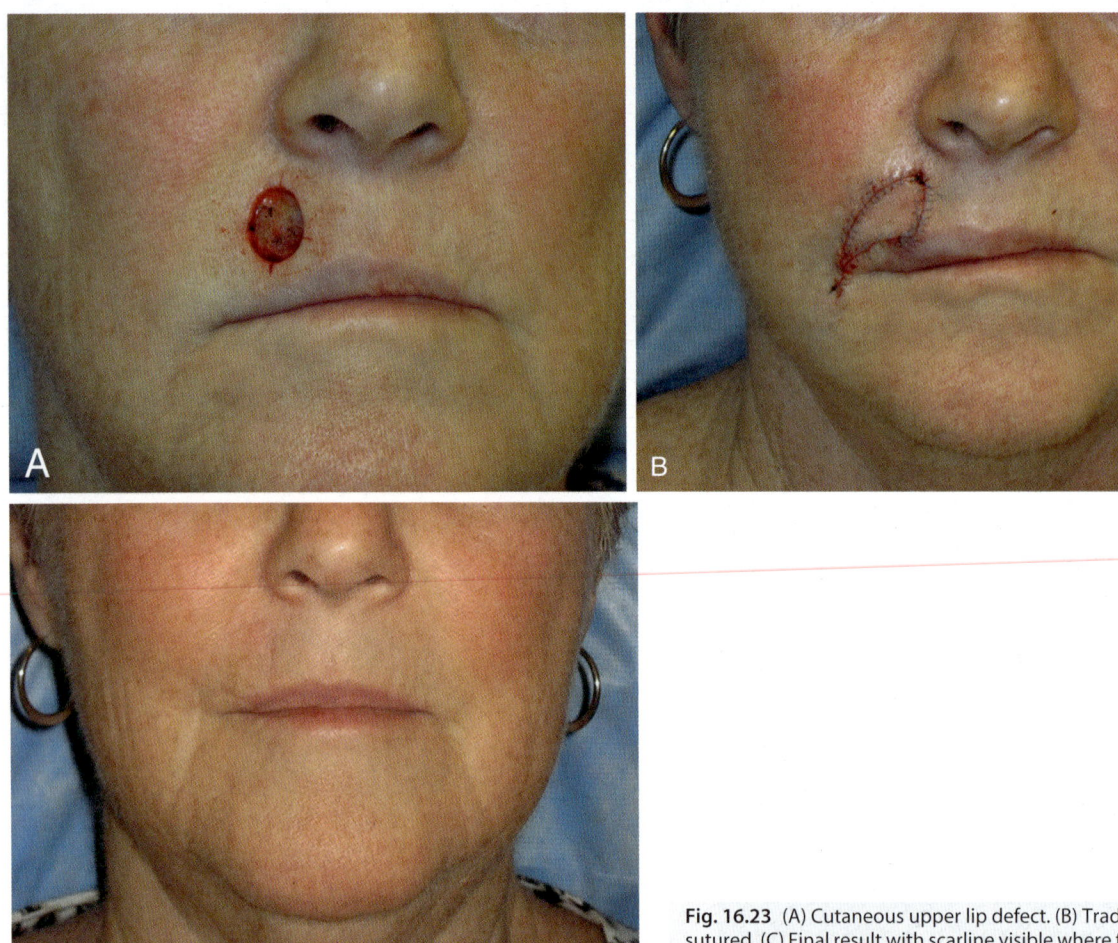

Fig. 16.23 (A) Cutaneous upper lip defect. (B) Traditional V-Y flap sutured. (C) Final result with scarline visible where flap borders do not align with cosmetic junction borders.

dermal and cuticular layers (Fig. 16.23). Crescentic modifications of the V-Y flap may be implemented for smaller defects located near the alar sill (Fig. 16.24). Traditional V-Y flap design is also a reliable method to reconstruct defects located in the apical portion of the upper lip located between the ala, cheek, and lip (Fig. 16.25).

The conventional design of the V-Y advancement flap has a number of limitations. First, one of the horizontal limbs of the flap diagonally transects the RSTLs in the middle of the subunit creating a conspicuous scar (Fig. 16.26). Second, medial advancement of the flap may be restricted because the base of the flap is tethered to the orbicularis oris. Finally, advancement of the flap may displace the lip inferiorly, and bunching of the orbicularis muscle may create a pincushioned appearance.

A modification to the traditional V-Y flap design addresses these challenges. Rather than incise the flap at the defect borders, columnar strips of skin are removed from the defect that extend to the cephalic border (e.g., alar sill) and caudal border (e.g., VCJ) of the subunit. This creates a rectangular defect that allows for flap limbs to be designed precisely in the VCJ and just outside the melolabial fold, so that this junction border is restored when the flap moves medially. This subunit restoration is analogous to that commonly employed in nasal reconstruction.[31] Inferior bulging and restriction of flap movement is obviated by blunt release of the orbicularis muscle at the pars marginalis, sharp release of the flap at the anterior and lateral edges of the flap, and suturing the flap into place with a superomedial vector (Figs. 16.27–16.29).

Full-Thickness Circumoral Flaps

Defects greater than one-fourth the upper lip and one-third the lower lip provide especially unique reconstructive challenges. Traditional wedge repairs and random-based flaps elevated above the muscle risk microstomia or free margin distortion because of an inability to restore tissue volume. Additionally, excessive tension risks ischemia or dehiscence. Full-thickness circumoral flaps address these challenges in three ways. They (1) harness the pliability and vascularity of the orbicularis muscle; (2) recruit sufficient amounts of tissue from the cheek; and (3) properly camouflage incisions along cosmetic junction borders. These flaps also have an advantage over other complex perioral reconstructive designs such as lip switch flaps, because they circumvent the need for suturing the mouth shut for 2 to 3 weeks.

Full-thickness, circumoral flap design originated in the 19th century with von Bruns,[32] and then evolved in the mid-20th century with Gillies and Millard.[33] Karapandzic later refined the flap execution to preserve tissue sensation,

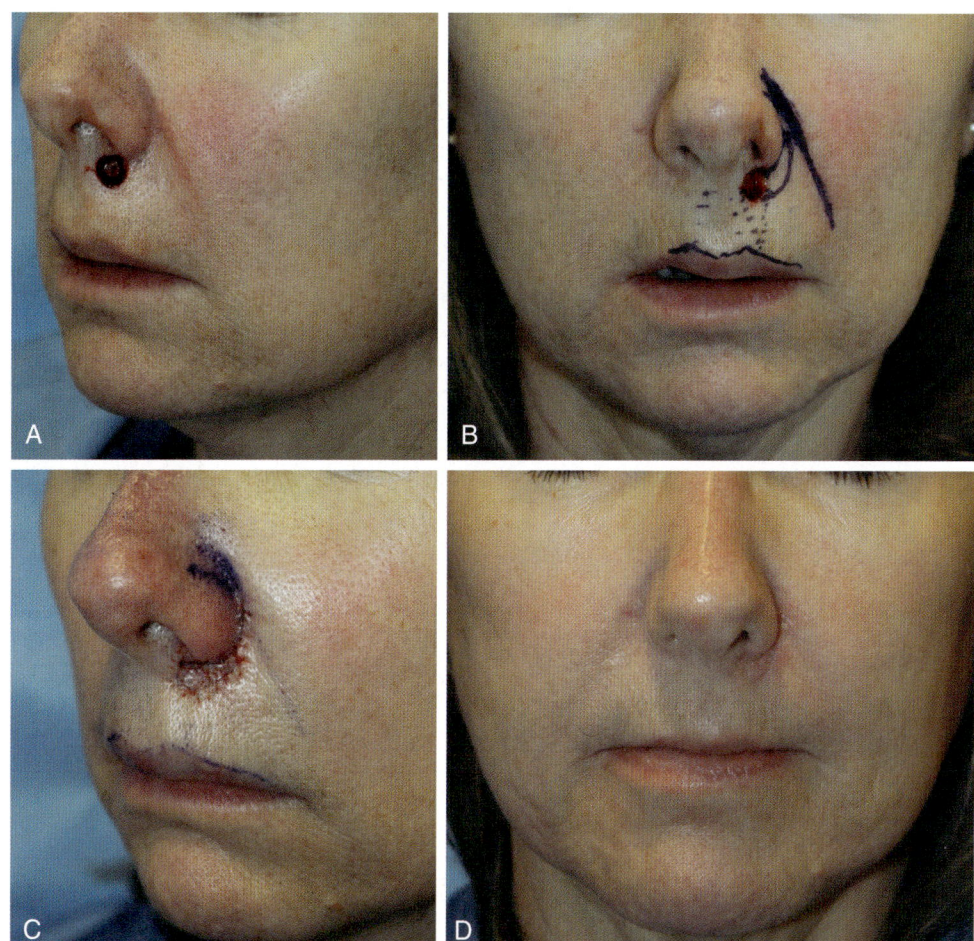

Fig. 16.24 (A) Alar sill defect. (B) Crescentic V-Y flap design. (C) Crescentic V-Y flap sutured. (D) Final result.

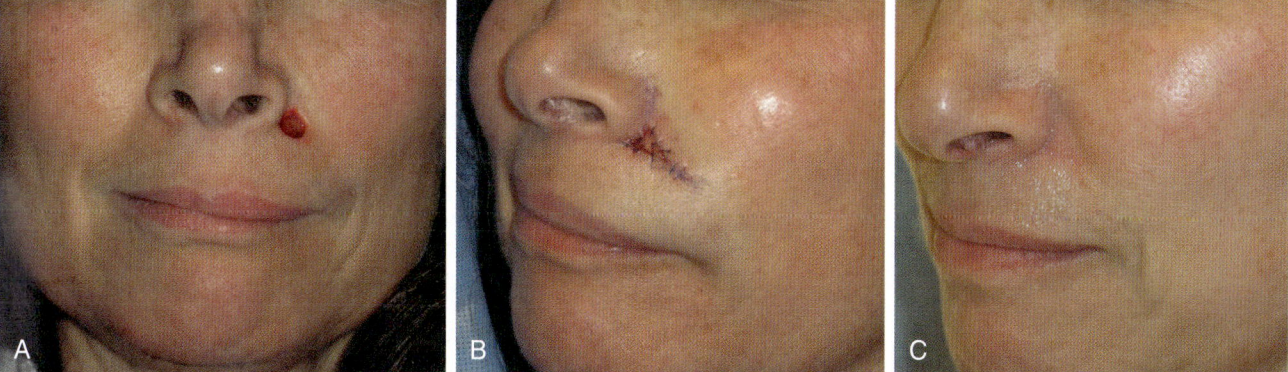

Fig. 16.25 (A) Apical triangle defect. (B) Traditional V-Y flap sutured. (C) Final result.

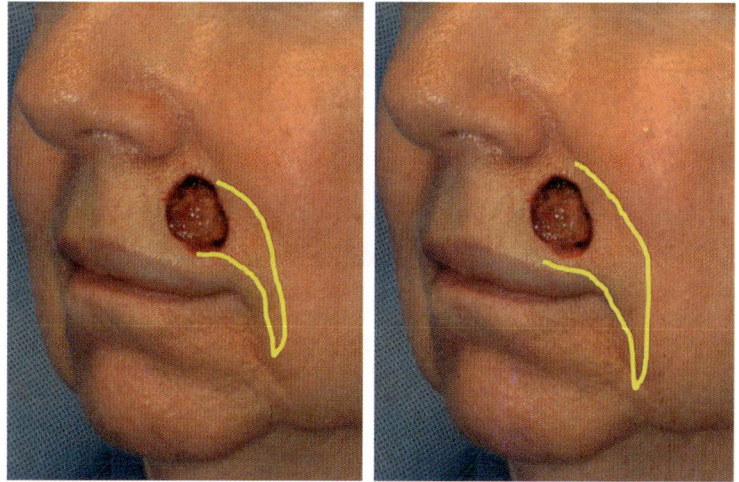

Fig. 16.26 Left side illustrates a traditional V-Y flap design for a lateral subunit defect. The upper and lower incisions are contained within the subunit and perpendicularly cross relaxed skin tension lines. The right side modification camouflages the flap's leading arms to the subunit borders.

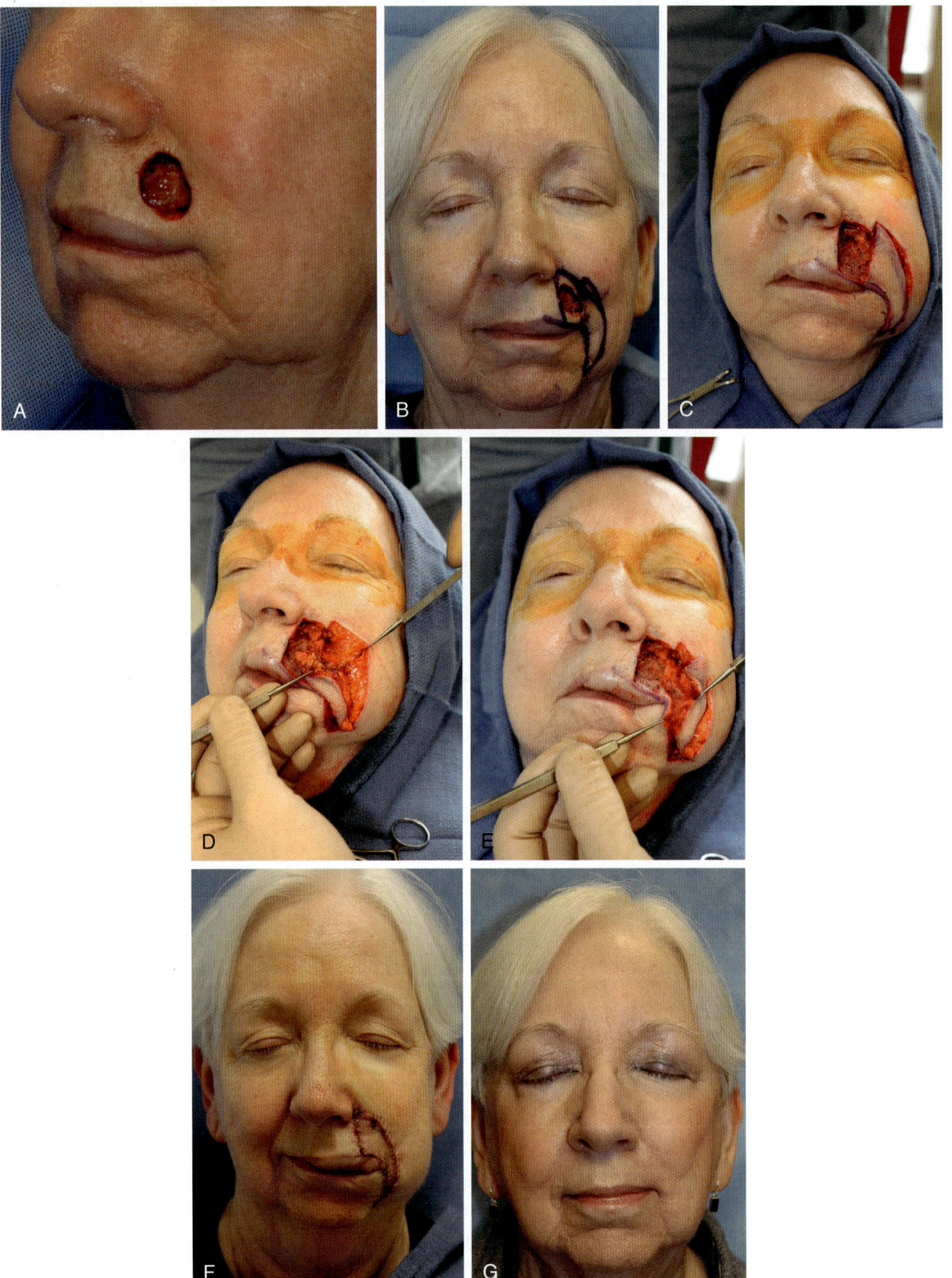

Fig. 16.27 (A) Cutaneous upper lip defect. (B) Subunit V-Y flap design. (C) Subunit V-Y flap incised. Note that a columnar strip of skin has been removed from above and below the defect to allow the flap to adhere to the subunit principle of reconstruction. (D) Subunit V-Y flap elevated in subcutaneous plane. (E) Subunit V-Y flap elevated above muscle prior to releasing incisions through orbicularis muscle. (F) Subunit V-Y flap sutured in place. (G) Final result with scarlines less visible within cosmetic junction borders.

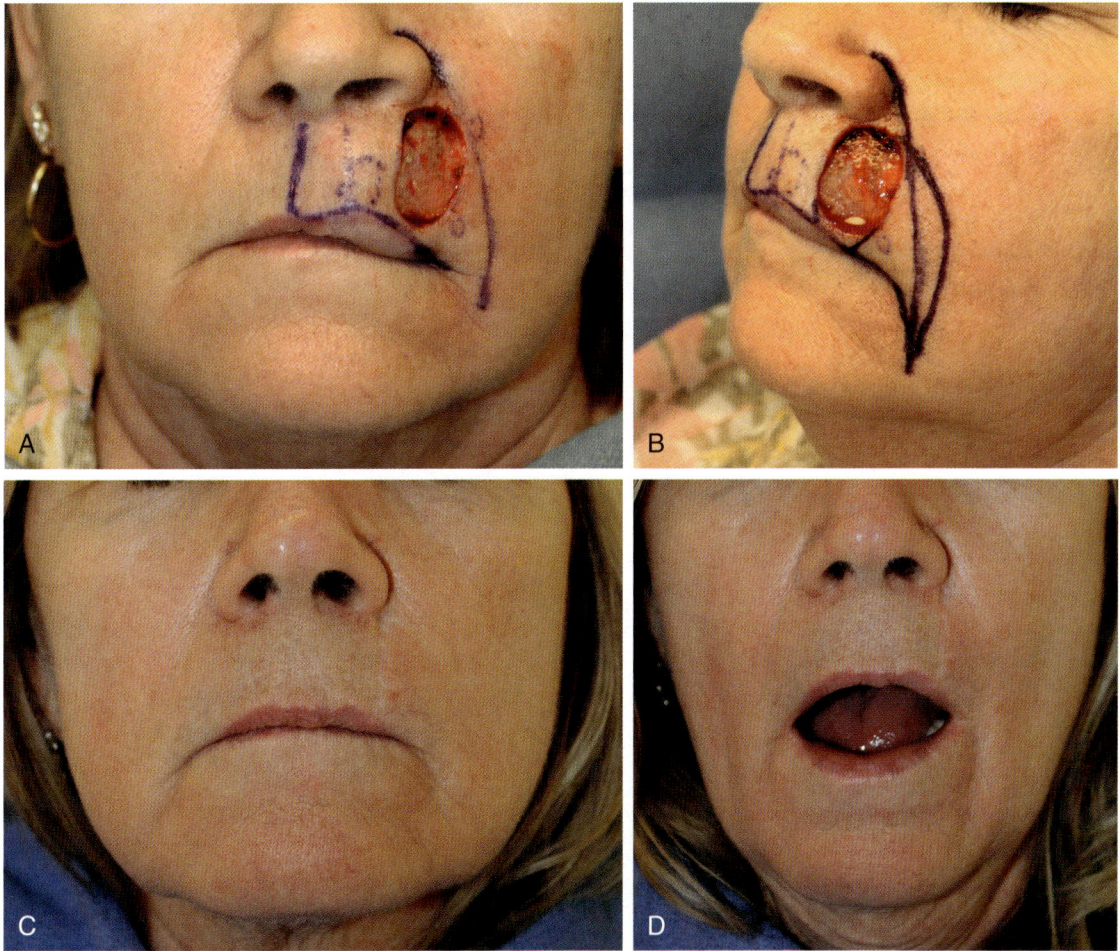

Fig. 16.28 (A) Cutaneous upper lip defect. (B) Subunit V-Y flap design. (C, D) Final result.

motor function, and oral competence.[34] Large upper or lower lip defects that extend substantially into or through orbicularis muscle are ideally reconstructed with a circumoral flap. The pliability of the lip allows for most closures to be designed unilaterally, but bilateral flaps may be used if excessive tension is anticipated with single-arm design. Contralaterally based flaps for paramedian or laterally located defects allow for better restoration of the lip anatomy.[35]

Flap execution begins with composite wedge resection of skin from the base of the defect to the subunit border (e.g., mental crease for lower lip, alar sill for upper lip). An incision through the skin into the subcutaneous tissue of the flap or flaps is carried from the subunit border into the melolabial fold. In order to maintain uniform lip height as the tissue advances and rotates into position, the flap incision should be carried outside of the fold, then mimicking its curvature. A back-cut to facilitate movement may be created in the melolabial fold at the proximal portion of the flap.

Once hemostasis has been achieved, the flap may be further mobilized with dissection of muscle fibers while still preserving the neural and vascular structures. What is most important is that the modiolus and buccinator muscle are not severed in order to preserve oral competence and dynamic expression. Thus full-thickness incision from the defect to the depressor anguli oris (for lower lip defects) or levator labii superioris (for upper lip defects) will allow for release of enough tissue to close almost any-sized lip defect while still allowing for the lip elevators and lip depressors to remain intact. Horizontal incisions in the subunit border up to the commissural area that preserve mucosa can be made to mobilize the flap, and full-thickness incision through mucosa may be reserved for instances where additional flap movement is required. Sensory nerve transection will produce anesthesia that improves over time. Similar to the wedge repair, the three tissue components (mucosa, muscle, skin) must be sutured in four layers, starting with the innermost layer first, and alignment of the VCJ is essential for aesthetic success (Figs. 16.30 and 16.31).

TRANSPOSITION FLAPS

While most perioral defects can be repaired with primary closures, wedge repairs, and sliding flaps, some defects are amenable to closure with lifting flaps such as the rhombic and bilobed flaps. The two main reasons to select a transposition design for the perioral area are to recruit extra tissue for closure of a larger defect and to change the tension vector of repair for preservation of free margin position.[36] The cheek provides the reservoir of skin for the upper lip

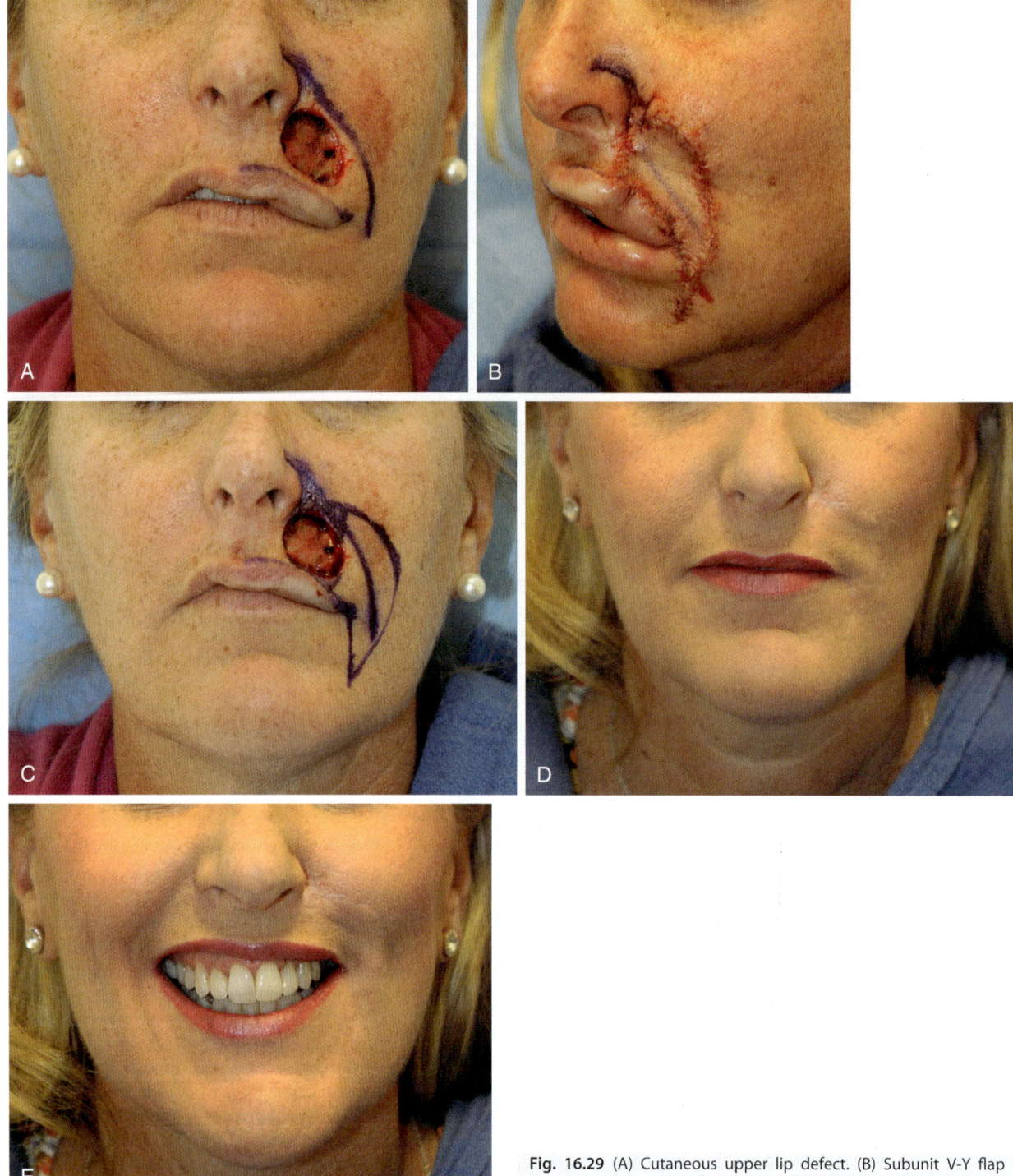

Fig. 16.29 (A) Cutaneous upper lip defect. (B) Subunit V-Y flap design. (C) Subunit V-Y flap sutured. (D, E) Final result.

and the cheek, submentum, and neck provide reservoirs of tissue for lower lip and chin reconstruction.

The rhombic flap is the commonly employed repair for facial defects, but its use in the perioral area is limited because it often requires movement of tissue over cosmetic borders that may leave pincushioning and broken line scars that rarely align with RSTLs and cosmetic junction boundaries. Although the rhombic flap has many nuances and variations to its design, perhaps the simplest conceptualization is to compare it to a musical note.[10] For laterally located defects, the leading limb of the flap is placed within or parallel to the melolabial fold with the width of the flap matching the height of the defect (Fig. 16.32). Flap design may need to extend onto the cheek to create a sufficient vascular pedicle and to avoid displacement of the commissure (Fig. 16.33). Rhombic flaps are elevated in the subcutaneous plane and are first closed by realigning the secondary defect. This pushes the flap toward the primary defect and

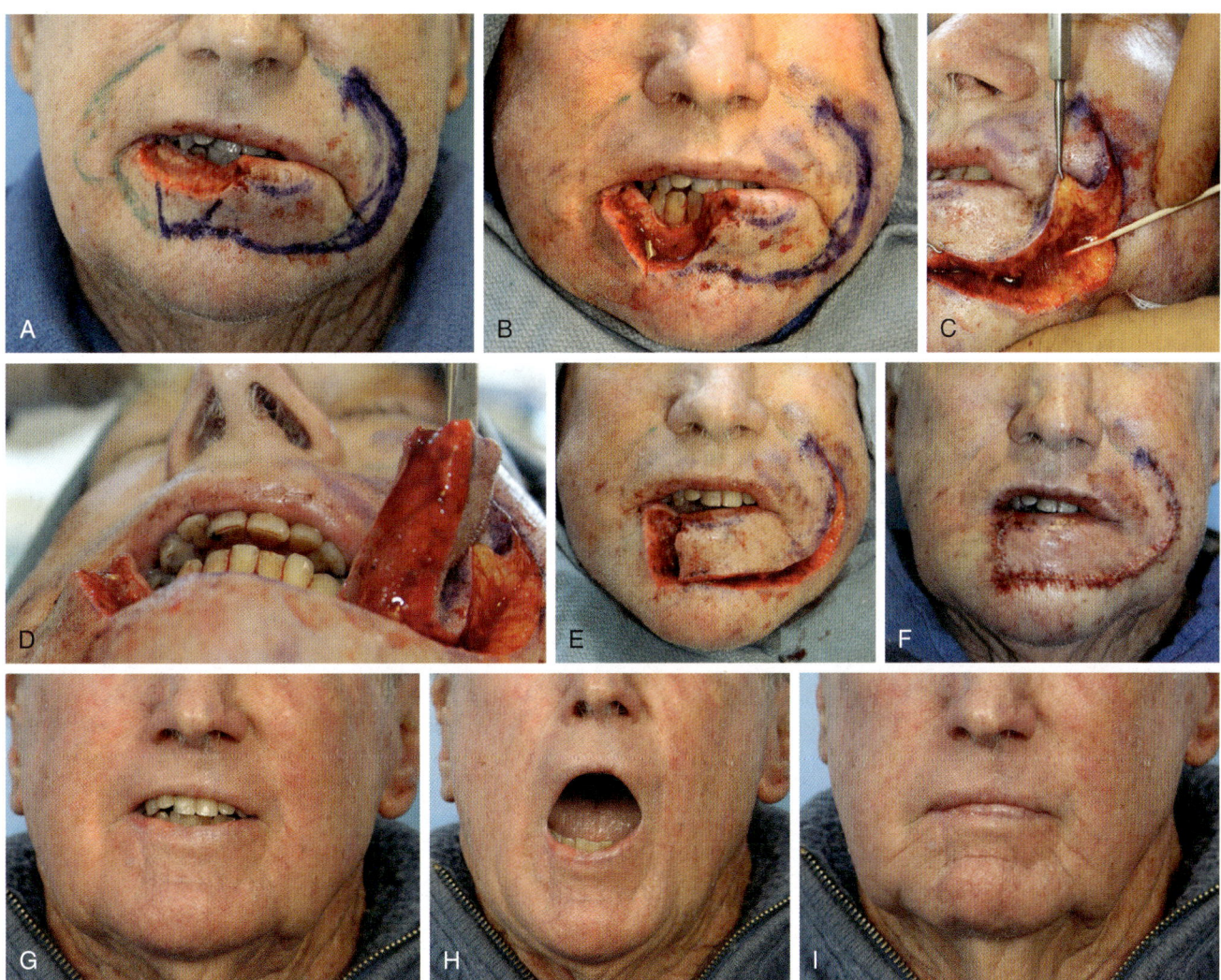

Fig. 16.30 (A) Full-thickness lower lip defect. (B) Defect extended to subunit border. (C) Circumoral flap incised through the skin, cotton tip applicator pointing toward depressor anguli oris muscle (DAO). (D) Full-thickness release of tissue to the DAO. (E) Flap approximated and mucosal layer sutured. (F) Flap fully sutured. (G–I) Final result.

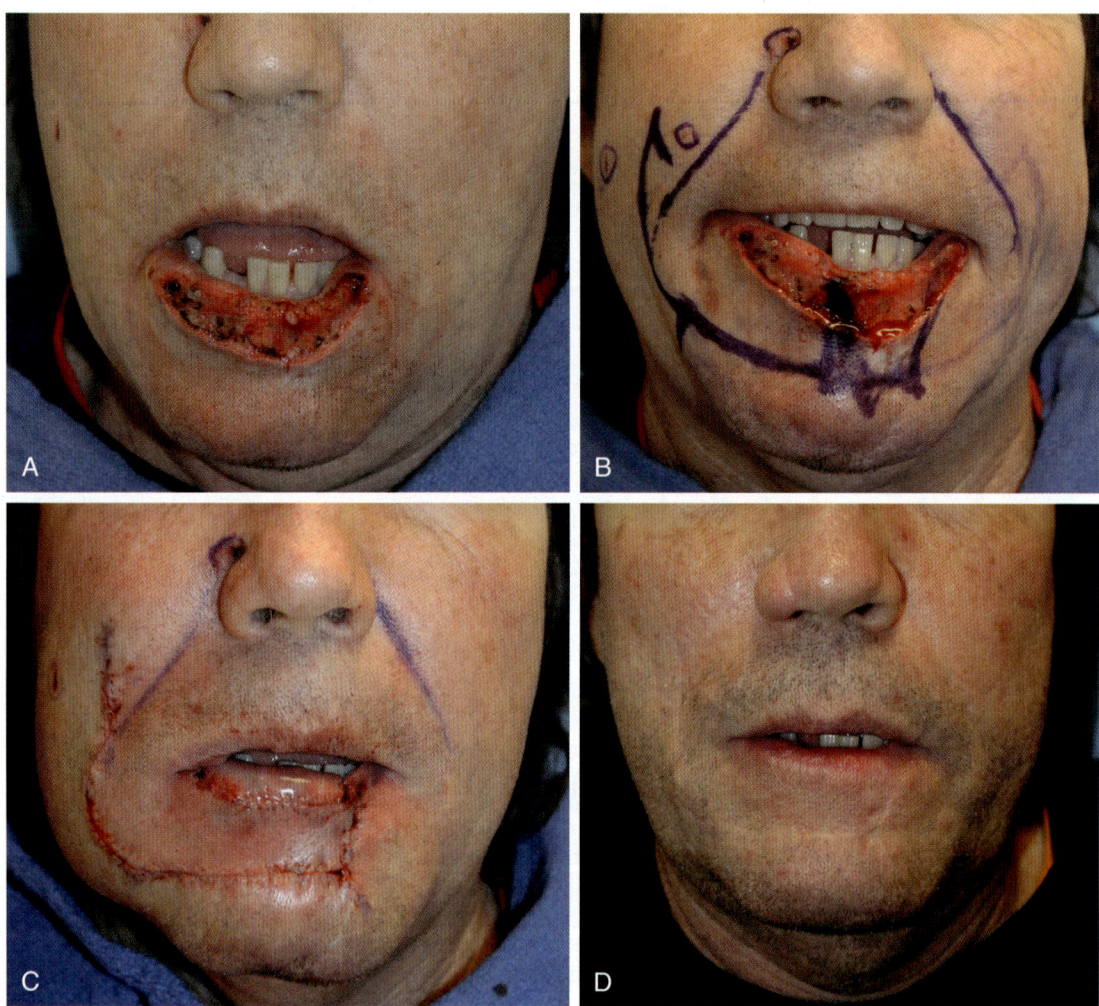

Fig. 16.31 (A) Full-thickness lower lip defect. (B) Unilateral circumoral flap design. (C) Flap sutured. (D) Final result.

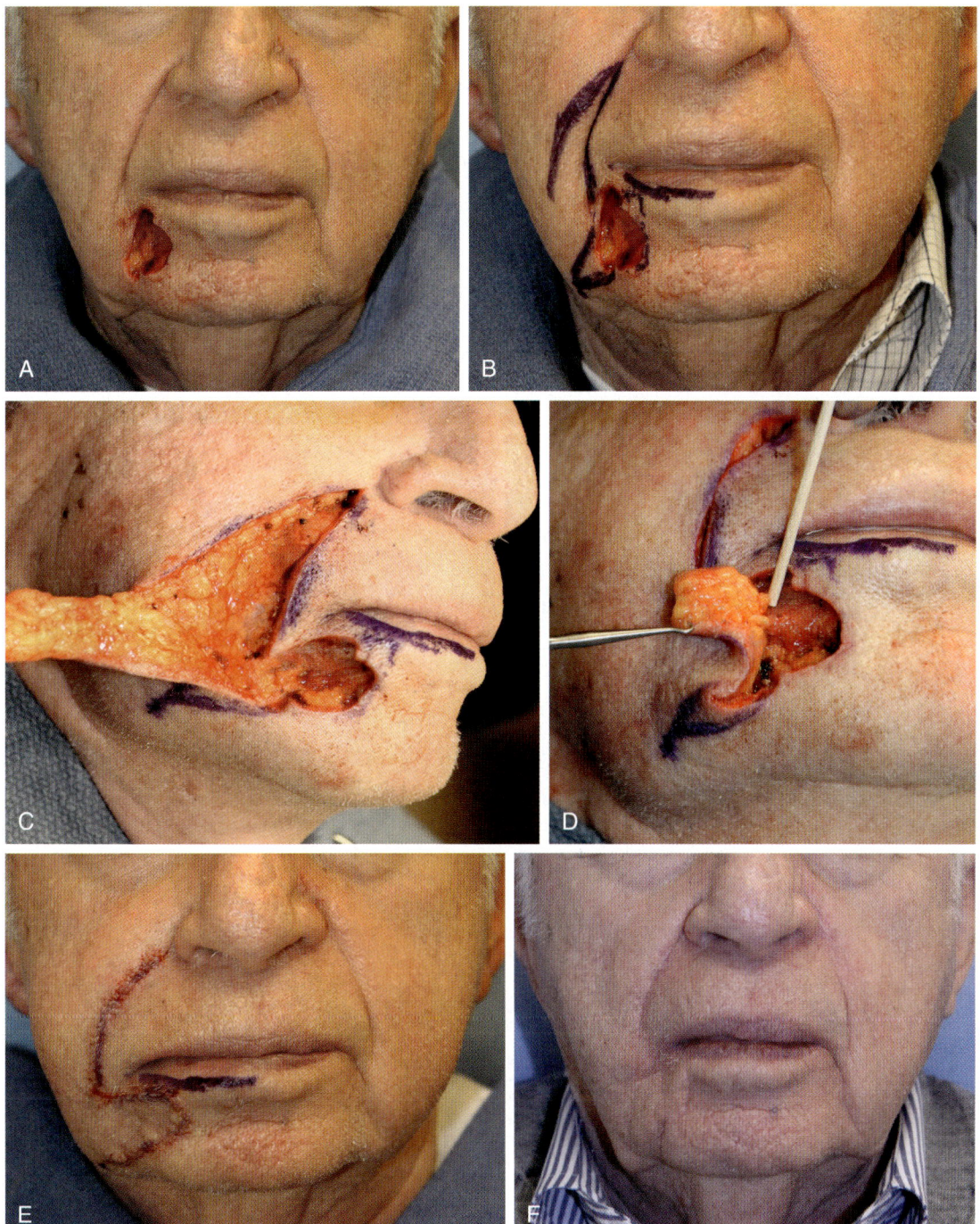

Fig. 16.32 (A) Cutaneous lower lip defect. (B) Inferiorly based rhombic flap design. (C) Flap elevated above lip elevator and depressor muscles. (D) Tacking suture in place. (E) Flap sutured. (F) Final result.

minimizes closure tension. Tacking sutures can be placed below the flap to further ensure correct free margin position and to minimize flap pincushioning.

A modification to the traditional rhombic flap allows for recreation of the upper cutaneous subunit with placement of scarlines within RSTLs and cosmetic junction lines (Fig. 16.34). Originally described by Burget and Hsiao[37] as a rotation flap, its motion may be better considered a subunit transposition of cheek skin onto the lip. A template of the upper lip is placed on the cheek off of the superolateral portion of the defect and the remaining skin of the ipsilateral lip subunit is removed. The flap is elevated above the SMAS with its blood supply based on the facial artery, superior labial artery, or angular artery.[38] Flap movement, as with traditional rhombic flaps, is facilitated by first closing the secondary defect. This may require wide undermining of the cheek, and thorough hemostasis is advised prior to suturing the flap into place under minimal tension.

Single-limb transposition flaps fail to deliver sufficient tissue for large upper and lower lip defects, particularly ones

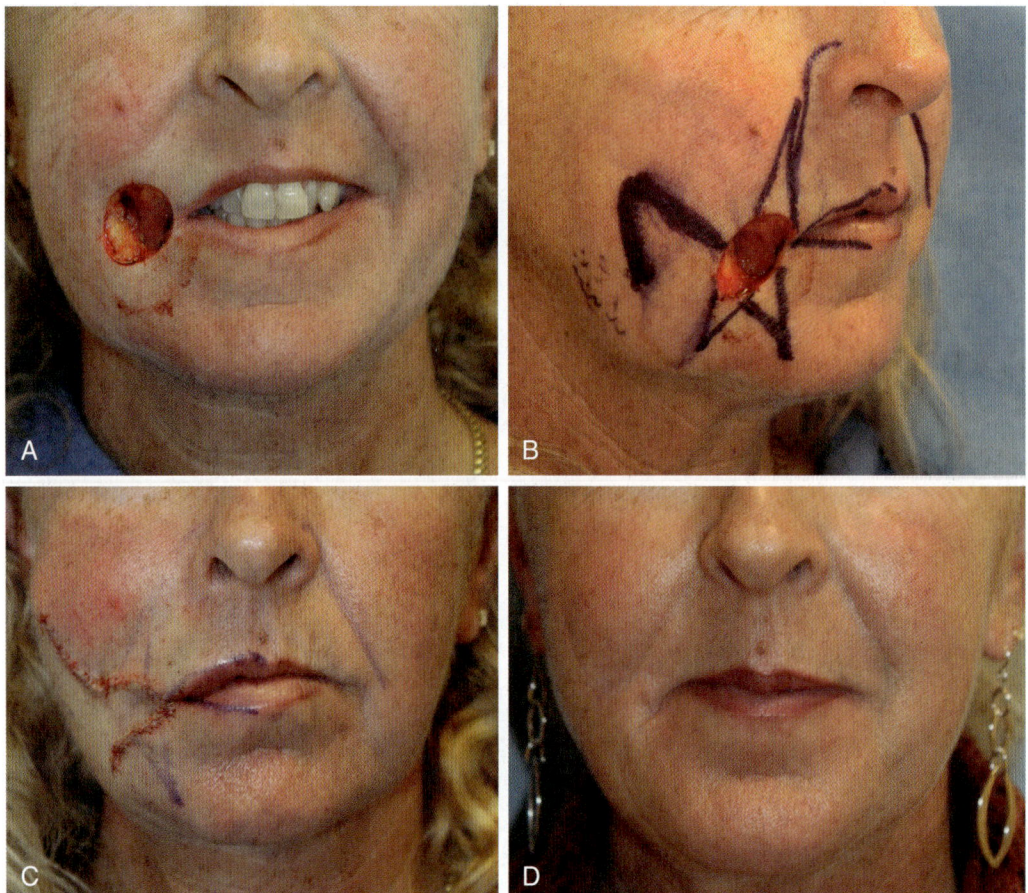

Fig. 16.33 (A) Lip commissure-cheek defect. (B) Rhombic flap design avoids commissure displacement that would likely occur with linear closure. (C) Flap sutured. (D) Final result revealing visible angulated scar but preserved free margin. Patient declined scar revision.

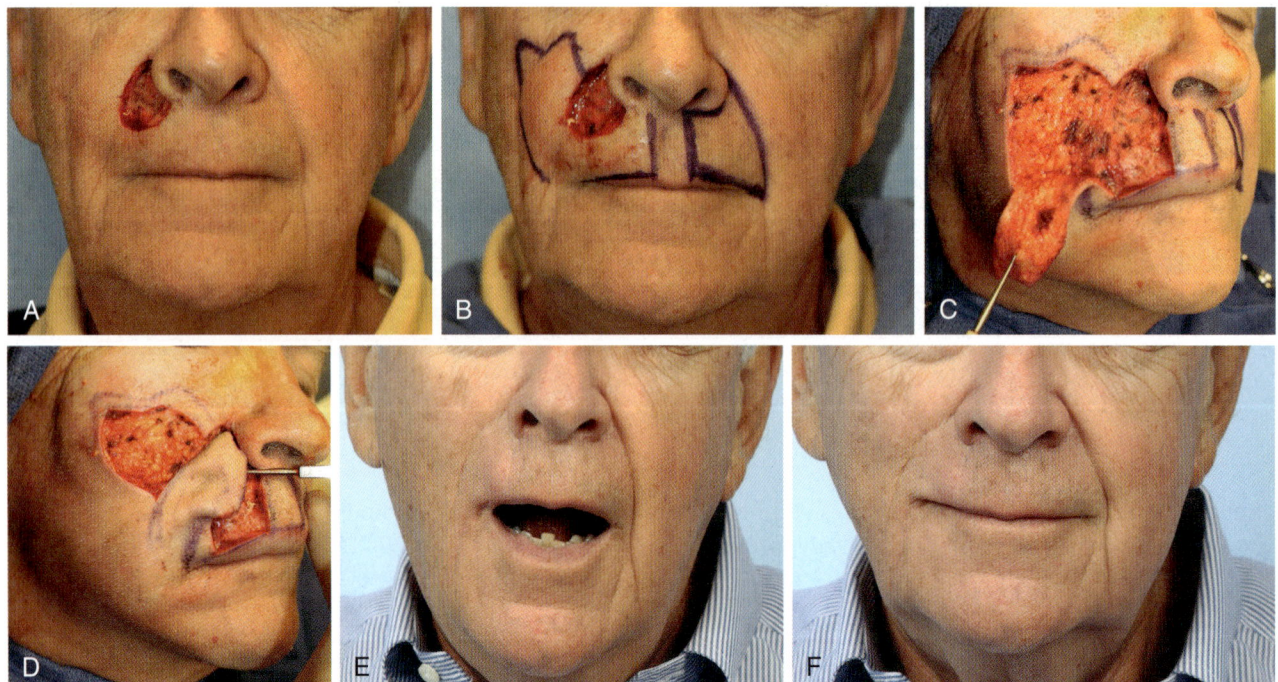

Fig. 16.34 (A) Defect spanning lip and cheek. (B) Subunit flap design. (C) Flap elevated above muscle and melolabial fat pad. (D) Flap being moved toward primary defect, and revealing large secondary defect that must be closed. (E, F) Final result with lip position preserved but notable melolabial fold asymmetry.

that span multiple cosmetic units. In such instances, bilobed flaps may be used (Fig. 16.35). When mobilized, the leading edge of the flap meets the philtrum and VCJ, while the triangular junction of the primary and secondary lobes helps recreate the melolabial fold. Tacking sutures placed at the zygoma minimize ectropion risk, and suturing the tertiary defect along the zygomatic cheek displaces tension away from the lip. For patients with concomitant alar deficits, this flap provides a stable platform for future alar recreation.[39] Bilobed flap reconstruction also eliminates the risk of microstomia that may be observed with other repairs such as the lip switch flap. Lower lip and chin bilobed flaps are executed in the same manner with the submentum and neck, providing the reservoir of skin (Fig. 16.36).

Rhombic and bilobed flaps come with inherent disadvantages. First, transferring skin between subunits can produce pincushioning of the flap and fullness of skin at the commissure. Second, unless the flap is delivered to subunit borders, scarlines can be conspicuous. Finally, melolabial fold displacement or ablation can happen despite precise

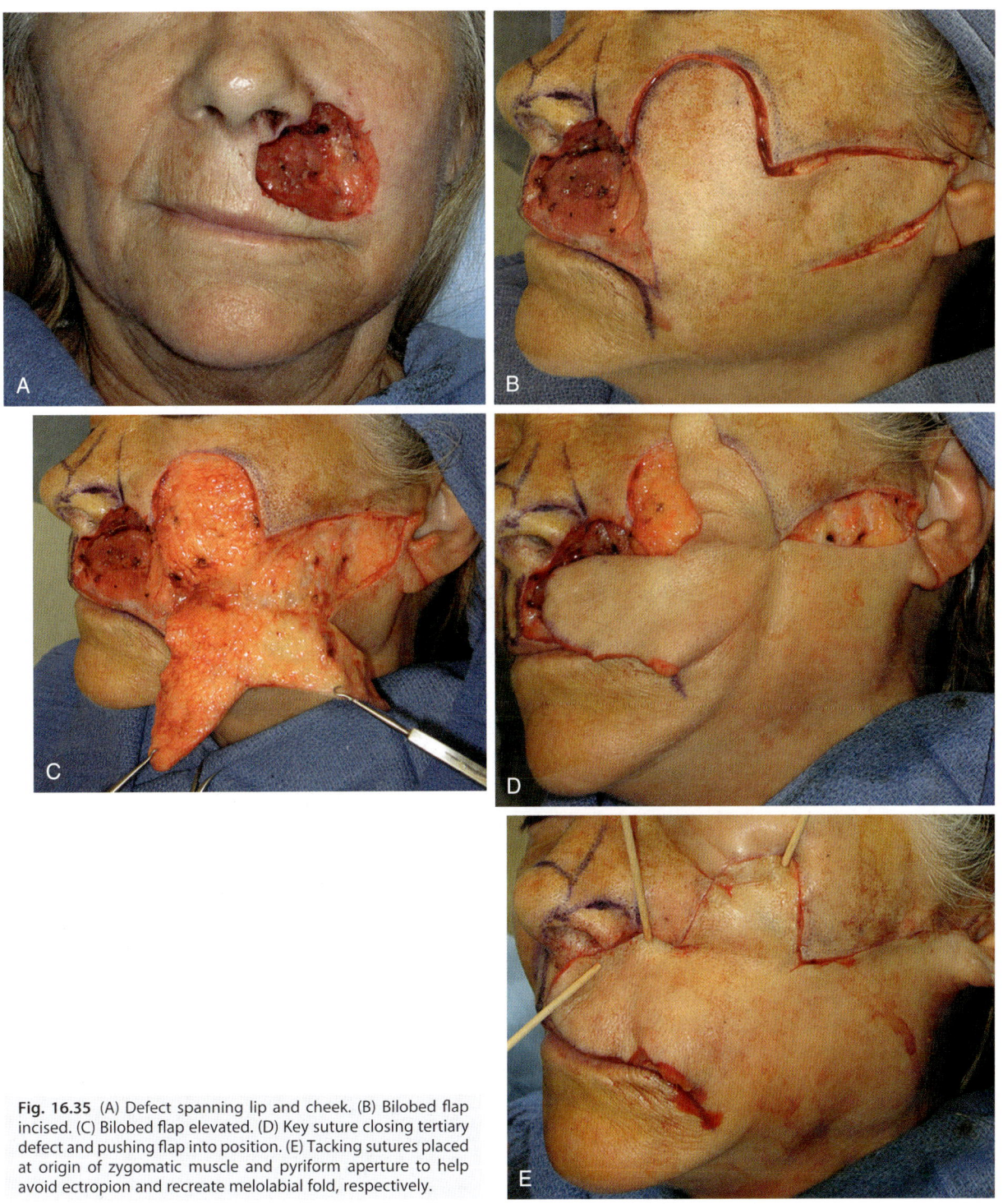

Fig. 16.35 (A) Defect spanning lip and cheek. (B) Bilobed flap incised. (C) Bilobed flap elevated. (D) Key suture closing tertiary defect and pushing flap into position. (E) Tacking sutures placed at origin of zygomatic muscle and pyriform aperture to help avoid ectropion and recreate melolabial fold, respectively.

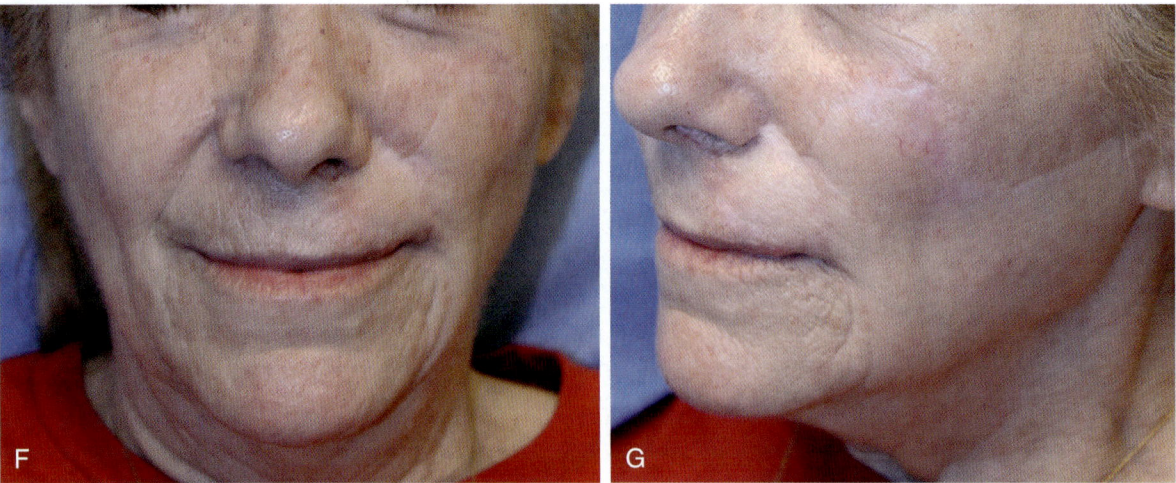

Fig. 16.35, cont'd (F, G) Final result.

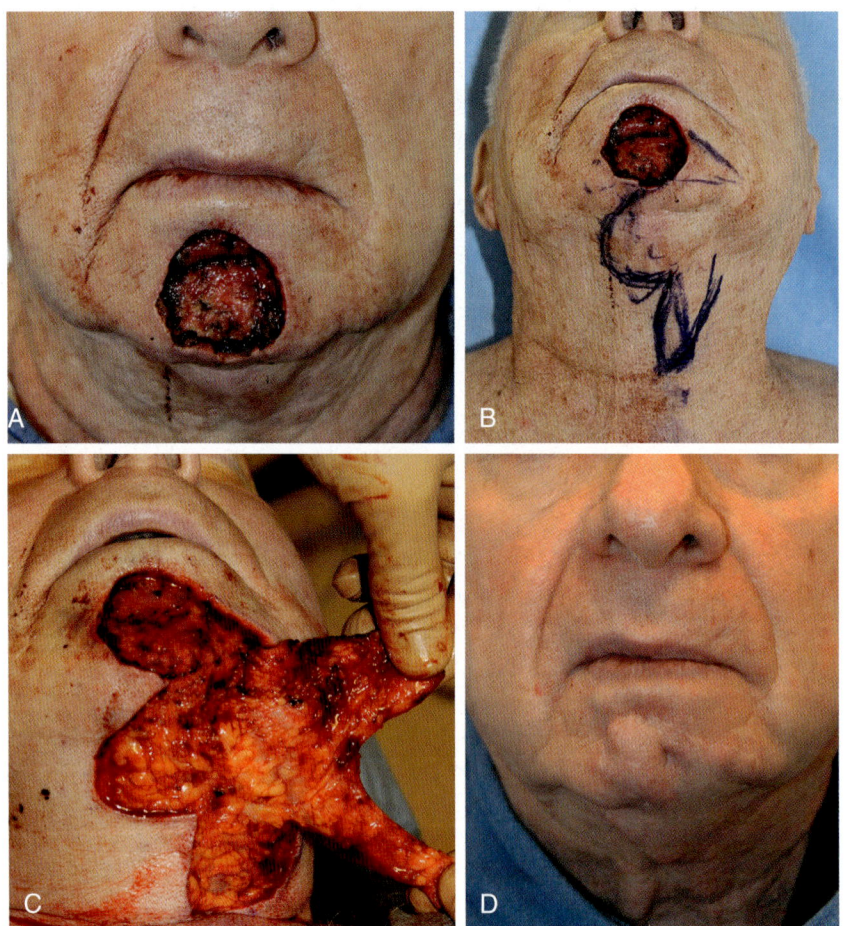

Fig. 16.36 (A) Chin defect. (B) Bilobed flap design. (C) Bilobed flap elevated. (D) Final result (tacking suture has resulted in prolonged dimpling).

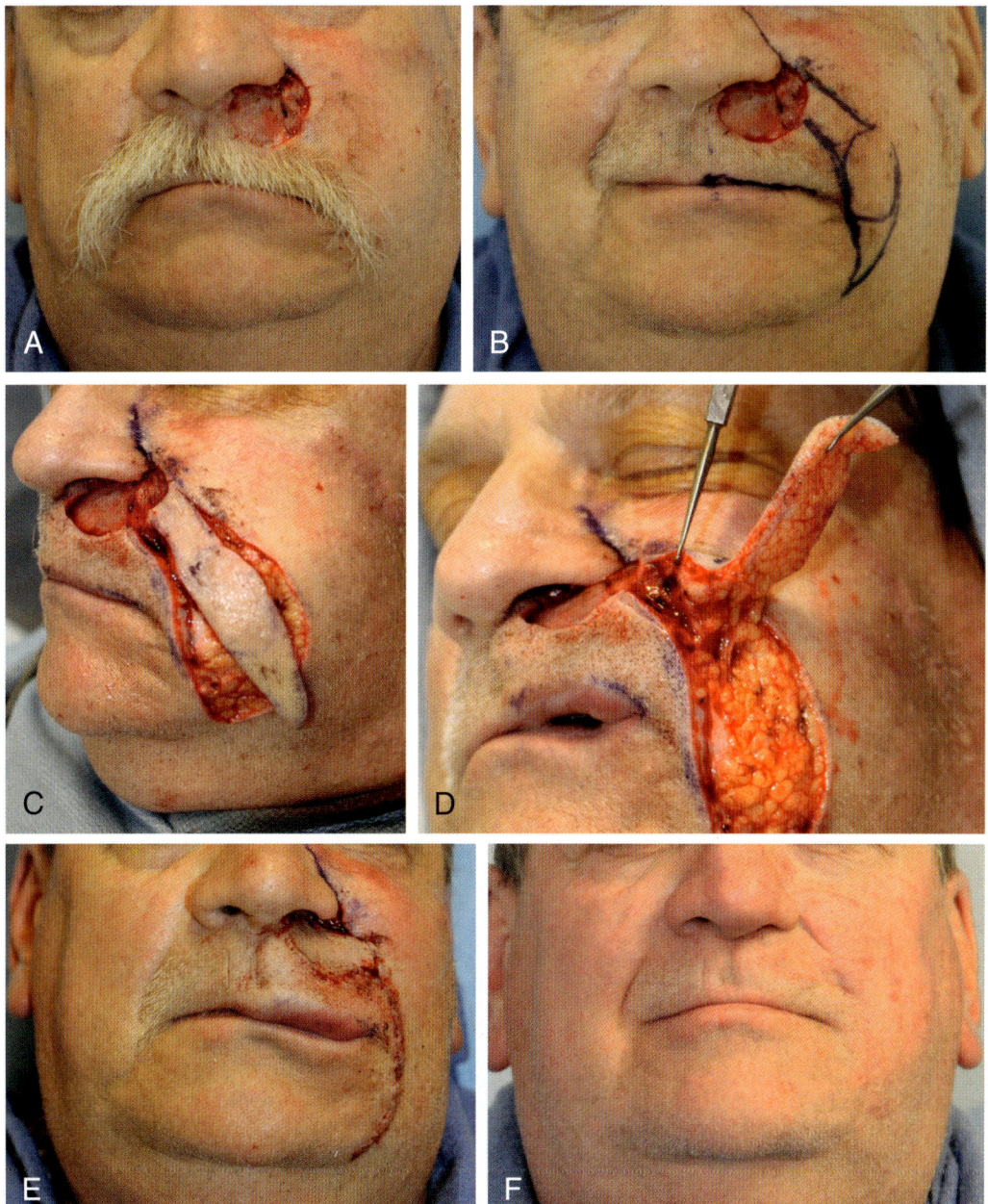

Fig. 16.37 (A) Alar sill-apical triangle defect. (B) Tunneled and transposed flap design. (C) Flap incised to subcutaneous fat. (D) Flap elevated above lip elevator muscles. (E) Flap sutured. (F) Final result.

tacking sutures. Because of these downsides, patients warrant counseling that transposition flap reconstruction may necessitate a subsequent revision for flap thinning and/or cosmetic border recreation.

Tunneling tissue provides another modification to the transposition flap that allows for delivery of distant, similar-appearing tissue. Lifting tissue and tucking it underneath cosmetic borders helps reduce displacement of the ipsilateral melolabial fold observed with other laterally based transposition flaps from the cheek.[40,41] Design, incision, and elevation of a tunneled flap for an upper cutaneous lip defect are analogous to that of a melolabial interpolation flap (Fig. 16.37). Prior to transposition and suturing the flap, skin proximal to the template is de-epithelialized.

Trapdoor deformation may be obviated with undersizing the flap.

Lip Switch Flap

Large lip defects can have trilaminar tissue restored with cross-lip flaps. These flaps have a robust axial blood supply based on the labial artery, and allow for sensory and motor nerve preservation. The ideal defect for a lip switch flap is deep-partial thickness or full-thickness and spans greater than one-third the width of the upper lip or half the width of the lower lip. Although each lip may be used to repair the contralateral side, use of the upper lip skin as a donor site should be restricted for lower lip defects that have few alternative means of reconstruction, because this risks alteration of the upper lip's delicate surface anatomy. Lip switch flaps that repair midline, paramedian, and laterally based defects are interpolated. These are often referred to as Abbe flaps[42] and require a second procedure to separate the lips (Fig. 16.38). Commissural defects repaired by switching lips are referred to as Estlander flaps.[43] Commissural lip switch flaps do not require a take-down procedure but frequently benefit from delayed commissuroplasty for aesthetic and functional improvement.

Correct sizing of the flap facilitates success. Elastic recoil of tissue creates an illusion of a larger defect when skin is resected for tumor clearance. This splaying is further exacerbated with tumescence from local anesthesia. Designing lip switch flaps to 50% to 75% the width of the defect accounts for this tissue effect, minimizes the donor site morbidity, and maintains balance between both lips. As with many other lip repairs, the VCJ must be clearly marked, and the vertical height of the upper lip defects is best extended to the alar sill, columella, and melolabial fold, while lower lip defects should be extended to the mental crease. Central lip defects may have a lateral or medial-based pedicle, and lateral defects should have a medial-based pedicle. The flap pedicle should be designed at the mid position of the defect so that it aligns with one end of the defect when the flap is transposed and donor site closed.[35] Nerve blocks are a helpful tool to minimize tissue swelling.

Once the defect has been squared off to the subunit border, the flap is incised through the epidermis, dermis, and fat circumferentially. Isolation of the labial arteries bordering the flap may be performed by blunt dissection through the muscle on each side. Use of tenotomy scissors to gently lift and individually spread orbicularis fibers is a helpful technique to isolate and visualize the vessels. Once the side of the pedicle is decided upon, the nonpedicle side has the labial artery ligated and is incised through the muscle and mucosa. The pedicled side of the flap is meticulously incised through the muscle in order to preserve the feeding labial artery. Release of tissue should preserve 1 cm of muscle and mucosa in order to avoid venous congestion. Hemostasis is carefully performed with indirect electrocoagulation, and the donor site is repaired in typical four-layered fashion. The flap then rotates 180 degrees and is also sutured into the defect four-layered fashion. Realignment of the upper and lower VCJ is essential for aesthetic success.

The patient is prescribed antibiotics, antiemetics, and analgesics in liquid form for the early postoperative period.

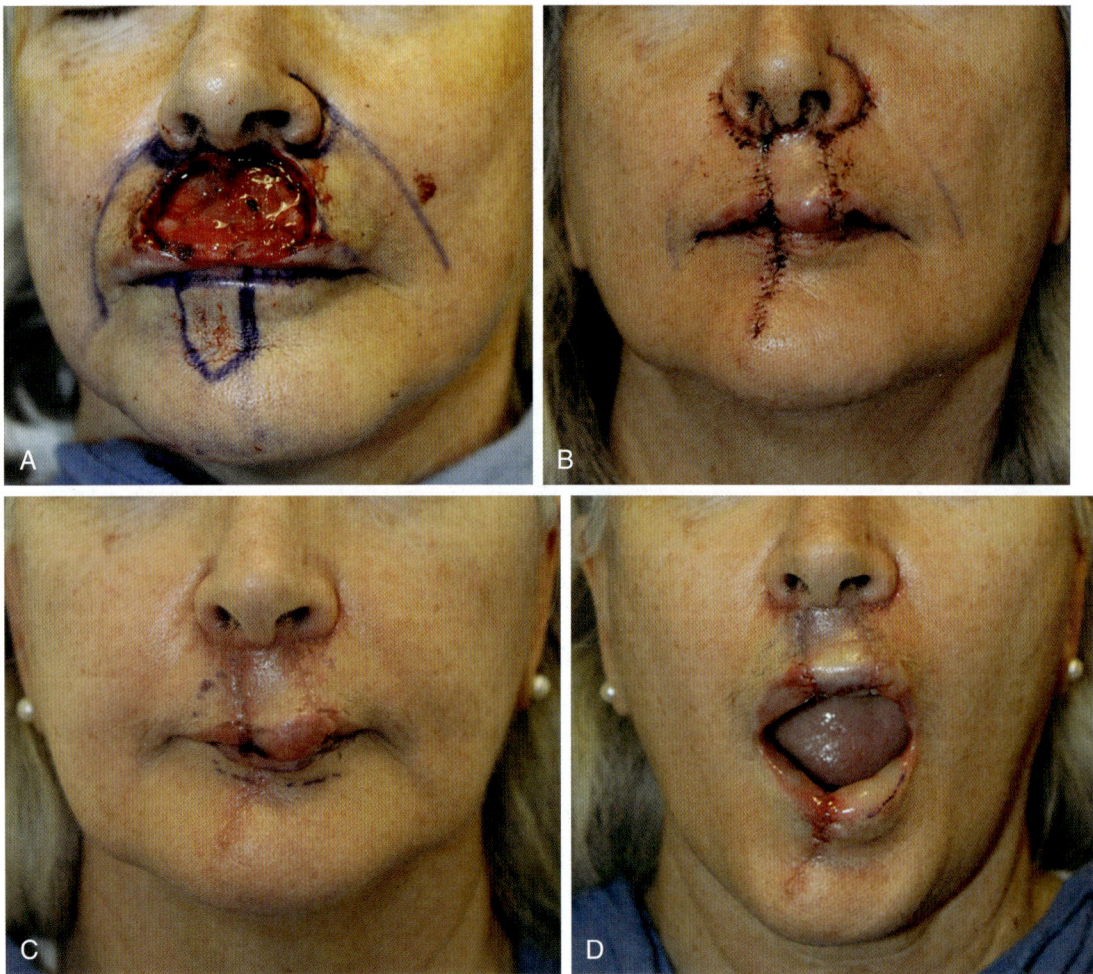

Fig. 16.38 (A) Defect of upper lip spanning philtrum and upper cutaneous subunits. (B) Lip switch flap sutured. (C) 3 weeks postoperative. (D) Lip switch flap divided and sutured.

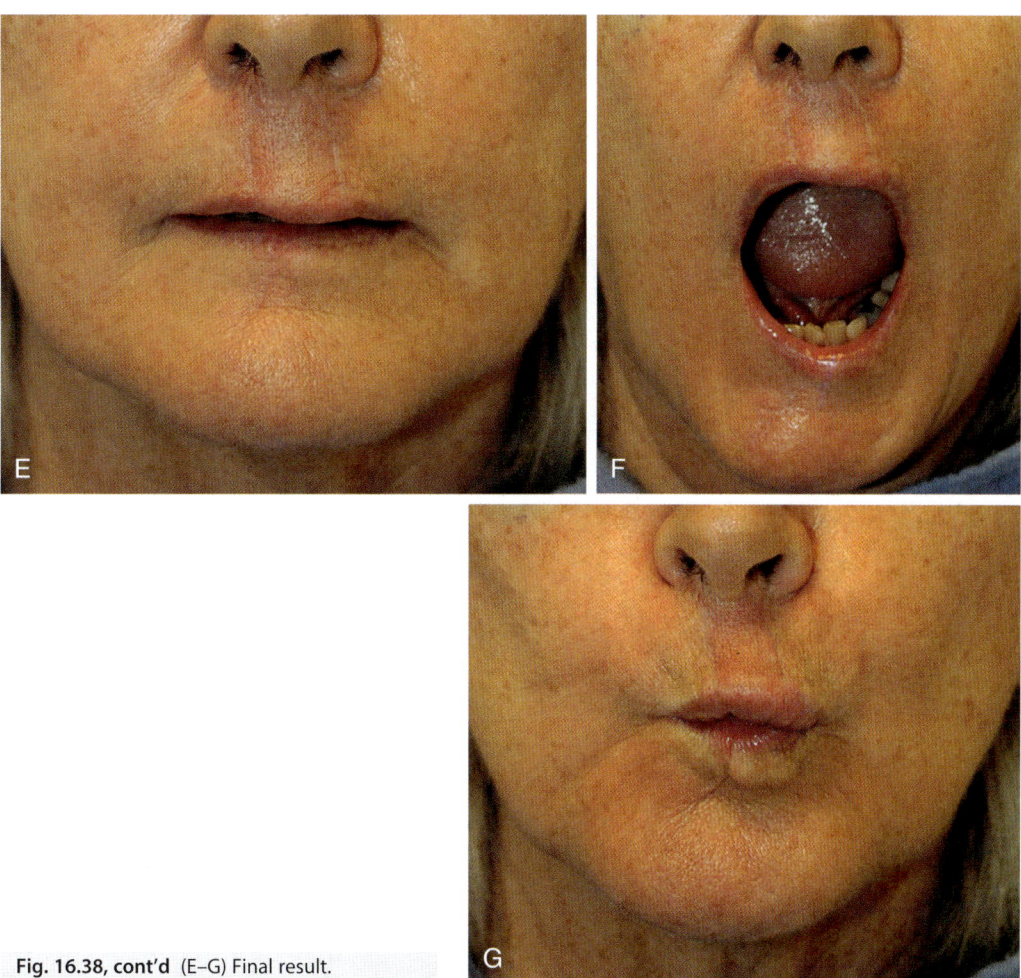

Fig. 16.38, cont'd (E–G) Final result.

Diligent counseling on a soft food and liquid diet helps ease the challenge oral aperture restriction. Division of the flap is performed 3 weeks from the time of inset. Patients should expect to have an edematous, pincushioned appearance that can take months to improve. Although permanent anesthesia is possible, patients usually regain pain sensation within a couple of months, and then tactile and temperature sensation in the months to follow.[44]

PHILTRAL RECONSTRUCTION

The philtral subunit is a highly visible area that warrants a dedicated section of discussion. It is uniquely positioned in the center of the upper lip with a concave body bounded by convex philtral columns laterally, Cupid's bow inferiorly, and columella superiorly. Although ascending philtral arteries perfuse the lateral aspect of this subunit,[16] the blood supply and reservoirs of available skin for reconstruction are limited compared with other parts of the perioral region. Furthermore, restoration of Cupid's bow, an anterior projection of pars marginalis and decussation of orbicularis oris fibers,[45,46] is particularly challenging because of its intricate three-dimensional contour.

Primary closure of small defects contained within the philtral subunit is possible if the caudal margin of the closure does not extend past the VCJ to eliminate Cupid's bow. This may be aided with the use of an M-plasty caudally. As noted earlier, central mucosal defects may be repaired with a gull wing design to restore the Cupid's bow.[20] If LC risks ablation of Cupid's bow, then an alternative repair option should be selected.

The V-Y advancement flap is a workhorse repair for defects less than 50% of the philtral height and up to 1.5 times the width of the philtrum.[47] Depending upon the location and size, flaps may be designed from cutaneous skin above (Fig. 16.39), mucosal skin below, or have both flaps meet to recreate the VCJ.[48] Flap design may need to extend onto the columella to recruit sufficient tissue and the lateral arms of the flap should align with the philtral columns in order for the scarline to camouflage properly. Movement of the flap is often restricted because of the muscular attachments, but undermining should be performed cautiously so as to not induce ischemia.

Larger philtral defects, particularly deep partial thickness and full-thickness defects, require donation of skin laterally or from the lower lip. If the width of a full-thickness defect is restricted to the central portion of the upper lip, then a lip switch flap may be the most appropriate repair, as it can restore the subunit's natural cosmetic borders (see Fig. 16.38). Larger philtral defects may also be repaired with use of Webster crescentic perialar excision[49] or nasolabial flaps that transpose-advance flaps bilaterally (Fig. 16.40).[50]

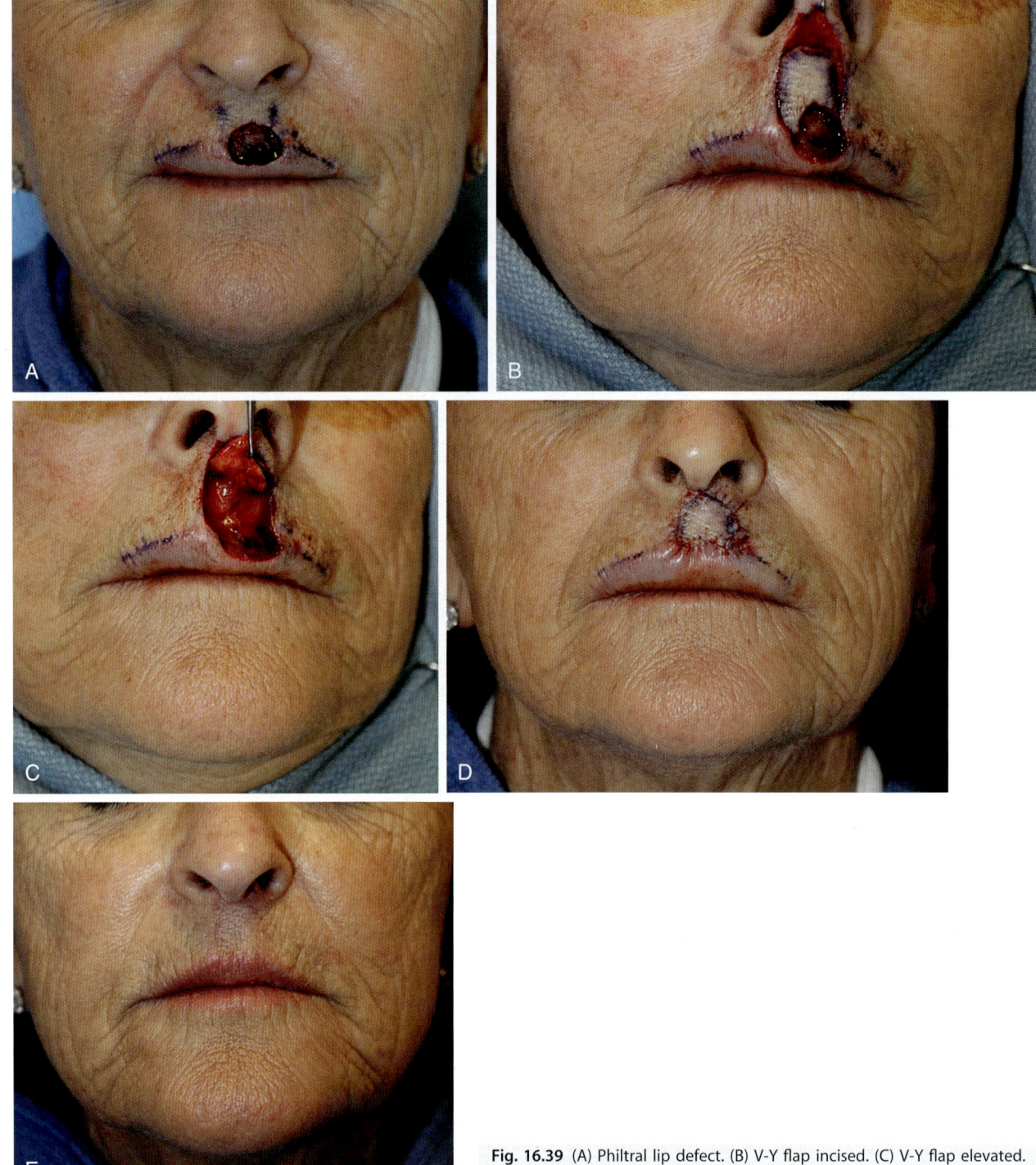

Fig. 16.39 (A) Philtral lip defect. (B) V-Y flap incised. (C) V-Y flap elevated. (D) Flap sutured. (E) Final result.

Upper lip flattening is an anticipated outcome of these latter repairs.

Summary

Detailed knowledge of lip anatomy, flap design, and tissue biomechanics permit the dermatologic surgeon to achieve desirable functional and aesthetic results for perioral defects. Many lip defects heal well with second intention, LCs, or wedge repairs. Larger defects and those that span multiple subunits often require flap reconstruction to minimize closure tension and avoid free margin distortion. Patients benefit from counseling that some repairs, especially those that transfer tissue across subunits, may require revision once fully healed.

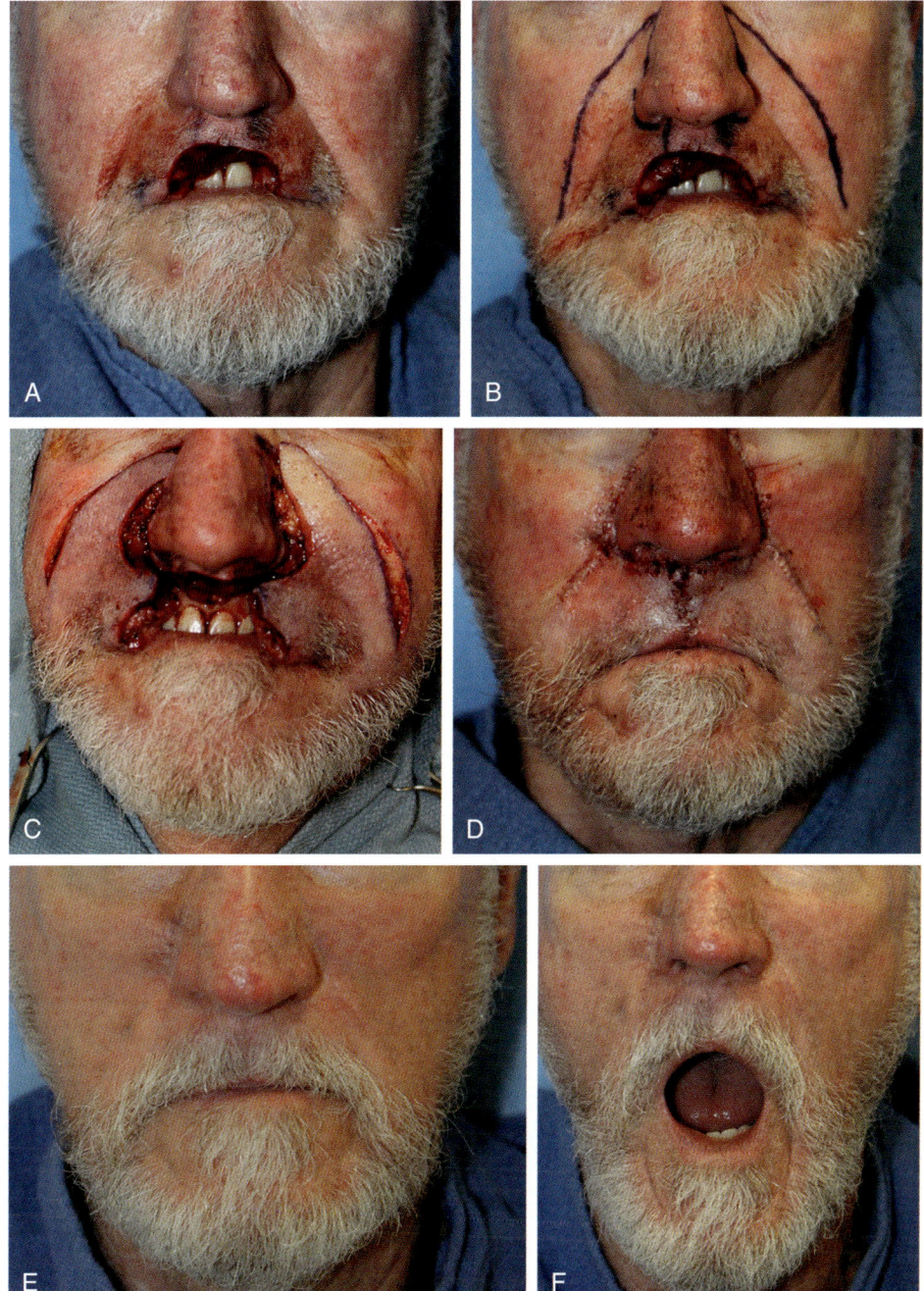

Fig. 16.40 (A) Full-thickness philtral lip defect. (B) Bilateral transposition-advancement flaps designed along melolabial folds and nasofacial sulcus. (C) Flaps incised to subcutaneous layer. (D) Flaps sutured. (E–F) Final result.

References

1. Richmond-Sinclair NM, Pandeya N, Ware RS, et al. Incidence of basal cell carcinoma multiplicity and detailed anatomic distribution: longitudinal study of an Australian population. *J Invest Dermatol*. 2009; 129:323-328.
2. Franceschi S, Levi F, Randimbison L, La Vecchia C. Site distribution of different types of skin cancer: new aetiological clues. *Int J Cancer*. 1996;67:24-28.
3. Ishii L, Carey J, Byrne P, Zee DS, Ishii M. Measuring attentional bias to peripheral facial deformities. *Laryngoscope*. 2009;119:459-465.
4. Springer IN, Wannicke B, Warnke PH, et al. Facial attractiveness: visual impact of symmetry increases significantly towards the midline. *Ann Plast Surg*. 2007;59:156-162.
5. Sobanko JF, Sarwer D, Miller CJ. The importance of physical appearance in skin cancer patients. *Dermatol Surg*. 2014;41(2):183-188.
6. Langstein HN, Robb GL. Lip and perioral reconstruction. *Clin Plast Surg*. 2005;32:431-445, viii.
7. Larrabee WF, Makielski KH, Henderson JL. *Surgical Anatomy of the Face*. 2nd ed. Philadelphia: Lippincott Williams & Wilkins; 2004.
8. Drake RL. *Gray's Atlas of Anatomy*. 2nd ed. London: Churchill Livingstone; 2014.
9. Ha RY, Nojima K, Adams WP Jr, Brown SA. Analysis of facial skin thickness: defining the relative thickness index. *Plast Reconstr Surg*. 2005;115:1769-1773.
10. Baker SR. *Local Flaps in Facial Reconstruction*. 2nd ed. Philadelphia: Mosby Elsevier; 2007.

11. Pilsl U, Anderhuber F, Neugebauer S. The facial artery-the main blood vessel for the anterior face? *Dermatol Surg.* 2016;42:203-208.
12. Schulte DL, Sherris DA, Kasperbauer JL. The anatomical basis of the Abbe flap. *Laryngoscope.* 2001;111:382-386.
13. Al-Hoqail RA, Meguid EM. Anatomic dissection of the arterial supply of the lips: an anatomical and analytical approach. *J Craniofac Surg.* 2008;19:785-794.
14. Pinar YA, Bilge O, Govsa F. Anatomic study of the blood supply of perioral region. *Clin Anat.* 2005;18:330-339.
15. Crouzet C, Fournier H, Papon X, Hentati N, Cronier P, Mercier P. Anatomy of the arterial vascularization of the lips. *Surg Radiol Anat.* 1998;20:273-278.
16. Garcia de Mitchell CA, Pessa JE, Schaverien MV, Rohrich RJ. The philtrum: anatomical observations from a new perspective. *Plast Reconstr Surg.* 2008;122:1756-1760.
17. Harris L, Higgins K, Enepekides D. Local flap reconstruction of acquired lip defects. *Curr Opin Otolaryngol Head Neck Surg.* 2012;20:254-261.
18. Gloster HM Jr. The use of second-intention healing for partial-thickness Mohs defects involving the vermilion and/or mucosal surfaces of the lip. *J Am Acad Dermatol.* 2002;47:893-897.
19. Leonard AL, Hanke CW. Second intention healing for intermediate and large postsurgical defects of the lip. *J Am Acad Dermatol.* 2007;57:832-835.
20. Paniker PU, Mellette JR. A simple technique for repair of Cupid's bow. *Dermatol Surg.* 2003;29:636-640.
21. Lane JE, Kent DE. Repair of vermilion Mohs defect with unilateral axial myocutaneous advancement flap. *Dermatol Surg.* 2007;33:1502-1504, discussion 4.
22. Sobanko JF. Optimizing design and execution of linear reconstructions on the face. *Dermatol Surg.* 2015;41(suppl 10):S216-S228.
23. Miller CJ, Antunes MB, Sobanko JF. Surgical technique for optimal outcomes: Part II. repairing tissue: suturing. *J Am Acad Dermatol.* 2015;72:389-402.
24. Etzkorn JR, Sobanko JF, Miller CJ. Free margin distortion with fusiform closures: the apical angle relationship. *Dermatol Surg.* 2014;40:1428-1432.
25. Wentzell JM, Lund JJ. Z-plasty innovations in vertical lip reconstructions. *Dermatol Surg.* 2011;37:1646-1662.
26. Johnson-Jahangir H, Stevenson M, Ratner D. Modified flap design for symmetric reconstruction of the apical triangle of the upper lip. *Dermatol Surg.* 2012;38:905-911.
27. Gormley DE. A brief analysis of the Burow's wedge/triangle principle. *J Dermatol Surg Oncol.* 1985;11:121-123.
28. Oberemok S, Eliezri Y, Desciak E. Burow's wedge flap revisited. *Dermatol Surg.* 2005;31:210-216, discussion 6.
29. Skouge JW. Upper lip repair–the subcutaneous island pedicle flap. *J Dermatol Surg Oncol.* 1990;16:63-68.
30. Ray TL, Weinberger CH, Lee PK. Closure of large surgical defects on the cutaneous upper lip using an island pedicle flap. *Dermatol Surg.* 2010;36:931-934.
31. Burget GC, Menick FJ. The subunit principle in nasal reconstruction. *Plast Reconstr Surg.* 1985;76:239-247.
32. Hauben DJ. Victor von Bruns (1812–1883) and his contributions to plastic and reconstructive surgery. *Plast Reconstr Surg.* 1985;75:120-127.
33. Gillies H, Millard D. *Principles and Art of Plastic Surgery.* Boston: Little, Brown; 1957.
34. Karapandzic M. Reconstruction of lip defects by local arterial flaps. *Br J Plast Surg.* 1974;27:93-97.
35. Neligan P, Rodriguez ED, Losee JE, EBSCOhost, Alumni and Friends Memorial Book Fund. *Plastic Surgery. Volume Three, Craniofacial, Head and Neck Surgery, Pediatric Plastic Surgery.* 3rd ed. London, New York: Elsevier Saunders; 2013:1. [Online resource (various pagings)].
36. Miller CJ. Design principles for transposition flaps: the rhombic (single-lobed), bilobed, and trilobed flaps. *Dermatol Surg.* 2014;40(suppl 9):S43-S52.
37. Burget GC, Hsiao YC. Nasolabial rotation flaps based on the upper lateral lip subunit for superficial and large defects of the upper lateral lip. *Plast Reconstr Surg.* 2012;130:556-560.
38. Magden O, Edizer M, Atabey A, Tayfur V, Ergur I. Cadaveric study of the arterial anatomy of the upper lip. *Plast Reconstr Surg.* 2004;114:355-359.
39. Sobanko JF, Miller CJ. Midface composite defect: laterally based bilobed flap as a platform for a 3-stage folded paramedian forehead flap. *Dermatol Surg.* 2014;40:327-332.
40. Hollmig ST, Leach BC, Cook J. Single-stage interpolation flaps in facial reconstruction. *Dermatol Surg.* 2014;40(suppl 9):S62-S70.
41. Cook JL. Tunneled and transposed island flaps in facial reconstructive surgery. *Dermatol Surg.* 2014;40(suppl 9):S16-S29.
42. Agostini T. The Sabattini-Abbe flap: a historical note. *Plast Reconstr Surg.* 2009;123:767, author reply 767–768.
43. Alvarez GS, Siqueira EJ, de Oliveira MP. A new technique for reconstruction of lower-lip and labial commissure defects: a proposal for the association of Abbe-Estlander and vermilion myomucosal flap techniques. *Oral Surg Oral Med Oral Pathol Oral Radiol.* 2013;115:724-730.
44. Smith JW. The anatomical and physiologic acclimatization of tissue transplanted by the lip switch technique. *Plast Reconstr Surg Transplant Bull.* 1960;26:40-56.
45. Mulliken JB, Pensler JM, Kozakewich HP. The anatomy of Cupid's bow in normal and cleft lip. *Plast Reconstr Surg.* 1993;92:395-403, discussion 4.
46. Briedis J, Jackson IT. The anatomy of the philtrum: observations made on dissections in the normal lip. *Br J Plast Surg.* 1981;34:128-132.
47. Kaufman AJ, Grekin RC. Repair of central upper lip (philtral) surgical defects with island pedicle flaps. *Dermatol Surg.* 1996;22:1003-1007.
48. Garces Gatnau JR, Ruiz-Salas V, Alegre Fernandez M, Puig L. Reconstruction for defects at the base of the philtrum affecting the upper lip vermilion. *Dermatol Surg.* 2016;42:677-680.
49. Webster JP. Crescentic peri-alar cheek excision for upper lip flap advancement with a short history of upper lip repair. *Plastic Reconstr Surg (1946).* 1955;16:434-464.
50. Cook JL. The reconstruction of two large full-thickness wounds of the upper lip with different operative techniques: when possible, a local flap repair is preferable to reconstruction with free tissue transfer. *Dermatol Surg.* 2013;39:281-289.

Videos for this chapter can be found online by accessing the accompanying Expert Consult website.

17 Neck Reconstruction

ANNA BAR, MD, and SPRING GOLDEN, MD

Introduction and Perioperative Consideration

The neck is the portion of the body that links the trunk to the head. As the neck is prone to sun exposure, it is a common location for dermatologic surgeons to remove skin cancers. The neck contains many vital structures, and one should therefore be familiar with the neck anatomy and potential reconstructive options.

The mobility and thickness of neck skin are dependent on location as well as the age of the patient. The posterior neck skin is usually thicker and less mobile than the skin on the anterior or lateral portions of the neck. With increasing age, the skin of the neck also becomes more pliable, which allows the neck to serve as a reservoir for tissue recruitment. The relaxed skin tension lines on the central anterior and posterior neck lie horizontally and transition to an oblique orientation on the lateral portions of the neck (Fig. 17.1). Placing scars within the relaxed skin tension lines whenever possible will lead to better cosmetic results.

Positioning a patient appropriately prior to surgery can have a great impact on the ease of performing the surgical procedure as well as overall cosmesis. When performing a surgery on the anterior or posterior neck, the patient should be positioned supine or prone respectively. When the surgical site is located on the lateral neck, the patient should be marked for closure while the patient is holding the neck in a neutral position. If the neck is turned far laterally for suturing, this may distort the relaxed skin tension lines and result in misplacement of scars and standing cones.

Anatomy of the Neck

CUTANEOUS ANATOMY

The anterior aspect of the neck is bound superiorly by the mandible of the jaw and inferiorly by the clavicle. The posterior aspect of the neck is bound superiorly by the hairline or base of the skull and inferiorly by the upper portion of the scapula.[1]

TRIANGLES

The sternocleidomastoid muscle divides the neck into the anterior and posterior triangles (Fig. 17.2). The anterior triangle is defined by the anterior border of the sternocleidomastoid, the inferior margin of the mandible, and the midline of the neck. This triangle contains the platysma muscle, which constitutes a major component of the superficial musculoaponeurotic system (SMAS) layer, and is continuous with the SMAS of the face.[2] This muscle overlays the investing cervical fascia and is approximately 0.6 mm thick, but becomes slightly thicker in the submental area.[1] The platysma is considered a muscle of facial expression, as contraction of the platysma muscle pulls down the lower lip and results in grimacing.

The posterior triangle is defined by the posterior border of the sternocleidomastoid muscle, the anterior border of the trapezius muscle, and the superior aspect of the clavicle. This triangle contains the spinal accessory nerve (cranial nerve XI) at its most superficial point, known as Erb's point. Erb's point describes the area where the spinal accessory nerve emerges from approximately one-third down the posterior border of the sternocleidomastoid muscle and courses through the posterior triangle inferiorly and diagonally along the levator scapulae muscle to penetrate a point two-thirds down the anterior edge of the trapezius muscle before it runs deep under the muscle.[2,3]

Erb's point can be easily located by finding the half-way point between the mastoid process and the angle of the jaw and drawing a perpendicular line 6.0 cm vertically down the neck to the point where it intersects the posterior aspect of the sternocleidomastoid muscle (Fig. 17.3).[2] Another way to identify Erb's point is by drawing a horizontal line from the thyroid notch to the posterior triangle on the neck. The area approximately 2 cm above and below where this line crosses the posterior border of the sternocleidomastoid is the where the nerve traverses the posterior triangle and is most prone to injury.

This point is particularly important for dermatologic surgeons given the superficial nature of the spinal accessory nerve lying just below the skin and subcutaneous tissue. Fig. 17.4A shows a basal cell carcinoma located over the posterior triangle of the neck, and the spinal accessory nerve is visible after removal of the tumor (see Fig. 17.4B). Damage to the spinal accessory nerve can cause significant morbidity including shoulder drop and the inability to abduct the shoulder past 80 degrees. Paresthesias and pain may also accompany damage to this nerve.[4] Given the superficial nature of this nerve, great care should be taken when operating in this area.

BLOOD SUPPLY

Arteries

The common carotid artery courses through the anterior triangle, and divides within the triangle into the external

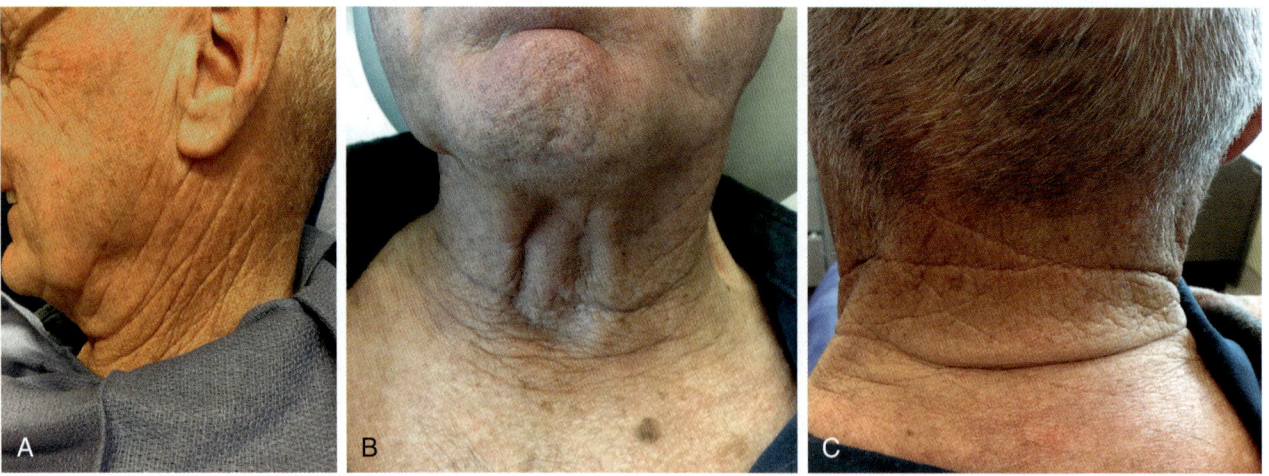

Fig. 17.1 Relaxed skin tension lines of the neck. (A) Lateral neck. (B) Anterior neck. (C) Posterior neck.

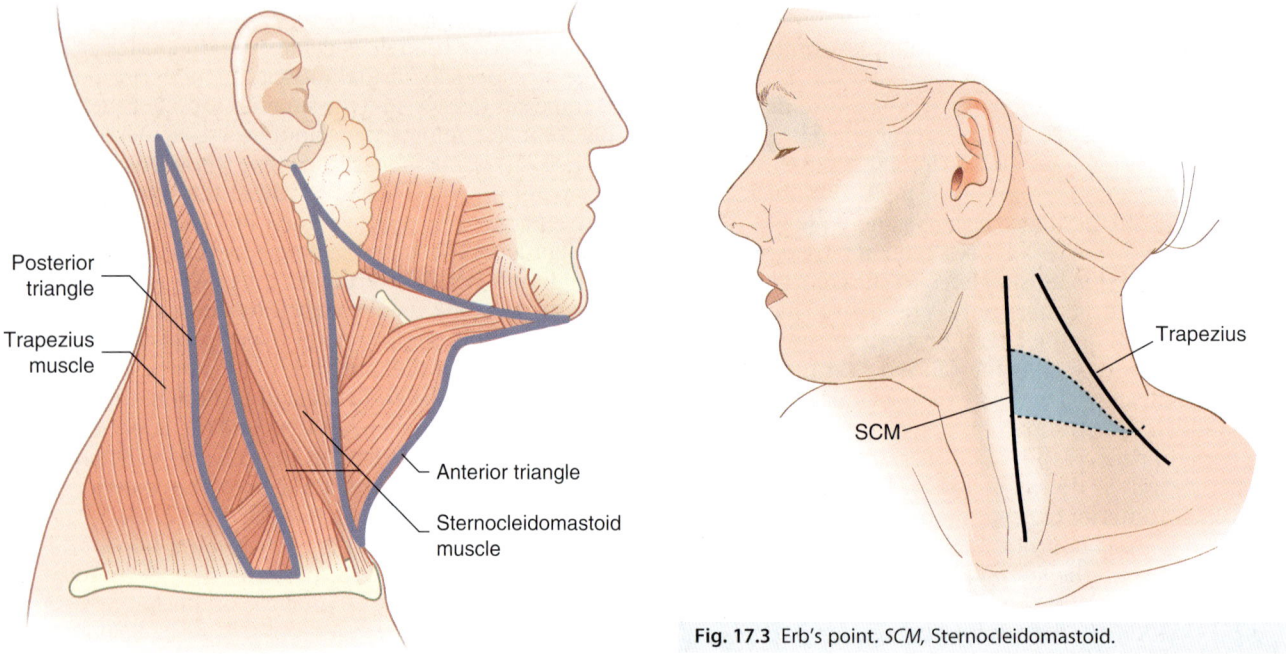

Fig. 17.2 Anterior and posterior triangles of the neck.

Fig. 17.3 Erb's point. *SCM*, Sternocleidomastoid.

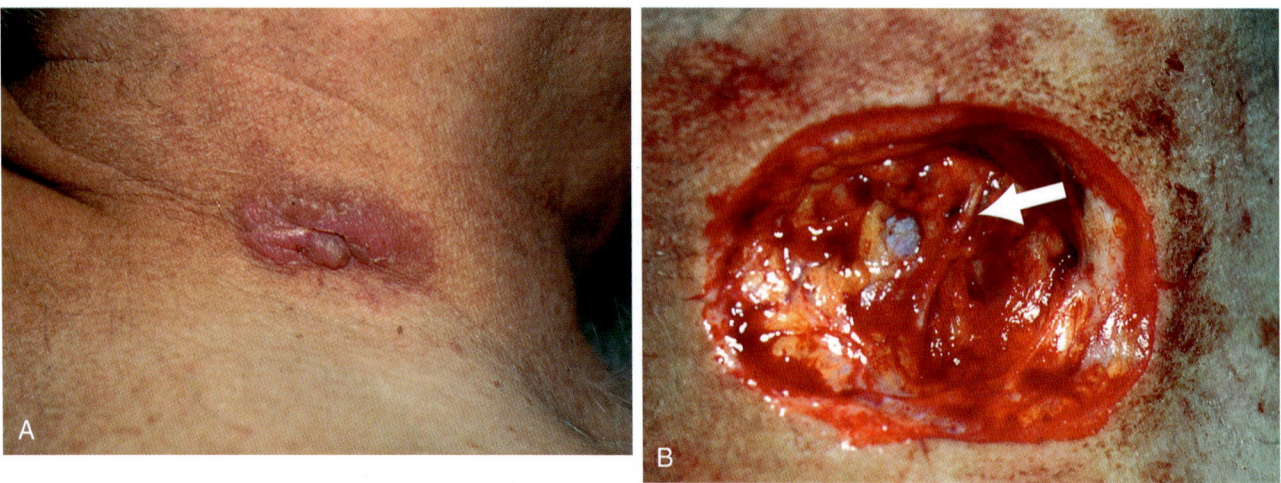

Fig. 17.4 (A) Basal cell carcinoma preoperatively. (B) Spinal accessory nerve visible after removal of tumor. *White arrow* indicates the spinal accessory nerve.

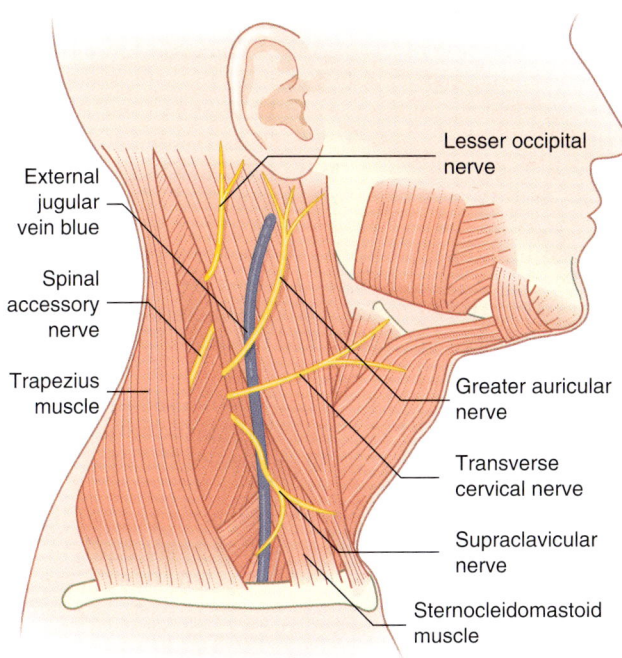

Fig. 17.5 Nerves of the neck.

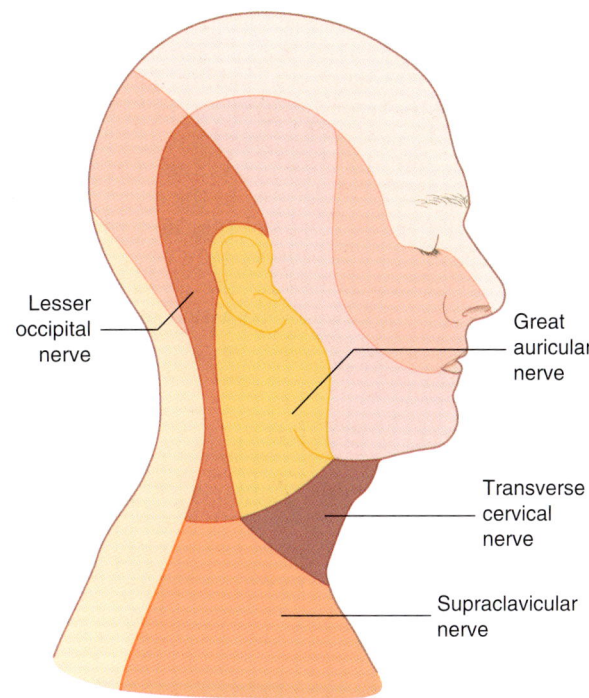

Fig. 17.6 Cutaneous nerve supply of the superficial cervical plexus.

and internal carotid arteries. After it leaves the neck, the external carotid artery branches extensively.[5] Branches of note are the facial and superficial temporal arteries that provide blood supply to the face and anterior scalp.

Veins

The external jugular vein (Fig. 17.5) is a major drainage point for the scalp and face. It begins near or in the parotid gland, travels underneath the platysma, and crosses above the sternocleidomastoid muscle before it empties into the internal jugular or subclavian vein. Additionally, the external jugular vein has tributaries that connect with the internal jugular vein and the anterior jugular vein that is located anterior in the neck.[2,5]

Nerves

Besides the major motor nerve, the spinal accessory nerve, which innervates the trapezius, a few important sensory nerves from the superficial cervical plexus also emerge near Erb's point (Fig. 17.5). The greater auricular nerve exits the posterior surface of the sternocleidomastoid and runs toward the earlobe and mastoid process. Damage to this nerve produces numbness to the earlobe.[4] This nerve is one of the most frequently injured nerves during face and neck lift surgery, and the resulting sensory deficit can be distressing for patients. The transverse cervical nerve and supraclavicular nerve similarly can be damaged in this area and result in a loss of sensation to the anterior and lateral neck (Fig. 17.6).

The cervical plexus also lies beneath the platysma and emerges behind the posterior border of the sternocleidomastoid muscle. The cervical plexus provides cutaneous innervation to the neck and auricular region, as well as motor innervation to muscles of the neck, back, and diaphragm.[1,5]

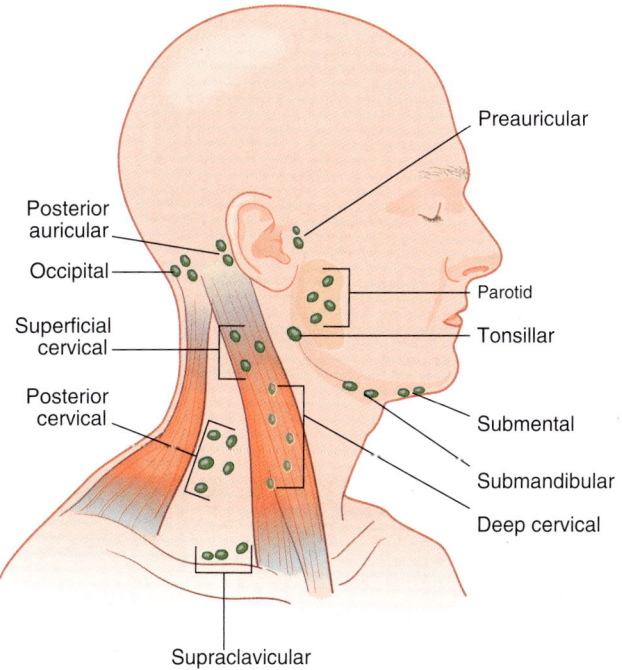

Fig. 17.7 Lymphatics of the neck.

Lymphatics

The most frequently encountered lymph nodes for dermatologic surgeons are the postauricular lymph nodes (Fig. 17.7), which are located in the upper neck region behind the ear in a relatively superficial location. The postauricular lymph nodes are located at the insertion of the sternocleidomastoid muscle into the mastoid process. They provide lymphatic drainage to the posterior neck, upper ear, and external auditory canal. Superficial cervical lymph nodes travel along the external jugular vein in the posterior triangle, and along the anterior jugular vein in the anterior triangle. These nodes collect lymph from the superficial portions of the anterior and lateral neck. Submental and submandibular nodes are also located in the anterior triangle and provide drainage to the local skin and oral cavity.[1,2] Metastasis to the submental nodes may occur with squamous cell carcinomas located on the lower lip, so these should be carefully assessed by palpation and/or imaging before surgery.

Neck Reconstruction

Primary closure is the most common type of closure in all subunits of the neck, given the laxity and mobility of the tissue. On the posterior and lower anterior subunits of the neck, primary closure is typically oriented horizontally, given the relaxed tension lines. In both of these locations, dermatologic surgeons must take into account the tension produced by flexion or extension of the neck, as these movements can cause great tension on wounds closed in a horizontal fashion. On the lateral neck, standing cones are oriented in an oblique fashion to place the final scar into relaxed skin tension lines, which can result in a near invisible scar.[6] Even large defects can be closed in this manner quite easily, as there is a large amount of laxity in the neck skin. Figs. 17.8 to 17.11 illustrate typical linear closures on the lateral and posterior neck. On the midline anterior neck, primary closure may be oriented horizontally or vertically, depending on the shape of the defect. Fig. 17.12 shows a vertically oriented closure on the anterior neck of this bearded gentleman. Occasionally this placement may result in scar contraction that would require lengthening or revision with Z-plasties.

When primary closure of the neck is not possible due to a large-sized defect or when the defect is approaching the immobile mastoid area, local flaps may be considered.

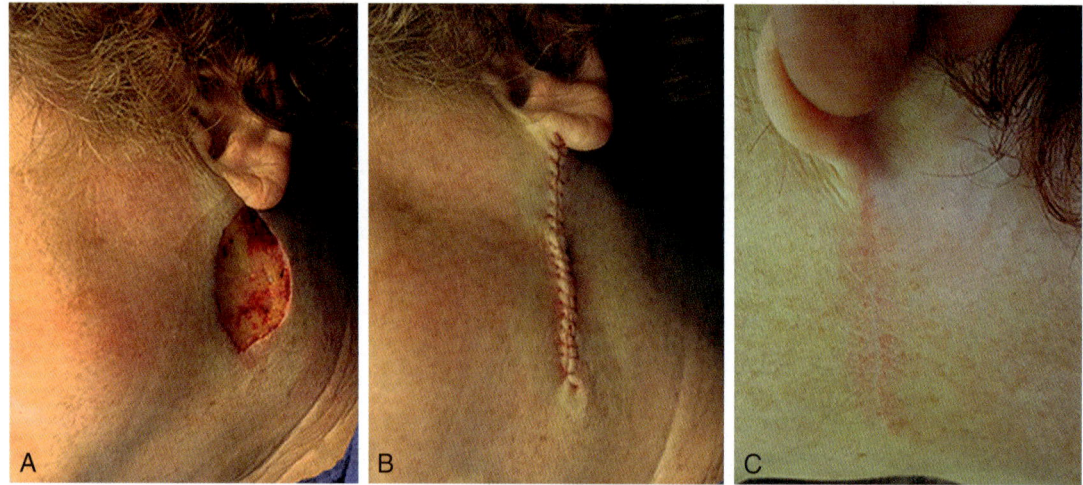

Fig. 17.8 (A) Defect after removal of basal cell carcinoma. (B) Primary closure designed along relaxed skin tension lines. (C) Healed result at 4 months.

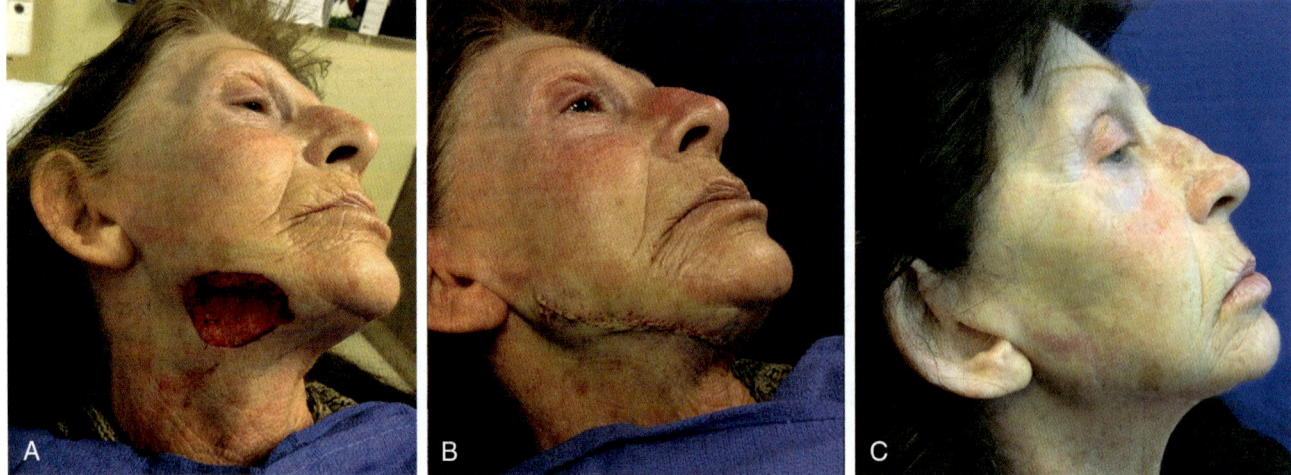

Fig. 17.9 (A) Lateral neck/mandible defect. (B) Closure along relaxed skin tension lines. (C) Healed result at 6 months.

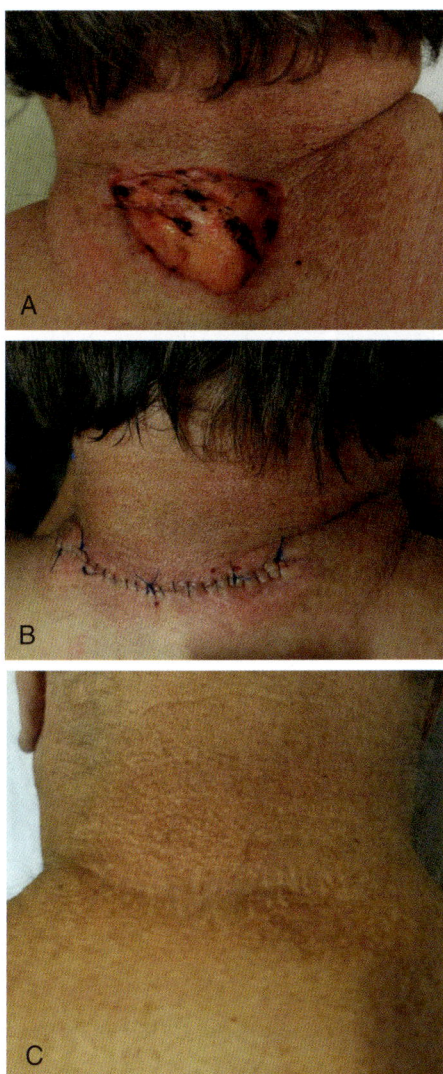

Fig. 17.10 (A) Large defect of posterior neck. (B) Linear closure. (C) Healed result at 1 year.

Transposition or advancement flaps can be used to recruit skin from the lower lateral neck to the mastoid area.[6,7] Fig. 17.13 shows the typical design of a rhombic transposition flap from the neck to the postauricular skin. Figs. 17.14–17.16 show typical rhombic flaps for defects of the postauricular area. The rhombic flap leads to a good cosmetic result, as portions of the scar of the rhombic flap can be placed in the creases of the neck.[7] Advancement flaps can be oriented similarly to place most of the scar in the relaxed skin tension lines (Fig. 17.17). Fig. 17.18 shows an advancement flap on the neck with excision of a tricone to facilitate tissue advancement of the flap. In Fig. 17.19, tricones were excised at the superior, inferior, and medial aspects of the defect to close a large defect.

When repairing a defect using primary closure or a flap, the wound can be undermined either superficial or deep to the platysma; however, care should be used if undermining in the deep plane.[6] Because of the laxity of the neck, a majority of wounds do not require extensive undermining. Typically deep subcutaneous and dermal absorbable sutures

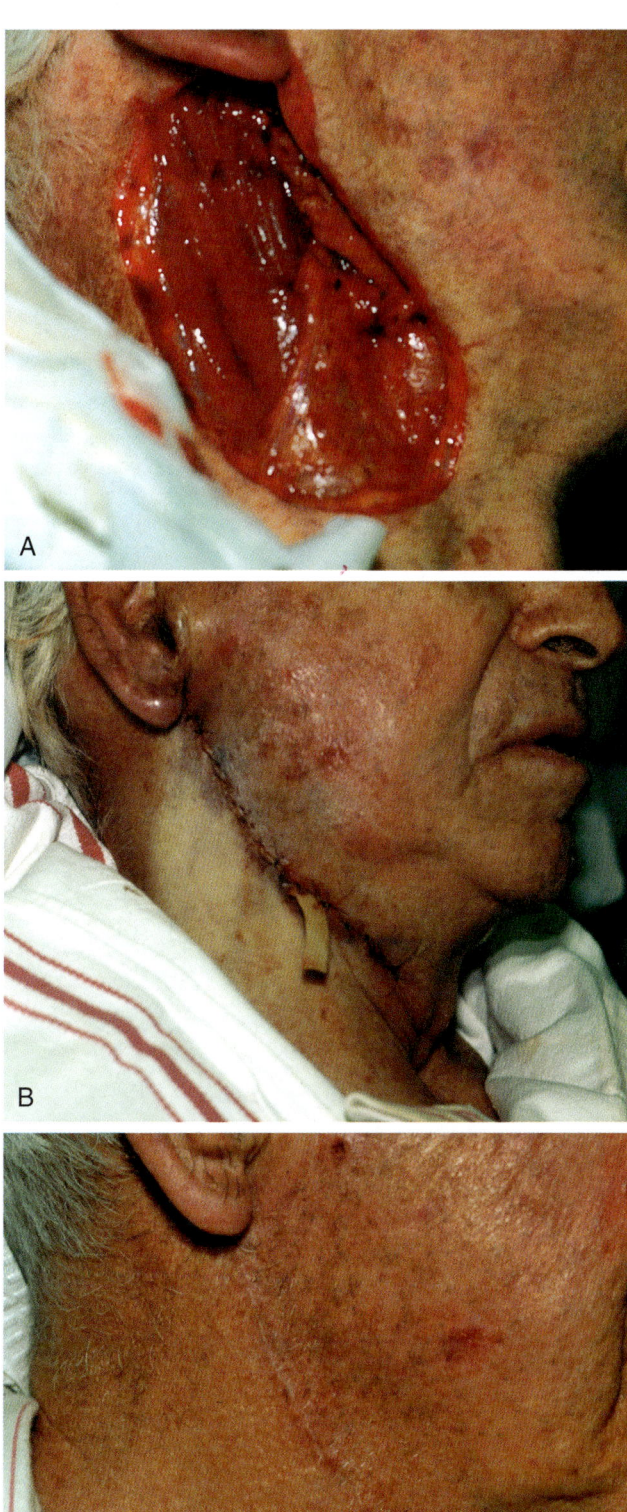

Fig. 17.11 (A) Large defect on the neck following Mohs surgery. (B) Primary closure of large neck defect. (C) Healed result at 6 months.

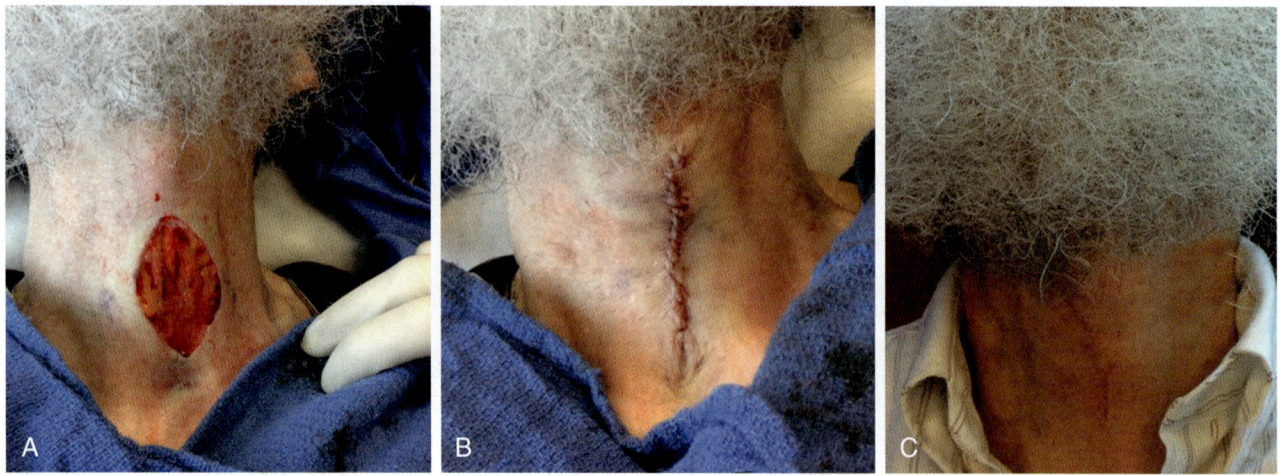

Fig. 17.12 (A) Defect on midline anterior neck. (B) Linear closure oriented vertically. (C) Healed result at 1 month.

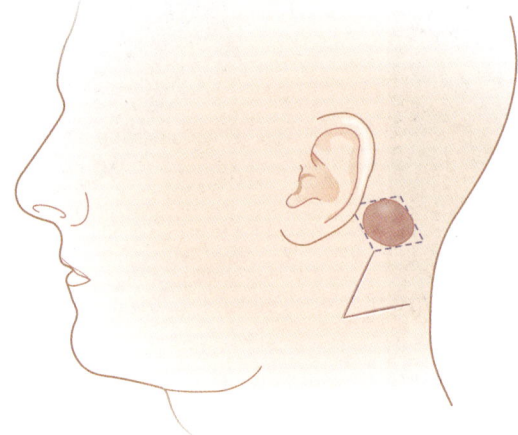

Fig. 17.13 Rhombic transposition flap design from neck to postauricular area.

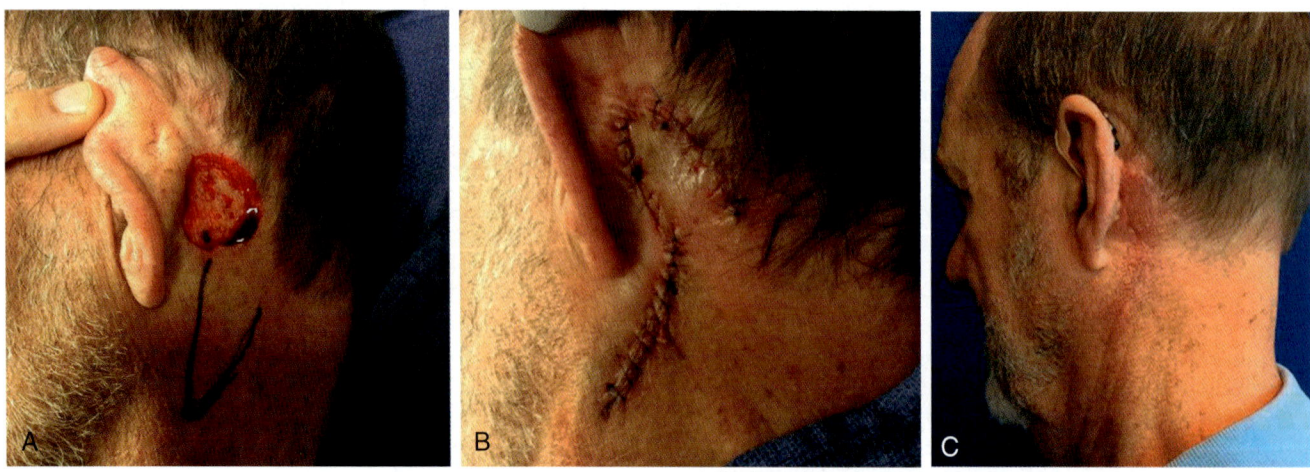

Fig. 17.14 (A) Defect after removal of tumor. (B) Rhombic transposition flap sutured into place. (C) Follow-up at 2 months.

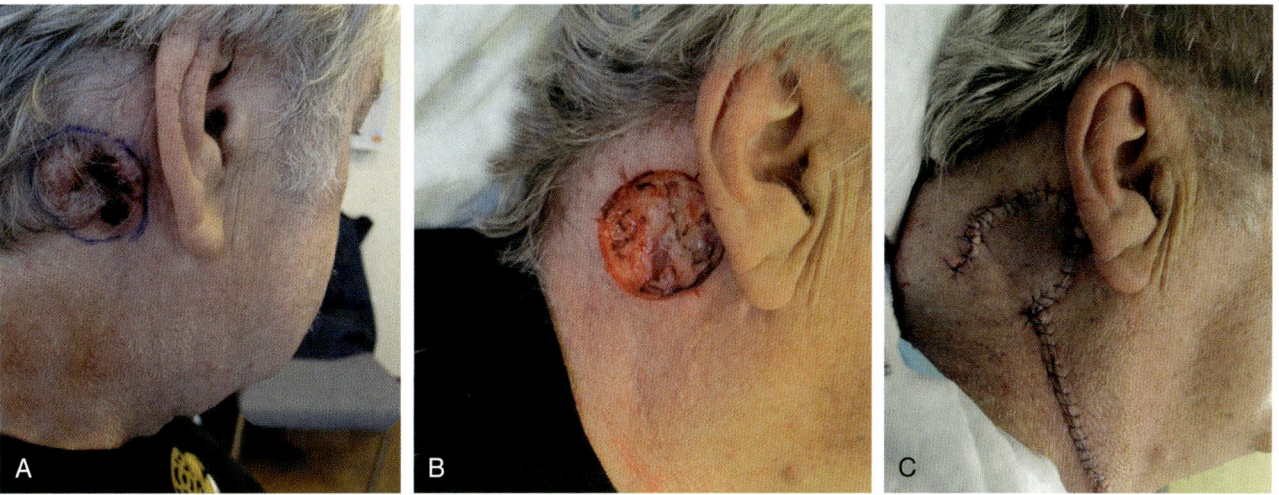

Fig. 17.15 (A) Large basal cell carcinoma of postauricular area. (B) Defect after Mohs surgery. (C) Closure with a rhombic transposition flap from the lateral neck.

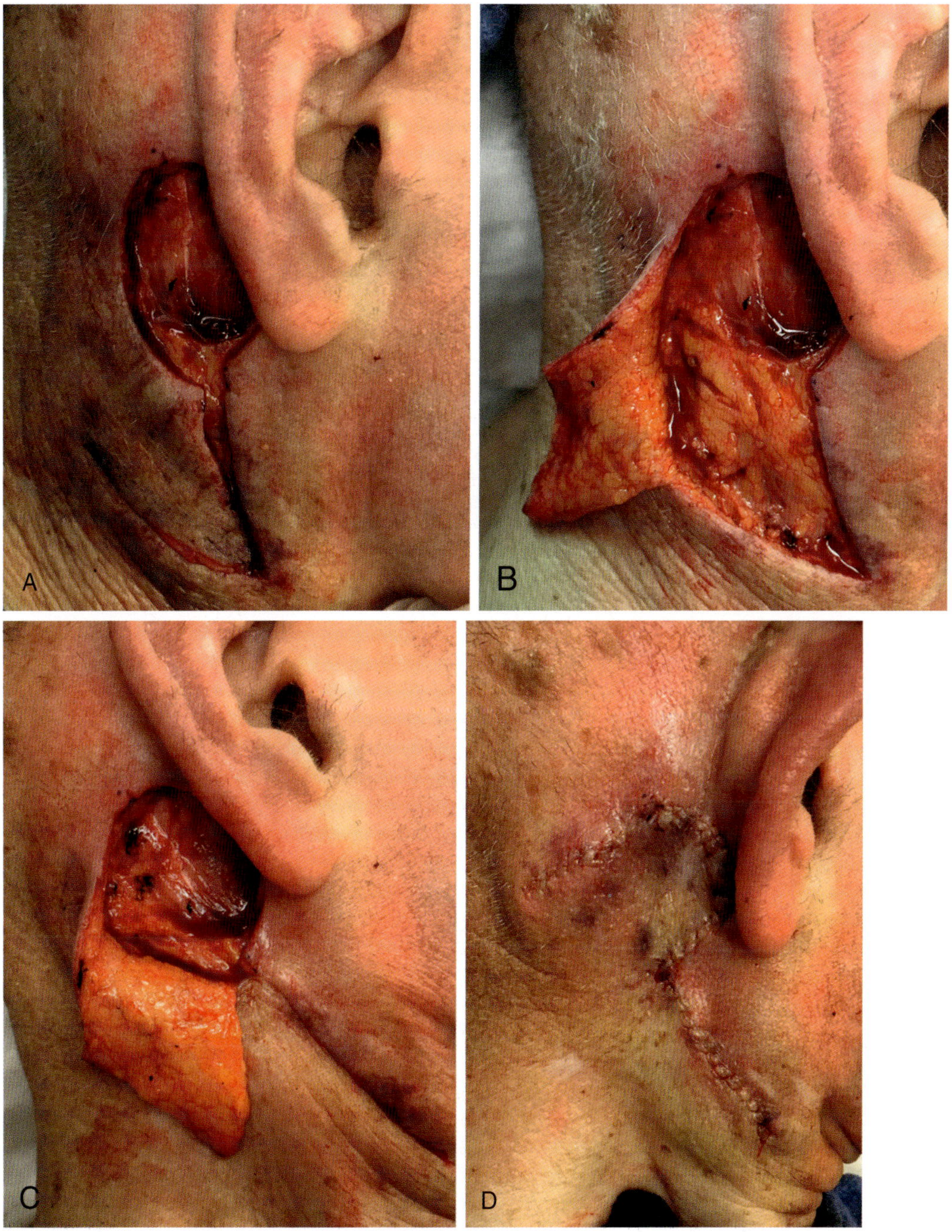

Fig. 17.16 (A) Defect of postauricular area after Mohs surgery. (B) Rhombic flap undermined. (C) Key stitch of rhombic flap closes the secondary defect. (D) Rhombic flap sutured into place.

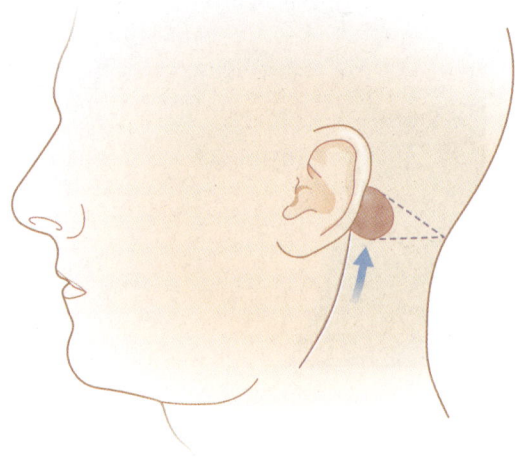

Fig. 17.17 Advancement flap design.

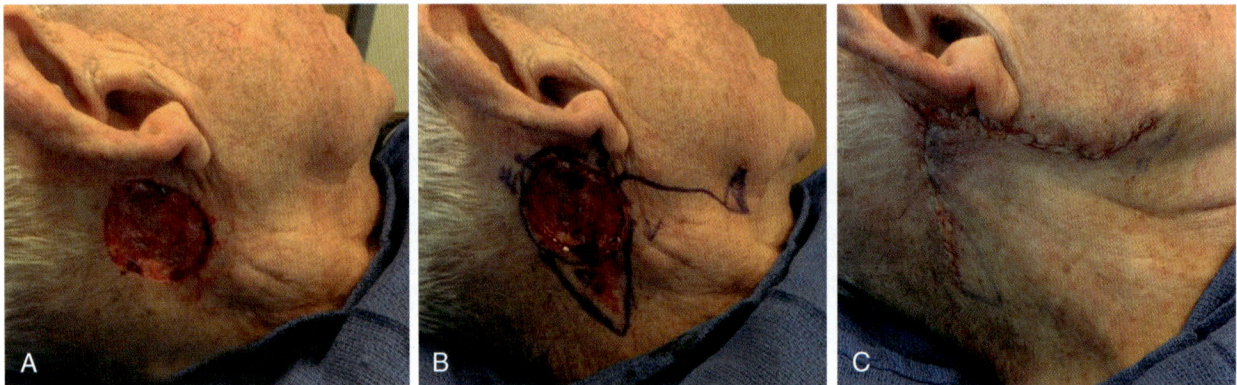

Fig. 17.18 (A) Defect after Mohs surgery. (B) Advancement flap design recruiting lateral neck skin inferior to the defect. (C) Advancement flap mobility enhanced by excision of a tricone and sutured into place.

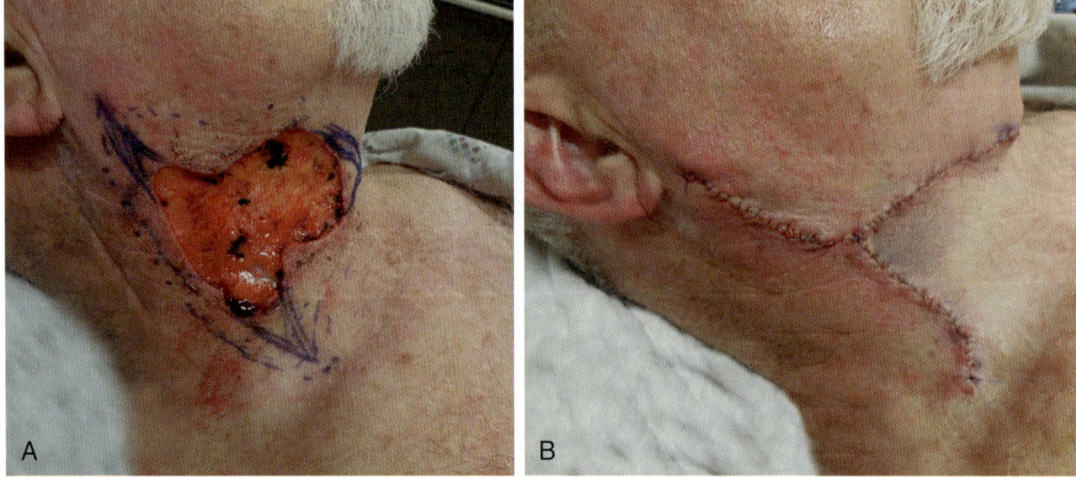

Fig. 17.19 (A) Large defect on lateral neck. (B) Advancement flap design recruits lax skin and places most of the incisions into relaxed skin tension lines.

are 4-0 or 5-0 in caliber, and superficial epidermal sutures are 4-0 or 5-0 in caliber when closing neck defects.

Healing by secondary intent is another option that can be utilized in certain locations on the neck. Defects near the mastoid region or defects on the posterior neck are areas that heal remarkably well when left to granulate. Fig. 17.20 shows excision of acne keloidalis nuchae on the posterior neck, a large excision that is typically allowed to heal by granulation with an excellent cosmetic result. Fig. 17.21 shows a large Mohs defect that was allowed to heal by secondary intention. Patients must be properly instructed on the care of a granulating wound, and must also be informed that healing by secondary intent often takes many months.

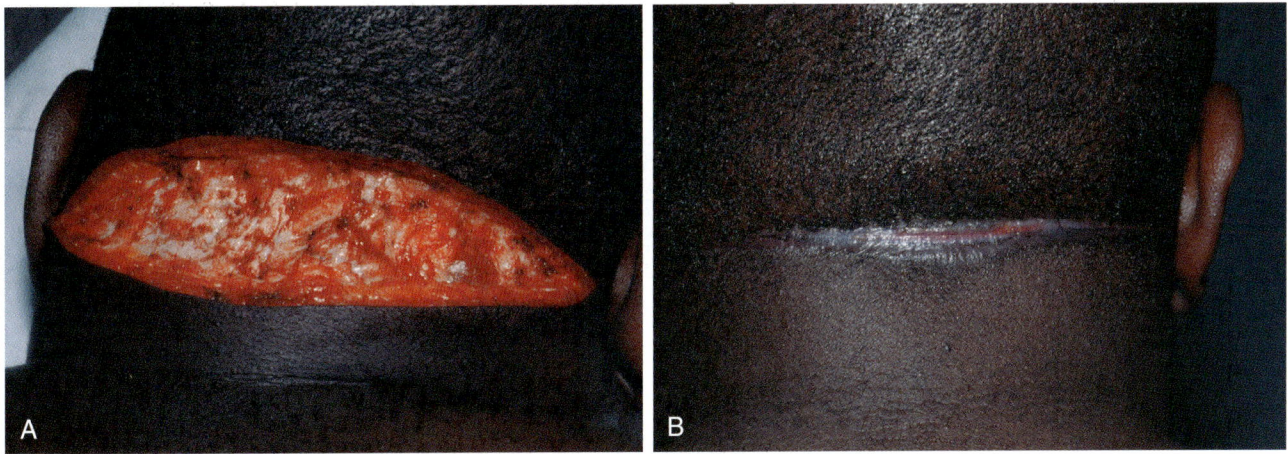

Fig. 17.20 (A) Posterior neck defect after excision of acne keloidalis nuchae. (B) Final scar after neck defect healed by secondary intention.

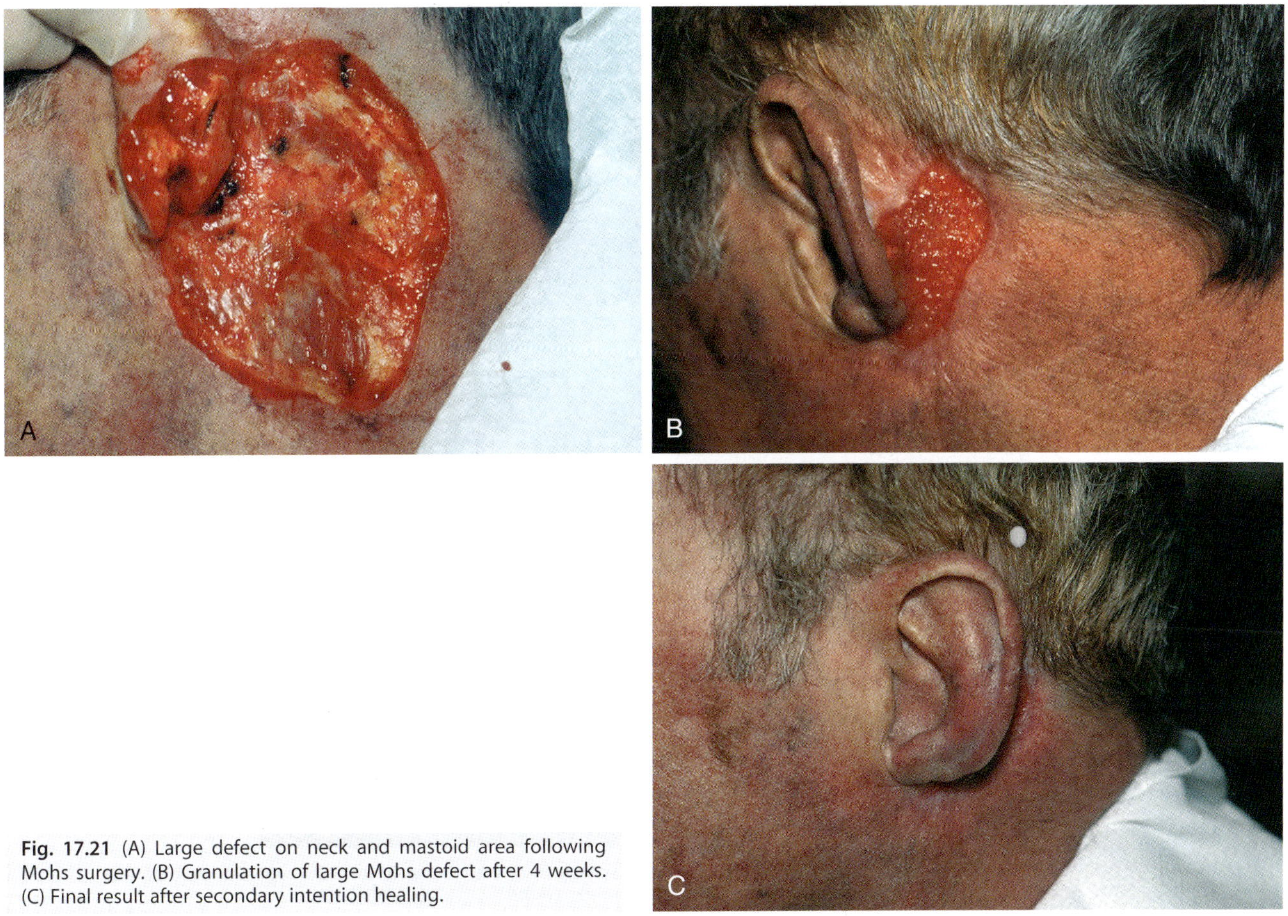

Fig. 17.21 (A) Large defect on neck and mastoid area following Mohs surgery. (B) Granulation of large Mohs defect after 4 weeks. (C) Final result after secondary intention healing.

Other Surgical Considerations

The neck can also be a reservoir for tissue when closing defects that are not located on the neck. A rhombic transposition flap from the neck may be used to cover lower cheek, chin, or mandibular area defects (Fig. 17.22). Bilobed flaps from the neck can be used for a similar purpose. With these repairs, the surgeon must be very mindful when designing the flap, to ensure adequate sizing and appropriate angles.[6]

The neck can also be used to repair defects on the ear as seen with this transposition flap to repair the lobule (Fig. 17.23). The flap is harvested as a banner-type transposition

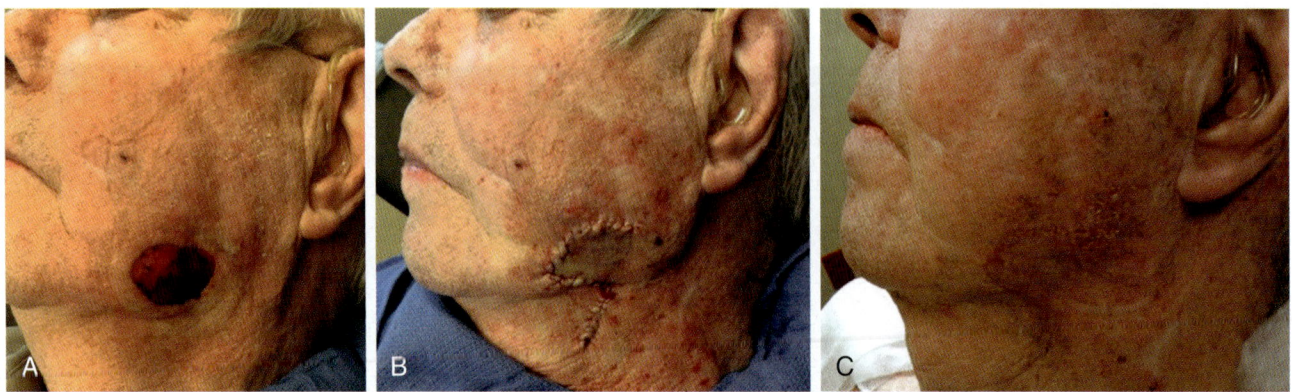

Fig. 17.22 (A) Defect on mandibular area after Mohs. (B) Rhombic designed from neck to mandible. (C) Healed result at 3-month follow-up.

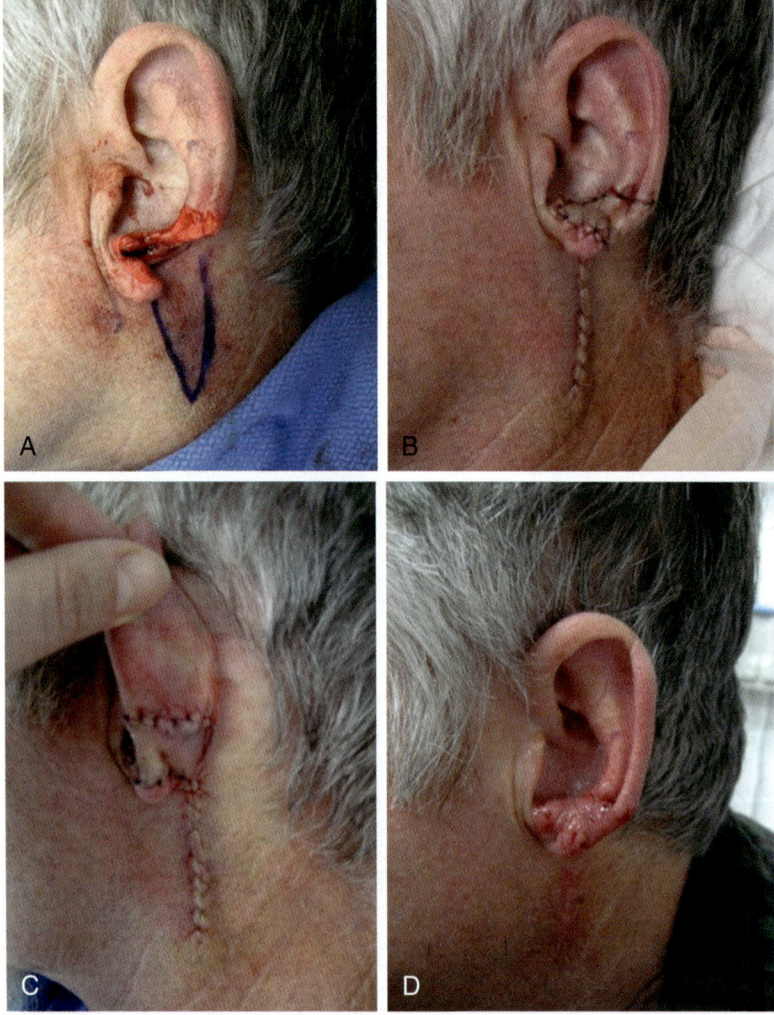

Fig. 17.23 (A) Full-thickness defect of earlobe after Mohs surgery. (B) Banner transposition flap designed from infraauricular area of neck to earlobe. (C) Flap is folded onto itself and sutured into place to create anterior and posterior earlobe. (D) Healed flap recreates a normal earlobe at 1 week.

flap and folded on itself to recreate both sides of the earlobe. Finally, the neck is an excellent area to harvest a full-thickness skin graft. Both the skin on the postauricular neck and the submental neck are relatively sun spared compared to other areas on the face, and can provide a great tissue match for facial defects where full-thickness skin grafting is used. The neck skin should therefore be considered for defects on adjoining facial subunits such as the cheek or the ear as well as an area to attain a full thickness skin graft.

Postoperative Considerations and Complications

When operating on the neck, it is important to consider and avoid postoperative complications. Dermatologic surgeons should take care when undermining on the neck to avoid injuring deeper structures. Furthermore, when working on the neck, it is important to ensure that adequate hemostasis is attained, especially given the neck is a highly mobile structure and neck movement postoperatively can lead to bleeding and hematoma formation.[4] Avoiding hematoma formation is critical, as this can lead to compression of vital structures in the neck. Therefore, postoperatively it is important that patients receive an appropriate pressure dressing to help prevent hematoma formation.

Summary

The neck is a very important surgical site to familiarize oneself with, as skin cancers are quite common in this location. Dermatologic surgeons should be aware of the location of the spinal accessory nerve when operating. Primary closure is the mainstay of repairing defects on the neck, given the laxity of skin in this area; however, other closure options such as sliding flaps and transposition flaps can be considered. The neck is a highly mobile surgical site and therefore can also be used in the closure of adjacent anatomic regions or used as a skin graft. The abundant skin on the neck makes it an ideal place to hide scars, and operating in this location can lead to excellent surgical outcomes.

References

1. Thomaidis VK. *Cutaneous Flaps in Head and Neck Reconstruction*. New York: Springer-Verlag Berlin Heidelberg; 2014:313-336.
2. Robinson J, Hanke CW, Seigel D, Fratila A, Bhatia A, Rohrer T. *Surgery of the Skin: Procedural Dermatology*. New York: Elsevier/Saunders; 2015:394-399.
3. Landers JT, Maino K. Clarifying Erb's point as an anatomic landmark in the posterior cervical triangle. *Dermatol Surg*. 2012;38:954-957.
4. Seckel BR. *Facial Danger Zones: Avoiding Nerve Injury in Facial Plastic Surgery*. Missouri: Quality Medical Publishing; 1994.
5. Chow S, Bennett RS. Superficial head and neck anatomy for dermatologic surgery: critical concepts. *Dermatol Surg*. 2015;41(suppl 10):S169-S177.
6. Ilankovan V, Ethunandan M, Seah TEe. *Local Flaps in Facial Reconstruction: A Defect Based Approach*. New York: Springer International Switzerland; 2015:315-336.
7. Blake BP, Simonetta CJ, Maher IA. Transposition flaps: principles and locations. *Dermatol Surg*. 2015;41(suppl 10):S255-S264.

18 Surgical Complications and Revision of Scars

CHERYL JANENE GUSTAFSON, MD, and C. WILLIAM HANKE, MD, MPH, FACP

Having a thorough knowledge of common dermatologic surgery complications is essential for physicians to develop a safe surgical practice. Overall, the incidence of complications in dermatologic surgery is very low. However, complications are to be expected, particularly in practices with a high volume of dermatologic surgical procedures. Therefore it is critical the physician know how to manage complications.

Before performing a surgical procedure, an experienced dermatologic surgeon should visualize the steps of the procedure from start to finish, including the management of potential side effects. By doing this, many complications can be prevented. For example, if a patient is on anticoagulant medication, the physician will recognize that the patient is at a higher risk for hematoma formation. Therefore the surgeon will take extra precautions to ensure adequate management of hemostasis, such as having the medical assistant hold firm pressure for 8–10 minutes following suture closure.

In this section the most common surgical complications will be reviewed, including their etiology, management, and prevention. Of note, specific complications associated with various surgical flaps are discussed throughout this textbook.

Hemorrhage

Postoperative bleeding is one of the most common complications of cutaneous surgery. A variety of factors contribute to postoperative hemorrhage, including medications, inadequate intraoperative hemostasis, suboptimal wound closure that fails to obliterate tissue dead space, poorly controlled hypertension, and patients overexerting themselves after surgery.

Although achieving adequate hemostasis during the surgical procedure is critical for preventing postoperative bleeding, the prevention of postoperative hemorrhage is primarily managed preoperatively and postoperatively. For example, when patients are scheduled for their surgical procedure, they should be provided with instructions regarding how to prepare for surgery, such as whether they should withhold any medications, vitamins, and/or supplements. Of note, certain over-the-counter vitamins and supplements, such as vitamin D, vitamin E, fish oils, garlic, ginseng, and St. John's wort, increase the risk of bleeding. Therefore many dermatologic surgeons recommend patients withhold these vitamins and supplements 2–3 weeks prior to the procedure. In addition, it is important for the physician to be familiar with the current guidelines for withholding anticoagulants and platelet inhibitors.

Among dermatologists there is a general consensus that continuation of anticoagulants, such as warfarin, is associated with a very low risk of surgical complications. Therefore continuing anticoagulant therapy is strongly favored, since a postoperative bleed is easier to manage and has a significantly lower morbidity/mortality risk compared with a stroke or embolus from discontinuation of the medication. There may be certain instances in which reduction or cessation of anticoagulation therapy is warranted. In such instances, this decision is best made on an individual basis. Moreover, the physician prescribing and managing the patient's anticoagulant therapy should be explicitly involved in the decision on whether to hold or continue the medication.

Following the procedure, a good pressure dressing should be placed. If the patient is on aspirin, warfarin, or other anticoagulant therapy, firm pressure should be held for 8–10 minutes before placing the surgical dressing. The pressure dressing should remain in place for 24 hours. Patients should be instructed on how to properly change the pressure dressing and care for the wound. Likewise, they should be provided with instructions regarding how to manage a postoperative bleed, including holding firm, continuous pressure for 20 minutes. In addition, patients should be advised to avoid vigorous activities (e.g., exercise, bending over, heavy lifting, pushing, pulling) for several weeks following surgery, since such activities can increase the risk of postoperative bleeding and wound dehiscence.

Early, active postoperative bleeding can often be successfully managed with direct pressure to the wound. First, any saturated, wet bandages should be discarded. A dry gauze bandage should then be applied to the wound and held in place with continuous, firm pressure for 20 minutes. If bleeding continues, patients should be advised to call the surgeon and return to the office or local emergency room promptly. Excessive postoperative bleeding and expanding hematomas are primarily treated via the following procedure: (1) partial or complete opening of the surgical wound, (2) identification of the culprit blood vessel(s), (3) hemostasis with electrosurgery and/or suture ligation, (4) possible irrigation and lavage of the surgical wound with sterile sodium chloride (if a hematoma needs to be evacuated), and (5) reclosure of the wound or allowing the wound to heal via second intention. The latter option is considered if the wound is contaminated or if the patient is at a high risk for additional postoperative bleeding.

For patients who present a few days postprocedure with a stable hematoma, one can consider monitoring the area versus evacuating the hematoma. Small, stable hematomas with no necrosis of the overlying skin can often be managed with observation. If the area is extremely tender or if the overlying skin exhibits features worrisome for necrosis, the hematoma should be evacuated. This can often be accomplished under local anesthesia by making a small incision and inserting a cannula attached to a syringe to evacuate the hematoma. To help break up the blood clot, one can irrigate the wound with normal saline and aspirate the fluid using the syringe. If the cannula/syringe technique is unsuccessful, then the sutures should be removed to enable adequate evacuation of the hematoma. The wound can subsequently be resutured or allowed to heal via second intention.

Infection

The risk of surgical site infection (SSI) following dermatologic surgery is usually less than 5%.[1] *Staphylococcus aureus* is the most common, isolated organism in SSIs.[2] When reviewing postoperative care instructions, patients should be thoroughly educated regarding the signs and symptoms of SSI, which include an increase in erythema, pain, warmth, and/or edema at the wound site. These signs and symptoms typically present 4–6 days postoperatively. Patients should be strongly encouraged to contact the clinic if they have any questions/concerns regarding the surgical wound.

Usually SSI associated with dermatologic surgery can be managed on an outpatient basis. If possible, exudate from the surgical wound should be collected for bacterial culture and sensitivity. Patients should be started on broad-spectrum antibiotics with close follow-up care to monitor clinical response. The potential sequelae of wound infection include pain, prolonged healing, and altered aesthetic outcome.

Infection control and prevention includes thoroughly reviewing the patient's medical history and medication list to identify patients at a higher risk of SSI. Risk factors include diabetes, poor nutrition, and immune suppression (e.g., transplant patients, patients undergoing chemotherapy, HIV). For patients undergoing dermatologic procedures around the lips, it is important to inquire about a history of herpes infection. If patients have a history of cold sores, they should be prescribed prophylactic oral antiviral therapy with acyclovir or a related medication.

Another important aspect of infection control/prevention is strict surgical aseptic protocol by the surgical team.

The use of oral postoperative antibiotics following dermatologic procedures remains a controversial topic. Surgical sites at higher risk for SSI include the lower extremities, genitals, ear, nose, eyelids, and lips. Thus when surgery is performed at these locations, the dermatologic surgeon may opt to prescribe a short 5–7 day course of oral antibiotics.

Wound Dehiscence

Wound dehiscence is the unintentional separation and reopening of the wound following surgery. This occurs when there is excessive tension and strain on the wound edges. For instance, inadequate undermining during surgery can result in increased tension on the wound edges. Surgical wounds located on highly mobile and high-tension areas, such as the hands, back, shoulders, or lower extremities, are at a higher risk for wound dehiscence. Other risk factors include tobacco use, previous scarring or radiation to the surgical site, and chronic use of topical or systemic corticosteroids. Poor patient compliance regarding wound care instructions, such as failure to avoid exertional activities for 1–2 weeks following surgery, can result in wound dehiscence. In addition, blunt trauma to the surgical site following suture removal can result in wound dehiscence, since scar tissue is weaker than surrounding, unaffected tissue, especially during the first 4 weeks postprocedure. At the time of suture removal, Steri-Strips can be placed to help decrease tension on the surgical wounds.

The management of wound dehiscence includes resuturing the wound edges versus allowing small dehiscent areas to heal by second intention. One should consider reclosure of the wound with sutures if dehiscence occurs within a few days following the initial procedure, if there is no evidence of infection, or if there is a deep dehiscent area. Oral antibiotics should be started if there are signs/symptoms of infection. Close follow-up care is critical to ensure assessment of the healing process and aesthetic outcome.

Eyelid Swelling/Lymphedema

Prolonged swelling of the lower eyelids due to lymphedema is a potential complication of procedures involving the lower eyelid and upper cheek. Lymphatic drainage of the eyelid primarily occurs laterally and inferiorly along the cheek. Excess wound closure tension, particularly on the lateral cheek and lower eyelid, results in temporary compression of the eyelid lymphatics, thereby impairing drainage of lymph fluid. In addition, lymphedema can result from disruption of the lymphatic system during tissue undermining. Therefore the surgeon can minimize the risk of lymphedema by doing minimal undermining in the lower eyelid region. To avoid exacerbating lymphedema, patients should be advised to avoid rubbing the lower eyelid and cheek, as this friction and blunt trauma can result in additional disruption of the eyelid lymphatic drainage system. Usually lymphedema will gradually resolve with time. However, if there has been extensive disruption of the lymphatics, the lymphedema may be chronic and persistent.

Ectropion

Ectropion is a condition in which the lower eyelid is turned outward, thereby leaving the inner eyelid surface exposed, resulting in irritation to the cornea. In addition, the lower eyelid eversion can result in an inability to fully close the eye. The most common cause of ectropion is wound closure tension vectors that result in downward displacement and eversion of the lower eyelid. Postoperative edema can cause temporary ectropion that gradually resolves with the swelling. In addition, injury to the branch of the facial nerve (CN VII) that innervates the orbicularis oculi muscle, which functions to close the eye, can result in ectropion.

To reduce the risk of ectropion, the surgeon should avoid placing sutures that result in wound tension creating downward pull on the lower eyelid. Therefore the orientation of the key sutures to close the primary defect is critical, since it determines the tension vector on the wound edges. Ideally the key sutures should be placed perpendicular to the lower eyelid margin. By doing this, the surgeon can avoid downward pull and eversion of the lower eyelid.

Patients with ectropion should be advised to use over-the-counter, lubricating eye drops several times a day to reduce dryness and irritation of the cornea. Options for surgical management of ectropion include canthopexy versus a full-thickness skin graft.

Motor Nerve Deficits

Prior to performing any procedure, the surgeon should consider if there are any major motor nerves within the surgical zone that could possibly be damaged. Before obtaining written, informed consent from the patient, the surgeon must educate the patient regarding potential complications, including possible nerve damage. To avoid nerve damage, it is critical for the surgeon to have a detailed knowledge of the anatomy of the head and neck and pay close attention to the tissue plane of undermining. Refer to the Chapter 1 discussion on anatomy for a detailed explanation of the danger zones and proper undermining plane for the various regions on the face.

Scars

Scar formation is an inevitable consequence of cutaneous surgery. The primary goals of surgical repair include (1) preserving/restoring function of anatomical units/subunits; (2) creating a minimally visible, fine-line scar; and (3) preserving/maintaining symmetry and contour of anatomical units. From the patient's perspective, one of the most significant factors determining the success of a cutaneous surgical procedure is the aesthetic appearance of the final scar. Therefore the surgeon should be familiar with various techniques to improve the appearance of the final surgical scar. This includes surgical techniques during the initial repair, as well as techniques for revising the scar.

There are several ways to classify scars. For instance, scars can be classified by their underlying cause, such as surgical scars, acne scars (which can be further subclassified into depressed scars, including boxcar, icepick, and rolling scars), raised scars (which are subclassified into hypertrophic and keloid scars), and scars secondary to trauma (e.g., lacerations, abrasions, thermal burns, chemical burns). Another means to classify scars is to categorize them as being either raised or depressed. The International Advisory Panel on Scar Management classifies scars via the following categories: mature, immature, linear hypertrophic, widespread hypertrophic, minor keloid, and major keloid.[3]

When evaluating and describing scars, one should note the following features: thickness, visibility, erythema, contour, texture, vascularity, hypopigmentation or hyperpigmentation, symmetry to contralateral side, and relation to relaxed skin tension lines (RSTLs). In addition, it is important to note whether the patient is experiencing functional impairment of the involved anatomical unit/subunits, such as inability to fully close or open the eyes, difficulty breathing through the nose due to nasal valve collapse, and inability to open or close the mouth. Successful scar revision is usually optimized with a combination approach to address these different features.

Scar Revision

The main goals of scar revision are to make scars less noticeable and more aesthetically acceptable. Prior to performing scar revision, the surgeon should discuss the realistic, expected outcomes and manage patient expectations.

Improving surgical outcomes and minimizing the visibility of scars entails the surgeon having a sound understanding of anatomical form, the function of anatomical subunits, and an appreciation for free margins. When assessing a scar, just as when assessing a surgical wound, the surgeon should note which cosmetic units and subunits the defect involves, have a good understanding of tissue recruitment and tension vectors, and determine the direction of the RSTLs. Meticulous surgical technique always plays a key role in surgical aesthetic outcomes. Important features of meticulous surgical technique include minimizing wound tension, good reapproximation of fresh wound edges, and wound edge eversion. Precise surgical technique is key, as failure to properly align wound edges will result in an irregular scar (Fig. 18.1).

Postoperative care also plays a major role on aesthetic outcomes. Patient compliance, in regard to wound care management, can significantly impact the final appearance of the scar. During the postoperative period, patients should be advised to keep the wound clean, as well as covered with emollients (e.g., petrolatum) and an occlusive dressing. Similarly, wearing compression dressings and avoiding exertional activities that place increased tension on the wound are important aspects of wound care. It is important for the nursing staff to counsel patients and their family/caregivers regarding postoperative wound care. In addition to providing verbal instructions, patients find printed handouts to be very helpful. Patients should have access and be encouraged to contact the clinic, should they have questions/concerns regarding their surgical wound and postoperative care. In addition, a postoperative follow-up visit is necessary to evaluate aesthetic and functional outcomes.

Surgeons should continuously review their outcomes to further improve their technique. We recommend taking photographs of the surgical site at various stages, including (1) prior to surgical closure, (2) immediately following repair, and (3) at subsequent follow-up visits. In addition, it is helpful to make notes regarding the types of sutures and closure techniques used, so the surgeon can further refine his or her surgical skills.

A variety of surgical and nonsurgical techniques exist for revising scars. We will start by reviewing nonsurgical options, which include intralesional injections, dermabrasion, microneedling, subcision, soft tissue fillers, and laser treatment.

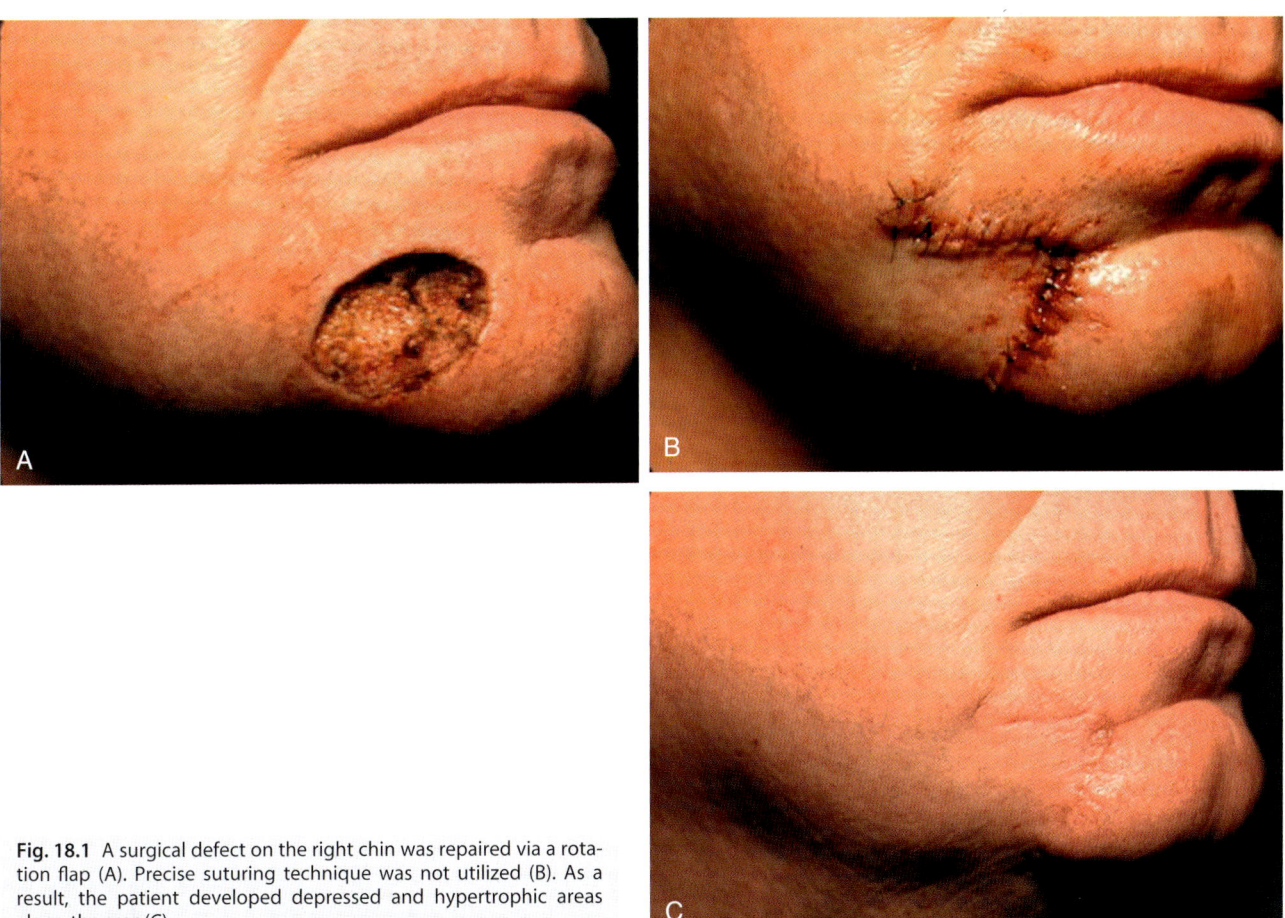

Fig. 18.1 A surgical defect on the right chin was repaired via a rotation flap (A). Precise suturing technique was not utilized (B). As a result, the patient developed depressed and hypertrophic areas along the scar (C).

Intralesional Injections

Intralesional triamcinolone (ILT) is frequently used for hypertrophic and keloid scars. ILT can be helpful for revising bulky, elevated skin caused by "trapdoor deformity" from skin flaps. Intralesional corticosteroids suppress inflammation, reduce collagen synthesis, and inhibit fibroblast growth. In addition, they also enhance fibroblast and collagen degeneration. The response rate varies widely, between 10% and 50% reduction, and is more effective on earlier rather than more mature scars.

A small amount of low-strength steroid is injected into the scar only, not any adjacent skin. A slight blanching of the scar is a good endpoint, as it is typically observed when an appropriate quantity of ILT has been injected. The procedure is generally repeated on a monthly basis to achieve optimal results. Caution must be taken with regard to the strength, quantity, and placement of the steroid dose, since aggressive treatment can result in skin atrophy, hypopigmentation, and telangiectasia. It is better to start with a lower concentration of steroids. Some surgeons use light cryotherapy prior to the steroid injection. Liquid nitrogen produces some edema to make injections easier and produces some vascular damage that leads to tissue anoxia and destruction.

In addition to ILT, the use of intralesional 5-fluorouracil (5-FU) has been reported to be beneficial in the treatment of hypertrophic scars. 5-FU is an antimetabolite that inhibits fibroblast proliferation. It inhibits thymidylate synthetase and therefore DNA synthesis. By inhibiting DNA synthesis, it increases fibroblast apoptosis. Injections are done in a similar fashion to that of ILT, filling the scar just enough to blanch it. The response rate varies but has been reported to be approximately 50% on keloids injected weekly. The primary benefit of 5-FU is the lack of atrophy or erythema associated with steroid injections. The use of combination ILT and 5-FU has been demonstrated to be at least as efficacious as ILT alone in the treatment of hypertrophic scars with fewer side effects.[4,5] Side effects reported from intralesional 5-FU include injection-site irritation, skin hyperpigmentation, and ulceration.[6] Treatment with 5-FU is contraindicated during pregnancy and in patients with bone marrow suppression.

Interferon and bleomycin have also been injected into keloidal scars with good results. Both interferon and bleomycin affect transforming growth factor β-1 and decrease collagen synthesis.

Dermabrasion

Dermabrasion entails the removal of the superficial layers of the skin using an abrasive tool. It may be performed with sterilized, very fine gauge sandpaper, or an electrically powered dermabrasion system utilizing a spinning diamond fraise or wire brush. Dermabrasion works best on scars with irregular texture, skin grafts, and elevated flaps (i.e., trapdoor deformity). In addition, dermabrasion is sometimes useful for depressed scars with sharp edges as it will soften the edges of the scar to reduce shadowing and make the scar less visible.

During dermabrasion the skin is abraded to the level of the papillary or reticular dermis. The endpoint is fine pinpoint bleeding. If dermabrasion extends too deeply into the dermis or subcutaneous adipose tissue, the scar can potentially increase in severity. Postoperative care is the same as any open wound, keeping the area clean and moist with a petrolatum ointment until complete healing is achieved.

Microneedling

Microneedling involves the use of a device with numerous small, minimally invasive needles that puncture the epidermis and superficial dermis. The punctures create a multitude of tiny wounds that in turn induce a wound healing response, which leads to neocollagenesis, dermal remodeling, and improvement in scar texture.

Recent anecdotal reports have described the application of topical steroids, platelet-rich plasma, and growth factors to the skin immediately following microneedling and fractionated lasers. The microscopic holes created by the needle or laser allow increased absorption of topical products. The long-term benefits of microneedling, with and without the use of topical products, need to be further investigated to assess the consistency and efficacy of these treatments for both atrophic and hypertrophic scars.

Subcision

Subcision is a revision technique to consider for atrophic, depressed scars, especially oval or circular scars (e.g., punch biopsy scars, acne scars, and postvaricella scars). The procedure entails insertion of a needle obliquely into the dermis to break up collagen bundles, thereby releasing the scar and triggering new collagen production. Subcision can be performed alone or in combination with soft tissue fillers.[6]

Soft Tissue/Dermal Fillers

Soft tissue/dermal fillers can be used to add volume and elevate depressed scars. While the majority of soft tissue fillers are not permanent and are degraded over time, most will result in some long-term improvement of depressed scars. This is likely a result of some neocollagenesis that occurs with the trauma of the injection itself (akin to microneedling), as well as the effect of the filler product. Patients should be counseled on the temporary effects of such treatment and that repeat injections would be required to keep the volume optimized. In addition, some scars that are more epidermal in nature and bound down do not respond to injections with filler products. A small and very slow test injection should be done to see how a scar responds to treatment.

Laser Treatment

A variety of laser devices can be utilized to improve surgical scars. Erythematous scars may be targeted with vascular devices such as the pulsed dye (585 or 595 nm) or potassium titanyl phosphate (KTP) (532 nm) lasers (Fig. 18.2).[7] Hypertrophic scars can be treated with pulsed dye laser (PDL), KTP, as well as ablative and nonablative fractional devices. Atrophic scars can be improved with ablative and nonablative fractional devices.

Alster first described the use of PDLs in hypertrophic and keloidal sternotomy scars back in 1995.[8] She noted significant improvement in the vascularity of the scar, as well as the scar height, texture, and pruritus. It was hypothesized that destruction of the microvasculature produced local ischemia and reduced collagen. Subsequent studies have exhibited significant and persistent improvement in scar thickness, pliability, and pruritus in hypertrophic and keloid scars treated with the PDL.[9,10] While the full mechanism by which PDL induces the regression of hypertrophic and keloid scars remains under investigation, in vitro studies have demonstrated that PDL inhibits the expression of connective tissue growth factor and inhibits the proliferation of keloid fibroblasts.[11] In addition, PDL has been demonstrated to suppress TGFB1 and upregulate matrix metalloproteinase, which helps facilitate the regression of hypertrophic scars.[12,13]

Treatment with the PDL is usually well tolerated and results in minimal downtime. Common side effects include a temporary increase in erythema, mild edema, and post-treatment purpura. These side effects typically resolve within 7–10 days. An alternative treatment option for scar erythema is KTP and intense pulsed light (IPL). Asilian showed that the combination of ILT, 5-FU, and PDL was more effective than any of the modalities alone. In a split scar study, Nouri also showed PDL treatment following suture removal of a surgical scar improved overall appearance over no treatment.

Prior to the advent of fractionated devices, a variety of nonablative lasers had been used to revise atrophic scars. These devices included the 1064 nm neodymium-doped-yttrium-aluminum garnet (Nd:YAG) and 1320 nm and 1450 nm diode lasers. However, the clinical outcomes were variable with these devices.[6]

Nonablative and ablative fractional resurfacing lasers (NAFR; AFR) have revolutionized the treatment of surgical scars. These laser devices thermally heat (nonablative) and or ablate (ablative) microscopic columns of epidermal and dermal tissue at regularly spaced intervals. Sufficient laser energy within the laser columns is required to induce local thermal damage without spreading to adjacent tissue. The thermal damage from these lasers helps promote wound healing by inducing collagen synthesis. The intact, unaltered skin between the microscopic treatment zones (MTZs) produces rapid healing of the treated areas and allows high energies to be used that create wounds far deeper than those seen with dermabrasion or traditional laser resurfacing. This increased depth of penetration allows remodeling to occur much deeper into scars than was possible with prior devices. The drawback is that since only a fraction of the surface area is affected in any given treatment, multiple treatments are generally required for optimal results.

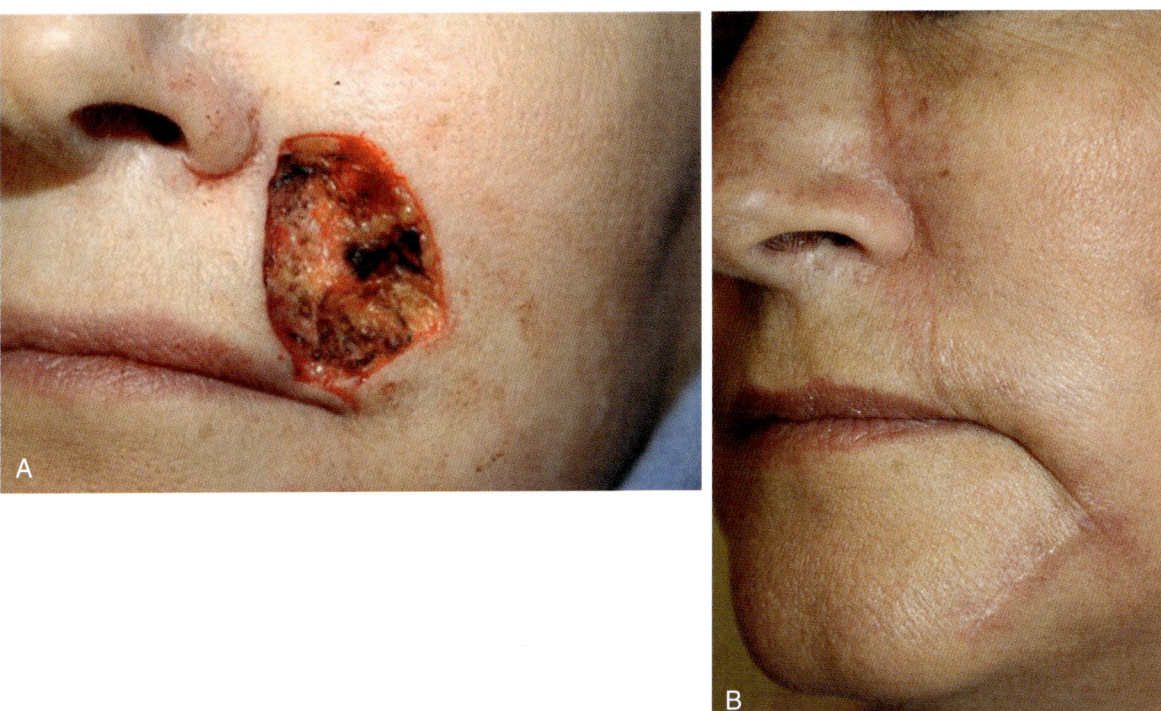

Fig. 18.2 An advancement flap was used to close the large defect (A). At the patient's 6-week postoperative visit, she was noted to have a red, slightly hypertrophic surgical scar (B). This type of scar can be treated with a pulsed dye laser or fractionated CO_2 laser.

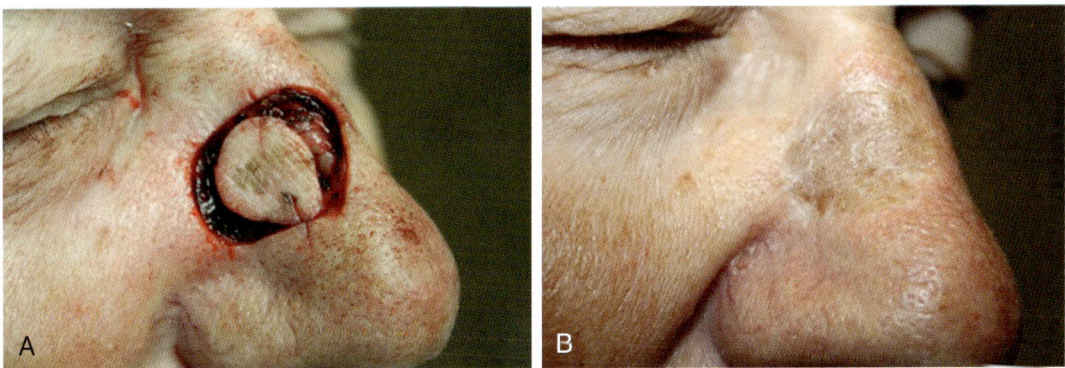

Fig. 18.3 (A) A full-thickness skin graft was used to repair a surgical defect on the nasal sidewall following removal of a melanoma in situ. (B) The irregular texture and pigmentation can be improved with fractionated CO_2 laser.

Fractional resurfacing can be utilized to improve a variety of scar features, including hyperpigmentation and hypopigmentation, hypertrophy, atrophy, contractures, and texture irregularity. In essence, fractional devices replace small amounts of damaged skin, and the body replaces them with more normal skin. They should be thought of as skin normalizing devices. Lax skin tightens, contracted skin relaxes, elevated areas flatten, and depressed areas elevate.

Fractional devices can be used alone or in combination with other treatment modalities to achieve cosmetic improvement in surgical scars. For example, non-AFR with the 1550 nm erbium-doped laser has been used alone or with bimatoprost to treat hypopigmented scars. Following two to four fractional resurfacing treatments using the 1550 nm erbium laser alone, the majority of patients exhibited 50%–75% improvement in hypopigmented scars.[14]

With topical bimatoprost, patients exhibited 50%–75% improvement in their hypopigmented scars.[15] AFR with the CO_2 laser has also demonstrated effectiveness in the management of hypopigmented scars.[16]

Fractional ablative lasers have also been used to treat hyperpigmented scars. The mechanism by which fractional laser resurfacing helps improve the pigmentation of scars is likely that the MTZs created by the laser promotes the extrusion of melanocytes and microscopic epidermal debris, thereby allowing more normal keratinocytes and melanocytes to repopulate these areas.[17–19]

Ablative and nonablative laser resurfacing can improve the appearance of full-thickness skin grafts (FTSGs) that do not match the recipient site perfectly (Fig. 18.3).

The concept of laser-assisted drug delivery is a rapidly evolving area of interest in the management of surgical scars. Waibel et al. demonstrated that fractional CO_2 laser therapy used in combination with delivery of topical triamcinolone may be a safe and effective for the management of hypertrophic scars.[20] The density of the fractional injuries seems to be more important than the depth of the column created by the device in the effectiveness of topical drug delivery. In fact, since the dermal vascular plexus is at a depth of approximately 100–300 μm, deeper fractional injuries may result in decreased effectiveness. Promising work is presently being done on stem cell delivery through fractional injuries.

Surgical Options for Scar Revision

A variety of surgical techniques can be utilized to revise cutaneous surgical scars. Fusiform excision is a good option for widened scars oriented within RSTLs that exhibit atrophy, hypertrophy, or irregular contour. The primary goal is to create a fine-line, minimally visible scar. The existing, linear scar tissue is excised with narrow margins and then resutured. Of note, the resulting scar may be slightly greater in length.

Z-plasty is a useful option to reorient visible scars that are not within RSTLs, or to elongate contracted scars, such as scars involving the medical canthus that result in webbing. Similarly, it is a good option for contracted scars involving free margins, such as the lips. Contracted scars of the upper and lower lip can result in impaired function of the mouth.

Z-plasty is technically a transposition flap (Fig. 18.4). The technique breaks up a linear scar into a zigzag, irregular line, thereby increasing the length of the scar and potentially decreasing the visibility of the scar. To perform Z-plasty, the original scar line is used as the common diagonal. Two triangles of the same size are extended in opposite directions with the base of the triangles being the common diagonal. Of note, the size of the angle between the arm of the triangle and the common diagonal determines the degree of lengthening of the scar. A 30-degree angle will lengthen the scar by 25%. Similarly, the following angles will increase the scar length by the following percentages: 45 degrees → 50%, 60 degrees → 75%, and 75 degrees → 100%. Of note, an angle greater than 60 degrees will increase the force needed to transpose the flaps, thereby increasing the tension needed for closure of the secondary defects.

Similar to Z-plasty, some surgeons use either W-plasty or geometric broken-line closures (GBLC) to help decrease the visibility of longer scars. Both of these techniques involve creating a zigzag, irregular scar line. The primary principle behind these irregular, broken-line scars is to reduce the visibility of the scar, since such scars are less perceptible to the eye compared with straight-line scars.[21] W-plasty is a good option for scars that are oriented at an angle greater than 35 degrees to RSTLs and scars located on convex, curved surfaces, such as the mandible and chin. In comparison, GBLC is good for long scars that are oriented at an angle 45 degrees or greater to RSTLs. GBLC is also useful for scars located over convex or concave surfaces.[22] Recent studies have cast doubt on this theory and shown that longer broken line closures may actually be more visibly and aesthetically displeasing than a linear closure.

To perform W-plasty, a marking pen is used to draw a series of equal-sized triangles along one side of the scar, with a mirror image on the other side (Fig. 18.5). The apex points of the triangles should be 3–5 mm from the scar. The angle of the triangular apex is usually 60–90 degrees. The distance between the apex points of adjacent triangles should be 5–6 mm. The limbs of the triangles should be 3–5 mm in length. The scar is then excised, incisions are made along the triangular lines of the W-plasty, and the

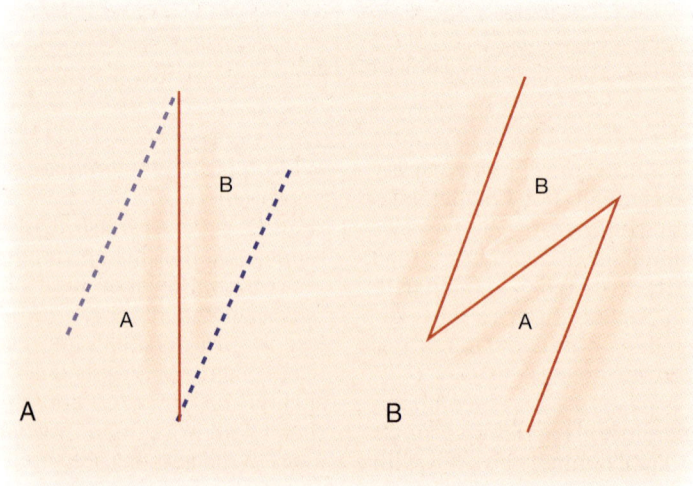

Fig. 18.4 Diagram of a Z-plasty. (A) The vertically oriented solid line represents the scar, which serves as the common diagonal for the Z-plasty. In this example, the angle between the common diagonal and arm of each triangle is 30 degrees. Hence this will lengthen the scar by 25%. (B) The two triangular flaps are subsequently transposed, resulting in a zigzag scar.

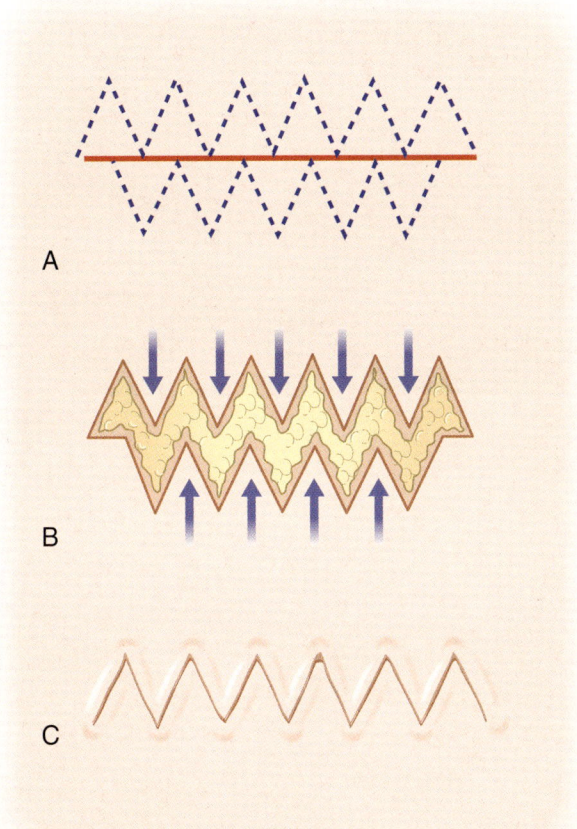

Fig. 18.5 Diagram of a W-plasty. (A) A series of equal-sized triangles are drawn along one side of the scar, with a mirror image on the other side. (B) Incisional cuts are made along the outline of the W-plasty, with subsequent excision of the central scar. (C) The wound edges are aligned by interdigitating the triangles, subsequently resulting in a single zigzag.

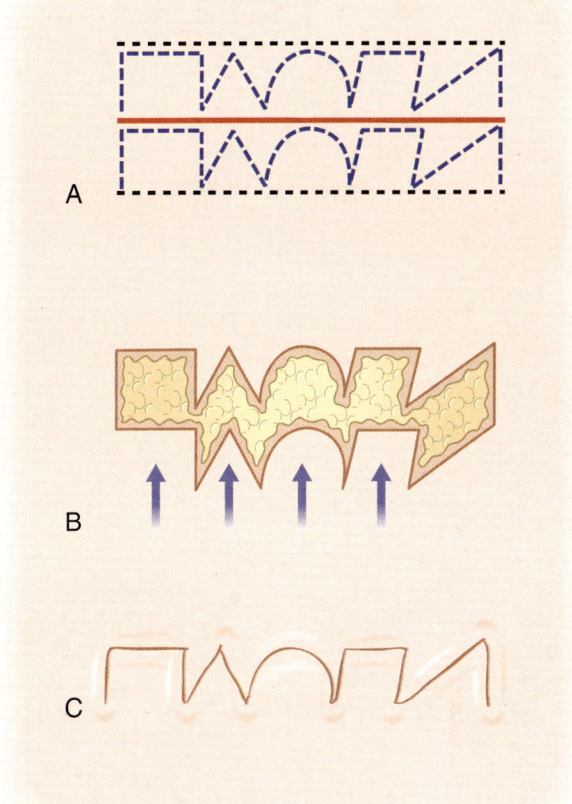

Fig. 18.6 Diagram of a geometric broken line closure. (A) Two dotted lines are drawn with a marking pen on either side of the scar. These lines should be of equal distance from the scar. On one side of the scar a series of random, geometric shapes is drawn. The shapes should extend to the margin of the dotted line. On the opposite side of the scar, a mirror image of the geometric pattern is made. (B) An incision is made along the outline of the geometric pattern, and the scar is excised. (C) The edges are aligned by advancing the interposed geometric shapes, thereby resulting in a single, irregular line.

underling tissue is undermined. The wound edges are subsequently realigned by interdigitating the triangles to form a single zigzag line.[22]

To perform GBLC, a marking pen is used to draw a dotted line at a distance of 3–6 mm on either side of the scar. On one side of the scar, an outline is drawn consisting of random, irregular geometric shapes, such as semicircles, triangles, rectangles, and squares. These shapes should extend to the margins of the dotted line. A mirror image of the geometric pattern is made on the other side of the scar, which will enable a succession of interposed flaps. Similar to W-plasty, the scar is excised, the geometric pattern is incised, and the wound edges are realigned by interposing the geometric shapes.

Certain surgical repairs, such as advancement and transposition flaps, can lead to "trapdoor deformity," which is characterized by a pronounced, elevated, thick skin flap (Fig. 18.6). Initially, "trapdoor deformity" can be treated conservatively with ILT and 5-FU injections. Often a series of injections, interspaced 4–6 weeks apart, is necessary. Injections can be used in combination with other scar revision procedures, such as laser resurfacing and dermabrasion. If these minimally invasive procedures do not yield satisfactory improvement, surgical debulking of the scar (Fig. 18.7) is generally performed. An incision is made along the scar to allow elevation of the flap. The bulky scar and adipose tissue is excised in thin layers, using a scalpel blade until it matches normal contour. It is better to conservatively excise the excess scar tissue, as too aggressive debulking will result in a depressed flap.

Timing of Scar Revision

The optimal timing of scar revision remains a debatable topic. Since surgical scars may require one or more years to fully mature, many physicians recommend waiting at least 6 months postprocedure before considering scar revision. However, the use of nonsurgical modalities can be considered earlier in the healing process. For instance,

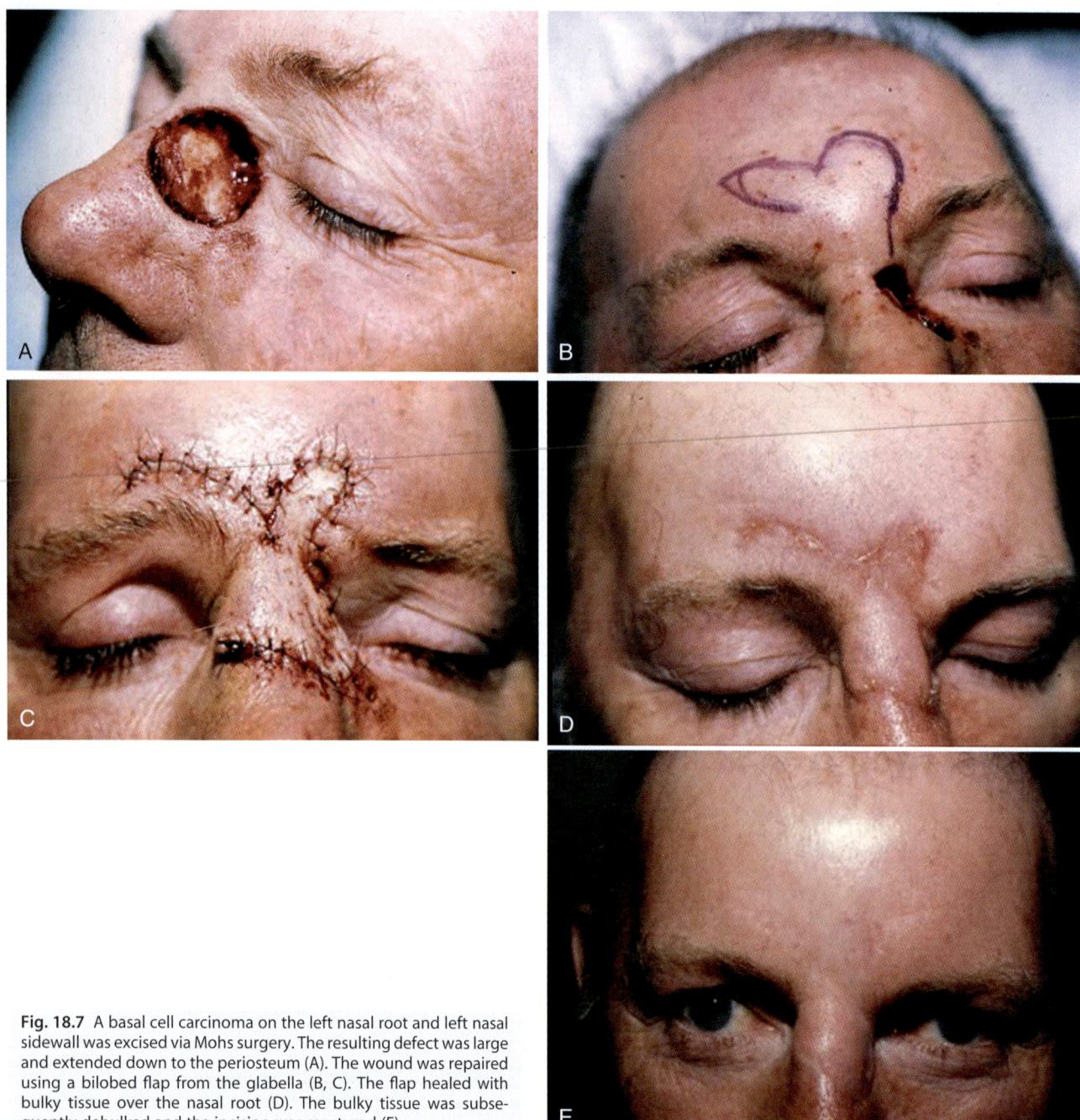

Fig. 18.7 A basal cell carcinoma on the left nasal root and left nasal sidewall was excised via Mohs surgery. The resulting defect was large and extended down to the periosteum (A). The wound was repaired using a bilobed flap from the glabella (B, C). The flap healed with bulky tissue over the nasal root (D). The bulky tissue was subsequently debulked and the incision was resutured (E).

laser treatments are generally most effective when initiated within a several weeks of the initial surgery. Dermabrasion has been shown to be most effective when performed 2–3 months following the initial surgical procedure.

Conclusion

All surgical procedures produce a scar. The goal is to produce the least noticeable scar possible. Surgical scars are influenced by a diversity of factors, including the surgeon's understanding of anatomy and wound healing, the surgeon's personal experience with reconstruction and scar revision, meticulous planning and surgical technique, and patient compliance in wound care.

Prior to proceeding with scar revision, it is important the physicians counsel the patient regarding the different revision options, including their risks, benefits, and expected outcomes. Understanding and managing patient expectations is a major component of patient counseling. Although two of the primary goals of scar revision are to improve the aesthetic appearance of the scar and reduce the visibility of the scar, the patient needs to understand that the scar cannot be completely erased. In addition, the patient should understand that two or more revision treatments may be required to obtain the desired outcome.

References

1. Dixon AJ, Dixon MP, Askew DA, Wilkinson D. Prospective study of wound infections in dermatologic surgery in the absence of prophylactic antibiotics. *Dermatol Surg.* 2006;32:819-826, discussion 26-27.
2. Saleh K, Schmidtchn A. Surgical site infections in dermatologic surgery: etiology, pathogenesis, and current preventatitive measures. *Dermatol Surg.* 2015;41:537-549.
3. Mustoe TA, Cooter RD, Gold MH, et al. International clinical recommendations on scar management. *Plast Reconstr Surg.* 2002;110:560-571.
4. Manuskiatti W, Fitzpatrick RE. Treatment response of keloidal and hypertrophic sternotomy scars: comparison among intralesional corticosteroid, 5-fluorouracil, and 585-nm flashlamp-pumped pulse dye laser treatments. *Arch Dermatol.* 2002;138:1149-1155.
5. Darougheh A, Asilian A, Shariati F. Intralesional triamcinolone alone or in combination with 5-fluorouracil for the treatment of keloid and hypertrophic scars. *Clin Exp Dermatol.* 2009;34:219-223.
6. Balaraman B, Geddes E, Friedman P. Best reconstructive techniques: improving the final scar. *Dermatol Surg.* 2015;41(suppl 10):S265-S275.
7. Eilers RE Jr, Ross EV, Cohen JL, Ortiz AE. A combination approach to surgical scars. *Dermatol Surg.* 2016;42(suppl 2):S150-S156.
8. Alster TS, Williams CM. Treatment of keloid sternotomy scars with 585 nm flashlamp-pumped pulsed-dye laser. *Lancet.* 1995;345:1198-1200.
9. Manuskiatti W, Fitzpatrick RE, Goldman MP. Energy density and numbers of treatment affect response of keloidal and hypertrophic sternotomy scars to the 585-nm flashlamp-pumped pulsed-dye laser. *J Am Acad Dermatol.* 2001;45:557-565.
10. Brewin MP, Lister TS. Prevention or treatment of hypertrophic burn scarring: a review of when and how to treat with the pulsed dye laser. *Burns.* 2014;40(5):797-804.
11. Zhu R, Yue B, Yang Q, et al. The effect of 595 nm pulsed dye laser on connective tissue growth factor (CTGF) expression in cultured keloid fibroblasts. *Lasers Surg Med.* 2015;47:203-209.
12. Kuo YR, Jeng SF, Wang FS, et al. Flashlamp pulsed dye laser (PDL) suppression of keloid proliferation through down-regulation of TGF-beta1 expression and extracellular matrix expression. *Lasers Surg Med.* 2004;34:104-108.
13. Kuo YR, Wu WS, Jeng SF, et al. Suppressed TGF-beta1 expression is correlated with up-regulation of matrix metalloproteinase-13 in keloid regression after flashlamp pulsed-dye laser treatment. *Lasers Surg Med.* 2005;36:38-42.
14. Glaich AS, Rahman Z, Goldberg LH, Friedman PM. Fractional resurfacing for the treatment of hypopigmented scars: a pilot study. *Dermatol Surg.* 2007;33:289-294.
15. Massaki AB, Fabi SG, Fitzpatrick R. Repigmentation of hypopigmented scars using an erbium-doped 1,550-nm fractionated laser and topical bimatoprost. *Dermatol Surg.* 2012;38(7 Pt 1):995-1001.
16. Tierney EP, Hanke CW. Treatment of CO_2 laser induced hypopigmentation with ablative fractionated laser resurfacing: case report and review of the literature. *J Drugs Dermatol.* 2010;9(11):1420-1426.
17. Manstein D, Herron GS, Sink RK, Tanner H, Anderson RR. Fractional photothermolysis: a new concept for cutaneous remodeling using microscopic patterns of thermal injury. *Lasers Surg Med.* 2004;34:426-438.
18. Laubach HJ, Tannous Z, Anderson RR, Manstein D. Skin responses to fractional photothermolysis. *Lasers Surg Med.* 2006;38:142-149.
19. Hantash BM, Bedi VP, Sudireddy V, Struck SK, Herron GS, Chan KF. Laser-induced transepidermal elimination of dermal content by fractional photothermolysis. *J Biomed Opt.* 2006;11:041115.
20. Waibel JS, Wulkan AJ, Shumaker PR. Treatment of hypertrophic scars using laser and laser assisted corticosteroid delivery. *Lasers Surg Med.* 2013;45:135-140.
21. Rodgers BJ, Williams EF, Hove CR. W-plasty and geometric broken line closure. *Facial Plast Surg.* 2001;17:239-244.
22. Garg S, Dahiya N, Gupta S. Surgical scar revision: an overview. *J Cutan Aesthet Surg.* 2017;7:3-13.

Index

A

Abbé (lip-switch) flap, 127–129
　anatomy of, 127, 127f
　execution for, 128, 129f, 129t
　flap design for, 127–128, 128f
　indications for, 127
　postoperative care for, 128–129
　stage II, 129–130, 130f
Ablative fractional resurfacing lasers (AFR)
　full-thickness skin grafts (FTSGs) and, 305, 305f
　for scar revision, 304
Adjacent tissue transfer, for ear reconstruction, 212–213, 213f–215f
Advancement flaps, 21–23, 21f, 24f–25f, 50–70, 82
　advantage of, 50
　design and considerations for, 50, 51f–52f
　disadvantages of, 68
　for forehead and temple repair, 158–162, 159f–161f, 160b
　mobilization and key sutures, 50–53, 52f
　modifications and applications, 53–68
　　Burow triangle flap, 58–61, 61f–63f
　　cheek, 60f, 61–63, 64f
　　crescentic, 64–68
　　helical rim, 63–64, 65f–66f
　　H-plasty or bilateral, 53–56, 54f–56f
　　L-plasty, 58, 59f–60f
　　Peng flap, 68, 69f
　　T-plasty, 56–58, 57f–59f
　in nasal reconstruction, 235–238, 236f–237f
　　Burow, 237, 237f
　　island, 238, 239f
　　V-Y, 237–238, 238f
　for neck reconstruction, 292–293, 296f
　for scalp reconstruction, 150, 151f
Advancement-rotation flaps, in perioral reconstruction, 267–275
　Burow wedge, 267, 268f–269f
　full-thickness circumoral flap, 272–275
　rotation flap, 269–270, 270f–272f
　V-Y advancement flap, 270–272, 272f–278f
Aesthetic subunits, nose, 223, 224f
Aesthetics, of ear, 210, 211f
Aging face, 3–4
Ala nasi, 13
Alar cartilage, 13
Alar collapse, in nasal reconstruction, 252–255
Anatomy, 1–15
　aging face, 3–4
　motor nerves, 7–8
　musculoaponeurotic system, 4–7
　perioral, 258–259
　special structures, 12–15
　surface landmarks, 1–3
　vascular, 10–12
　see also individual procedures
Anchoring suture, 3
Anesthesia, 118–119

Page numbers followed by f indicate figures; t, tables; b, boxes.

Angular artery, 10–11, 10f–11f
Anterior ethmoid nerve, 9–10
Antibiotics, oral, postoperative, 301
Anticoagulant therapy, continuation of, before surgery, 300
Antihelix, 15
Arnold nerve, 212
Arterial flaps, 16
Arteries
　angular, 10–11, 10f–11f
　carotid. see Carotid system
　facial, 2f, 10–11, 12f, 259
　internal maxillary, 11
　labial, 10–11
　lacrimal, 11f
　of neck, 289–291
　occipital, 11
　ophthalmic, 10–11
　postauricular, 11
　posterior auricular, 211
　superficial temporal, 11, 145, 211
　supraorbital, 11
　supratrochlear, 11
　temporal, 11, 157f
Artificial dermal grafts, scalp reconstruction and, 149
Auricular defects, 92
Auriculotemporal nerve, 212
Axial dorsal nasal rotation flap, 75
Axial flaps, 16
Axial vessel, 84

B

Banner-type flaps, 103, 103f–105f
Bilateral advancement flap, 53–56
　see also H-plasty
Bilateral rotation flaps, 73, 74f
Bilobed flap, 25, 28f, 105–108, 106f–109f
　for nasal reconstruction, 242–243, 244f–245f
Bleeding, postoperative, 300
　excessive, treatment of, 300
Bleomycin, for keloidal scars, 303
Blepharoplasty advancement flap, for defects below lid margin, 174f
Blood supply, flaps defined by, 16–18, 17f–18f
Buccal fat pad, 184
Buccal nerve, 7f, 8
Burow advancement flap, in nasal reconstruction, 237, 237f
Burow triangle, 21f, 23, 26f, 51f, 53, 53f
　for ear reconstruction, 212
　flap, 58–61, 61f–63f
Burow grafts, 231
　scalp reconstruction and, 149–150
Burow wedge flap, 58
　as cutaneous advancement flap, in perioral reconstruction, 267, 268f–269f

C

Canthus
　inner, tenting, 206
　lateral, 110, 111f

medial, 110, 111f
　anatomy of, 175
　defects of, 93f–94f, 175–176, 175f–178f
　wounds of, second intention healing and, 34–35, 37f
　rhombic flap for, 111f
　transposition flap for, 110, 111f
Carotid system
　external, 10–11, 11f
　internal, 11–12
Cartilage, 213–214, 216f
　alar (lower lateral), 13
　nasal septum, 13
　upper lateral, 13
Cartilage grafts, 140
Cervical nerve, 7f, 8
Cervicofacial rotation flaps, 80
Cheek, transposition flap for, 111, 112f
Cheek advancement flap, 60f, 61–63, 64f, 167, 173f
Cheek reconstruction, 183–209
　advancement flap for, 185–188, 189f
　complications of, 202–206
　　anesthesia and, 206
　　dehiscence as, 203–206
　　ectropion as, 203
　　eyelid swelling as, 202–203
　　flap necrosis as, 203
　　hematoma as, 202
　　hypertrophic scarring and keloid formation as, 206
　　infection as, 203
　　inner canthus tenting as, 206
　　motor nerve deficits as, 206
　　parotid fistula as, 206, 208f
　　telangiectasia as, 206
　flaps by cheek region for, 185–201
　　anterior cheek, 192–194, 194f–197f
　　buccal cheek, 201
　　infraorbital cheek, 194–196
　　malar cheek, 196–201, 198f–202f
　　mandibular cheek, 201, 207f
　　medial cheek, 185–192, 186f–194f
　　preauricular cheek, 201, 203f–206f
　flaps to avoid in, 185
　procedure for, 184, 185f
　relaxed skin tension lines and, 183
　rhombic transposition flap for, 186, 188f
　skin texture and, 183–184
　special anatomic structures and, 184
　subcutaneous anatomy and, 184
　surface anatomy and, 183
　see also Periocular reconstruction
Cheek rotation flap, for defects below the lid margin, 172f
Cheek-to-nose interpolation flaps, 123–126
　anatomy of, 124
　execution for, 125, 125f, 125t
　flap design of, 124–125, 124f
　indications for, 124, 124f
　postoperative care for, 125–126
　stage II, 126–127, 126f–127f
Chin
　rotation flaps for, 80, 80f
　transposition flap for, 111, 113f
Chondrocutaneous flap, composite, 215–216, 217f

311

Cilia, 15
Circular defect, 23
Circumoral flaps, full-thickness, 272–275
Collagen, 19–20
Composite chondrocutaneous grafts, 137–138, 138f–139f
Composite grafts, 232–233, 235f
Compression dressing, for scars, 302
Concavities, second intention healing, 3
Conchal grafts, 231
Contour, normal, preservation and restoration of, primary closure and, 40–41
Convexities, second intention healing, 3
Corneal shields, 165
Corrugator supercilii muscle, 6, 155, 156f
Corticosteroids, intralesional, 303
Cosmetic subunit junction lines, scar orientation, primary closure and, 41–42, 42f
Cosmetic units, 1–2, 2f
　of forehead, 156f
　periocular, 167
　perioral reconstruction, 259f
Creep, 20
Crescentic advancement flap, 64–68
　modifications of, 64–68, 68f
　Webster perialar, 50, 52f, 64, 67f
Crescentic excision, primary closure and, 43, 44f
Cupid's bow, 258
Curvature, of rotation flaps, 71–73, 73f
Cutaneous flaps, 82, 87f

D

Defect depth, 259–260
Dehiscence, cheek reconstruction and, 203–206
Delayed knot tying technique, in full-thickness skin grafts, 138–140
Depressor labii inferioris muscle, 7
Depressor supercilii muscle, 6, 156f
Depressors, in perioral reconstruction, 258–259
Dermabrasion, for scar revision, 303–304
Dermal fillers, for scar revision, 304
"Dog ears." see Standing cone deformities
Donor sites, for full-thickness skin grafts, in nasal reconstruction, 231
Dorsal nasal rotation flap, 23, 74–75, 76f–77f
　in nasal reconstruction, 238–242, 240f–241f
　variants of, 75–76, 78f
Double 30-degree angle flap, 102, 102f
Drug delivery, laser-assisted, 305–306
DuFourmentel flap, 25, 27f, 101–102, 101f

E

Ear, 15, 15f
　composite chondrocutaneous grafts of, 137–138, 138f–139f
　wounds of, full-thickness skin grafts for, 133–134
Ear reconstruction, 210–222
　adjacent tissue transfer for, 212–213, 213f–215f
　aesthetics, 210, 211f
　cartilage in, 213–214, 216f
　embryology and, 210
　innervation and, 212
　principles, 212
　prosthetics, 222
　regional reconstruction, 214–222
　　composite chondrocutaneous flap, 215–216, 217f
　　concha, 221, 222f
　　lobule, 220–221, 221f
　　lower auricle, 220
　　middle auricle, 216–220, 218f–220f
　　posterior auricle, 221–222
　　upper auricle, 215
　skin grafts for, 212, 212f
　topography and, 210–212, 211f
　vasculature and, 211, 211f
Ectropion
　cheek reconstruction and, 203
　as surgical complication, 301–302
Elastin, 20
Elliptical excisions, 45, 47f
Erb's point, 289, 290f
External auditory meatus, 15
External jugular vein, 291
Eye, 14f
　anatomy of, 166f
Eyelids, 5–6, 13–15
　anatomy of, 165
　defects of, full-thickness skin grafts for, 134–135, 135f
　full-thickness lid defects, 176–180
　　lateral canthotomy, 178
　　primary repair, 176–178, 179f
　　tarsoconjunctival flap, 179–180, 181f
　　Tenzel semicircle flap, 178–179, 180f
　margin, defects below, flap repairs for, 167, 168f–173f
　muscles acting around, 5–6
　swelling of
　　cheek reconstruction and, 202–203
　　as surgical complication, 301
　upper, defects on, flap repairs for, 167–175, 174f
　see also Periocular reconstruction

F

Facial artery, 2f, 10–11, 12f
Facial expression, muscles of, 6f
Facial fat compartments, retaining ligaments and, 5f
Facial nerve, 7, 7f
Facial skeletal resorption, 3f
Facial vein, 184
Flaps, 3, 16–33
　advancement, 21–23, 24f–25f, 50–70, 82
　　advantage of, 50
　　design and considerations for, 50, 51f–52f
　　disadvantages of, 68
　　mobilization and key sutures, 50–53, 52f
　　modifications and applications, 53–68
　arterial, 16
　base of, 16
　basic terminology, 16, 17f
　biomechanics, 20–21, 20f
　for cheek reconstruction, 185–201
　　anterior cheek, 192–194, 194f–197f
　　buccal cheek, 201
　　infraorbital cheek, 194–196
　　malar cheek, 196–201, 198f–202f
　　mandibular cheek, 201, 207f
　　medial cheek, 185–192, 186f–194f
　　preauricular cheek, 201, 203f–206f
　composite chondrocutaneous, 215–216, 217f
　cutaneous, 82, 87f
　definition of
　　by blood supply, 16–18, 17f–18f
　　by movement, 21–27, 21f–22f
　dorsal nasal rotation, 23
　flip-flop, 92
　for forehead and temple repair, 158–162
　interpolation, 27, 116–131
　island, 82–98
　　complications, 92–98
　　modifications, 88–92, 89f–97f
　　technique, 84–88
　island pedicle, 23
　mastoid pull-through, 97f
　mucosal advancement, 87f
　for nasal reconstruction, 234–252
　　advancement, 235–238, 236f–237f
　　cutaneous, 234–235
　　interpolation, 244–252
　　rotation, 238–242, 239f
　　transposition, 242–244
　necrosis, cheek reconstruction and, 203
　pedicle of, 16
　for periocular reconstruction, 167–180, 167f
　　defects below lid margin, 167, 168f–173f
　　full-thickness lid defects, 176–180
　　medial canthal defects, 175–176, 175f–178f
　　upper lid defects, 167–175, 174f
　for perioral reconstruction
　　advancement-rotation, 267–275
　　full-thickness circumoral, 272–275
　　Karapandzic, 272–275
　　for linear closure, 265–267
　　lip switch, 283–285, 284f–285f
　　mucosal advancement, 260–262, 260f–261f
　　rotation, 269–270, 270f–272f
　　transposition, 275–285, 279f–283f
　　V-Y advancement, 270–272, 272f–278f
　physiology, 18–20
　practical points in, 27–29, 30f–31f
　primary defect in, 16
　rotation, 23, 26f, 71–81
　secondary defect and, 16
　temporoparietal, 216, 218f
　transposition, 23–27, 27f–29f, 99–115
　　on cheeks, 111, 112f
　　on chin, 111, 113f
　　complications of, 112–114, 114b
　　design and considerations for, 99
　　in dorsum of the nose, 109–110, 110f
　　general application of, 109–111, 109f
　　on medial and lateral canthi, 110, 111f
　　in nasal sidewall, 109–110, 110f
　　on nasal tip, 110
　　perioral area, 111, 113f
　　rhombic, 99–100
　　single-lobed, 99–100
　　on temple, 110–111
　　Z-plasty effect of, 100
　tubed, 215, 216f
　tunneled island, 95f
　two-stage, 215
　V-Y, 82–98, 84f–87f
　　classical, 82–84, 83f
　　complications, 92–98
　　modifications, 88–92, 89f–97f
　　technique, 84–88
　　traditional, 82–84, 83f
　see also individual types
Flip-flop flap, 92
5-Fluorouracil (5-FU), intralesional, for scar revision, 303
Folded paramedian forehead flap, 121–123, 123f
Forehead, 155
　flap for, in nasal reconstruction, 248, 250f–251f, 251–252, 254f–256f
　paramedian, 253f
　three-staged, 252, 252f
　two-staged, 252
　sensory innervation of, 157f

Forehead and temple repair, 155–164
  advancement, rotation, and transposition flaps for, 158–162, 159f–163f, 160b
  complications of, 162–163, 163b
  primary linear closure for, 157–158, 158f, 160b
  reconstructive principles of, 156–162
Free cartilage, simultaneous, full-thickness skin grafting and, 140
Free margins, 2–3
Frontalis muscle, 5–6, 155, 156f
FTSGs. see Full-thickness skin grafts (FTSGs)
Full-thickness circumoral flaps, in perioral reconstruction, 272–275
Full-thickness lid defects, 176–180
  lateral canthotomy, 178
  primary repair, 176–178, 179f
  tarsoconjunctival flap, 179–180, 181f
  Tenzel semicircle flap, 178–179, 180f
Full-thickness skin grafts (FTSGs), 3, 132
  ablative and nonablative laser resurfacing for, 305, 305f
  complications and management of, 137
  for ear reconstruction, 212, 212f
  modifications of, 137–140, 138f–139f
  for nasal reconstruction, 229f, 231–233, 232f–235f
    donor sites for, 231
  for periocular reconstruction, 167
  physiology of, 132
  for scalp reconstruction, 149–150
  selection for, 132–136, 133f–136f
  simultaneous free cartilage and, 140
  technique for, 136–137, 137f
Fusiform excision, for scar revision, 306

G
Galea aponeurotica, 145, 146f, 155
Galeotomy, 146–147
Geometric broken-line closures (GBLC), for scar revision, 306–307, 307f
Granulation. see Second intention healing
Greater auricular nerve, 212

H
Hatchet rotation flaps, for medial canthal defects, 175–176, 175f
  Island pedicle flaps and, 177f
Helical rim advancement flap, 63–64, 65f–66f
Hematoma
  cheek reconstruction and, 202
  stable, postprocedure, 300–301
Heminasal rotation flap, 75–76
Hemorrhage, as surgical complication, 300–301
  excessive, treatment of, 300
H-plasty, 53–56, 54f–56f
Hughes tarsoconjunctival flap, 181f
Hyperpigmented scars, fractional ablative lasers for, 305
Hypertrophic scarring
  cheek reconstruction and, 206
  intralesional triamcinolone for, 303

I
Indian flap, 23–25
Infection
  cheek reconstruction and, 203
  as surgical complication, 301
Infraorbital nerve, 10
Infraorbital rotation flaps, 78–79, 79f
Infratrochlear nerve, 10

Inner canthus tenting, 206
Intense pulsed light (IPL), for scar revision, 304
Interferon, for keloidal scars, 303
Internal maxillary artery, 11
Interpolated island flap, 88–92, 92f–94f, 97f
Interpolated nasolabial flap, 244–247
Interpolation flaps, 18f, 27, 29f, 116–131
  Abbé (lip-switch) flap, 127–129
    anatomy of, 127, 127f
    execution for, 128, 129f, 129t
    flap design of, 127–128, 128f
    indications for, 127
    postoperative care for, 128–129
    stage II, 129–130, 130f
  cheek-to-nose, 123–126
    anatomy of, 124
    execution for, 125, 125f, 125t
    flap design of, 124–125, 124f
    indications for, 124, 124f
    postoperative care for, 125–126
    stage II, 126–127, 126f–127f
  complications with, 131
  for nasal reconstruction, 244–252
    forehead, 248, 250f–256f, 251–252
    nasolabial, 244–247
    pedicled melolabial, 244, 248, 248f–250f
  paramedian forehead flap
    stage I, 116–121
    stage II, 121, 121f–122f
    variations of, 121–123
Intralesional injections, for scar revision, 303
Island flaps, 82–98
  complications, 92–98
  modifications, 88–92, 89f–97f
  technique, 84–88
Island pedicle flap, 23, 84
  for medial canthal defects, 176
    hatchet flap and, 177f
  in nasal reconstruction, 238, 239f

J
Junction lines, 1–2, 2f

K
Karapandzic, flap and, 272–275
Keloid
  formation of, cheek reconstruction and, 206
  intralesional triamcinolone for, 303

L
Lacrimal nerve, 9–10
Lacrimal system, 14f, 15
Laser treatment, for scar revision, 304–306, 305f
Lateral canthotomy, 178
Lateral cheek advancement flap, for cheek reconstruction, 188, 191f–192f
Lesser occipital nerve, 212
Levator anguli oris muscle, 7
Levator labii superioris alaeque nasi muscle, 6–7
Levator palpebrae superioris muscle, 13–15
Lid advancement flap, medial canthal defects, 176, 178f
Lid margin, defects below, flap repairs for, 167, 168f–173f
Limberg flap, 25, 27f
Linear closure (LC), in perioral reconstruction, 262–267, 263f–265f
  flaps, 265–267
  wedge repair, 263–265, 265f–267f

Lip defect, full-thickness skin grafts for, 135–136, 136f
Lip reconstruction. see Perioral reconstruction
Lip switch flap, 283–285, 284f–285f
Lips, 12–13, 13f
  arterial supply to, 259f
  cutaneous skin of, 258
  rotation flaps on, 80, 80f
  sensor innervation to, 259f
Lower lip defects, in perioral reconstruction, 269–270
  cutaneous subunits, 258
  full-thickness defects, 260
L-plasty, 58, 59f–60f
Lymphatics/lymphatic system, 12, 12f
  of neck, 291–292, 291f
Lymphedema, as surgical complication, 301

M
Mandibular nerve, 7f, 8, 10
Marginal nerve, 8
Masseter muscle, 1, 2f
Mastoid pull-through flap, 97f
Maxillary nerve, 10
Medial cheek rotation flaps, 79–80, 80f
Melolabial interpolation flap, 27, 29f
Melolabial transposition flap, 25
Mental nerve, 10
Mentalis muscle, 7
Microneedling, for scar revision, 304
Midpupillary line, 1
Modiolus, 7
Mohs excision, in nasal reconstruction, 225f, 227f, 228–229, 232f, 236f, 239f, 241f, 246f–247f, 251f, 256f
  defect in, 237f–238f
Mohs micrographic surgery, tumor extirpation with, for ear reconstruction, 212
Moll, glands of, 15
Motor nerve deficits
  cheek reconstruction and, 206
  as surgical complication, 302
Motor nerves, 7–8
  facial nerve, 7, 7f
  temporal nerve, 8
  see also Nerves
Mouth
  muscles acting around, 7
  see also Perioral reconstruction
M-plasty, 23, 24f–25f, 56, 60f
  primary closure and, 44–45, 45f–46f
  for temple repair, 157–158, 158f
Mucosal advancement flap, 87f
  for lip defects, 260–262, 260f–261f
Muller's muscle, 13–15
Multilobe transposition flaps, 105
Muscles
  corrugator supercilii, 6
  depressor labii inferioris, 7
  depressor supercilii, 6
  of facial expression, 6f
  frontalis, 5–6
  levator anguli oris, 7
  levator labii superioris, 7
  levator labii superioris alaeque nasi, 6–7
  levator palpebrae superioris, 13–15
  lip elevators in, 258–259
  masseter, 1, 2f
  mentalis, 7
  Muller's, 13–15
  orbicularis oculi, 6, 165
  orbicularis oris, 258
  risorius, 7

Musculoaponeurotic system, 4–7, 4f, 6f
  eyelids, 5–6
  mouth, 7
  nose, 6–7
  superficial, 6f
    forehead, 155, 156f
    neck, 289
Mustarde rotation flaps, 76–79, 79f

N

Nasal bones, 13
Nasal reconstruction, 223–257, 224f–229f
  aesthetic subunit concept, 224f–226f
  complications of, 252–257, 256f
  flaps for, 234–252
    advancement, 235–238, 236f–239f
    interpolation, 244–252, 248f–256f
    rotation, 238–242, 239f–242f
    transposition, 242–244, 243f–247f
  full-thickness skin grafts in, 231–233, 232f–235f
  primary closure in, 229–231, 230f
  repair alternatives for, 229–252
Nasal tip defects, repair of, transposition flap for, 110
Nasolabial (melo-labial) transposition flap, in nasal reconstruction, 243–244, 246f–247f
Nasolacrimal duct, 15
Neck, anatomy of, 289–292
  blood supply, 289–292
  Erb's point, 289, 290f
  lymphatics, 291–292, 291f
  nerves, 291, 291f
  triangles, 289, 290f
Neck reconstruction, 292–297
  complications in, 299
  other surgical considerations for, 298–299, 298f
  perioperative consideration for, 289
  postoperative considerations for, 299
  primary closure in, 292, 292f–294f
  secondary intention healing in, 297, 297f
Necrosis
  as full-thickness skin graft complication, 137
  in nasal reconstruction, 252–255, 256f
  as split-thickness skin graft complication, 142–143
Nerves
  anterior ethmoid, 9–10
  Arnold, 212
  auriculotemporal, 212
  buccal, 7f, 8
  cervical, 7f, 8, 212
  facial, 7, 7f
  greater auricular, 212
  infraorbital, 10
  infratrochlear, 10
  lacrimal, 9–10
  lesser occipital, 212
  mandibular, 7f, 8, 10
  marginal, 8
  maxillary, 10
  mental, 10
  of neck, 291, 291f
  oculomotor, 13–15
  ophthalmic, 9–10
  sensory, 8–10, 9f
  temporal, 8
  trigeminal, 8–10, 9f, 145, 212
  vagus, 212
  zygomatic, 8
Neuromuscular anatomy, of perioral reconstruction, 258–259

Nonablative fractional resurfacing lasers (NAFR)
  full-thickness skin grafts (FTSGs) and, 305, 305f
  for scar revision, 304
Nose, 13, 13f
  division of, into aesthetic subunits, 223, 224f
  muscles acting around, 6–7
  reconstruction of. see Nasal reconstruction
  wound of, full-thickness skin grafts for, 132–133, 133f

O

Occipital artery, 11
Oculomotor nerve, 13–15
Offset bias suturing, 3
180-degree transposition flap, for cheek reconstruction, 189, 193f–194f
Ophthalmic artery, 10–11
Ophthalmic nerve, 9–10
Opsite, 141–142
Oral commissure, defects at, 262f
Orbicular oculi, 155, 156f
Orbicularis oculi muscle, 165
O-to-T advancement flap, 150, 151f
O-Z rotation flap, 73, 75f

P

Paramedian forehead flap, 88–92, 91f
  folded, 121–123, 123f
  in nasal reconstruction, 253f
  stage I, 116–121
    anatomy of, 116, 117f
    anesthesia for, 118–119
    cartilage and lining restoration in, 119, 119f
    defect preparation in, 120
    donor site closure in, 120, 120f–121f
    execution for, 119–120
    flap design of, 116–118, 117f, 117t
    flap harvesting and pedicle mobilization in, 118t, 119–120, 120f
    flap preparation and inset in, 120, 120f
    indications for, 116
    postoperative care for, 120–121
  stage II, 121, 121f–122f
  variations of, 121–123
Parotid fistula, cheek reconstruction and, 206, 208f
Partial-thickness lip defects, 259
Pedicle, of flap, 16
Pedicled melolabial flap, in nasal reconstruction, 244, 248, 248f–250f
Peng flap, 68, 69f
Perfusion pressure, 16–17
Periocular reconstruction, 165–182
  anatomy of, 165–166
  flap repairs for, 167–180, 167f
    defects below lid margin, 167, 168f–173f
    full-thickness lid defects, 176–180
    medial canthal defects, 175–176, 175f–178f
    upper lid defects, 167–175, 174f
  linear repairs, 166–167, 167f
  periocular repairs, 166, 167f
  postoperative considerations for, 181–182
  principles of, 166
  skin grafts, 167
  specialized instrumentation, 165
  tension and, 166
Perioral area, transposition flaps in, 111, 113f

Perioral reconstruction, 258–288
  anatomy of, 258–259
  cosmetic subunits, 259f
  evaluation of patient and defect, 259–260
  general principles of, 260, 260b
  lower lip defects, 269–270
    cutaneous subunits, 258
    full-thickness defects, 260
  methods of closure, 260–286
    advancement-rotation flaps, 267–275
    linear closure, 262–267, 263f–265f
    mucosal advancement flap, 260–262, 260f–261f
    philtral reconstruction, 285–286, 286f–287f
    second intention healing, 260, 260f–261f
    transposition flaps, 275–285, 279f–283f
  neuromuscular anatomy, 258–259
  relaxed skin tension lines, 259
  surface anatomy, 258
  upper lip defects, 259
  vascular anatomy, 259
Philtral reconstruction, lip defect and, 285–286, 286f–287f
Pinch grafting, in split-thickness skin grafts, 141
Platysma, 289
Postauricular artery, 11
Posterior auricular artery, 211
Preauricular grafts, in nasal reconstruction, 231
Pressure dressing, for hemorrhage, 300
Primary closure, 39–49
  complications of, 48–49
  defined, 34
  elliptical, 39
  fusiform excision variations, 42–45
    crescentic excision, 43, 44f
    M-plasty, 44–45, 45f–46f
    serial elliptical excisions, 45, 47f
    S-plasty, 43–44, 44f–45f
  in nasal reconstruction, 229–231, 230f
  in neck reconstruction, 292, 292f–294f
  phases of wound healing in, 39
  reconstruction principles, 39–42
    contour preservation and restoration, 40–41
    cosmetic subunit junction lines, scar orientation along, 41–42, 42f
    free margin position, preservation and restoration of, 39–40, 42f–43f
    relaxed skin tension lines, scar orientation along, 42
  scalp reconstruction and, 147–148, 148f
  standing cone deformities and, 45–48, 48f
Primary defect, 16
Primary lid repair, 176–178, 179f
Primary linear closure, for forehead and temple repair, 157–158, 158f, 160b
Procerus, 155, 156f
Prosthetics, in ear reconstruction, 222
Pulsed dye laser (PDL), for scar revision, 304
  side effects of, 304

R

Reconstructive surgery, second intention healing as adjunct to, 37–38, 40f
Rectangular advancement flap, 50, 51f–52f
Regional reconstruction, for ear, 214–222
Relaxed skin tension lines (RSTLs), 1, 2f, 27–29, 302
  cheek reconstruction and, 183
  of forehead and temple, 155, 156f
  of neck, 289, 290f
  periocular, 166–167, 167f

Relaxed skin tension lines (RSTLs) (cont'd)
  perioral reconstruction, 259
  scars oriented along, primary closure and, 42
Retaining ligament, 4f
  sagittal section of, 6f
Rhombic flaps, 99–100
  for cheek reconstruction, 186, 188f
  for defects below lid margin, 168f–169f
  design of, 99–100
  modified, 100f–101f, 101–103
    in cheeks, 111, 112f
    in chin, 111, 113f
    in dorsum of the nose, 109–110, 110f
    double 30-degree angle flap in, 102, 102f
    DuFourmentel flap in, 101–102, 101f
    flap mobilization and key sutures in, 102–103
    in medial and lateral canthi, 110, 111f
    in nasal sidewall, 109–110, 110f
    in nasal tip, 110
    in perioral area, 111, 113f
    single-lobed, 99–100
    in temple, 110–111
    Webster 30-degree angle flap in, 102, 102f
  for nasal reconstruction, 242, 243f
  for neck reconstruction, 292–293, 294f–295f
Rhomboid transposition flaps, 25, 27f
Rieger flap, 23
Rintala flap, 50, 51f
Risorius muscle, 7
Rotation flaps, 21, 22f, 23, 26f, 71–81
  bilateral, 73, 74f
  cervicofacial, 80
  on chin, 80, 80f
  classic, 72f
  curvature of, 71–73, 73f
  design of, 71–73, 72f–73f
  dorsal nasal, 74–75, 76f–78f
    axial, 75
  flap elevation and surgical undermining in, 80–81
  for forehead and temple repair, 158–162, 162f
  heminasal, 75–76
  length of, 71
  on lip, 80, 80f
  medial cheek, 79–80, 80f
  Mustarde, 76–79, 79f
  in nasal reconstruction, 238–242, 239f
    dorsal nasal, 238–242, 240f–241f
    traditional, 242f
  O-Z, 73, 75f
  for perioral reconstruction, 269–270, 270f–272f
  for scalp reconstruction, 150–153, 151f–153f
  spiral, 76, 78f
  Tenzel, 76–79, 78f

S
Scalp reconstruction, 145–154
  anesthesia for, 146
  basic concepts in, 146–147, 146f–147f
  evaluation of scalp defect in, 145–146
  full-thickness skin grafts for, 149–150
  primary closure for, 147–148, 148f
  random pattern cutaneous flaps for, 150–154
    advancement flaps as, 150, 151f
    rotation flaps as, 150–153, 151f–153f
    transposition flaps as, 153–154, 154f
  second intention healing for, 147
  with skin substitute, 149
  split-thickness skin grafts for, 148–149, 149f
  surgical anatomy for, 145, 146f
  tissue laxity and, 146
Scapha, 15, 15f
Scars, 302
  aesthetic outcomes of, postoperative care for, 302
  appearance of, in second intention healing, 34
  classification of, 302
  features of, 302
  revision of, 302, 303f
    dermabrasion for, 303–304
    intralesional injections for, 303
    laser treatment for, 304–306, 305f
    microneedling for, 304
    soft tissue/dermal fillers for, 304
    subcision for, 304
    surgical options for, 306–307
    timing of, 307–308
  surgical debulking of, 307, 308f
  surgical repair of, goals of, 302
Second intention healing, 3, 34–38
  as adjunct to reconstructive surgery, 37–38, 40f
  complications of, 38, 41f
  defined, 34
  in forehead and temple repair, 156–157, 157f
  in neck reconstruction, 297, 297f
  patient factors affecting decisions about, 36
  in perioral reconstruction, 260, 260f
    of vermilion-cutaneous defect, 261f
    from vermilionectomy, 261f
  phases of wound healing in, 34, 35f
  in scalp reconstruction, 147
  scars from, appearance of, 34
  wounds
    care of, 38
    ideal, 34–36, 36f–38f
    suboptimal, 36, 38f–39f
Secondary defect, 16
Sensory nerves, 8–10, 9f
  see also Nerves
Serial elliptical excisions, primary closure and, 45, 47f
Side-to-side closure, 2–3, 183
Simple wedge excision, for ear reconstruction, 212
Simultaneous free cartilage, full-thickness skin grafting and, 140
Single-lobed transposition flaps, 99–100
  design of, 99–100
  in nasal reconstruction, 242
Skeletal resorption, facial, 3f
Skin flap, 16
Skin grafts, 132–144
  for ear reconstruction, 212, 212f
  full-thickness, 132
    complications and management of, 137
    modifications of, 137–140, 138f–139f
    physiology of, 132
    selection for, 132–136, 133f–136f
    simultaneous free cartilage and, 140
    technique for, 136–137, 137f
  full-thickness, for periocular reconstruction, 167
  for nasal reconstruction
    full-thickness, 229f, 231–233, 232f–235f
    split-thickness, 231–233
  for periocular reconstruction, 167
  physiology of, 132
  split-thickness, 140
    complications and management of, 142–143
    selection for, 140
    technique for, 141–143, 142f
Soft tissue fillers, for scar revision, 304
Spinal accessory nerve (cranial nerve XI), 289, 290f
Spiral flap, 76, 78f
S-plasty, 43–44, 44f–45f
Split-thickness skin grafts (STSGs), 140
  for cheek reconstruction, 184
  complications and management of, 142–143
  for nasal reconstruction, 231–233
  for scalp reconstruction, 148–149, 149f
  selection for, 140
  technique for, 141–143, 142f
Standing cone deformities, 45–48, 48f
Staphylococcus aureus, surgical site infection and, 301
Stenson duct, 184
Steroid, low-strength, for scar revision, 303
Stress-strain curve, 20, 20f
STSGs. *see* Split-thickness skin grafts (STSGs)
Subcision, for scar revision, 304
Subgaleal space, scalp reconstruction and, 146, 146f–147f
Sub-muscular aponeurotic system (SMAS), 184
Superficial cervical plexus, 291
Superficial musculoaponeurotic system (SMAS), 4f, 6f
Superficial temporal arteries, 11, 145, 211
Superior labial artery, 10
Superior palpebral fold, 13–15
Supraorbital artery, 11
Supratrochlear artery, 10–11
Surface landmarks
  cosmetic units and junction lines, 1–2, 2f
  free margins, 2–3
  masseter muscle and midpupillary line, 1, 2f
  skin tension lines, relaxed, 1, 2f
Surgery, complications of, 300–309
  ectropion as, 301–302
  eyelid swelling as, 301
  hemorrhage as, 300–301
  infection as, 301
  lymphedema as, 301
  motor nerve deficits as, 302
  wound dehiscence, 301
Surgical debulking, of scar, 307, 308f
Surgical site infection (SSI), after surgery, 301
  risk factors for, 301
Suspension suture, 3
Sutures
  advancement flaps, 50–53, 52f
  Frost, 134–135
  for rhombic flap, 102–103
  suspension (or tacking), 81

T
Tarsoconjunctival flap, 179–180, 181f
Telangiectasia, cheek reconstruction and, 206
Temple
  repair, 155–164
  rotation flap for, for defects below the lid margin, 171f
  transposition flap for, 110–111
  see also Periocular reconstruction
Temporal artery, 11, 157f
Temporal fat pad, 5f
Temporal nerve, 8
Temporoparietal flap, 216, 218f

Tension, periocular reconstruction and, 166
Tension vector of closure, 2–3
Tenzel rotation flaps, 76–79, 78f
Tenzel semicircle flap, 178–179, 180f
Three-staged forehead flap, in nasal reconstruction, 252, 252f
Tie-over bolster, 137
Tissue mobility, in ear, 214–215
Topography, of ear, 210–212, 211f
T-plasty, 56–58, 57f–59f
Transposition flaps, 21, 22f, 23–27, 27f–29f, 99–115
　on cheeks, 111, 112f
　on chin, 111, 113f
　complications of, 112–114, 114b
　design and considerations for, 99
　in dorsum of nose, 109–110, 110f
　for forehead and temple repair, 158–162, 163f
　general application of, 109–111, 109f
　on medial and lateral canthi, 110, 111f
　for nasal reconstruction, 242–244
　　bilobed, 242–243, 244f–245f
　　nasolabial (melo-labial), 243–244, 246f–247f
　　rhombic, 242, 243f
　　single-lobe, 242
　　trilobed, 243, 245f
　in nasal sidewall, 109–110, 110f
　on nasal tip, 110
　perioral area, 111, 113f
　for perioral reconstruction, 275–285, 279f–283f
　rhombic. *see* Rhombic flaps
　for scalp reconstruction, 153–154, 154f
　single-lobed, 99–100
　on temple, 110–111
　Z-plasty effect of, 100
Trapdoor deformity, 114b, 256, 307, 307f
Triamcinolone, intralesional, 303
Triangular fossa, 15
Trigeminal nerve, 8–10, 9f, 212
Trilobed flaps, 108
　for forehead and temple repair, 162, 162f
　for nasal reconstruction, 243, 245f
Trippier flap, for defects below lid margin, 170f
Tubed flap, 215, 216f
Tumor extirpation with Mohs micrographic surgery, for ear reconstruction, 212
Tunneled island flap, 95f
Two-stage flap, 215
Two-staged forehead flap, in nasal reconstruction, 252

U

Undermining, 80–81, 88, 260
U-plasty, 50
　see also Rectangular advancement flap
Upper lip defects, in perioral reconstruction, 259

V

Vagus nerve, 212
Vascular system, 10–12
Veins
　external jugular, 291
　facial, 184
　of neck, 291
Venous drainage, 211
Venous system, of face, 12, 12f
Vermilion-cutaneous defect, second intention healing for, 261f
Vermilionectomy, second intention healing from, 261f
V-Y advancement flaps, 82–98, 84f–87f
　classical, 82–84, 83f
　complications with, 92–98
　modifications of, 88–92, 89f–97f
　for nasal reconstruction, 237–238, 238f
　for perioral reconstruction, 270–272, 272f–278f
　technique, 84–88
　traditional, 82–84, 83f

W

Webster 30-degree angle flap, 102, 102f
Webster perialar crescentic flap, 50, 52f, 64, 67f
Weck blade, for split-thickness skin grafts, 141
Wedge repair, for linear closure, 263–265, 265f–267f
Wound
　dehiscence, as surgical complication, 301
　depth of, scalp reconstruction and, 145
　second intention healing for
　　care during, 38
　　contraction of, 34, 36f
　　ideal, 34–36, 36f–38f
　　phases, 34, 35f
　　suboptimal, 36, 38f–39f
Wound healing, phases of
　primary closure, 39
　second intention healing, 34, 35f
W-plasty
　for donor site closure, 120
　for scar revision, 306, 307f

Z

Zeis, glands of, 15
Zimmer dermatome, for split-thickness skin grafts, 141
Z-plasty, 53–56, 56f
　double, 185, 187f, 196f
　for ear reconstruction, 212
　for neck reconstruction, 292
　for scar revision, 306, 306f
Z-plasty effect, of transposition flap, 100
Zygomatic arch, 11–12
Zygomatic nerve, 7f, 8
Zygomaticotemporal artery, 11f